Small Animal Toxicology Essentials

Small Animal Toxicology Essentials

Editors
Robert H. Poppenga, DVM, DABVT, PhD
Sharon Gwaltney-Brant, DVM, PhD, DABVT, DABT

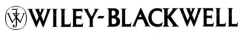
WILEY-BLACKWELL

A John Wiley & Sons, Inc., Publication

Registered office: John Wiley & Sons Ltd, The Atrium, Southern Gate, Chichester, West Sussex, PO19 8SQ, UK

Editorial offices: 2121 State Avenue, Ames, Iowa 50014-8300, USA
The Atrium, Southern Gate, Chichester, West Sussex, PO19 8SQ, UK
9600 Garsington Road, Oxford, OX4 2DQ, UK

For details of our global editorial offices, for customer services and for information about how to apply for permission to reuse the copyright material in this book please see our website at www.wiley.com/wiley-blackwell.

Library of Congress Cataloging-in-Publication Data
Small animal toxicology essentials / editors, Robert H. Poppenga, Sharon Gwaltney-Brant.
     p. ; cm.
   Includes bibliographical references and index.
   ISBN 978-0-8138-1538-1 (pbk. : alk. paper) 1. Veterinary toxicology.   2. Pet medicine.   I. Poppenga, Robert H.   II. Gwaltney-Brant, Sharon.
   [DNLM: 1. Poisoning–therapy.   2. Poisoning–veterinary.   3. Pets. SF 757.5]
   SF757.5.S63 2011
   636.089′59—dc22
                                                     2010049403

A catalogue record for this book is available from the British Library.

Set in 9.5/12 pt Times by Toppan Best-set Premedia Limited

Printed and bound in Singapore by Fabulous Printers Pte Ltd

1   2011

Dedication

A special thank-you to my wonderful family (Amy, Mia, and Zoe), to all the pets who depend on us to provide them with a safe and healthy environment, and to all of the dedicated veterinary technicians who enrich the veterinary profession.
–Robert H. Poppenga

This book is dedicated to my husband, Tom Brant, who provides unwavering support to all of my endeavors.
–Sharon Gwaltney-Brant

Contents

This book is accompanied by a companion website at www.wiley.com/go/poppenga.
The website includes review questions and answers and color images available for download in PowerPoint.

Preface

As vital members of their veterinary medical teams, veterinary technicians are routinely involved in managing potential or real animal poisonings in several ways. In many cases, veterinary technicians are asked for information about the safety of a product, food, or plant. They may be the first to talk to a distraught client on the telephone and make initial decisions regarding the severity of a situation and the need for immediate action. They may perform the initial triage of a poisoned animal or initiate decontamination procedures when a poisoned patient is presented to a veterinary hospital. They may provide initial stabilization of a critically ill patient or collect samples to submit to a laboratory for confirmation of exposure or intoxication. For all of these reasons, veterinary technicians need to have a resource to help them in these tasks. Although several textbooks pertaining to veterinary toxicology have been published over the last several years, none were specifically targeted to veterinary technicians. *Small Animal Toxicology Essentials* is a valuable resource for you. We have enlisted the help of veterinary toxicologists, emergency service technicians, and animal poison control specialists to help make this textbook as useful as possible. Our focus is on pet animals and the most common poisons that they are likely to encounter. Because of their inquisitive natures, pets may be exposed to a wide variety of agents with varying levels of toxicity. However, only a small fraction of exposures have the potential to cause clinically significant effects, and an even smaller fraction of exposures require extensive medical intervention. In order to assist in differentiating between significant and insignificant exposures, it is imperative that veterinary technicians have a handy resource available to provide information and guidance when needed. This is our objective in formulating and compiling *Small Animal Toxicology Essentials*.

Robert H. Poppenga
Sharon Gwaltney-Brant

Contributors

Mindy Bough, CVT, BA
ASPCA Animal Poison Control Center
Urbana, IL, USA

Rhian Cope, BVSc, BSc, PhD, DABT
ERMA New Zealand
New Zealand

Camille DeClementi, DVM, DABVT, DABT
ASPCA Animal Poison Control Center
Urbana, IL, USA

Joanna Delaporte, CVT
ASPCA Animal Poison Control Center
Urbana, IL, USA

Kiran Dhakal
Interdisciplinary Graduate Program in Human Toxicology
The University of Iowa
Iowa City, Iowa, USA

Eric Dunayer, DVM, MS, DABVT, DABT
St. Matthews University School of Veterinary Medicine
Grand Cayman, Cayman Islands

Joyce Eisold, DVM
ASPCA Animal Poison Control Center
Urbana, IL, USA

Tamara Foss, CVT
ASPCA Animal Poison Control Center
Urbana, IL, USA

Erin Freed, CVT
ASPCA Animal Poison Control Center
Urbana, IL, USA

Sharon Gwaltney-Brant, DVM, PhD, DABVT, DABT
Veterinary Information Network
Mahomet, IL, USA

Safdar A. Khan, DVM, PhD, DABVT
ASPCA Animal Poison Control Center
Urbana, IL, USA

Carrie Lohmeyer, CVT
ASPCA Animal Poison Control Center
Urbana, IL, USA

Bridget McNally, CVT, VTS
University of Pennsylvania
Philadelphia, PA, USA

Irina Meadows, DVM, DABT
ASPCA Animal Poison Control Center
Urbana, IL, USA

Charlotte Means, DVM, MLIS, DABVT, DABT
ASPCA Animal Poison Control Center
Urbana, IL, USA

Michelle Mostrom, DVM, DABVT, DABT
North Dakota State University
Fargo, ND, USA

Lisa Murphy, DVM, DABT
University of Pennsylvania
Kennett Square, PA

Elisa Petrollini-Rogers, CVT, VTS
University of Pennsylvania
Philadelphia, PA, USA

John Pickrell, DVM, PhD, DABT
Kansas State University
Manhattan, KS, USA

Robert H. Poppenga, DVM, DABVT, PhD
CAHFS Toxicology Laboratory
Davis, CA, USA

Mary M. Schell, DVM, DABT, DABVT
ASPCA Animal Poison Control Center
Urbana, IL, USA

Karla R. Smith, DVM
ASPCA Animal Poison Control Center
Urbana, IL, USA

Petra A. Volmer, DVM, MS, DABVT, DABT
Summit VetPharm
Champaign, IL, USA

Tina Wismer, DVM, DABT, DABVT
ASPCA Animal Poison Control Center
Urbana, IL, USA

Small Animal Toxicology Essentials

Section 1

Fundamentals of Veterinary Clinical Toxicology

General Toxicologic Principles

Sharon Gwaltney-Brant and Robert H. Poppenga

INTRODUCTION

Toxicology is the study of the nature, effects, and detection of poisons and the treatment of poisoning. Although the broad definition of toxicology encompasses "clinical" toxicology, for the purposes of this textbook, we define *clinical toxicology* as the diagnosis and treatment of the poisoned patient. Many of the basic principles of toxicology, such as the inherent toxicity of various forms of a chemical, variations in dose-response curves, different mechanisms of toxic action, variations in individual and species sensitivities to chemicals, and how differences in kinetics of chemicals (sometimes referred to as "toxicokinetics") need to be applied to the successful diagnosis and treatment of poisoning. In addition, in many instances, in clinical toxicology there is a need for the application of good critical care and medical practices (e.g., stabilizing, monitoring, and treating a patient) to achieve a successful outcome.

DEFINITIONS

All special areas of study have unique terminology that is important to master in order to fully appreciate the discipline. The following definitions provide some needed terminology in order to more effectively utilize this textbook.

Toxicant

A poison or poisonous agent; an intoxicant; any solid, liquid or gas that, when introduced into or applied to the body, can interfere with the life processes of cells or the organism by its own inherent qualities (toxicity) without acting mechanically and irrespective of temperature.

Toxin

A poisonous material that is synthesized or derived from an animal or plant; also referred to as a *biotoxin*. Zootoxins, bacterial toxins, and phyto (or plant) toxins are subcategories of toxins.

Toxicity

The poisonous characteristics of a substance; the degree to which something is poisonous. Perhaps the best known measure of toxicity of a chemical is its lethal dose or LD_{50} (Table 1.1).

Acute Toxicity

Intoxication that results from the effects of a single dose or multiple doses of a toxicant given during a 24-hour period (e.g., dog got into a box of chocolates or dog was left in a room contaminated by chemical fumes overnight). The LD_{50} of a chemical is most often determined during acute exposure studies in which a single dose of a chemical is given.

Subacute Toxicity

Exposure to multiple doses of a toxin or toxicant given for greater than 24 hours but no longer than 30 days (e.g., animal owner administers ibuprofen to dog for a week).

Small Animal Toxicology Essentials, First Edition. Edited by Robert H. Poppenga, Sharon Gwaltney-Brant.

Table 1.1. Classification scheme for relative toxicity

Classification	Toxicity (LD$_{50}$ in mg/kg body weight)
Extremely toxic	<1 mg/kg
Highly toxic	1 to 50 mg/kg
Moderately toxic	50 to 500 mg/kg
Slightly toxic	0.5 to 5.0 g/kg
Practically nontoxic	5 to 15 g/kg
Relatively harmless	>15 g/kg

Subchronic Toxicity

Repeated or continuous exposures to toxicants for a duration of 1 to 3 months (e.g., patient on weekly chemotherapy for cancer).

Chronic Toxicity

Intoxication that results from prolonged exposure, with the duration of exposure being 3 months or longer (e.g., repeated exposure of a cat to low levels of lead as a result of environmental contamination and grooming of contaminated paws or hair).

Dose

The quantity of drug or toxicant administered at one time irrespective of body weight.

Dosage

The regimen governing the size, amount, frequency, and number of doses of a therapeutic agent to be administered to a patient.

Lethal Dose (LD)

The lowest dose that causes death. An LD can be expressed as a percentage of individuals dying (e.g., an LD$_{10}$, or, most commonly, an LD$_{50}$)

Median Lethal Dose (LD$_{50}$)

The quantity of an agent that will kill 50% of the test subjects to which it is administered.

ppm

Abbreviation for parts per million; a weight-for-weight (w/w) concentration equal to 1 mg/kg or 1 g/tonne. Used most commonly to express the concentration of toxicants or trace elements in water, feeds, solvents, and tissues. Note that mg/kg can refer to either a concentration or a dosage; its meaning is dependent on the context of its use.

Parts per million (ppm), parts per billion (ppb), and parts per trillion (ppt) are the most commonly used terms to describe very small amounts of contaminants in our environment. They are measures of concentration or the amount of one material in a larger amount of another material; for example, the weight of a toxic chemical in a certain weight of food. The following example might help conceptually. If you divide a pie equally into 10 pieces, each piece would be one part per ten or one-tenth of the total pie. If, instead, you cut this pie into a million pieces, each piece would be very small and would represent a millionth of the total pie or one part per million of the original pie. If you cut each of these million pieces into a thousand little pieces, each of these new pieces would be one part per billion of the original pie. To give you an idea of how little this would be, a pinch of salt in ten tons of potato chips is also one part (salt) per billion parts (chips). In the pie example, the pieces of the pie are made up of the same material as the whole. However, if there were a contaminant in the pie at a level of one part per billion, one of these invisible pieces of pie would be made up of the contaminant and the other 999,999,999 pieces would be pure pie. Similarly, one part per billion of an impurity in a biological or environmental sample represents a tiny fraction of the total amount of the sample (e.g., water, food, whole blood, urine, or tissue).

Hazard (Risk)

The likelihood that a chemical will cause harm under certain conditions. The hazard can vary for the same chemical. For example, the hazard or risk of intoxication is greater if a potentially toxic product or chemical is not stored properly and thereby the chance for accidental exposure is increased due to greater accessibility.

Other relevant definitions are provided below (i.e., toxic dose, effective dose, margin of safety).

CLASSIFICATION OF TOXICANTS

Toxins and toxicants are classified in a variety of ways; no one way is better than another and a combination of classification schemes is used in this textbook. Poisons can be classified based upon the organ systems that are primarily affected (e.g., hepatotoxicants, neurotoxicants, nephrotoxicants, etc.). The limitation to this scheme is that many toxins or toxicants affect more than one organ system. Alternatively, poisons can be classified based upon their chemical structure. For example, alkaloids are cyclic compounds that contain a nitrogen molecule within the ring.

Toxic alkaloids are common in plants (e.g., nicotine in *Nicotiana* spp. or coniine in *Conium maculatum*). A third classification scheme categorizes poisons according to their use or location. For example, pesticides are subcategorized into rodenticides, insecticides, herbicides, fungicides, avicides, parasiticides, etc. based upon the type of target organism for which they were developed. Poison categories based upon location might include those found in homes, yards, or industrial sites. Within each of these categories are chemically diverse compounds with quite distinct target organs or mechanisms of toxic action. Finally, poisons can also be categorized according to their mechanism of toxic action. For example, some poisons cause damage via free radical formation or lipid peroxidation of cellular membranes and others inhibit protein synthesis.

SPECTRUM OF UNDESIRED EFFECTS

Toxicants cause damage through a variety of mechanisms including altering cell and organelle membrane integrity, altering cell energy production, inhibiting protein synthesis or enzyme activity, or damaging DNA (Osweiler 1996). Other undesired effects that need to be considered are discussed below.

Idiosyncratic Reactions

Idiosyncratic reactions to chemicals are defined as genetically determined abnormal reactivity to a chemical (Eaton and Gilbert 2008). Most commonly, this is caused by an acquired or congenital enzyme deficiency that prevents a toxicant from being processed properly. In some cases, the reason for an idiosyncratic reaction is unknown. See the discussion on *Genetic Polymorphisms* below.

Immediate vs. Delayed Reactions

Immediate effects can be defined as those that occur rapidly after a single exposure to a chemical. In contrast, delayed toxic effects are those that occur after some period of time (often, but not always, following repeated exposures). For example, many chemicals can induce cancer, but only after a long latency period of years (Osweiler 1996) (Eaton and Gilbert 2008). The focus of this textbook is on immediate adverse effects.

Reversible vs. Irreversible Damage

If a chemical damages a tissue, the ability of that tissue to regenerate largely determines whether the effect is reversible or irreversible. Tissues such as the gastrointestinal tract and the liver, which have high regenerative capabilities, are less likely to suffer irreversible damage than other tissues, such as nervous tissue, which has much more limited regenerative capacity. However, it is important to point out that even highly regenerative tissues such as the liver can suffer irreversible damage, particularly as a result of fibrosis in response to chemically induced damage.

Local vs. Systemic Effects

Local effects of a chemical are those that typically occur at the site of first contact between the biological system and the chemical. Good examples of chemicals with primarily local effects include acid and alkali corrosives. Systemic effects require the absorption and distribution of a chemical to a distant site where damage occurs. Most chemicals discussed in this textbook have systemic effects. It is possible for some chemicals to have both local and systemic effects. A good example of this occurs following exposure to iron salts. The reactivity of iron damages mucosal cells along the gastrointestinal tract; systemic absorption of iron results in more systemic and widespread damage.

INTERACTION OF CHEMICALS

Because animals and people are exposed to multiple chemicals at any given time, it is necessary to consider how different chemicals might interact with each other to modify toxic responses. Chemical interactions occur by a number of mechanisms that can include alterations of absorption, biotransformation, protein binding, or elimination (Eaton and Gilbert 2008). An example of two chemicals interacting to affect toxicity of one involves the combination of piperonyl butoxide and pyrethrin/pyrethroid insecticides. Piperonyl butoxide interferes with the metabolism, and therefore the detoxification, of the insecticides (Volmer 2004).

In general, types of interactions between chemicals that can influence the toxicity of one or more of the chemicals are classified as additive, synergistic, or antagonistic. Additive interaction means the effect of two chemicals is equal to the sum of the effect of the two chemicals taken separately (e.g., 2 + 3 = 5). This is usually due to the two chemicals acting on the body in the same way. An example of additive toxicity would be exposure to two different organophosphorus insecticides at the same time. Both have the same mechanism of toxic action (i.e., inhibition of acetylcholinesterase activity). Synergistic interaction means that the effect of two chemicals taken together is greater than the sum of their separate effect at the same doses (e.g., 2 + 2 = 20). One example of synergism is simultaneous exposure to the hepatotoxicants ethanol and carbon tetrachloride. In this case the damage to the liver is greater than that expected from summing the toxicities of each individual chemical. Antagonistic interaction means that the effect of two chemicals is less than the sum of the effect of the individual chemicals (e.g., 4 + 6 = 8). This can be due to the second chemical increasing the excretion of the first or perhaps as a result of the first directly blocking the toxic actions of the second. Antagonism forms the basis for many antidotal drugs. For example, atropine blocks cholinergic receptors that are stimulated following exposure to organophosphorus or carbamate insecticides.

One other term, *potentiation*, is used to describe chemical interactions. Potentiation occurs when one substance does not have a toxic effect on a certain organ or system but, when added to another chemical, makes the second chemical much more toxic (Eaton and Gilbert 2008). For example, isopropanol is not hepatotoxic. However, when combined with carbon tetrachloride, the hepatoxicity of carbon tetrachloride is greatly enhanced.

Finally, *tolerance* is another term worth noting. It is defined as the state of decreased responsiveness to the toxic effect of a chemical as a result of prior exposure to that chemical or to a structurally related chemical (Eaton and Gilbert 2008). Tolerance can occur either as a result of a decreased amount of a chemical reaching its site of toxic action or as a result of reduced responsiveness of a target to the chemical. The former can occur, for example, when a chemical induces metabolic enzymes in the liver that results in enhanced metabolism and detoxification of that chemical with subsequent exposures. The latter can occur as a result of down-regulation of receptor numbers for chemicals that cause adverse effects due to receptor stimulation.

CHARACTERISTICS OF EXPOSURE

Every day, animals (including humans) are exposed to poisons in the air they breathe, the food they eat, and the water they drink. Even agents necessary for life such as oxygen, water, and sodium can be toxic under certain circumstances. The fact that we don't all develop signs of poisoning on a daily basis underscores the basic concept of toxicology: the dose makes the poison. However, many factors are involved in determining whether a sufficient dose of a poison reaches its site of action in order to invoke a toxicosis. Agent factors to consider include the toxicant, its physical properties (i.e., liquid vs. solid vs. gas, pH, etc.), its chemical structure, and its stability or reactivity. Host factors to consider include species and/or breed of animal, age, weight, and general health status. The most

important factors that must be considered in determining whether a toxicosis will develop are those surrounding the introduction of toxicant to host: the exposure. Without an exposure to a poison, there will be no poisoning, so it is important to understand the characteristics of exposures to toxicants that help to determine whether a toxicosis will develop.

Route and Site of Exposure

When a poisoning occurs, most people automatically assume that the exposure was via ingestion (gastrointestinal tract), and, indeed, the gastrointestinal tract is the site of exposure for the majority of toxicoses dealt with in a veterinary setting. However, exposures to toxicants can occur via other routes, including inhalation (lungs), transdermal (skin), injection, ocular, and other minor parenteral routes (intramammary, etc.) Toxicants injected intravenously produce the most rapid response, with inhalation, intraperitoneal, subcutaneous, intramuscular, intradermal, oral, and dermal following in descending order of speed of response (Eaton and Gilbert 2008). Not all poisons are toxic by all routes of exposure; in fact most toxicants have a narrow range of routes by which they can gain access to the body. For instance, elemental mercury (quicksilver) is virtually nontoxic by dermal or oral routes; however, inhalation of the vapors can result in respiratory irritation as well as systemic absorption of mercury vapors via the lungs, which can, over time, result in central nervous system dysfunction from mercury toxicosis (Merrill et al. 2008).

Duration and Frequency of Exposure

Some toxicants can cause clinical effects with a single exposure, but others may require repeated exposures over time before a toxicosis develops; the clinical syndromes of each of these types of exposures may be quite different. In small animal medicine, most toxicoses that present to the veterinary hospital are acute because they are most often due to a single exposure to a toxicant.

There can be significant differences between clinical syndromes demonstrated by patients, depending on whether the exposure was acute or chronic. For example, acute arsenic toxicosis causes severe gastrointestinal hemorrhage, shock, and, often, death in dogs, whereas chronic toxicosis is expected to cause renal failure.

The frequency of exposure also can dictate the degree and severity of a toxicosis. For instance, a cat given 10 mg/kg of aspirin on a daily basis will quickly develop a toxicosis, but if the same dose is given every third day, toxicosis is unlikely.

DOSE-RESPONSE RELATIONSHIP

As mentioned, the basic concept in toxicology is "the dose makes the poison." This concept is essential in assessing the risks of exposures to toxicants, and it is often overlooked by the lay public, who typically perceives substances as either "toxic" or "nontoxic." Virtually any substance can be toxic under the appropriate circumstances. A veterinary technician who understands and is able to apply the basic concepts of toxicology to clinical situations will be able to provide objective and rational input into development of risk assessments for patient exposures to potential toxicants.

The dose-response relationship is the correlation between the characteristics of the exposure with the spectrum of toxic effects that a particular toxicant can produce. Knowing the dose-response relationship allows us to predict what type of reaction might be expected from a potential exposure. For example, methylxanthines in chocolate can cause serious clinical effects if sufficient amounts are ingested (Gwaltney-Brant 2001). A patient ingesting chocolate equal to 5 mg/kg of methylxanthines is not expected to have any serious clinical problems, but a dosage of 50 mg/kg could put the dog at risk for serious cardiovascular effects.

There are two components to the dose-response relationship: the population component and the individual component. Most dose-response relationships are made by grouping the responses of individuals to develop a population dose-response curve. As with all statistical studies of populations, the curve is bell-shaped, and the majority of individuals (the "normal" population) fall under the middle area of the curve. However, there are always individuals on the lower or upper limits of the curve (i.e., *outliers*), meaning they are more or less sensitive, respectively, to the toxicant and they will respond at lower or higher levels than the "normal" population (Figure 1.1). For instance, most dogs ingesting 20–30 mg/kg of methylxanthines from chocolate will develop agitation, restlessness, polydipsia, and gastrointestinal upset (Gwaltney-Brant 2001). However, at this dose, some dogs will show none of these clinical effects and appear clinically normal (less sensitive), while other dogs may develop signs at doses below 20 mg/kg (more sensitive). So, while knowing the dose-response relationship for a toxicant, it is important to also realize that there will be occasions when an individual patient fails to "read the same book" as the rest of us and responds differently than the norm. Some potential reasons

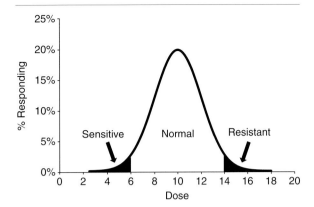

Figure 1.1. Illustration of dose-response curve. The majority of responders fall into the "Normal" range, but a small percentage of "Sensitive" individuals will respond at lower doses and another small percentage of "Resistant" individuals will not respond until the dose is much higher.

for these individual variations will be discussed later in the chapter.

Therapeutic Index

Medications provide an excellent example of the dose-response relationship. If too small a dose of medication is taken, it will not have the desired therapeutic effect, and if too high a dose is taken, signs of toxicosis may be seen. The goal is to find a dose that is effective and yet carries a low risk of intoxication. When comparing the relative safety of two similar drugs, a measurement called the *therapeutic index* is often used. This index is a ratio of the dose known to produce a toxic effect in 50% of the population (TD_{50}) to the dose known to produce a desirable therapeutic dose in 50% of the population (ED_{50}) (Eaton and Gilbert 2008). The larger the ratio, the greater the relative safety.

Another parameter that also compares a toxic dose (TD_1; the dose at which 1% will experience toxic effect) with an effective dose (ED_{99}; dose that is effective in 99% of the population) is the *margin of safety*. A drug with a wide margin of safety will have low risk of adverse effects in the vast majority of patients.

Variation in Toxic Responses

In discussing dose-response, one must keep in mind that there will always be individuals who do not respond to a xenobiotic in the same fashion as the majority of the population. An individual may show a higher or lower sensitivity to toxicosis than expected or may not show a therapeutic effect from a medication. Some reasons for these individual variations have been elucidated, but others still remain to be discovered (see *idiosyncratic* definition above).

Species Differences

Response to toxicants can vary tremendously between different species, with compounds that are relatively nontoxic to one species being quite toxic in a different species. These species differences can be the result of differences in physiology or toxicant absorption, metabolism, and/or elimination. For instance, cats evolved as true carnivores that did not need to metabolize plant-derived compounds such as phenols, and they did not evolve the necessary enzymes required to eliminate phenolic compounds from the feline body. As a result, cats have diminished ability to metabolize certain phenolic compounds, making them more susceptible to toxicosis from xenobiotics (such as acetaminophen) that contain phenols. Cats are also highly susceptible to developing methemoglobinemia and Heinz body anemia because their hemoglobin contains 8 reactive sulfhydryl groups (compared to 4 in dogs and 2 in humans), which can bind to oxidative agents that can denature hemoglobin. Additionally, a relative deficiency of methemoglobin reductase in their red blood cells makes it difficult for them to reverse the hemoglobin damage (Osweiler 2006). Because species differences are common and many are not fully elucidated, care must be taken when attempting to extrapolate toxicity data from one species and apply it to another.

Genetic Polymorphisms

The influence of genetics on an individual's response to xenobiotics is the subject of much study in the human pharmaceutical world. *Genetic polymorphism* is the term for hereditary differences in a single gene that occur in more than 1% of the population (Eaton and Gilbert 2008). Genetic polymorphisms are significant causes of individual variation in response to toxicants. Although a large number of genetic polymorphisms relating to xenobiotics have been identified in humans, less study has been done in companion animals. Perhaps the best known toxicology-related genetic polymorphism in the veterinary world is the sensitivity of dogs to macrolide antiparasitic agents (e.g., ivermectin, moxidectin, etc.). Individuals within certain genetic lines of collies, Shetland sheepdogs, Old English sheep dogs, and several other related breeds carry an autosomal recessive defect in a gene that codes for a blood-brain barrier P-glycoprotein (Mealey 2006; Lanusse

et al. 2009). This defect results in a faulty "pump" that normally excludes certain xenobiotics (including macrolides) entering from the central nervous system. As a result, macrolide agents are able to enter the CNS and cause clinical signs of intoxication at dosages that are not toxic to dogs without this defect. Likewise, other drugs that are normally excluded from the CNS by this pump but can gain access to the CNS in P-glycoprotein–defective dogs include digoxin, doxorubicin, and vincristine (Mealey 2006).

Age

Age-related responses to toxicants must be considered when dealing with pediatric and geriatric patients, because behavioral, physiological, and pathological differences in these special populations can have a profound influence on sensitivity to toxicants. When assessing the risk of an exposure to a toxicant, pediatric and geriatric animals should be considered at increased risk, and treatment should be considered at lower levels of exposure than would occur with a young adult animal.

Pediatric Patients

Nursing puppies and kittens may be exposed to toxicants not only through ingestion or inhalation of toxicants in their environments but are also subject to exposure to toxicants that the nursing dam may have ingested if these toxicants are passed through the milk (Boothe and Peterson 2006). By their inquisitive nature, young animals are more inclined to be exposed to toxicants in their environment that adult animals have learned to avoid (e.g., skunk spray). Younger animals have a variety of physiological differences making them more susceptible to toxicosis, including

- Increased intestinal permeability to some toxicants (e.g., lead)
- Increased gastric pH, which enhances the absorption of some toxicants
- Decreased intestinal motility, which allows toxicants to stay in the gastrointestinal tract longer and provides more opportunity for absorption of toxicants
- Decreased plasma protein concentrations to bind toxicants, allowing more free toxicant in the blood to reach target tissues
- Less body fat to sequester lipid soluble toxicants
- Decreased glomerular filtration rate, which results in decreased excretion of toxicants and their metabolites
- Decreased hepatic function and metabolic enzymes to detoxify toxicants

Geriatric Patients

As animals age, they experience physiological and metabolic changes that can alter the way that they respond to toxicants. Additionally, these animals may be on medications for degenerative disorders typical of elderly animals (e.g., arthritis), and interaction with the medication and toxicant may occur. Aging results in decreased renal and hepatic function. Because these two organ systems are the predominant means of toxicant elimination, the aging animal has a decreased capacity to efficiently remove toxicants from the body. Geriatric animals share some of the same metabolic derangements seen in pediatric animals, including decreased intestinal motility, decreased plasma protein production, decreased glomerular filtration rate, and decreased hepatic function. Additionally, elderly animals may have decreases in cardiovascular function, making them less able to handle the stresses of intoxication. Concurrent disease processes are more common in older patients and may increase the susceptibility to organ damage by toxicants (e.g., preexisting renal dysfunction may make a patient more susceptible to the toxic effects of NSAIDs) or compromise the animal's ability to respond to a toxicant. The behavior of a geriatric patient on some medications might be altered such that there is an increased risk for toxicant exposure (e.g., dogs on corticosteroid therapy often experience polyphagia and may ingest something they normally would avoid).

DEVELOPMENTAL AND REPRODUCTIVE TOXICITY

Pregnant animals exposed to toxic agents represent a special case when doing a risk assessment. Not only do the immediate needs of the patient need to be considered, but the potential effects of the toxicant (and any agents used to treat the mother) on the fetuses must be taken into account before a treatment plan is initiated. Pregnancy itself can cause some physiological changes in the mother, including decreased intestinal motility, decreased plasma protein concentrations, and alterations in renal and hepatic function (Kutzler 2006). These changes can impact the absorption, distribution, metabolism, and elimination of toxic compounds, making the dam more or less susceptible to a particular toxicant. Pregnant animals may spontaneously abort their pregnancies due to stress, direct effects of toxicants on the reproductive organs, or fetal death from hypoxia secondary to hypotension or other hemodynamic aberrations.

Toxicants may have minimal effect on the pregnant female but result in significant harm to the fetuses.

Whether a toxicant has a direct effect on the fetuses will depend on several factors. Most importantly, in order for a toxicant circulating in the blood to directly impact the fetus, it will need to cross the placenta in sufficient quantities to cause fetal damage. Whether a toxicant can pass the placenta will depend on the physical and biochemical properties of the toxicant as well as the structure of the placenta, which varies according to species. Toxicants reaching the fetuses can result in fetal death, fetal malformation (teratogenesis), or functional abnormalities (e.g., behavioral abnormalities), depending on the toxicant, species involved, and stage of gestation when the exposure occurs. Throughout gestation, there are peak times of susceptibility for organ malformation, generally coinciding with organogenesis. Organ-specific teratogens introduced prior to or after organogenesis may have little or no impact on the developing fetus, (Rogers and Kavlock 2008). Toxicants administered during gestation may cause a wide range of fetal defects. For example, feeding carbaryl (Sevin®) to dogs during gestation resulted in abdominal-thoracic fissures, intestinal agenesis, brachygnathia, and a variety of appendicular skeletal abnormalities (Smalley et al. 1968).

Unfortunately, the potential effects of many toxicants on pregnant animals or their offspring are not known. When presented with a pregnant patient who has been exposed to a potential toxicant, it is always safest to err on the side of caution and attempt decontamination when it can be performed safely.

TOXICOKINETICS

Toxicokinetics refers to the movement of a toxicant through the body. The principles of toxicokinetics are the same as pharmacokinetics (the movement of drugs in the body) with the exception that the agent moving through the body is considered a toxicant rather than a therapeutic agent. The ultimate disposition of a toxicant in the body depends on the four components of toxicokinetics: absorption, distribution, metabolism (also called *biotransformation*), and elimination (Evans 2006). These components are often abbreviated as ADME for ease of use. The ADME characteristics will vary with the toxic agent, species, and individual.

Absorption

Other than caustic and corrosive agents that inflict their damage locally, most toxicants must enter the body to exert their effects (Evans 2006). *Absorption* is the process by which toxicants pass through the various barriers to enter the systemic circulation. The degree and extent to which a toxicant will be absorbed is dependent upon the physical and chemical characteristics of the toxicant (molecular weight, pH, lipid solubility, etc.), the route of exposure, and species of animal. With the exception of intravenous injection, it is unlikely that 100% of a toxicant to which an animal is exposed will be absorbed. *Bioavailability* is a term that refers to the fraction of a toxicant that is actually absorbed.

The passage of toxicants into the body requires transport across cellular membranes to reach the general circulation; this transport can be passive (e.g., simple diffusion) or active, requiring energy to facilitate absorption (Evans 2006). Passive transport mechanisms do not require energy expenditure and include simple diffusion and filtration across membranes. Both of these processes require a concentration gradient for the toxicant to move along. The rate of toxicant movement is determined by the degree of difference in concentration between the two sides of the membrane, i.e., the larger the concentration differential, the faster the rate of movement. Simple diffusion is the primary means of toxicant passage across cell membranes, and it is most effective with small, lipid-soluble, nonionized molecules. Filtration is the movement of molecules through pores in cellular membranes and is dependent upon the size of the pores and size of the toxicant molecule. Facilitated diffusion is mediated by carrier molecules, which assist in carrying molecules across membranes. Active transport processes are energy-dependent and do not depend on a concentration gradient; in fact, most active transport mechanisms work against concentration gradients (i.e., take a molecule from an area of low concentration to an area of high concentration). Examples of active transport "pumps" include the Na^+–K^+ ATPase transporter in nerve cell membranes and the P-glycoprotein–dependent multidrug-resistant "pumps" in the blood-brain barrier. Pinocytosis is another active transport system that involves internalization of molecules through the "pinching off" and engulfment of fragments of cell membranes.

Absorption can be influenced by a variety of factors including route of exposure and the chemical and physical properties of the toxicant. The route of exposure plays a major role in determining how and to what extent a toxicant will be absorbed. In the gastrointestinal tract, the majority of molecules are absorbed by passive diffusion or carrier-mediated processes (Lehman-McKeeman 2008). Gastrointestinal absorption is highly dependent on the pH of the toxicant, with weak acids being better absorbed in the stomach and weak bases being better absorbed in the proximal small intestine. Absorption of toxicants across the skin requires that the toxicant pass through the lipophilic stratum corneum (the major barrier to absorption of toxicants via the skin) and then through the hydrophilic dermis to reach the bloodstream. Solvents such as dimethyl sulfoxide (DMSO) greatly enhance absorption of topically applied agents by increasing the permeability of the stratum corneum. Absorption of toxicants (primarily gases, vapors, and aerosols) via the lungs is second only to intravenous injection in regard to the speed and efficiency of absorption. Toxicants reaching the alveoli have only a thin wall to pass through in order to reach the systemic circulation. Fortunately, the structure of the respiratory tract can filter out many toxicants and prevent them from reaching the alveoli.

Some toxicants undergo what is termed a *first pass effect* whereby toxicants absorbed from the gastrointestinal tract are taken via portal circulation to the liver, where a fraction of toxicant is removed from the blood prior to reaching the systemic circulation. The first pass effect can dramatically decrease the bioavailability of toxicants. For example, a dog ingesting its owner's nitroglycerine sublingual tablets will be at low risk of toxicosis as long as the dog swallows all of the tablets. The nitroglycerine absorbed from the stomach will be largely removed by the liver and will not enter the systemic circulation. However, if the dog has one or more tablets that remain in the oral cavity (e.g., adhered to the oral mucosa), absorption across the oral mucosa will allow the nitroglycerine to enter the systemic circulation and the dog will develop signs of hypotension because compounds absorbed from the oral cavity do not enter the portal circulation.

Distribution

Once a toxicant enters the body it may remain within the systemic circulation, or it may distribute to organs and tissues. *Distribution* is the translocation of the toxicant to various organs and tissues throughout the body. The degree and extent to which a particular toxicant will distribute to tissues is dependent upon a variety of toxicant properties, including lipid solubility, molecular weight, and the affinity of the toxicant for various tissues (Evans 2006; Lehman-McKeeman 2008). The body has several physiologic barriers that may limit the distribution of certain xenobiotics, such as the blood-brain barrier, which excludes a large number of molecules from the central nervous system. The distribution characteristics of a toxicant are important in determining the clinical effects that a toxicant will produce. For example, the herbicide paraquat selectively concentrates in the lungs, where it is converted into toxic metabolites that induce severe lung damage and fibrosis. A related compound, diquat, has a similar mechanism of action, but does not selectively locate to the lung and therefore does not cause the pulmonary lesions that are seen with paraquat.

The storage of some toxicants within the body can actually aid in decreasing the acute toxicity of the compound. Some common storage depots for toxicants include bone (e.g., lead, cadmium), fat (e.g., organochlorine pesticides such as DDT), liver (e.g., copper) and kidney (e.g., cadmium). The toxicants in these *storage depots* are in equilibrium with the plasma, but certain metabolic situations can sometimes disrupt the equilibrium. For example, in chronic, low-level exposure to lead, much of the lead is stored in the bones, which may protect the animal from manifestations of acute toxicosis; blood lead concentrations may be only slightly above the normal range in these cases. However, any condition that causes an increase in bone remodeling (e.g., lactation, fracture) may result in a sudden release of lead from the storage depot and precipitate an acute toxicosis.

Plasma proteins are a special storage depot for toxicants and are important in determining the toxicity of an agent. There are a large number of proteins in the blood that can bind toxicants, but albumin is the major protein responsible for the binding of xenobiotics (drugs and toxicants). Because only a free (unbound) toxicant can reach its site of action, plasma proteins essentially "bind up" the toxicant, preventing it from exerting its toxic effect. Toxicants that are highly protein-bound have a lower level of toxicity than similar toxicants, which have poor protein binding. Species differences in types and amounts of plasma proteins are one reason for species differences in toxicity of various toxicants. An important consideration when dealing with a highly protein-bound compound is the potential interaction that may occur with other highly protein-bound agents. For instance, a dog that is on carprofen (a highly protein-bound drug) for arthritis is exposed to a warfarin-based rodenticide. Because warfarin is also highly protein-bound, the two xenobiotics are in competition for plasma proteins, resulting in higher unbound concentrations of both, which may result in clinical signs of warfarin toxicosis at doses lower than those normally associated with warfarin. Additionally, there also might be increased risk of adverse effects from the carprofen (i.e., gastrointestinal upset or bleeding).

Metabolism

Metabolism refers to the fate of a toxicant within the body and is often used synonymously with the term *biotrans-*

formation, which more correctly refers to the metabolic processes involved in creating a more water-soluble form of xenobiotics (Evans 2006). In order to prepare toxicants for elimination from the body, they must be converted into forms that are excretable. In most circumstances, this entails making the toxicant more water-soluble so that it can be eliminated by the kidneys; less commonly, compounds are made more lipid-soluble and eliminated via the bile into the feces. The body has a limited range of metabolic enzymes that can act on a wide range of substrates. These enzymes are present in most tissues but are most concentrated in organs with highest exposure to xenobiotics, including the liver, gastrointestinal tract, kidneys, and lung.

There are two levels of biotransformation, termed *Phase I* and *Phase II* reactions, used to make toxicants more excretable. Not all toxicants undergo both reactions; some toxicants are eliminated with little or no metabolism, and others undergo one of the two reactions. Phase I reactions generally involve hydrolysis, oxidation, or reduction and are designed to make a compound more water-soluble and/or expose a functional group for a subsequent Phase II reaction. Phase I reactions include the oxidation reactions mediated by cytochrome P450 enzymes, which are the basis for much of the individual variation in susceptibility to adverse drug reactions (Parkinson and Ogilvie 2008). Phase II reactions involve attachment (conjugation) of a functional group (sulfate, glucuronide, amino acid, glutathione, methyl group, acetyl group) to a parent compound or one of its metabolites that results in a compound that has greatly increased water solubility. Species differences in Phase II reactions include the defective glucuronidation in cats that makes them sensitive to phenolic compounds such as acetaminophen.

Bioactivation

Although biotransformation is generally thought of as a detoxifying process, allowing the body to eliminate potential toxicants, in some instances Phase I or Phase II reactions might result in a compound that is more toxic than the parent compound. This conversion of a low or nontoxic parent compound to a toxic metabolite is termed *bioactivation*. Examples include the conversion of ethylene glycol to metabolites that induce acidosis and renal failure and the conversion of acetaminophen to a highly reactive intermediate that causes liver damage.

Elimination

Elimination is the process of removing toxicants and their metabolites from the body. As has been mentioned, most biotransformation reactions are geared toward making toxicants more water-soluble so that they can be excreted via the kidneys. Renal excretion is the most common means by which the body eliminates waste. Other elimination pathways include fecal (via bile), exhalation (via lungs), saliva, sweat, and milk. Toxicants and their metabolites can be eliminated by more than one route (e.g., fecal and urinary).

The elimination half-life of a toxicant is the amount of time it takes for the original absorbed dose to be reduced by one-half. Compounds with shorter half-lives will be eliminated from the body more quickly than those with longer half-lives. Two processes that can prolong half-lives of a toxicant include enterohepatic recirculation and saturation of metabolic enzymes. Enterohepatic recirculation is the repeated cycling of a toxicant between the liver and the gastrointestinal tract. The toxicant passes from the systemic circulation into the liver, where it is excreted via the bile duct into the small intestine from where it is reabsorbed to reenter the systemic circulation. This continued cycling can greatly prolong the amount of time that a toxicant stays in circulation. For example, in dogs, the nonsteroidal anti-inflammatory drug naproxen undergoes extensive enterohepatic recirculation and has a half-life of 74 hours, whereas in humans naproxen does not undergo enterohepatic recirculation, is eliminated primarily via the urine, and has a half-life of 6 hours (Frey and Rieh 1981; Lees 2009; Talcott 2006).

Toxicants that must be metabolized through enzyme-mediated processes can have their half-lives increased if the dose of toxicant exceeds the capacity of the enzyme system to catalyze the conversion of toxicant to metabolite. In these situations, the toxicant "backs up" as the enzyme system becomes saturated with substrate. For toxicants that can be eliminated as parent compound as well as metabolites (e.g., ethanol), saturation may only mildly affect half-life, but for compounds that cannot be eliminated without first being converted to metabolites, the half-life can be significantly impacted. An example is aspirin, which requires glucuronidation for elimination. In cats, the half-life of aspirin ranges from 22 to 45 hours depending on the dose administered. As the dose increases, the half-life increases due to saturation of the cat's defective glucuronidation system. This is why the dosing interval of aspirin for cats is every 48 to 72 hours compared to every 8 to 12 hours for dogs.

CHAPTER 1 STUDY QUESTIONS

1. Banjo, a 2-year-old, 25-pound, neutered male dachshund mix ingested a 25 mg propranolol tablet that his owner accidentally dropped on the floor. When researching this drug, which of the following information would be LEAST helpful to you in determining whether Banjo is at risk for serious clinical effects?
   a. The minimum toxic dose for dogs
   b. The maximum tolerated dose for dogs
   c. The LD_{50} for dogs
   d. The minimum lethal dose for dogs
   e. The therapeutic index for dogs
2. Ranger, a 3-year-old golden retriever, was just prescribed phenobarbital to control his epilepsy. Ranger's owner called later that day to say that Ranger was acting groggy and wants to know whether this is expected with the phenobarbital. Ranger's veterinarian tells you to relay to the owner that this is an expected event and that Ranger should adapt to his medication after several days. A call back to the owner a week later finds that Ranger is no longer acting groggy after receiving his phenobarbital. Ranger's decreased sensitivity to the sedative effects of phenobarbital over time is an example of
   a. Potentiation
   b. Tolerance
   c. Synergism
   d. Antagonism
   e. Additivity
3. The fundamental principle of toxicology is "the dose makes the poison." When determining whether the dose of a particular compound poses a risk of toxicosis to an animal, which of the following must be taken into account?
   a. Physical properties of the compound (e.g., physical state, pH, reactivity, etc.)
   b. Species exposed to the compound

c. Route of exposure

d. Age, sex, and weight of the patient

e. All of the above must be considered.

4. In general, the most rapid response to a toxicant will occur if it is administered

a. Intravenously

b. Intradermally

c. Orally

d. Intramuscularly

e. Subcutaneously

5. The dose-response curve represents the characteristics of a xenobiotic within a _____, but _____ variation can result in increased or decreased response at a particular dose.

a. Species, normal

b. Population, individual

c. Species, individual

d. Population, normal

e. Class, statistical

6. When compared to humans, the increased susceptibility of cats to acetaminophen toxicosis is related primarily to species differences in which of the following:

a. Absorption of acetaminophen

b. Distribution of acetaminophen

c. Metabolism of acetaminophen

d. Elimination of acetaminophen

e. Bioavailability of acetaminophen

7. Some Doberman pinschers have an increased susceptibility to liver injury when they receive sulfonamide antibiotics at therapeutic doses. Because this susceptibility in Doberman pinschers is familial (i.e., runs in families), it is suspected that this trait is inherited. If so, this would be an example of

a. Species difference

b. Genetic polymorphism

c. Age-related response

d. Gender difference

e. Fetal toxicity

8. In cats, organogenesis is complete in the first trimester (first 3 weeks) of pregnancy. At week 8 of pregnancy, a queen was exposed to a medication known to adversely affect fetuses. Which of the following would NOT be a potential outcome of this exposure?

a. Anencephaly

b. Abortion

c. Stillborn kittens

d. Mummified fetuses

e. Premature parturition

9. The percentage of an ingested toxicant that is absorbed into the circulation is a measure of its

a. Toxicity

b. Distribution

c. Metabolism

d. Teratogenesis

e. Bioavailability

10. Select the incorrect statement.

a. Distribution refers to the movement of xenobiotics throughout the body and includes binding of xenobiotics to plasma proteins and storage of xenobiotics in various tissues including bone, liver, and kidney.

b. The "first pass effect" refers to the inability of some toxicants to cross the gastrointestinal mucosal barrier and enter the systemic circulation.

c. Metabolic activity that results in a metabolite that is more toxic than the parent compound is referred to as bioactivation.

d. The predominant goal of metabolism is to make xenobiotics more water-soluble so that they can be more easily excreted via the urine.

e. Enterohepatic recirculation of a xenobiotic can result in prolongation of the xenobiotic's half-life.

ANSWERS

1. c. The LD_{50} identifies the dose at which 50% of dogs will die but does not give an indication of the dose at which dogs can tolerate propranolol without showing clinical signs (maximum tolerated dose), the dose at which clinical signs may be expected to develop (minimum toxic dose), or the lowest dose at which death might be possible (minimum lethal dose). All of these parameters are far more helpful in determining the risk following an acute exposure than is the LD_{50}.

2. b. Tolerance is the reduced responsiveness to a chemical due to prior exposure to that chemical (or a similar chemical). In the case of phenobarbital, the enzymes that metabolize the drug are

induced in the liver, resulting in increase in phenobarbital metabolism, lower blood levels, and decreased adverse effect.

3. e. All of these factors are important in determining the risk of toxicosis from a toxicant.

4. a. Intravenous administration will produce the most rapid distribution of a toxicant to its site of action in the body.

5. b. The dose-response curve represents the characteristics of a xenobiotic within a population, but individual variation can result in increased or decreased response at a particular dose.

6. c. Cats lack essential enzymes for metabolizing acetaminophen into nontoxic compounds and instead produce metabolites that are highly reactive, resulting in toxicosis at relatively low doses of acetaminophen.

7. b. Genetic polymorphisms are inherited traits that result in differences in response to xenobiotics.

8. a. Anencephaly (absence of brain) would not occur because the exposure occurred after the brain had formed (i.e., after completion of organogenesis).

9. e. Bioavailability

10. b. The first pass effect refers to the hepatic removal of a fraction of a xenobiotic that has been absorbed into the portal circulation before the xenobiotic can reach the systemic circulation.

REFERENCES

Boothe, Dawn M. and Peterson, Michael E. 2006. Considerations in pediatric and geriatric poisoned patients. In *Small Animal Toxicology*, 2nd edition, edited by Michael E. Peterson and Patricia A. Talcott, pp. 165–177. St. Louis: Saunders.

Eaton, David L. and Gilbert, Steven G. 2008. Principles of toxicology. In *Casarett and Doull's Toxicology, the Basic Science of Poisons*, 6th edition, edited by Curtis D. Klaasen, pp. 11–43. New York: McGraw-Hill Medical.

Evans, Tim J. 2006. Toxicokinetics and toxicodynamics. In *Small Animal Toxicology*, 2nd edition, edited by Michael E. Peterson and Patricia A. Talcott, pp. 18–28. St. Louis: Saunders.

Frey, H.H. and Rieh, B. 1981. Pharmacokinetics of naproxen in the dog. *American Journal of Veterinary Research* 42(9):1615–1617.

Gwaltney-Brant, Sharon M. 2001. Chocolate intoxication. *Veterinary Medicine* 96(2):108–110.

Kutzler, Michelle A. 2006. Considerations in pregnant or lactating patients. In *Small Animal Toxicology*, 2nd edition, edited by Michael E. Peterson and Patricia A. Talcott, pp. 178–190. St. Louis: Saunders.

Lanusse, Carlos E., Lifschitz, A.L., and Imperiale, F.A. 2009. Macrocyclic lactones: endectocide compounds. In *Veterinary Pharmacology and Therapeutics*, 9th edition, edited by Jim E. Riviere and Mark G. Papich, pp. 1119–1144. Ames, Iowa: Blackwell.

Lees, Peter. 2009. Analgesic, antiinflammatory, antipyretic drugs. In *Veterinary Pharmacology and Therapeutics*, 9th edition, edited by Jim E. Riviere and Mark G. Papich, pp. 457–492. Ames, Iowa: Blackwell.

Lehman-McKeeman, Lois D. 2008. Absorption, distribution, and excretion of toxicants. In *Casarett and Doull's Toxicology, the Basic Science of Poisons*, 6th edition, edited by Curtis D. Klaasen, pp. 131–159. New York: McGraw-Hill Medical.

Mealey, Katrina L. 2006. Ivermectin: Macrolide antiparasitic agents. In *Small Animal Toxicology*, 2nd edition, edited by Michael E. Peterson and Patricia A. Talcott, pp. 785–794. St. Louis: Saunders.

Merrill, Jill C., Morton, Joseph, and Soileau, Stephen D. 2008. Metals. In *Principles and Methods of Toxicology*, 5th edition, edited by A. Wallace Hayes, pp. 841–896. New York: Informa Health Care.

Osweiler, Gary D. 1996. *Toxicology. The National Veterinary Medical Series*, Philadelphia: Williams and Wilkins.

———. 2006. General toxicological principles. In *Small Animal Toxicology*, 2nd edition, edited by Michael E. Peterson and Patricia A. Talcott, pp. 2–17. St. Louis: Saunders.

Parkinson, Andres and Ogilvie, Brian W. 2008. Biotransformation of xenobiotics. In *Casarett and Doull's Toxicology, the Basic Science of Poisons*, 6th edition, edited by Curtis D. Klaasen, pp.161–304. New York: McGraw-Hill Medical.

Rogers, John M and Kavlock, Robert J. 2008. Developmental toxicology. In *Casarett and Doull's Toxicology, the Basic Science of Poisons*, 6th ed., edited by Curtis D. Klaasen, pp.415–451. New York: McGraw-Hill Medical.

Smalley, H.E., Curtis, Jack M., and Earl, F.L. 1968. Teratogenic action of carbaryl in beagle dogs. *Toxicology and Applied Pharmacology* 13(3):392–403.

Talcott, Patricia A. 2006. Nonsteroidal antiinflammatories. In *Small Animal Toxicology*, 2nd edition, edited by Michael E. Peterson and Patricia A. Talcott, pp. 902–933. St. Louis: Saunders.

Volmer, Petra A. 2004. Pyrethrins and pyrethroids. In *Clinical Veterinary Toxicology*, edited by K.H. Plumlee, pp. 188–190. St. Louis: Mosby.

Incidence of Poisoning in Small Animals

2

Sharon Gwaltney-Brant

INTRODUCTION

Animals are exposed to potentially toxic products every day, yet the actual incidence of poisoning in animals is relatively low when compared to other causes of illness, such as infectious and metabolic diseases, allergy, trauma, neoplasia, etc. Animals presenting with signs that pet owners may suspect are related to poisoning need to be fully evaluated in order to rule out the possibility of an unrelated illness. Veterinary technicians can assist in sorting out the cause of illness by obtaining thorough details on the suspected exposure as well as a complete medical history of the patient (see Chapter 4). With this information and the results of a thorough physical examination, the determination as to the likelihood of a poisoning can be made.

Recall from Chapter 1 that the fundamental tenet of toxicology is "the dose makes the poison," meaning that only when a sufficient amount of a toxicant is involved will a poisoning take place. Obviously the dose required to induce a poisoning will depend on a variety of factors, including the agent in question, route of exposure, and species, age, and weight of the animal. Most of the information on animal poisonings comes from human and animal poison control center data; because there is no reporting requirement nor is there a central reporting agency for animal poisonings, the actual incidence of animal poisonings is not known. However, information from poison control centers is still helpful in understanding the most common features of animal poisonings, which can aid in instituting measures that may help in minimizing exposures of animals to toxicants.

DEMOGRAPHICS

Demographic information on companion animal poisonings has largely come from calls to human or animal poison control centers contacted about exposures of the animal to potentially toxic agents (Forrester and Stanley 2004; Haliburton and Buck 1983; Hornfeldt and Murphy 1992, 1997, 1998; Hornfeldt and Borys 1985) or from surveys of veterinary emergency centers or teaching hospitals (Cope et al. 2006; Osweiler 1975). In all these reports, dogs and cats are the species for which assistance is most commonly sought regarding potential poisonings, accounting for 95%–98% of all reported calls (Forrester and Stanley 2004; Guiliano Albo and Nebbia 2004; Xavier et al. 2002; Hornfeldt and Murphy 1998). These percentages have changed considerably since 1983, when dogs and cats accounted for only 44% of calls to an animal poison control center (Trammel et al. 1985).

Dogs account for up to 80% of animal-related calls to human poison control centers (Hornfeldt and Murphy 2006) and up to 85% of calls to animal poison control centers (ASPCA Animal Poison Control Center unpublished data, 2009). Calls regarding cats comprise another 12%–15% of the total, with the remaining cases involving food animals, horses, birds, pocket pets, wildlife, etc. (Gwaltney-Brant 2007). Exposures of animals to potentially toxic agents are more common in the summer, although peaks around the winter holiday seasons have been noted (Gwaltney-Brant 2007). The majority of poisonings are accidental in nature and occur at or near the animal owner's home (Hornfeldt and Murphy 1992, 1998; Khan et al. 1999). Malicious poisonings are relatively rare,

Small Animal Toxicology Essentials, First Edition. Edited by Robert H. Poppenga, Sharon Gwaltney-Brant.

accounting for less than 1% of all exposures to potentially toxic agents (Gwaltney-Brant 2007). In most (>75%) poisonings of dogs and cats, the route of exposure is due to ingestion of the toxicant, with dermal exposures accounting for 4%–15% (Hornfeldt and Murphy 1997). Less than 1% of exposures are by routes other than oral or dermal, including inhalation, bites/stings, injection, or ocular. Ninety-nine percent of reported exposures are acute in nature and 97% involve a single toxicant (Hornfeldt and Murphy 1998).

Dogs are inquisitive creatures with a propensity for investigating the world with their mouths, which makes it easy to understand why dogs far outrank other species in reports of exposures to potentially toxic agents. There is no gender predisposition to poisoning exposures, with males and females being equally represented (Gwaltney-Brant 2007). The average age for cases involving dogs is approximately 4 years, suggesting that young adults are most often involved in potential poisonings. Some breeds, particularly Labrador retrievers, are considered to be more "poison-prone" than others, and a review of over 68,000 animal poison control center cases involving purebred dogs showed that cases involving Labrador retrievers were three times higher than the next most common breed (Gwaltney-Brant 2007). However, the overall percentage of cases involving Labradors (17.6%) was not significantly different than the overall popularity of Labradors based on American Kennel Club registrations (15%). In other words, it may very well be that there are three times more cases involving Labradors because there are three times more Labradors in the population. Some breeds that do appear to be overrepresented in these poisoning cases compared to their overall popularity include cocker spaniels and bichon frises (Gwaltney-Brant 2007).

Unlike dogs, cats have discriminating habits and appetites, making them less likely to ingest things that are not good for them. Calls to poison centers involving cats occur at less than onethird the rate of calls involving dogs (Hornfeldt and Murphy 2006), even though cat ownership exceeds dog ownership in the United States, with over 81 million owned cats vs. 72 million owned dogs in 2007 (AVMA 2007). There are no gender or age differences reported in cat poisoning cases (Gwaltney-Brant 2007), and the most commonly reported purebreds were Siamese, Persians, Maine coon, and Himalayan. Because of their grooming habits, cats are more at risk than dogs from agents that come into contact with their fur. For example, many ethylene glycol exposures in cats are thought to occur when cats walk through or lie in puddles and then groom the ethylene glycol off their hair.

AGENTS

There is a virtually unlimited number of agents to which animals may be exposed, and the potential for an exposure to turn into an actual poisoning depends on a number of factors, including the inherent toxicity of the agent, the sensitivity of the animal to the effects of the agent, the amount of the agent to which the animal is exposed, and the route of exposure (e.g., ingestion vs. dermal). The potential for exposure to specific agents may vary with the time of the year; for instance, chocolate exposures increase around holidays where chocolate is traditionally featured and pesticide exposures are more frequent during the spring and summer, when use of these products increases.

Based on reports from human and animal poison control centers, the most frequent exposures of companion animals tend to involve rodenticides, chocolate, and pharmaceuticals (Gwaltney-Brant 2007). The most common pharmaceutical agents to which pets are exposed include analgesics (especially nonsteroidal anti-inflammatory agents) and central nervous system drugs (e.g., antidepressants, sedatives, stimulants, etc.) Exposures to pesticides, once the most common cause of animal-related calls, have declined significantly, possibly due to the introduction of newer, less toxic products and better public awareness of the potential hazards of pesticides to pets. Plant exposures are also common both inside and outside the house. Household cleaning agents, automotive products, and food products are other common causes of animal-related calls to poison control centers.

SIGNS AND OUTCOMES

In spite of the wide range of potentially toxic agents to which animals may be exposed, the vast majority of exposures result in no signs for the patient, based on poison control center data (Gwaltney-Brant 2007). In many cases, the animal may not have been exposed to a sufficient amount to cause toxicosis, while in other cases successful decontamination by animal caretakers may have prevented the development of clinical signs. Mild signs that develop are expected to be self-limiting and generally do not require treatment (e.g., mild vomiting), and they occur in ~25% of poison control center cases involving animals. Moderate signs occur in about 7% of exposures; these signs generally require some form of treatment (e.g., antiemetics for persistent vomiting), but are not expected to be life threatening. Major signs are those in which life-threatening conditions occur or there is potential for significant residual disability or disfigurement following recovery; fortunately, toxicoses associated with major signs generally account for about

1% of animal poisoning cases. The overall mortality rate for animal cases reported to human poison control centers ranges from 2%–3% (Hornfeldt and Murphy 2006). Agents most commonly associated with severe signs and deaths include rodenticides, pesticides, pharmaceuticals, plants, and ethylene glycol.

CONCLUSION

Poisoning is a serious cause of morbidity and mortality in animals, particularly in dogs and cats. Based on information obtained by veterinary clinics and human and animal poison control centers, the incidence of animal poisoning does not appear to be waning, although the agents to which animals are exposed does appear to change with time. While significant pesticide exposures may be on the decline due to the development of newer and less toxic pesticides, exposures to other agents, such as chocolate and pharmaceutical agents, may be on the rise. Knowing what agents have the potential to be involved in serious toxicoses should allow veterinary technicians to better educate clients on means of preventing animal poisonings through the appropriate use of household products and the removal of potential hazards from the animals' environments.

CHAPTER 2 STUDY QUESTIONS

1. Which of the following best characterizes the most common scenario for animal poisonings with regard to species involved, time of year, location of exposure, intent, and route of exposure?
   a. Feline, fall, veterinary clinic, malicious, intramuscular injection
   b. Canine, summer, home, accidental, oral ingestion
   c. Feline, summer, home, malicious, oral ingestion
   d. Canine, fall, home, malicious, oral ingestion
   e. Canine, spring, accidental, dermal exposure
2. Which one of the following includes toxicants most often involved in pet poisonings?
   a. Pool chemicals, insecticides, and chocolate
   b. Plants, chocolate, and lawn chemicals
   c. Antifreeze, rodenticide, and chocolate
   d. Rodenticides, pharmaceuticals, and chocolate
   e. Pharmaceuticals, automotive products, and lawn chemicals
3. Which of the following statements is incorrect?
   a. The majority of exposures of animals to potentially toxic agents result in no clinical signs.
   b. Most animals developing clinical signs following exposure to potentially toxic agents develop mild effects only.

   c. Toxicants most commonly associated with mortality in dogs and cats include pharmaceuticals, rodenticides, and ethylene glycol.
   d. The incidence of poisoning due to exposure of pets to pesticides has increased dramatically over the past 25 years.
   e. According to cases reported to poison control centers, deaths occur in less than 5% of all reported animal poisonings.

ANSWERS

1. b. Most poisonings occur in the summer and involve dogs that most commonly accidentally ingest poisons in or near the home.
2. d.
3. d. The incidence of pesticide poisoning of pets has declined significantly.

REFERENCES

AVMA (American Veterinary Medical Association). 2007. *U.S. Pet Ownership & Demographics Sourcebook*, Schaumburg: AVMA.
Cope, Rhian, White, K.S., More, E., Holmes, K., Nair, A., Chauvin, P., and Oncken, A. 2006. Exposure-to-treatment interval and clinical severity in canine poisoning: a retrospective analysis at a Portland veterinary emergency center. *Journal of Veterinary Pharmacology and Therapeutics* 29:233–236.
Forrester, Mathias and Stanley, Sharilyn K. 2004. Patterns of animal poisonings reported to the Texas Poison Center Network: 1998–2002. *Veterinary and Human Toxicology* 46:96–99.

Guiliano Albo, A. and Nebbia C. 2004. Incidence of poisonings in domestic carnivores in Italy. *Veterinary Research Communications* 28:83–88.

Gwaltney-Brant, Sharon M. 2007. Epidemiology of animal poisonings. In *Veterinary Toxicology: Basics and Clinical Principles*, edited by Ramesh C. Gupta, pp. 67–73. New York: Academic Press Elsevier.

Haliburton, John C. and Buck, William B. 1983. Animal poison control center: summary of telephone inquiries during the first three years of service. *Journal of the American Veterinary Medical Association* 182(5):514–515.

Hornfeldt Carl S. and Borys, Douglas J. 1985. Review of veterinary cases received by the Hennepin Poison Center in 1984. *Veterinary and Human Toxicology* 27(6):525–528.

Hornfeldt, Carl S. and Murphy, Michael J. 1992. 1990 report of the American Association of Poison Control Centers: Poisonings in animals. *Journal of the American Veterinary Medical Association* 200(8):1077–1080.

———. 1997. Poisonings in animals: The 1993–1994 report of the American Association of Poison Control Centers. *Veterinary and Human Toxicology* 39(6):361–365.

———. 1998. American Association of Poison Control Centers report on poisonings of animals, 1993–1994. *Journal of the American Veterinary Medical Association* 212(3):358–361.

———. 2006 Summary of small animal poison exposures. In *Small Animal Toxicology, Second Edition*, edited by Michael E. Peterson and Patricia A. Talcott, pp. 563–577. St. Louis: Elsevier Saunders.

Khan, Safdar A., Schell, Mary M., Trammel, Harold L., Hansen, Steven K., and Knight, Michael W. 1999. Ethylene glycol exposures managed by the ASPCA National Animal Poison Control Center from July 1995 to December 1997. *Veterinary and Human Toxicology* 41(6):403–406.

Osweiler, G.D. 1975. Sources and incidence of small animal poisoning. *Veterinary Clinics of North America* 5(4):589–604.

Trammel, Harold, Buck, William, and Beasley, Val. 1985. National Animal Poison Control Center: Seven years of service. *29th Annual Proceedings of the American Association of Veterinary Laboratory Diagnosticians*, pp. 183–191.

Xavier, F.G. and Kogika, M.M., de Sousa, Spinosa H. 2002 Common causes of poisoning in dogs and cats in a Brazilian veterinary teaching hospital from 1998 to 2000. *Veterinary and Human Toxicology* 44, 115–116.

Toxicology Information Resources 3

Sharon Gwaltney-Brant

INTRODUCTION

In the past several years, the amount of toxicology information has grown tremendously, as has the ability to access this information, whether through peer-reviewed publications, textbooks, or computer-based resources. The primary challenge is determining which sources provide the most up-to-date, accurate, and reliable information. Additionally, diagnostic laboratories and poison control centers can provide invaluable information when dealing with a toxicological problem. This chapter provides an overview of toxicology information resources that are available to assist in dealing with toxicology questions.

EVALUATION OF RESOURCES

When choosing a toxicology information resource, it is important that the veterinary technician be aware of any potential issues regarding quality or bias of the information. In general, peer-reviewed resources (e.g., veterinary journals) that outline the methods by which conclusions are reached are more reliable than non–peer-reviewed resources (lay journals, nonfiction literature, the Internet) which tend to summarize data, often adding personal opinion to, or in place of, scientific theory or facts. Even peer-reviewed resources may show some bias, because the research may have been sponsored by a corporation or group with a particular agenda. It is wise to check the institutions from which the author(s) came to determine whether there might be some conflict of interest. That is not to imply that all research funded by industry or other interest groups is suspect; the reader should keep an open mind while reading the material critically.

Computer-based resources, such as bibliography searches (e.g., Medline, offered by the National Institutes of Health) can be extremely valuable and reliable, whereas personal or corporate web pages may be fraught with inaccurate, outdated, biased, or outright damaging information, depending on the agenda of the page owner. Because anyone can post a well-designed website full of misinformation, close scrutiny of the source of the information is imperative. In general, sites sponsored by reputable governmental, educational, and institutional agencies will contain information that is up-to-date, is accurate, and tends to provide balanced views, even on controversial subjects. Sites that engage in polarized, emotional, or dogmatic discourse should be read with skepticism; in these cases, attempting to verify the statements made on these sites through other independent resources is highly recommended.

Items to consider in evaluating the information available on websites include

- The author's credentials and institutional affiliations
- The date the material was posted
- The clarity and comprehensiveness of the information provided
- The relevance of hyperlinks to other sites
- The inclusion of clear references, preferably peer-reviewed

"Internet rumors" are reports with little to no basis in fact, often with outrageously exaggerated claims, and they have the unfortunate tendency to become widely disseminated, usually via email, in a very short period of time. Not surpris-

Small Animal Toxicology Essentials, First Edition. Edited by Robert H. Poppenga, Sharon Gwaltney-Brant.
© 2011 John Wiley and Sons, Inc. Published 2011 by John Wiley and Sons, Inc.

ingly, many of these rumors involve poisonings of humans or pets, often by seemingly innocuous agents, such as shampoos, household cleaners, and the like. An example of an Internet rumor that has had wide dissemination (and several resurrections over the years) is the 2004 rumor that Swiffer WetJet cleaning solution poses a hazard to dogs because it contains an ingredient that is "one molecule away from antifreeze" and has caused liver failure in dogs and deaths in cats. The ingredient in question, propylene glycol n-propyl ether, is of low toxicity especially at the concentrations present in cleaning agents (it is present in a large number of common household cleaners) and it will not cause liver injury. The rumor has been discredited by a variety of sources, but it still crops up every now and then (Oehme and Hare 2009). In general, a good rule of thumb is to treat unsolicited warnings received via email or fax with skepticism until further research can be done to verify their authenticity. The Urban Legends References Page (www.snopes.com) is a good first stop in the search for the truth of a particular story. This website has compiled and researched thousands of rumors, Internet or otherwise, and rates them on their veracity as true, false, or undetermined.

TYPES OF RESOURCES

Peer-Reviewed Journals

Peer-reviewed journals provide detailed accounts of recent studies being done in a variety of specialized areas. They have the advantage of providing the most up-to-date information as well as describing the study in detail, allowing the reader to assess the conclusions drawn from the work. One disadvantage to this type of resource is that the information is new and may be revised over time based on the results of subsequent studies or scientific review.

There are no veterinary toxicology journals currently being published; however, animal toxicology information may be found in a variety of human toxicology journals as well as select veterinary journals. See Table 3.1 for a listing of some journals that publish clinically relevant toxicology articles.

Textbooks

In the past several years, the number of available veterinary toxicology texts and toxicology-related chapters in veterinary medical texts has expanded greatly. In general, these resources focus on the most commonly encountered toxicology issues, making them useful and convenient for those in clinical practice who lack the time to do detailed searches on individual topics. Textbooks are an economical and effective means of having toxicology information readily available. On the downside, texts may present

Table 3.1. Journals with veterinary toxicology articles

American Journal of Veterinary Research
Canadian Journal of Veterinary Research
Canadian Veterinary Journal
Clinical Techniques in Small Animal Practice
Compendium: Continuing Education for Veterinarians
Journal of the American Animal Hospital Association
Journal of the American Association of Veterinary Laboratory Diagnosticians
Journal of the American Veterinary Medical Association
Journal of Medical Toxicology
Journal of Small Animal Practice
Journal of Veterinary Emergency and Critical Care
Journal of Veterinary Internal Medicine
Journal of Veterinary Pharmacology and Therapeutics
Journal of Zoo and Wildlife Medicine
North American Veterinary Conference Clinician's Brief
Preventive Veterinary Medicine
Veterinary Clinics of North America, Small Animal Practice; Exotic Animal Practice
Veterinary and Human Toxicology (discontinued 2005)
Veterinary Journal
Veterinary Medicine
Veterinary Pathology
Veterinary Quarterly
Veterinary Record

abbreviated information due to limited space, some information may be outdated by the time the text is published, and newer discoveries must await the publication of newer editions. Table 3.2 provides a short list of some currently available toxicology textbooks applicable to small animal veterinary medicine.

Computer Databases and Internet Sites

A large number of computer databases exist that can provide quick access to a wide variety of toxicology information. Some of these are more geared toward human toxicology, but there often will be some animal information included. At the very least they can give the reader a rough estimate of potential for toxicity based on how hazardous some products are for humans. Proprietary databases such as Poisindex® or Tomes® (both by Micromedex) are available by subscription and would be of minimal availability to those working in veterinary practice. However, Poisindex® is used by all U.S. poison control centers, so the information would be available through a regional poison control center.

Table 3.2. Veterinary toxicology textbooks

Title, Author/Editor, Year	Publisher
Blackwell's Five-Minute Veterinary Consult Clinical Companion: Small Animal Toxicology, Osweiler, Hovda, Brutlag and Lee, 2011.	Wiley-Blackwell
Clinical Veterinary Toxicology, Plumlee, 2003	Mosby
Field Guide to Common Animal Poisons, Murphy, 1996	Iowa State Press
Handbook of Small Animal Toxicology and Poisonings, Gfeller, 2003	Mosby
Handbook of Toxic Plants of North America, Burrows and Tyrl, 2006	Blackwell
Natural Toxicants in Feeds, Forages and Poisonous Plants, Cheeke, 1998	Interstate Publishers
Small Animal Toxicology, Peterson and Talcott, 2006	Saunders
Toxicology (National Veterinary Medical Series), Osweiler, 1996	Williams & Wilkins
Toxic Plants of North America, Burrows & Tyrl, 2001	Iowa State Press
Veterinary Toxicology, Gupta, 2007	Academic Press
Veterinary Toxicology, Roder, 2001	Butterworth-Heinemann

Other accurate and up-to-date databases are accessible via the Internet, and many of these are provided for low to no cost. Other websites maintained by government agencies, academia, and organizations can provide a wealth of toxicology information, and most are available at no cost to the web surfer. As stated earlier, the veracity of the information available on websites can be in question, so some degree of healthy skepticism is merited when browsing information on websites maintained by individuals or organizations that may have underlying agendas (e.g., selling a product). Table 3.3 includes some websites providing reliable toxicology information.

Poison Control Centers

There are approximately 66 poison centers in the United States that provide 24-hour/7-day assistance to the public and health care providers in cases of human exposures to potentially toxic agents (McNally et al. 2006). These centers are generally staffed by nurses and pharmacists, many with specialized training in toxicology (Specialists in Poison Information or SPIs), and are funded through tax dollars. Most are members of the American Association of

Poison Control Centers, an organization that oversees the education and training of poison control specialists and provides public education by promoting awareness of the importance of poison prevention. Individuals can reach their regional poison control center by calling 1-800-222-1222 from anywhere in the United States; callers using land lines (not cell phones) will automatically be routed to the appropriate poison control center for their region.

Human poison control centers can be of assistance to veterinary staff in helping to identify unknown human medications through their database of imprint codes. Although some centers permit their staff to manage animal cases, most lack the information and financial resources to be primary resources for veterinary patients. Extrapolation of information from the human poison database to animals can sometimes result in erroneous treatment recommendations and is not generally recommended.

The American Society for the Prevention of Cruelty to Animals (ASPCA) Animal Poison Control Center (APCC) was the first animal oriented poison control center in the United States. The Center provides 24-hour/7-day assistance and is staffed by 30 veterinarians, 15 of whom have achieved specialty-board certification in general and/or veterinary toxicology. In addition to their extensive experience in dealing with animal toxicology emergencies, the veterinary staff at the APCC has access to a database that incorporates over 30 years of cases of animal poisonings to assist them in managing animal toxicoses. The APCC is a member of the American Association of Poison Control Centers and works with human poison control centers, governmental agencies, zoos, and other organizations to provide accurate and up-to-date information on newly discovered hazards to animals. The ASPCA-APCC can be contacted by telephone at 1-888-426-4435; in most cases a per-case consultation fee will apply, but there is no cost if the product involved is covered by the manufacturer through the Animal Product Safety Service division of the APCC.

Pet Poison Helpline is another 24-hour/7-day animal poison control center in North America. This poison control center is staffed by a large group of veterinarians who are board certified in veterinary toxicology (ABVT), internal medicine (ACVIM) and emergency and critical care (ACVECC) with the added benefit of having experts in human toxicology (PharmDs). Pet Poison Helpline is operated by SafetyCall International, the world's largest industry poison control center providing poison control services to consumers of veterinary and human pharmaceuticals, household goods, pesticides, personal care products, agricultural products and dietary supplements; it is also affiliated with the University of Minnesota. Pet Poison

Table 3.3. Internet websites with toxicology information

Name	URL	Description
General Search Engines		Utilize a variety of indexing programs to search and return websites based on keywords.
AllTheWeb	www.alltheweb.com	
Alta Vista	www.altavista.com	
Ask.com	www.ask.com	
Bing	www.bing.com	
Dogpile	www.dogpile.com	
Goodsearch	www.goodsearch.com	
Google	www.google.com	
Hotbot	www.hotbot.com	
Lycos	www.lycos.com	
MetaCrawler	www.metacrawler.com	
WebCrawler	www.webcrawler.com	
Yahoo	www.yahoo.com	
Toxicology Information		
American Academy of Clinical Toxicology (AACT)	www.clintox.org	Multidisciplinary organization uniting scientists and clinicians in the advancement of research, education, prevention and treatment of diseases caused by chemicals, drugs, and toxins
American Association of Poison Control Centers (AAPCC)	www.aapcc.org	Provides oversight and coordination of U.S. poison control centers
American Board of Veterinary Toxicologists (ABVT)	www.abvt.org/public/index.html	Certifying body for veterinary toxicologists
American Board of Toxicologists (ABT)	www.abtox.org	Certifying board for general toxicology
Agency for Toxic Substances & Disease Registry (ATSDR)	www.atsdr.cdc.gov	Health agency of the U.S. Department of Health and Human Services (USDHHS) providing public health information on science related to toxic substances
National Toxicology Program (NTP)	ntp-server.niehs.nih.gov	Evaluates agents of public health concern by developing and applying tools of modern toxicology and molecular biology Division of National Institutes of Health
Veterinary/Medical Information		
Centers for Disease Control and Prevention (CDC)	www.cdc.gov	Primary U.S. federal agency for conducting and supporting public health activities within the U.S.
PubMed	http://www.ncbi.nlm.nih.gov/PubMed	Search engine for biomedical literature from MEDLINE, life science journals, and online books
Veterinary Information Network (VIN)	www.vin.com	Online community of veterinarians with board-certified specialist consultants, diagnostic tools, and research materials
Veterinary Support Personnel Network (VSPN)	www.vspn.org	Online community for veterinary support staff providing expert consultants and continuing education

Table 3.3. *Continued*

Name	URL	Description
WHO	www.who.org	Directing and coordinating authority for health within the United Nations System
Pesticide Information		
Extension Toxicology Network (ExToxNet)	extoxnet.orst.edu	Collaborative effort by several U.S. universities to provide objective, science-based information about pesticides, written for nonexperts
National Pesticide Information Center (NPIC)	npic.orst.edu	Provides objective, science-based information about pesticides and pesticide-related topics; operates toll-free telephone service for questions related to pesticides
US Environmental Protection Agency	www.epa.gov	U.S. agency charged to protect human health and the environment by working for a cleaner, healthier environment
Food/Drug Information		
Food Animal Residue Avoidance Databank (FARAD)	www.farad.org	Computer-based decision system designed to provide information on avoiding drug, pesticide, and environmental contaminant residue problems in food animals
Internet Drug Index(RxList)	www.rxlist.com	Provides information on prescription drugs
US Food and Drug Administration	www.fda.gov	USHHS agency charged with overseeing safety of food, drugs, and medical devices
FDA Safety Portal	www.safetyreporting.hhs.gov	Portal for reporting safety issues regarding foods (human or pet), animal drugs, or NIH gene-transfer research
Dietary Supplements Labels Database	http://dietarysupplements.nlm.nih.gov/dietary/	Offers information about ingredients in >3000 selected brands of dietary supplements
Plant/Mushroom Information		
ASPCA Animal Poison Control Center plant list	www.aspca.org/pet-care/poison-control/plants/	Searchable site that outlines plants that are toxic and nontoxic to animals
MushroomExpert.Com	www.mushroomexpert.com/index.html	Website listing information on toxic and nontoxic mushrooms

Helpline's toxicologists have been serving the veterinary community for over 30 years and have managed 2.5 million poisonings. The Pet Poison Helpline can be consulted by telephone at 1-800-213-6680. All consultation fee of $35 per case may apply; this consultation fee includes unlimited follow-up. The website for Pet Poison Helpline is www.petpoisonhelpline.com.

Veterinary Diagnostic Laboratories

Veterinary diagnostic laboratories are invaluable tools in dealing with animal poisonings (Galey and Talcott 2006). Most states have their own veterinary diagnostic laboratories, often associated with veterinary colleges. Many are staffed with veterinary toxicologists, who can assist in case management (treatment, prognosis, etc.) as well as offer suggestions on which tests to perform and samples to submit in order to obtain a diagnosis of toxicant exposure or intoxication. Even if the diagnostic laboratory within a particular state is unable to perform a specific toxicologic analysis, samples often can be sent to other state laboratories for testing. Typically there are fees that are charged for such analytical tests, but in general they are relatively modest compared to the actual expense to the diagnostic laboratory performing the test.

Contrary to popular belief, there is no one "poison screen" that will test for all known toxic agents. Because there are a variety of tests available to detect various toxicants, it is important that the most appropriate test be selected in order to minimize the time and cost associated with testing. When presented with a sample for testing, the toxicologist will weigh all of the available information, including history, clinical signs, and any physical characteristics of the agent in question in order to determine which analysis is most appropriate. For this reason, the more information provided to the toxicologist the more likely it will be that he/she will be able to determine the most appropriate testing for that case. The veterinary technician can assist in this regard by ensuring that the submission forms are filled out as completely and legibly as possible.

Summary

A wide range of toxicology information resources is available to assist veterinary staff in the identification, diagnosis, and management of animal poisonings. Judicious care should be taken to confirm the reliability of information sources, particularly those found in the lay literature or on the Internet.

CHAPTER 3 STUDY QUESTIONS

1. A dog owner calls to say that Sarge, her 70-pound German shepherd dog, has just ingested an herbal supplement containing valerian. Which of the following would be the LEAST desirable source of information on this supplement?
   a. Peer-reviewed veterinary journal article on valerian use in dogs
   b. Veterinary herbal medicine text book
   c. Animal poison control center
   d. Internet website selling valerian for use in dogs
   e. Veterinary diagnostic laboratory toxicologist
2. Which of the following would be the least reliable source of information on potential toxicants for pets?
   a. U.S. Environmental Protection Agency website
   b. U.S. Food and Drug Administration website
   c. Medline literature search
   d. University website
   e. Pet owner's personal website
3. Poison control centers can provide vital, life-saving information in cases of animal poisonings. Which of the following is false regarding the use of poison control centers by veterinary professionals?
   a. In the U.S., there are currently two animal poison control centers staffed by veterinary professionals on a 24-hour/7-day basis.
   b. Human poison control centers are just as capable of managing animal poisonings because both animal and human poison control centers employ veterinary professionals and use information from the same databases.
   c. Poison control centers can assist in the identification of unknown medication through their database of imprint codes.
   d. The National Poison Control Hotline number is 1-800-222-1222 and will route land line callers to their appropriate regional poison control center.

ANSWERS

1. d. Internet websites selling products may overstate benefits and downplay risks in order to sell a product. In addition, such sites have rarely have information on accidental exposure or overdose.
2. e.
3. b. Human poison control centers rarely employ veterinary professionals and use a human-oriented database; animal poison control centers employ veterinarians and veterinary technicians and use their own animal-oriented databases.

REFERENCES

Galey, Francis D. and Talcott, Patricia A. 2006. Effective use of a diagnostic laboratory. In *Small Animal Toxicology*, 2nd edition, edited by Michael E. Peterson and Patricia A. Talcott, pp. 154–164. St. Louis: Elsevier Saunders.

McNally, Jude, Boesen, Keith, Tong, Theodore G. 2006. Toxicological information resources. In *Small Animal Toxicology*, 2nd edition, edited by Michael E. Peterson and Patricia A. Talcott, pp. 29–37. St. Louis: Elsevier Saunders.

Oehme, Fred W. and Hare, William R. 2009. Urban legends of toxicology: Facts and fiction. In *Current Veterinary Therapy XIV*, edited by John D. Bonagura, pp. 109–111. St. Louis: Elsevier Saunders.

Taking a Toxicologic History

4

Carrie Lohmeyer

INTRODUCTION

Obtaining a thorough history is critical in effectively treating patients that have been or are suspected of being exposed to a toxic agent. The history-taking process begins from the moment the client walks through the front door of the veterinary hospital or calls in on the telephone. The most important reason for obtaining a thorough history though is to provide the safest and most appropriate care for the patient (Fitzgerald 2006). It is the veterinary technician's responsibility to acquire a reliable and accurate history to prevent the loss of money, time, energy, and resources in the hospital setting. This chapter offers guidelines to assist veterinary technicians in developing the skills necessary to be successful in obtaining a toxicological history.

PATIENT PRESENTATION

Depending on the circumstances, the technician may not know that the patient has been exposed to a toxic agent upon its presentation to the veterinary hospital. When dealing with toxic exposures the case will reflect one of four situations: the agent is known and the patient is asymptomatic, the agent is known and the patient is symptomatic, the agent is not known and the patient is symptomatic (aka "mystery poisoning"), the agent is not known and the patient is asymptomatic. The general history-taking process will be the same for all four cases but may need adjustment according to the current situation at hand.

As with any medical emergency, it is important to be prepared and organized in the event a toxicology case presents. Some toxicants can act very quickly; therefore, time plays a key role in treatment implementation. Patients that present with clinical signs need to be assessed and stabilized as needed. Identifying ahead of time which staff member will assist in emergent patient care and which will obtain the historical information can save time and confusion. Having a predetermined protocol established for toxicological exposures enables the hospital staff to stabilize and treat the patients efficiently and effectively.

MEDICAL RECORD

The medical record for a toxicology case is composed of six sets of required data: client information, patient information, clinical status, agent information, exposure information, and implemented treatment. The first three categories are usually a component of any history-taking process, whether a poisoning is involved or not. Agent information, exposure information, and implemented treatment are going to be additional elements. A written protocol can be very helpful in guiding veterinary technicians through the history-taking process to avoid overlooking important information relating to a toxicological exposure. Each protocol is going to vary from veterinary hospital to veterinary hospital due to individual preferences, but the six key components of a toxicological history should be incorporated into the protocol and documented in a medical record. Once a written protocol is developed, it should be readily available to everyone in the hospital setting; this will prevent miscommunication when a toxicity case presents.

Small Animal Toxicology Essentials, First Edition. Edited by Robert H. Poppenga, Sharon Gwaltney-Brant.
© 2011 John Wiley and Sons, Inc. Published 2011 by John Wiley and Sons, Inc.

Client Information

The first component of any medical record is the client information. This should include the name of client, a billing address, and a telephone number where the client can be reached. If the client is not the owner of the patient (e.g., extended family member or pet sitter), the contact information for both parties should be obtained. When obtaining contact information, it is important to ensure that the record includes all possible means of contacting the client to assure that veterinary staff will be able to communicate changes in clinical status in a timely fashion.

Patient Information

Patient signalment is the second component of the medical history. The patient's name, breed, age, reproductive status, and weight should all be noted in the medical record. The vaccination status, environment, date of last veterinary visit, current medications and supplements (including dosage), diet, and preexisting health conditions should also be included. Each item of patient signalment has a purpose. Breed identification is important because some breeds can be more or less sensitive to certain agents. A dose of ivermectin considered nontoxic for a Labrador retriever could potentially be problematic for a collie because some collies possess a defective P-glycoprotein in the blood-brain barrier that makes them more sensitive to ivermectin. Similarly, the age of the patient is going to play a role in determining toxicity and recommended treatments. Very young or very old patients may have limited organ function, which can influence absorption, metabolism, and elimination of toxicants. For instance, a dog that is 14 years old may be at higher risk of developing kidney failure from an overdose of naproxen than a healthy 3-year-old dog ingesting the same dose. The reproductive status of a patient is also an essential element in a toxicological history. Pregnant or lactating females exposed to toxic agents may require additional or alternative treatment than males or nonpregnant, nonlactating females. The potential effects of the toxicant, as well as any drugs used to treat the toxicosis, on the fetuses must be considered when the case involves a pregnant animal. Some toxicants (e.g., some anticoagulant rodenticides) can be passed to offspring through the milk; an important consideration when dealing with lactating animals is whether they have nursed their young subsequent to being exposed to the toxic agent.

The basic tenet of toxicology is "the dose makes the poison," meaning that some exposures will result in no toxic consequences because a toxic dose is not achieved. For instance, a 0.5 oz bar of a 0.01% bromethalin rodenticide will not pose a toxic hazard for an 80 lb dog, but the same bar ingested by a 5 lb dog has potential to cause marked clinical signs if treatment is not implemented. Obviously, a current, accurate weight of the patient is critical for calculating doses of active ingredients of toxicants as well as for calculating appropriate medication dosages.

The patient's vaccination status, date of last veterinary visit, current medications and supplements, diet, and preexisting health conditions can be grouped into the general category of overall health. Knowing the vaccination status of the patient gives the veterinary technician an idea of how well the patient is cared for and may aid in ruling in or out infectious causes of a patient's clinical signs. For example, a 5-month-old, unvaccinated puppy presents to the veterinary hospital with severe vomiting and diarrhea. A toxicological history was obtained, but the vaccination status of the patient was not asked. According to the owners, the dog ingested a few crystals from a silica gel packet that came out of a shoebox a few hours before the signs began. Silica gel is a minimally toxic agent that may, at worst, cause mild and self-limiting stomach upset. Without knowing that silica gel exposures do not cause serious toxicosis, the assumption may be made that the puppy's signs are related to the ingestion of the silica gel while overlooking a more serious potential cause, such as parvoviral enteritis.

The date of the patient's last veterinary visit also provides information on the patient's prior health care. The prior health of patients that have not been examined by veterinarians for many years is going to be relatively unknown compared to patients that receive regular veterinary care. The results of any prior clinical pathology evaluations may be useful to determine whether any significant changes have occurred that may be attributable to the current exposure. Conversely, the lack of prior clinical pathology information may make it difficult to determine whether, for example, an elevation in liver enzyme values is due to the patient's current issue or whether preexisting liver disease is present.

Current medications and preexisting health conditions are two other components of a toxicological history that should not be overlooked. Medications that the patient is taking can influence a toxicology case in several ways. Some medications may increase sensitivity to certain toxicants. For instance, a dog that is being treated with a nonsteroidal anti-inflammatory drug for arthritis pain and then ingests ibuprofen may be at a higher risk for the development of gastrointestinal ulcers and acute renal failure. Medications may also influence the treatment plan for a given case, because possible interaction of the medication with a drug in a treatment protocol may result in the need to alter the protocol for that patient. Although less common, it is also possible that the patient's clinical signs in a "mystery poisoning" are due to an adverse reaction to a prescribed medication. Preexisting health conditions also come into play when deciding what treatment to implement. A patient that has a heart murmur, megaesophagus, or seizure disorder may require different or additional treatment and monitoring than a healthy patient. Decontamination is indicated in many exposures to toxicants; however, emesis may be contraindicated in a patient that has a history of seizures, heart problems, or megaesophagus. Patients with histories of prior organ dysfunction may be at increased risk from toxicants affecting those organs, and may therefore require more aggressive treatment at lower dosages than would healthy animals.

Clinical Status

Some patients may present to the hospital showing no clinical signs, but signs may have occurred prior to the presentation. Careful questioning of the client can help identify the signs that the patient has developed, when the signs began, and their severity. For example, a 10 lb dog ingested 3 oz of semisweet chocolate approximately 1.5 hours prior to presentation to the veterinary hospital. Upon presentation the dog is BAR and the physical exam is unremarkable. Since the dog is asymptomatic, the veterinary staff wishes to initiate treatment by administering a dose of apomorphine to induce emesis. However, the history indicates that the patient had already vomited 5 times at home, recovering a large amount of chocolate. Since the patient has already spontaneously vomited, induction of emesis is not indicated because additional vomiting is unlikely to result in significant further decontamination.

Environmental Information

The environment in which the patient lives is important when identifying possible contributing causes of clinical signs a patient has developed. A domestic animal that is indoor/outdoor or strictly outdoors will have additional opportunities to be exposed to toxic substances, infectious agents, trauma, and other hazards when compared to patients that live strictly indoors. Environmental information is especially essential in determining the cause of a patient's clinical signs when dealing with an unknown toxicant. For example, a previously healthy 2-year-old German shepherd presents to a veterinary hospital with severe vomiting and lethargy. Diagnostic testing indicates that the dog is in liver failure. The owner is unaware of

any toxic exposure that may have occurred and is certain that the dog was not exposed to anything inside the home. When questioned more thoroughly, the owner remembers that the dog was unattended in the yard for approximately 6 hours on the previous day. The owner has a wide variety of plants in the yard as well as occasional mushrooms growing in the grass. The plant varieties in the yard include juniper, sago palm, daffodils, rosebushes, and tulips. From this information, the possibility that the sago palm or a hepatotoxic mushroom may be the cause of the dog's signs must be considered. Without questioning the owner about possible exposures that may have occurred outside the home, the potential exposure to sago palm or mushrooms would have been overlooked.

For indoor animals, information that may be useful includes the areas of the house to which the animal has access, including recent access to areas the pet does not normally go (e.g., attic). The types of medications/herbal products (human and veterinary, prescription, illicit and OTC) in the household, and whether there have been recent visitors who may have dropped medication are important queries to make. It is best to ask for a list of all medications/herbals that are in the household, even if the client is sure that the patient did not have access to it. The types of houseplants in the home should be listed; and it is best to try to obtain the scientific name of the plant whenever possible because many different plants share common names. The presence of children or teenagers in the household is important to know, because the youngsters may have left items in the pet's reach or allowed the pet access to a toxicant; sometimes children on medication will feed the medication to a pet to avoid taking it themselves. The presence of rodenticides or insecticides in the home is an important bit of historical information. Recent redecorating or renovation may expose toxicants (e.g., old bags of rodenticide, lead in paint chips or flakes) that were not previously accessible to the animal. The presence of other pets and whether the other pets in the house appear normal should also be ascertained.

For outdoor animals confined by fences or other means, identification of potentially toxic agents in outbuildings, garages, or sheds to which the pet may have access is important. Other potential hazards found in yards include compost piles, plants, and yard treatments (especially some systemic insecticides and crabgrass killers). For free-roaming animals, the challenge is much greater because the number of potentially toxic agents available is quite large. Determining whether the animal is in an urban, suburban, or rural environment and identifying the nature of the animal's immediate surroundings (e.g., wooded areas vs. parks and lawns) may help in narrowing down the agents to which the roaming animal may have been exposed. The presence of livestock in the pet's environment should stimulate questioning to determine the pet's access to the barns or feed bins; whether medicated feeds, fly baits, or feeds with growth promoters (e.g., ionophores) in them are present; whether the livestock have recently been medicated or dewormed; or whether any livestock have recently been euthanized and buried on the property.

Agent Information

The next data set required for the toxicological medical record is the toxic agent, if known. The trade name of the product or medication, active and inactive ingredients, ingredient concentrations, scents or flavors, EPA registration numbers, and manufacturer contact information should all be documented in the medical record. This information is easy to obtain if the packaging (prescription bottles, containers, boxes, etc.) is brought to the veterinary hospital with the patient. In many cases, clients may not have that information with them because the package may have been ingested, discarded, or destroyed or may never have been available. In some cases it may be necessary to send clients back home or to the store where the agent was purchased to obtain package information. Imprint codes from individual medication tablets or capsules can be used to identify a drug in cases where prescription bottles are not available. A copy of *Physician's Desk Reference* can help to decipher imprint codes; if a *PDR* is not available, there is a variety of Internet resources (e.g., drugs.com) to obtain this information, or a poison control center could be contacted. Rodenticide exposures provide excellent examples of why ingredient information is essential. There are three main types of commonly used rodenticides, and each has a different level of toxicity and treatment protocol. Bromethalin exposure and bromadiolone exposures will not be managed in the same manner, because these rodenticides have different mechanisms of action and toxic dosages (bromethalin affects the central nervous system, but bromadiolone inhibits the normal blood coagulation process). Knowing the name brand of the product is often not sufficient to determine the active ingredient, because products with the same brand name may have different active ingredients (e.g., Rampage® rodenticide may contain either cholecalciferol or bromethalin as an active ingredient). Rodenticide pellets and bars come in a variety of colors, but, unfortunately, there is no way to identify the active ingredient by color or shape.

Exposure Information

Once the identity of an agent has been confirmed, the next step in the history-taking process is to obtain a detailed account of events surrounding the exposure. Knowing only the name of the agent, or the active ingredients, may not provide sufficient information to determine whether an exposure is likely to result in problems for the patient. The veterinary staff needs to have an accurate picture of what occurred before, during, and after the exposure. Information to be documented in the medical record includes amount of the agent ingested (count, volume or weight); physical form of the agent; calculated doses of active ingredients in mg/kg body weight; route, time, and location of the exposure; location of the owner when the exposure occurred; reason that the agent was administered (if applicable); original source of the agent; person(s) responsible for administering the agent (if applicable); and potential for other animals to be exposed. Many clients may initially feel they have "no idea" as to the amount of toxicant to which the patient may have been exposed, but patient questioning can sometimes help to get an approximation. For medication, if the original prescription amount is known, remaining pills (if any) can be counted out and subtracted from the original prescribed amount; calculating the dose taken and the number of days from the time that the prescription was filled may enable the veterinary technician to estimate the maximum number of pills that may be missing. For other products (e.g., rodenticide pellets, granulated material, liquids, etc.), information be gleaned by asking how much might be missing from the original and subtracting out a worst-case-scenario amount: "Complete this question: I know it could not have been more than (blank)." Narrowing down the amount with questions (i.e., "Was it as much as a tablespoon? Less? How about a teaspoon? More? Maybe two teaspoons?") can sometimes help to get an idea of how much might have been ingested. When estimating in this way it is important to err on the side of caution, so slightly overestimating the amount is better than underestimating.

Other questions to consider for "mystery poisonings" include:

How long has it been since the last time the animal appeared normal?
Was the onset of signs gradual or sudden?
What was the location of the animal in the last few hours prior to the development of clinical signs?
Is there any history of administration of medications/ herbal products/flea or tick control products to this

animal or other animals in the household in the past 24 hours?

The answers to these questions may assist in narrowing down the possible toxicants to which the patient might have been exposed.

Implemented Treatment

Once the where, how, and why of the exposure is known, the next step for the history-taker is to determine whether the owner had already implemented any treatment at home before calling the vet hospital or bringing the patient into the hospital setting. Implemented treatment may include induction of emesis, bathing the patient for dermal exposures, or giving over-the-counter medications to help prevent the development of signs or to treat current signs. Some owners will be knowledgeable about treatment that can be implemented at home, such as inducing emesis. If an owner has already been successful at inducing vomiting, this is an important piece of information to note in the medical record. What the owner gave to induce vomiting, how much, when it was given in relation to time of exposure, and the results (including what was observed in the vomitus) also need to be documented. In certain instances the agent administered as treatment by an owner can complicate the case. For example, salt and syrup of ipecac are sometimes used to induce vomiting at home. Administration of salt can cause serious electrolyte abnormalities, and large doses of syrup of ipecac can cause prolonged gastrointestinal upset and possible cardiac effects.

TELEPHONE TRIAGE

Some clients may call seeking advice about a toxicological exposure before bringing the patient into the veterinary hospital. In these cases, having a telephone questionnaire for obtaining a toxicological history may help to determine which patients need to be treated at a veterinary hospital and which patients can be monitored at home. The largest disadvantage to taking a history over the phone is that the clinical status of the patient may be unknown or inaccurate. Unlike when a patient is presented to the hospital, the components of a physical exam cannot be implemented over the phone. To the owner, the patient may look normal, and subtle clinical signs such as mydriasis or abnormal mucous membrane color can be overlooked. Heart rate, blood pressure, temperature, and respirations are generally unavailable, as many animal

owners are unaware of or lack the equipment to accurately obtain these vital statistics.

Another disadvantage to taking a history over the phone is determining the reliability of the owner; indeed, this can often be a challenge when dealing with clients in person. When speaking with a client over the phone, the veterinary technician has to rely solely on verbal communication. Observing a client's body language can at times provide more information about a particular situation than what is communicated verbally. Reliability can be poor due to a number of reasons. Clients may purposely withhold pertinent information as a result of feeling ashamed that their animal was exposed to a potentially toxic agent, whether by accident or simply due to a lack of knowledge as to what might be toxic. Clients may also feel they might be reprimanded by veterinary professionals for applying a product incorrectly or by attempting to treat a condition at home by giving over-the-counter human medications to their animal. Clients sometimes withhold information merely to avoid having to bring their patients into a veterinary hospital due to finances or inconvenience. When illicit substances are involved, clients may be reluctant to provide information due to fear of being "turned in" to law enforcement by veterinary staff. Tactful questioning and reassurance that the primary concern of the veterinary staff is the well-being of the patient can sometimes help to elicit truthful answers. A gentle reminder that knowing what the toxicant is will allow the patient to be treated much more effectively and cheaply, because knowing the toxicant may well reduce the number of diagnostic tests that may need to be performed. Veterinary technicians should be aware of reasons that client information may be less than accurate and use their common sense and instinct to try to determine whether the historical information provided does not seem to fit the circumstances.

CONCLUSION

It is a veterinary technician's responsibility to provide an accurate history to their veterinarians so that appropriate treatment decisions can be made. Taking an accurate history requires patience and attention to detail. In situations where aggressive patient care is required, it is sometimes tempting to skip parts of the history-taking process. However, if details in the history are overlooked, the patient's overall welfare could be compromised, and that key piece of information that could be vital to the case may be overlooked.

CHAPTER 4 STUDY QUESTIONS

1. The veterinary medical record is composed of basic data sets, including client information, patient signalment, and clinical status of the patient. When dealing with a suspected poisoning case, additional data that should be obtained for the medical record include which of the following?
   a.   Agent information
   b.   Exposure history
   c.   Implemented treatments
   a and b only
   a, b, and c

2. Patient signalment includes all of the following except:
   a. Breed
   b. Age
   c. Reproductive status
   d. Vaccination history
   e. Weight

3. Give three reasons why the patient's age and prior health history are important information to obtain when dealing with a poisoning case.

4. Sparky, a 5-year-old, neutered male, 12-pound Jack Russell terrier presents to the emergency clinic with a history of vomiting. According to the owner, Sparky has a habit of "eating everything within reach," but was not witnessed ingesting anything out of the ordinary by the owner. In spite of his history of dietary indiscretion, the owner reports that Sparky has never been ill and is current on his vaccination and heartworm status. What questions that should be asked about Sparky's clinical status?

5. Referring to the patient in Question 4, what questions should be asked about Sparky's environment?

ANSWERS

1.e. All of the listed data should be obtained for the medical record.

2.d. Signalment includes all of the "personal" information on the patient but does not include medical record.

3. Prior medical conditions may affect how the patient is managed (e.g., whether emesis is induced); patients may be more or less susceptible to toxicosis due to age-related differences in response to certain toxicants; medications that the patient is currently taking may alter how the toxicant affects the patient.

4. How long has Sparky been vomiting? Have there been any other clinical signs that are not currently apparent? Did he appear lethargic before he began to vomit?

5. Can you please outline Sparky's activities over the 24-hour period before he became ill? What is Sparky's normal diet and have there been any recent changes? Have there been any major household changes in the past few days (visitors, renovation, etc.)? Is Sparky on any medications, supplements, or herbal products? Is Sparky an indoor or outdoor dog? To what areas of the house, yard, and neighborhood does Sparky have access? Has he been allowed access to any areas that he normally doesn't go? Has Sparky traveled or been boarded in the past week? What type of plants are in Sparky's environment? Have any new weeds or mushrooms been noted in the yard? What type of medications, over-the-counter products, and herbals/supplements are in use in the house? Are there any children in the house; if so, do they have any medications/supplements, paintballs, sugar-free gums, or candies, etc.? Are there other pets in the household; if so, are any of them acting abnormally? Does Sparky have access to animals other than household cohorts? Are any rodenticides or insecticides used in the house or yard?

REFERENCE

Fitzgerald KT. 2006. Taking a toxicological history. In *Small Animal Toxicology*, 2nd edition, edited by Michael E. Peterson and Patricia A. Talcott PA, pp. 38–44. St. Louis: Saunders.

Essential Calculations

5

Camille DeClementi

INTRODUCTION

Dosage calculation is critical to clinical veterinary toxicology. This process allows one to answer two very important questions about an exposure. First, is the exposure going to cause adverse effects? And second, if adverse effects develop, how serious will they be? The relationship between the dosage and the effect or response to a poison is a crucial concept in toxicology (Osweiler 1996). Dosage is the most important factor in determining response (Osweiler 2006). As the amount or dosage of the toxicant increases, the toxic response is also expected to increase in degree or severity (Osweiler 1996).

Philipus Aureolus Theophrastus Bombastus von Hohenheim (Paracelsus), a sixteenth-century physician-alchemist said "All substances are poisons; there is none which is not a poison. The right dose differentiates a poison from a remedy" (Osweiler 2006). Water illustrates this concept well. Having adequate water is a requirement for animals; however, ingesting too much water leads to water intoxication and can be deadly. Another example is carprofen, a nonsteroidal anti-inflammatory (NSAID) medication commonly used in veterinary medicine. At therapeutic doses, this medication improves the quality of life of dogs suffering from osteoarthritis (Jenkins and Kanara 1998). But if a dog receives an overdose, one needs to determine whether the dosage can cause the adverse effects potentially associated with an overdose of any NSAID. These include gastrointestinal irritation and ulceration and adverse renal effects (Talcott 2006).

Determining the dosage helps one decide how to proceed with the case and to answer the following questions:

Is any treatment needed?
What, if any, method of decontamination should be performed?
Should this patient be hospitalized for monitoring?
What clinical signs may develop?
Is there an antidotal therapy and if so, is this patient a good candidate?
What are the likely costs associated with treatment?

DEFINITIONS

Understanding a few definitions will make it easier to comprehend the concepts and examples presented in this chapter. *Dose* is the total amount of toxicant that is received per animal, whereas *dosage* is the amount of toxicant per unit of body weight (Spoo 2004). For example, if a 13 lb dog is given a 25 mg pill of antibiotic, the dose is 25 mg and the dosage is 25 mg/13 lb or 1.9 mg/lb. In most cases, dosage will be expressed in mg/kg, so in this example, the dosage is 4.2 mg/kg.

A few additional commonly used definitions in toxicology are toxicity, threshold dose, LD_{50}, and NOEL. *Toxicity* is the amount of a toxicant that, under a specific set of conditions, causes toxic effects or results in detrimental biologic changes. (see Chapter 1, Table 1.1 for classifications of relative toxicities.) The *threshold dose* is the highest dose of a toxicant at which toxic effects are not

Small Animal Toxicology Essentials, First Edition. Edited by Robert H. Poppenga, Sharon Gwaltney-Brant.
© 2011 John Wiley and Sons, Inc. Published 2011 by John Wiley and Sons, Inc.

observed (Spoo 2004). The *lethal dose 50%* (LD$_{50}$) is the dose at which 50% of the animals die during an acute toxicity study (Spoo 2004). This value is used to compare the toxicity of compounds with one another (Osweiler 2006). The *no observable adverse effect level* (NOAEL) is the highest dose at which significant effects could not be found (Spoo 2004).

DETERMINING EXPOSURE AMOUNTS

Taking a thorough history is an important step in effectively calculating the dosage of an exposure. Find out when the exposure occurred and the largest amount to which the patient may have been exposed. It can sometimes be difficult for owners to determine the worst case scenario when they are upset and worried about their pet. One can be of assistance by asking certain questions. It may be helpful to ask them to read the label to determine the amount originally in the container. This is especially helpful with over-the-counter medications. If it can be determined how many were originally in the container, how many have been taken previously and how many are left, one can come to a good approximation of the largest possible amount of the exposure.

If the agent is a prescription medication, the following questions are also often helpful:

When was the prescription filled?
How often are the pills taken?
Are they taken as scheduled or are doses sometimes missed?

Sample Calculation 1

An owner contacts you on the phone and is frantic. Her Pomeranian ingested some of her Adderall capsules 1 hour ago and now is racing all over the house and is hyperactive. She just had the prescription refilled a few days ago and has used 5 capsules from the 60 capsules originally prescribed. She is able to count out 30 intact capsules on the floor and in the bottle. The capsules are 20 milligrams each and the dog weighs 15 pounds. Calculate the dosage in mg/kg.

Determine dog's weight in kilograms:
　15 lbs/2.2 kg = 6.8 kg
Determine the total milligrams ingested:
　60 capsules in original prescription minus 5 taken by owner minus 30 found capsules = 25 capsules missing

If these questions are not effective, it is sometimes useful to ask a question to help narrow down the possible amount. For example, is the amount likely to be closer to 100 or 10? Once they answer that question, one can attempt to narrow it down further. These types of questions are also helpful with other products including candies, gum, granular baits, fertilizer, insecticides, and pesticides. If the product is a liquid, ask whether it was spilled. If it was spilled, ask whether the spill was on a soft surface like a carpet or bedding that would absorb the liquid making it less available for ingestion, whether the area is still wet, and, if the liquid spilled on a hard surface, whether there is any liquid on the surface now. All these questions will help determine a worst case amount that can be used to calculate a possible dosage.

SAMPLE AND PRACTICE CALCULATIONS

In the following boxes some sample dosage calculations are shown. There will be an example that has been solved followed by a practice question. The answers to the practice questions can be found at the end of the chapter. It will be tempting just to read the samples, but to get the most from this chapter work through the practice questions. When following along with the examples and working through the practice questions, refer to Table 5.1, which contains commonly used conversions.

Calculating dosages involving medication in tablet or capsule form is fairly straightforward as long as the dose in each tablet/capsule is known and a worst case scenario can be determined as to the number of tablets/capsules ingested.

　25 pills × 20 mg/pill = 500 mg
Determine the mg/kg dosage:
　500 mg/6.8 kg = 73.6 mg/kg

Discussion

Adderall is a combination medication containing four amphetamines. It is used for the treatment of attention-deficit hyperactivity disorder in humans. Clinical signs, including cardiovascular and central nervous system (CNS) stimulation, can be seen at doses at or below 0.5 mg/kg (Youssef 2006). Since the dosage is very high and the patient is symptomatic, you advise the owner to bring her dog in immediately for treatment.

Table 5.1. Useful conversion factors

Unit	Abbreviation	Equivalent	Unit	Abbreviation	Equivalent
			1 cup	C	8 oz
Concentration			1 teaspoon	tsp	5 g
1 part per million	ppm	1 mg/kg or 1 µg/g (solids) 1 mg/l (liquid)	1 tablespoon	T	15 g
			Liquid		
1 percent	%	10,000 ppm 10 mg/g (solid) 10 mg/ml (liquid)	1 fluid ounce	fl oz	29.6 ml
			1 quart	qt	0.946 L
			1 gallon	gal	4 qt
1 proof (alcohol)		0.5% 5 mg/ml			8 pt
					128 fl oz
Dry					3785 ml
1 ounce	oz	28.35 g			3.785 liter
1 gram	g	15.43 grains 1000 mg			8.53 lb_
			1 cup	C	237 ml
1 grain	gr	65 mg			8 fl oz
1 pound	lb	454 g 0.454 kg 16 oz			16 T
			1 liter	L	1.057 qt
1 kilogram	kg	2.2 lb 1000 g	1 teaspoon	tsp	5 ml
			1 tablespoon	T; Tbsp	15 ml
1 milligram	mg	0.001 g 1000 µ	1 milliliter	ml	0.034 oz 1 g

Sources: Osweiler 2006; Spoo 2004.

Practice Calculation 1

An owner brings her cat into your clinic. She had dropped 1 500 mg acetaminophen tablet and her cat ran over and ingested it before the owner could get the pill from the cat. The cat weighs 12 pounds. The exposure happened only 10 minutes ago. You are aware that any dosage of acetaminophen is a concern in a cat. Doses of 10 mg/kg have produced toxicosis in cats (Richardson 2000a). Potential clinical effects include depression, weakness, methemoglobinemia, dyspnea, and facial or paw edema. Calculate the dosage in mg/kg. Will this cat need treatment?

When dealing with solid toxicants such as foods, it is best to try to get an estimate of how many ounces were ingested. In the case of exposures to chocolate, it is important to know what type of chocolate was ingested because the various forms of chocolate (white, milk, dark, etc.) have different amounts of chocolate in them, with the darker forms of chocolate being more toxic (see Chapter 24). When there is a mixture of chocolate types, use the darkest form in the mix and calculate the dosage using the worst case scenario. Although this will somewhat overestimate the dosage of methylxanthines, it is definitely better to err on the side of caution.

Sample Calculation 2

It is the day after Halloween and an owner calls your clinic for assistance. Her rottweiler ingested 2 candy bars and she has heard that chocolate is poisonous for dogs. The ingestion occurred up to 3 hours ago and the dog seems fine now. The dog weighs 90 pounds. The candy bars are solid milk chocolate and weigh 1.5 ounces each. Chocolate contains two methylxanthine stimulants:

Continued

caffeine and theobromine. Although the exact amounts of the methylxanthines vary in different types and brands of chocolate, a good estimate of the methylxanthine content in milk chocolate is 64 mg/oz (58 mg theobromine and 6 mg caffeine). Calculate the dosage in mg/kg.

Determine the weight of the dog in kilograms:
    90 lbs/2.2 kg = 41 kg
Determine the total milligrams of methylxanthines ingested:
    3 oz × 64 mg/oz = 192 mg
Determine the mg/kg dosage:
    192 mg/41 kg = 4.7 mg/kg

Discussion

Mild signs of methylxanthine intoxication can occur at dosages of 20 mg/kg and severe effects can occur at 40–50 mg/kg (Gwaltney-Brant 2001). Since this patient's

With exposure to rodenticide pellets or bars, it is important to try to estimate the amount ingested as closely as possible. Again, it is better to slightly overestimate the exposure than to underestimate. Bars of rodenticide can be examined to determine how much of the bar is missing, and pellets often come in packets with the amounts stated

Sample Calculation 3

One hour ago, a 16 lb pug chewed on two small packages of a pelleted rodenticide containing 0.01% bromethalin. Each package originally contained 0.75 oz. The owner brought in the remains of the packages, and the remaining pellets weighed 0.5 oz. Calculate the dosage in mg/kg. Will this patient require decontamination?

Determine the weight of the dog in kilograms:
    16 lbs/2.2 kg = 7.3 kg
Calculate the amount ingested:
    (0.75 oz/packet × 2 packets) = 1.5 oz
    1.5 oz minus 0.5 oz (weighed) = 1 oz missing
Convert to amount ingested to grams:
    1 oz × 28.35 g = 28.35 g
Convert rodenticide % to mg/g by moving the decimal point one place to the right:
    0.01% = 0.1 mg/g
Determine the milligrams ingested:
    0.1 mg/g × 28.35 g = 2.84 mg
Determine the mg/kg dosage:
    2.84 mg/7.3 kg = 0.39 mg/kg

dosage is <5 mg/kg, no treatment is warranted at this time. You advise the owner to monitor the dog at home for gastrointestinal upset and signs of pancreatitis.

Practice Calculation 2

On a weekend, a dog is presented to your hospital for treatment. The dog is pacing, panting, and agitated on presentation and the owners believe he may have ingested some semisweet chocolate morsels a few hours ago. Twenty-four ounces of the morsels are missing. The dog weighs 42 pounds. Although the exact amounts of the methylxanthines vary in different types and brands of chocolate, a good estimate of the methylxanthine content in semisweet chocolate is 160 mg/oz (138 mg theobromine and 22 mg caffeine) (Gwaltney-Brant 2001). Calculate the dosage in mg/kg. Could the chocolate be causing the signs the dog is exhibiting?

on the packaging. If the ingestion was witnessed, attempt to get the person who witnessed the exposure to estimate how much may have been ingested (e.g., 1 tsp vs. 1 Tbsp vs. 1/4 cup. etc.). Packets or bars brought into the veterinary clinic can be weighed if no packaging is available.

Discussion

Bromethalin is a neurotoxin. Signs of intoxication are most pronounced in the CNS and can include hindlimb weakness, ataxia, depression, tremors, paralysis, seizures, and death. In canine patients ingesting dosages between 0.1–0.49 mg/kg emesis or one dose of activated charcoal is recommended (Dunayer 2003). In this case, emesis is recommended with 3% hydrogen peroxide and is very successful. The dog vomits up many pellets, which weigh 1.2 oz. The extra weight is likely due to absorption of liquid by the pellets while they were in the stomach. No additional treatment is required.

Practice Calculation 3

A 75 lb Labrador retriever is observed ingesting 4 ounces of a rodenticide bait containing 0.005% brodifacoum. The dog has had no previous access to the bait. Calculate the dosage in mg/kg. Will this patient require decontamination if a toxic dose of brodifacoum for dogs is 1 mg/kg body weight? What other treatments may be needed?

Sample Calculation 4

An owner calls your clinic and informs you her 32 lb mixed breed dog ingested approximately 1/2 cup of snail bait containing 2.75% metaldehyde 15 minutes ago. Calculate the dosage in mg/kg. Is decontamination required?

Determine the weight of the dog in kilograms:
    32 lbs/2.2 kg = 14.5 kg
Convert % to mg/g by moving the decimal point one place to the right:
    2.75% = 27.5 mg/g
Convert amount ingested to grams:
    1/2 cup = 4 oz × 28.35 g = 113.4 g
Determine the milligrams ingested:
    27.5 mg/g × 113.4 g = 3118.5 mg
Determine the mg/kg dosage:
    3118.5 mg/14.5 kg = 215 mg/kg

Discussion

The dosage for this dog is well above the LD_{50} in dogs of 100 mg/kg. The clinical signs that may develop include tachycardia, hyperesthesia, mydriasis, hypersalivation, vomiting, ataxia, metabolic acidosis, tremors, seizures, and hyperthermia (Dolder 2003). Since the exposure was recent and the owner lives 30 minutes from the clinic, emesis was recommended at home but the owner was instructed to bring the dog in immediately if the dog began to act anxious or excited. Emesis was successful at home. Since the dosage was so large, the owners brought the dog in for activated charcoal and overnight monitoring.

Practice Calculation 4

Your dog is at work with you and finds one ant bait station in the bathroom. You find her chewing the bait. She has ripped open the bait and ingested the contents. She weighs 60 pounds and the bait is 1.98 g and contains 0.01% fipronil. Calculate the dosage in mg/kg. What treatments, if any should be considered?

Calculating dosages for topical (dermal, ocular, otic) exposures is done in the same manner as oral exposures although the risk for intoxication is dependent on bioavailability.

Sample Calculation 5

A 2-year-old, 7 lb neutered male domestic short-haired cat presents at your clinic with muscle fasciculations and tremors. The owner applied a dermal flea spot-on product, labeled for dogs, 10 hours earlier. The active ingredient in the product is 45% permethrin and the applicator contained 2 ml. Calculate the dermal dosage in mg/kg. Is this exposure the likely cause of the cat's clinical signs? What treatments should be performed?

Determine the weight of the cat in kilograms:
    7 lbs/2.2 kg = 3.2 kg
Convert liquid % to mg/ml by moving the decimal point one place to the right:
    45% = 450 mg/ml
Determine the milligrams placed on the skin:
    2 ml × 450 mg/ml = 900 mg
Determine the mg/kg dosage:
    900 mg/3.2 kg = 281 mg/kg

Discussion

Even a small amount of a concentrated permethrin product applied dermally to a cat can cause significant effects including tremors and seizures. Methocarbamol is very helpful in controlling these adverse effects. This cat was admitted to the hospital and given methocarbamol intravenously. The tremors resolved and then the cat was decontaminated by bathing with a liquid dishwashing detergent (Richardson 2000b).

Practice Calculation 5

A cat in your practice is being treated for ear mites with ivermectin. The cat is to receive a subcutaneous dose of 0.1 ml of a 1% ivermectin injectable product. The cat weighs 12 pounds. By mistake, the cat is given 1 ml instead. Calculate the dosage in mg/kg. What decontamination methods should be considered if any?

For some toxicants, toxic doses have been determined for a reference compound, and toxicants that are similar need to be converted to an equivalent in order to determine the risk based on the reference compound. For instance, most toxic doses for iron are based on elemental iron, and iron containing compounds must be converted to an elemental iron equivalent before calculating a dosage so that comparison with known toxic dosages of iron can be made. Table 5.2 lists the elemental iron level of various iron-containing compounds. Similarly, vitamins are frequently listed as international units (IU) rather than milligrams and a conversion to milligrams will need to be performed in order to determine the risk of a given exposure. Table 5.3 lists conversion factors for vitamins. Other toxicants requiring conversion include salicylate-containing compounds such as bismuth subsalicylate, which are converted to "aspirin-equivalent" dosages to determine the risk.

Sample Calculation 6

An owner brings her 65 lb boxer into your clinic. He has vomited twice but is normal on presentation. Earlier in the day the owner was gardening and was using a fertilizer. Her dog was outside with her and she caught him playing with the fertilizer bag. The contents were spilled all over the ground but she estimates 2 cups are missing and is concerned the dog may have ingested them. His vomit contained material that looked like the fertilizer. The fertilizer contains 0.4% ferrous sulfate (anhydrous). Calculate the elemental iron dosage in mg/kg (see Table 5.2 for conversion factor). Is the vomiting expected with this ingestion? What is the best treatment plan?

Determine the weight of the dog in kilograms:
  65 lbs/2.2 kg = 29.5 kg
Convert % to mg/g by moving the decimal point one place to the right:
  0.4% = 4 mg/g
Convert amount ingested to grams:
  2 cups = 16 oz × 28.35 g = 453.6 g
Determine the millligrams ingested:
  4 mg/g × 453.6 g = 1814 mg

Not all calculations in toxicology relate to calculating exposure dosages. Often, calculations need to be done when administering symptomatic or antidotal medications.

Convert ferrous sulfate to elemental iron =
  1814 mg × 37% (0.37) = 671 mg
Determine the mg/kg dosage:
  671 mg/29.5 kg = 22.7 mg/kg

Discussion

Doses of elemental iron approximately 20 mg/kg can cause mild clinical effects including vomiting and anorexia; therefore, the vomiting is likely due to the exposure (Albretsen 2004). The treatment plan should include managing the vomiting if needed and preventing dehydration. Life-threatening signs are not expected.

Practice Calculation 6

A 45 lb basset hound got into his owner's vitamins and ingested up to 85 of each of the following: emulsified vitamin A capsules (2500 IU/capsule), vitamin D capsules (1000 IU/capsule), and vitamin E capsules (1000 IU/capsule). Calculate the dosages in mg/kg by using the conversion factors in Table 5.4. What clinical signs may develop? What treatments should be considered?

Most frequently, this entails diluting solutions to a given concentration prior to administration to the patient.

Sample Calculation 7

A veterinarian needs 7% ethanol solution to treat a cat for ethylene glycol exposure. The veterinarian has 60 proof ethanol (30%) available for dilution. Calculate the "recipe" for mixing the ethanol with the fluids to produce 1 L of 7% solution (Plunkett 2001).

Discussion

Use the following equation: $Concentration_1 \times Volume_1 = Volume_2 \times Concentration_2$
(% stock ethanol solution)(X ml) = (1000 ml)(7%) where X ml is how much ethanol needed
(30%)(X ml) = (1000 ml)(7%) or (0.3)(X ml) = (1000 ml)(0.07)
Solve for X: X ml = ((1000 ml)(.07))/(.3)

X ml = 233 ml
Remove 233 ml from a liter bag of fluids and replace it with 233 ml of the ethanol.

Practice Calculation 7

A 70 lb dog has been admitted to your hospital for treatment of acetaminophen toxicosis. The dog will be receiving a loading dose of 140 mg/kg of a 5% solution of n-acetylcysteine (NAC) followed by seven additional doses of 70 mg/kg given every 6 hours (Plumb 2005). You are starting with 20% NAC and will be diluting it with 5% dextrose. How much 20% NAC will you need? How much 5% dextrose will you mix it with?

Table 5.2. Percentage of elemental iron in various iron salts

Iron Form	% Elemental Iron
Ferric Hydroxide	63
Ferrous Carbonate (Anhydrous)	48
Ferric Phosphate	37
Ferrous Sulfate (Anhydrous)	37
Ferric Chloride	34
Ferrous Fumarate	33
Ferric Pyrophosphate	30
Ferrous Lactate	24
Ferrous Sulfate (Hydrate)	20
Peptonized Iron	17
Ferroglycine Sulfate	16
Ferric Ammonium Citrate	15
Ferrous Gluconate	12
Ferrocholinate	12

Source: Albretsen 2004.

Table 5.3. Conversion of vitamin International Units to milligrams

Vitamin	Milligrams (mg)	International Units (IU)
Vitamin A	1	3333_
Vitamin D3	1	40,000_
Vitamin E	1	0.67_

Source: Debraekeleer 2000.

CHAPTER 5 REVIEW EQUATIONS

1. Max, an 80-pound Labrador retriever ingested the entire contents of a 6.8 g tube of horse dewormer paste. The concentration of ivermectin in the paste is 1.87%. Calculate a dosage (mg/kg) of ivermectin.

2. Mrs. Garner is concerned because the report from the county extension office indicated that the level of the herbicide atrazine in her well water, which was measured at 0.010 ppm, exceeds the EPA recommended upper limits of .003 ppm. She wants to know if this level will be a problem for her 45-pound, female spayed German shorthaired pointer named Sissy. We know that the no observable adverse effect level (NOAEL) of atrazine for dogs is 5 mg/kg/day and that dogs drink approximately 30 ml/lb/day. Does the level of atrazine in the water pose a hazard for Sissy?

3. Theo, a 12-pound domestic shorthair cat was given 1 tablet of Percocet by its owner. The medication contains 5 mg of oxycodone and 500 mg acetaminophen per tablet. What is the dosage in mg/kg for each of the ingredients? What types of clinical signs might be expected from each ingredient in the Percocet? (*Hint:* see Chapter 25, "Drugs of Abuse," and Chapter 26, "OTC Drugs.")

4A. Billy and Banjo are bloodhounds. Billy is a neutered male, 9 years old, and 90 pounds; Banjo is an intact male, 18 months old, and 95 pounds. Billy is on chewable carprofen for arthritis. The dogs' owner came home to find Billy's carprofen bottle chewed up on the floor and all of the tablets missing. What information do you need to know to help determine whether this exposure is serious?

4B. The owner is sure that Banjo is the culprit because Billy's arthritis would not have allowed him to get to the medication, which was on the kitchen counter. Which of the following is the best way to handle this situation?

  a. Assume Banjo got all of the medication since the owner thinks he is the most likely culprit. Calculate a dose for Banjo only, assuming he got all of the tablets.

  b. Assume the dogs shared the medication and calculate a dosage for each dog based on each eating ½ of the missing tablets.

  c. Assume each dog may have ingested the medication and calculate dosages as if each dog got the entire amount of medication.

4C. Seventy-five days ago, Billy's owner refilled his carprofen prescription and received 180 100 mg

Continued

tablets. The owner has administered 1 tablet twice daily since the refill, and there are now no remaining tablets. Calculate a worst-case-scenario dosage for each dog.

5. Bailey, a 3-year-old, 16-pound Cavalier King Charles spaniel chewed up three ant baits, ingesting the contents. The ant baits contained abamectin b_1 at 0.01% and the package indicates each bait station contains 0.07 oz of bait. Calculate a dosage (mg/kg) for Bailey's exposure.

6. A veterinarian needs 585 ml of 7% ethanol solution to treat a cat for ethylene glycol exposure. The veterinarian has 60 proof vodka available for dilution. Calculate the "recipe" for mixing the ethanol with fluids to produce 585 ml of 7% solution.

7. Hooch, a 62-pound golden retriever got into the owner's garden shed and was found eating out of the bag of cocoa bean mulch. The owner estimates that no more than 1–2 cups of mulch could have been eaten based on what's left in the bag and the amount of time the dog was alone in the shed.

What is the approximate dosage of methylxanthines that the dog ingested? (Hint: Cocoa beans contain from 0.5%–0.85% theobromine.)

8. Buddy, a 25-pound beagle mix ingested 1.5 oz of an unknown rodenticide. Calculate the dosage if the rodenticide was:
0.01% bromethalin
0.005% brodifacoum
0.075% cholecalciferol

9. Two miniature schnauzers, Click and Clack, ingested no more than 3 Tbsp of fire ant killer granules containing 0.04% lambda cyhalothrin. Calculate the dosages if the dogs weigh 14 and 17 pounds, respectively.

10. Mara is an 8-pound, 12-year-old Siamese cat whose owner applied 5% minoxidil solution to an area of alopecia on Mara's back. Now the owner is concerned that she should not have done that. She estimates she used no more than 1/10 tsp of liquid. The area where the minoxidil was applied is an area that Mara cannot reach to groom. Calculate a topical dosage of minoxidil.

ANSWERS

1. Convert Max's weight to kilograms:
80 pounds/2.2 kg/pound = 36.4 kg
Calculate the dose of ivermectin ingested:
1.87% = 18.7 mg/g
6.8 g × 18.7 mg/g = 127.16 mg
Calculate the dosage ingested:
127.16 mg/36.4 kg = 3.49 mg/kg

2. Determine Sissy's daily water intake:
30 ml/lb × 45 lb = 1350 ml per day = 1.35 liter/day
Determine the daily exposure to atrazine:
0.010 ppm = 0.010 mg/l
0.010 mg/l × 1.35 liter/day = 0.0135 mg/day
0.0135 mg/day
Determine Sissy's daily "dosage" of atrazine:
0.0135 mg/day divided by 20.5 kg = .00066 mg/kg/day

Discussion

Comparing our results to the known NOAEL for dogs (5 mg/kg/day) shows us that this concentration of atrazine in the well water will not pose a hazard to Sissy, even though it exceeds the EPA's recommended maximum level for drinking water for humans.

3. Convert the cat's weight to kg:
12 lb/2.2 kg/lb = 5.5 kg
Calculate the dosages for each ingredient:
500 mg acetaminophen/5.5 kg = 91 mg/kg
5 mg oxycodone/5.5 kg = 0.9 mg/kg

Discussion

This level of acetaminophen is sufficient to cause methemoglobinemia and liver injury in Theo. Although the oxycodone could cause sedation, it is not likely to cause any life-threatening issues.

4A. Milligram strength of the carprofen, the number of tablets missing, and any health issues the dogs have.

4B. The correct answer is c; often the least likely suspect is the guilty party.

4C. Calculate the weight of each dog in kilograms:
Billy: 90 lb/2.2 kg/lb = 41 kg
Banjo: 95 lb/2.2 kg/lb = 43 kg
Calculate the maximum number of tablets ingested:
180 tablets minus 75 days worth (150 tablets) = 180 – 150 = 30 tablets missing
30 tablets × 100 mg/tablet = 3000 mg
For Billy: 3000 mg/41 kg = 73 m/kg
For Banjo: 3000 mg/43 kg = 69 mg/kg

Discussion

Doses of carprofen over 40 mg/kg have the potential to cause gastrointestinal ulceration and renal injury in dogs. Both Billy and Banjo need to come in for treatment.

5. Convert Bailey's weight to kilograms:

16lb/2.2kg/lb = 7.3 kg

Calculate the amount of abamectin b_1 ingested:

(0.07 oz) × 28.35 g = 1.98 g per bait station

1.98 g × 3 baits = 5.95 g

0.01% = 0.1 mg/g

5.95 g × 0.1 mg/g = 0.595 mg abamectin b_1 ingested

0.595 mg/7.3 kg = 0.082 mg/kg

Discussion

Abamectin b_1 is a macrolide antiparasiticidal agent related to compounds such as ivermectin, milbemycin, and moxidectin. It is thought to be about 4 times as potent as ivermectin, although kinetic information is lacking to determine how well it is absorbed. If we assume it is well absorbed, this dose is equivalent to about 0.326 mg/kg of ivermectin. This dose of ivermectin is within the therapeutic range and would not cause clinical problems in dogs unless they were P-glycoprotein deficient (e.g., collies, Shetland sheepdogs, etc.). Because Bailey is not a breed wherein P-glycoprotein deficiency has been documented, this dose is unlikely to cause any serious problems.

6. Use this formula: $\text{Concentration}_1 \times \text{Volume}_1 = \text{Volume}_2 \times \text{Concentration}_2$

60 proof vodka is 30% ethanol

30% (xml) = 7% (585 ml)

X ml = (7 × 585 ml)/30 = 136.5 ml

Add 136.5 ml of vodka to 448.5 ml stock fluids to obtain 585 ml of 7% ethanol.

7. Assume a worst-case scenario of 2 cups and 0.85% theobromine.

Convert Hooch's weight to kilograms:

62lb/2.2kg/lb = 28.2kg

Convert 2 cups to grams:

2cups = 16oz × 28.35 g/oz = 453.6 g

Convert 0.85% to mg/g:

0.85% = 8.5 mg/g

Calculate mg theobromine ingested:

8.5 mg/g × 453.6 g = 3855.6 mg theobromine

Calculate Hooch's dosage of theobromine:

3855.6 mg/28.2kg = 136.7 mg/kg

Discussion

Doses of theobromine over 60 mg/kg can cause serious cardiovascular and central nervous system effects. Hooch will need decontamination, monitoring, and symptomatic care for any signs that develop.

8. Convert Buddy's weight to kilograms:

25lb/2.2kg/lb = 11.4kg

Convert 1.5 ounces to grams:

1.5 oz × 28.35 g/oz = 42.5 g

Convert percentages to mg/g:

0.01% bromethalin = 0.1 mg/g

0.005% brodifacoum = 0.05 mg/g

0.0075% cholecalciferol = 0.75 mg/g

Calculate dosages:

Bromethalin: (0.1 mg/g × 42.5 g)/11.4kg = 0.37 mg/kg

Brodifacoum:(0.05 mg/g × 42.5 g)/11.4kg = 0.19 mg/kg

Cholecalciferol: (0.75 mg/g × 42.5 g)/11.4kg = 2.8 mg/kg

Discussion

This ingestion merits decontamination regardless of the kind of bait it was. Since the type of rodenticide is not known, Buddy should be managed as if he ingested all three types. For bromethalin, induction of emesis alone would be sufficient, but for the other two activated charcoal administration is needed. Baseline prothrombin time (PT), serum calcium, and serum phosphorus should be obtained. PT can be repeated in 48 and 72 hours and the dog placed on vitamin K if the PT becomes elevated. Serum calcium and phosphorous should be monitored every 12–24 hours for 4 days and Buddy should be started on treatment for hypercalcemia the levels elevate.

9. Convert weight from kilograms to pounds:

Click: 14 pounds/2.2kg/pound = 6.4kg

Clack: 17 pounds/2.2kg/pound = 7.3 kg

Convert percent lambda cyhalothrin to mg/g:

0.04% = 0.4 mg/g

Convert 3 tablespoons to grams

3Tbsp × 15 g/tbsp = 45 g

Calculate milligrams ingested

45 g × 0.4 mg/g = 18 mg

Calculate dosages for each dog:

Click: 18 mg/6.4kg = 2.8 mg/kg

Clack: 18 mg/7.3kg = 2.5 mg/kg

Continued

Discussion

Lambda cyhalothrin is a synthetic pyrethroid with a moderate degree of toxicity. In chronic feeding studies in dogs, 2.5 mg/kg/day caused diarrhea; 3.5 mg/kg/day resulted in neurological signs. Although it is unlikely that signs more serious than gastrointestinal upset would occur with this exposure, decontamination would be prudent to prevent diarrhea.

10. Convert Mara's weight to kilograms:

    8 pounds/2.2 kg/pound = 3.6 kg

    Convert percentage minoxidil to mg/g:

    5% = 50 mg/g

    Convert 1/10 tsp to grams:

    1 tsp = 5 grams, so 1/10 tsp = 0.5 grams

    Calculate the dose of minoxidil:

    $0.5\,g \times 50\,mg/g = 25\,mg$

    Calculate Mara's topical dosage:

    $25\,mg/3.6\,kg = 6.9\,mg/kg$

Discussion

Minoxidil is a drug that is used for increasing hair growth, but it can also have profound cardiovascular effects in cats. Although toxic doses have not been established for cats, and it is not clear whether dermal absorption carries a risk of systemic involvement, the safest course of action would be to bathe the area of application and monitor Mara for hypotension.

REFERENCES

Albretsen, Jay C. 2004. Iron. In *Clinical Veterinary Toxicology*, edited by Konnie H. Plumlee, pp. 202–204. St. Louis: Mosby.

Debraekeleer, Jacques. 2000. Appendices. In *Small Animal Clinical Nutrition*, 4th ed., edited by Michael S. Hand, Craig D. Thatcher, Rebecca L. Remillard and Philip Roudebush, p. 1001. Topeka: Mark Morris Institute.

Dolder, Linda K. 2003. Metaldehyde toxicosis. *Veterinary Medicine* 98(3):213–215.

Dunayer, Eric K. 2003. Bromethalin: The other rodenticide. *Veterinary Medicine* 98(9):732–736.

Gwaltney-Brant, Sharon. 2001. Chocolate intoxication. *Veterinary Medicine* 96(2):108–111.

Jenkins, C.C. and Kanara, E.W. 1998. First-year clinical experience with Rimadyl (carprofen): Assessment of product safety. *Pfizer Animal Health Technical Bulletin*, May 1998. Exton, Pennsylvania.

Osweiler Gary D. 1996. *Toxicology*. Philadelphia: Lippincott Williams & Wilkens.

———. 2006. General toxicological principles. In *Small Animal Toxicology*, 2nd ed., edited by Michael E. Peterson and Patricia A. Talcott, pp. 2–17. St. Louis: Elsevier Saunders.

Plumb, Donald C. 2005. Acetylcysteine. In *Plumb's Veterinary Drug Handbook*, 5th ed., pp. 9–10. Ames, Iowa: Blackwell Publishing Professional.

Plunkett, Signe J. 2001. Ethylene glycol intoxication. In *Emergency Procedures for the Small Animal Veterinarian*, 2nd ed., pp. 319–326. Philadelphia: WB Saunders.

Richardson, Jill A. 2000a. Management of acetaminophen and ibuprofen toxicoses in dogs and cats. *Journal Veterinary Emergency and Critical Care* 10(4):285–291.

———. 2000b. Permethrin spot-On toxicoses in cats. *Journal Veterinary Emergency and Critical Care* 10(2):103–106.

Spoo, Wayne. 2004. Concepts and terminology. In *Clinical Veterinary Toxicology*, edited by Konnie H. Plumlee, pp. 2–7. St. Louis: Mosby.

Talcott, Patricia A. 2006. General nonsteroidal antiinflammatories. In *Small Animal Toxicology*, 2nd ed., edited by Michael E. Peterson and Patricia A. Talcott, pp. 902–933. St. Louis: Elsevier Saunders.

Youssef, Hany. 2006. Hyperactivity and disorientation in a cat. *NAVC Clinician's Brief* 4(12):49–56.

Initial Management of Acute Intoxications

6

Elisa Petrollini-Rogers and Bridget McNally

TELEPHONE TRIAGE

The initial contact with a patient client is often over the telephone. It is imperative that reception asks the appropriate questions to better instruct the client on what further steps need to be taken. One of the first queries should be to obtain the animal's signalment: species, breed, age, and approximate body weight. The information obtained from this question can greatly impact the course of treatment. A toxicant that may not affect a 100-pound Great Dane could greatly harm a 5-pound Devon Rex. Other information that should be obtained includes the type of exposure or ingestion, the length of time elapsed since the said exposure or ingestion, and the amount of potential toxicant. It is also important for reception to ask about the patient's mental state (i.e., alert, disoriented, reduced responsiveness, unresponsive). Although a client's estimation of the pet's mentation may not be completely accurate, a general idea about the pet's level of consciousness can be formulated. After this information is obtained, reception can then ask a veterinary medical staff member on duty whether the patient should seek medical attention. If there is a doubt on the patient's stability, the client should be advised to seek medical attention immediately.

Clients should be advised to bring any material or packages to which the patient may have had access. It is also advised that any vomitus from the patient be collected in a sealed container and brought into the hospital.

HOSPITAL PRESENTATION

Triage and History

An emergency can be described as any situation that arises suddenly and unexpectedly resulting in a sudden need for action. Upon presentation to the hospital/clinic, a member of the medical team should triage the patient. Triage refers to an initial, brief assessment of the emergency patient. It is performed immediately on presentation and should take less than 5 minutes. Triage involves a cursory evaluation of the four major organ systems (cardiovascular, respiratory, neurological, and renal) while simultaneously obtaining an abbreviated history. Conversation should be limited to significant points only, avoiding unrelated details. The history should include the primary complaint, duration of the problem, and any current drug therapy. The basic principles of emergency patient assessment should be applied even in the face of a potential poisoning.

The goal of triage is to determine whether the patient can be categorized as stable or unstable, allowing appropriate prioritization of care. A stable patient is one that is not in an immediate life-threatening condition. An unstable or emergent patient is one that is experiencing life-threatening signs and requires quick judgment and timely action. If any of the major body systems are significantly abnormal, the patient should immediately be

Small Animal Toxicology Essentials, First Edition. Edited by Robert H. Poppenga, Sharon Gwaltney-Brant.
© 2011 John Wiley and Sons, Inc. Published 2011 by John Wiley and Sons, Inc.

taken to the main treatment room of the emergency room to be assessed by the veterinarian.

In the emergent patient who has been exposed to a toxicant, the history is one of the most valuable pieces of information (Fitzgerald, 2006). Acquiring a detailed history can be the most difficult step, and further information on history-taking is found in Chapter 4. It is not uncommon for clients to be unaware that the patient was exposed to a toxicant. Recognizing clinical signs of common toxicants is an important skill in emergency medicine. The diagnosis of toxicant ingestion is generally based on a history of a witnessed exposure and/or suspicious clinical signs exhibited by the patient. It is not an uncommon occurrence for clients to believe that the patient has been poisoned in the face of an acute illness. Common diseases may imitate toxicant ingestion, and vice versa

If a toxic substance is known or suspected, but treatment options are not known or are immediately unavailable, a poison control center should be contacted. The ASPCA Animal Poison Control Center (1-800-548-2423) has the largest accumulation of veterinary toxicologists specializing in the effects of toxicants in animals (rather than people). Pet Poison Helpline (800-213-6680) is staffed with an array of board specialized veterinarians (toxicology, critical care, internal medicine) as well as toxicologists specializing in human toxicology (PharmDs). Both poison control centers charge consultation fees. More information on this and other toxicology information resources can be found in Chapter 2. Treatment can then be initiated in accordance with the recommendations provided for the specific toxicant.

Initial Assessment

The initial assessment should include assessment of the major organ systems and vital signs, obtaining vascular access, and an initial database followed by development of the emergency plan.

Respiratory System

One always determines the patency of the airway first. Ideally, patent and clear breath sounds should be heard. If the patient is in distress, upper airway noise (stridor/stertor) and/or distress with inspiration associated with stridor may be noted. This can be assessed without the use of a stethoscope.

The respiratory rate should be also be noted; normal for dogs and cats is considered to be 12–32 respirations per minute (rpm). If tachypnea (increased respiratory rate); slow, prolonged breathing; or apnea (no respiration) is noted, the patient should be immediately assessed by a veterinarian. Other abnormal findings include labored inspiration and/or labored expiration or paradoxical respiration (chest wall and abdominal wall do not move synchronously). Postural adaptations associated with respiratory distress may be seen is distressed patients as well (e.g., standing rather than sitting, abducted elbows, abdominal effort, extended neck, head lifted, etc.).

Cardiovascular System

Assessment of the cardiovascular system includes determination of mucous membrane color, capillary refill time, heart rate, and rhythm and pulse quality.

Normal mucous membrane color should be pink. Muddy or gray color suggests poor perfusion. Pale or white color suggests anemia, shock or pain; brick red mucous membrane color (hyperemic) is seen in situations including sepsis, hyperdynamic states, and hyperthermia. Dark blue (cyanotic) mucous membranes suggest hypoxemia from a variety of causes (cardiac dysfunction, pulmonary insufficiency, etc.). Yellow or icteric mucous membranes occur in cases of hepatic dysfunction, hemolysis, or biliary obstruction. Brown mucous membranes and blood are seen in cases of methemoglobinemia, which in companion animals is most commonly seen with acetaminophen toxicosis.

Normal capillary refill time (CRT) is 1–2 seconds. If the CRT is prolonged, this indicates poor perfusion. Rapid CRT indicates a hyperdynamic state or hemoconcentration.

Normal pulse rates for canines are 80–120 beats per minute (bpm) with <70 bpm suggesting bradycardia and >140 bpm suggesting tachycardia (Plumb 2005). For felines, normal pulse rates range from 130–140 bpm with <100 bpm suggesting bradycardia and >180 bpm suggesting tachycardia. When assessing heart rate, it is important to consider the animal's mental status, because excitement from being transported and handled may spuriously elevate the rate, and sleeping or comatose animals may have lower heart rates.

The pulse quality should be strong and synchronous with heart rate. Weak pulses indicate poor perfusion. Pulse quality feels "tall and thin" when associated with anemia; "bounding" pulses suggest hypertension.

Central Nervous System

The patient's central nervous system can initially be assessed by the evaluation of its gait (ataxia, loss of motor function), level of consciousness, and pupil size and position. Muscle twitching may be observed with some toxic exposures such as pyrethroid, chocolate, or ethylene glycol toxicoses. The following levels of consciousness can be observed:

Alert: Normal

Depressed: Quiet, unwilling to perform normally; responds to environmental stimuli

Obtunded: Minimally responsive to auditory or tactile stimuli

Stuporous: Unresponsive to environmental stimuli; responds to painful stimuli

Comatose: No response to environmental and painful stimuli

Renal System

On triage, the renal system is assessed with abdominal palpation when urinary blockage is suspected. Other emergencies affecting the renal system are identified while assessing the patient's cardiovascular status.

VASCULAR ACCESS AND THE EMERGENCY DATABASE

Intravenous access should be obtained in any critically ill patient for administration of fluids and drugs. The most common vessels used for intravenous catheterization are the cephalic or lateral saphenous veins. Central venous access the medial femoral or jugular vein allows for a larger diameter catheter to be placed, which is ideal for allowing achievement of higher drug concentrations in the coronary vessels as well as rapid fluid administration. These vessels are not as accessible as the peripheral vessels. In neonates, the easiest and most expeditious way to obtain vascular access is via intraosseous catheter placement. Ideally, at this time a blood sample may be collected and stored for future toxicological analysis, because some medications that may subsequently be administered may interfere with diagnostic tests (e.g., propylene glycol in diazepam injectable solutions will cause a false positive on ethylene glycol tests (Thrall et al. 2006)).

After the patient has been stabilized and decontaminated (if appropriate) and vascular access obtained, a medical problem list should be generated in the order of most to least life-threatening. Each problem should then be addressed in that order. Categories that should be covered include fluid therapy, medications, diagnostics, and treatment orders.

Emergency Database

Most modern veterinary hospitals are well equipped and have the ability to provide in-house diagnostics. Using these tools, rapid evaluation of the poisoned patient's metabolic and hydration status can be performed. This information will aid in the overall approach to and outcome for these patients. If the exact toxicant has already been determined, the direct effects and any secondary consequences of it can be predicted. In situations where the toxicant is not known, the diagnostic approach must be based upon clinical signs, a thorough history, and response to symptomatic therapy.

Once the patient has been appropriately triaged and vital signs stabilized, a systematic approach to diagnostics should be taken. If possible, during venous access, blood samples should be collected. A serum chemistry/electrolytes, blood gas, and complete blood cell count (CBC) should be analyzed as a baseline assessment. Depending on the history and clinical signs, ECG, blood smear, coagulation panel, and urinalysis may also reveal further evidence of a toxicosis. Other diagnostics that may provide useful information include radiographs, illicit drug screening, or ethylene glycol testing.

Blood Gases

Blood gas analysis is a great tool used to assess the patient's acid-base status. Many intoxicated patients will present with a history of vomiting, diarrhea, respiratory distress, or seizures. Although these clinical signs may be secondary, patients will likely present with some degree of acid-base derangement. The rapid evaluation of blood gas parameters is highly useful and can provide great insight to the patient's acid-base status.

Metabolic acidosis is characterized as a pH of <7.2 with a base excess of <4 (Waddell 2004). Mild acidosis may be corrected with intravenous fluid therapy and management of the underlying disease, whereas more severe metabolic acidosis may require sodium bicarbonate therapy.

Respiratory acidosis may be present in the intoxicated patient, this is characterized by a pH of <7.2 and PCO_2 of >45 (Waddell 2004). Respiratory acidosis may be due to the effect of the toxicant on the respiratory center in the central nervous system (CNS) as well as interference with innervation of the intercostal muscles. There is also the potential for respiratory acidosis to occur with the use of medications causing respiratory depression, resulting in hypoventilation. This is especially important with patients treated with high doses of anticonvulsants or opioids.

Lactic acidosis is due to the large amounts of lactic acid produced in response to excessive muscle activity. This can occur with seizure activity or with toxicants causing tremorgenic activity such as pyrethroid toxicosis or tremorgenic mycotoxin ingestion. This type of acidosis will generally resolve on its own once the seizures or tremors have been controlled. In other situations, hypoperfusion may result in lactic acidosis, requiring intravenous fluid therapy to resolve.

If a patient presents with severe vomiting or diarrhea, a blood gas may reveal a metabolic alkalosis (pH >7.4, base excess >4). In the case of ongoing gastrointestinal losses (i.e., potassium, chloride), it is important to treat the underlying cause and provide appropriate therapy for the vomiting and diarrhea to resolve the metabolic alkalosis.

Hyperventilation can cause a respiratory alkalosis. Based on a blood gas, this can be defined as a PCO_2 of <35 mmHg. This type of disturbance is most commonly seen in patients presenting hypoxemic or who have ingested something causing excitement, therefore stimulating the respiratory system. Respiratory alkalosis can also result from excessive ventilation in the patient that is being mechanically ventilated.

Hematocrit and Total Solids

The packed cell volume (PCV; aka hematocrit [Hct]) and total solids (TS) are generally interpreted in conjunction with each other. The changes in the two parameters often parallel each other in situations of free water loss or hemorrhage. Decrease in both PCV and TS suggests hemorrhage. Acute blood loss will not immediately affect PCV and TS because it takes time for interstitial fluid to move into the vascular space and dilute out the remaining red blood cells and proteins. In canines, splenic contractions secondary to catecholamine release may actually cause a transient increase in PCV in the face of acute hemorrhage. The changes in packed cell volume will become immediately apparent with intravenous fluid replacement. Because of this phenomenon, some consider TS to be a more sensitive indicator of blood loss than PCV. A decreased PCV with normal TS indicates red blood cell destruction or decreased red blood cell production. Anemia of chronic disease is characterized by a decreased PCV with normal TS. The foremost clinical significance to a decreased PCV is reduced oxygen-carrying capacity of the blood. Decreased total solids may occur due to loss from hemorrhage, protein loss into third spaces, or external loss through the intestines or kidneys. Hypoproteinemia results in decreased intravascular oncotic pressure. This may result in loss of fluid from the intravascular space and decreased ability to maintain vascular volume and blood pressure. Increases in both TS and PCV are most commonly due to dehydration.

Blood Glucose

Blood glucose readings are an essential portion of the emergency data base. Normal blood glucose ranges from 80–120 g/dl, and severe aberrations (either elevations or depressions) can be life-threatening to the patient. Hypo-

glycemia can occur due to conditions such as sepsis, liver dysfunction, neonatal/juvenile hypoglycemia, insulin or insulin-like factor secreting tumors, xylitol ingestion (dogs) or alpha-lipoic acid ingestion. A transient hyperglycemia can occur in overly stressed patients (particularly felines). True hyperglycemia is most commonly due to diabetes mellitus.

Blood Urea Nitrogen

Determination of the BUN provides an estimate of renal and hepatic function as well as hydration status. Low BUN concentration may be the result of fluid diuresis. Other causes can be polydipsia/polyuria or decreased production of BUN due to liver disease or a portal-caval vascular shunt. BUN can be elevated due to prerenal, renal, or postrenal mechanisms, and all of these should be considered when an increase in BUN is detected.

The amount of information obtained from the emergency database in regard to the patient's status should not be underestimated. This information combined with a solid history and thorough physical exam can often assist in confirming a diagnosis or providing direction for further investigation.

Serum Chemistry and Electrolytes

Serum chemistry and electrolyte panels are important to assess because some alterations in these measurements may be a direct result of the toxicant. Many toxicants affect renal function (i.e., ethylene glycol). If there is evidence of azotemia or acute renal failure, one then can move forward with diuresis and other appropriate therapy. Some toxicants (e.g., xylitol) may result in acute hepatic failure or necrosis, which will be reflected in the liver enzymes. Blood glucose, calcium, sodium, potassium, or chloride concentrations can also be altered by various toxicants, such as calcium channel blockers, digitalis, or vitamin D–based rodenticides. Evaluation of serum chemistry and electrolyte results can provide clues into the original cause of the abnormalities and provide feedback on response to therapy.

Hematology

Complete blood cell count (CBC) and peripheral blood smear analysis are useful tools in diagnosing hematological abnormalities. The CBC provides information on the oxygen-carrying capacity of the blood by measuring red blood cell parameters. The CBC helps classify anemia as acute or chronic as well as determine whether regeneration is occurring, all of which can assist in formulating a list of differential diagnoses. Measurement of white blood cell parameters can assist in identifying and characterizing inflammatory or infectious mechanisms.

Peripheral blood smear analysis is performed to evaluate the appearance of the cellular components of the blood (red blood cells, white blood cells, platelets), identify the presence of hematologic infectious agents (e.g., *Dirofilaria* or *Babesia*) and identify any other changes that may assist in diagnosis. For example, the presence of Heinz bodies and methemoglobinemia can put acetaminophen toxicosis on the list of differential diagnoses. During acute toxicosis, some changes may not be evident in the first 24–48 hours and it may be necessary to reevaluate a CBC at a later time. For patients who may need a transfusion, blood typing should be performed and potential appropriate donor animals identified. If blood typing is unavailable, the "universal donor" blood may be administered (DEA 1.1 Negative in dogs and Type A in cats).

Urinalysis

Urine should be collected for a baseline screening in the toxic patient, especially in patients who have ingested or have been exposed to nephrotoxic substances such as ethylene glycol or lilies. A complete urinalysis will provide useful information in determining the ability of the kidneys to concentrate urine. The presence of hemoglobinuria, glucosuria, proteinuria, cellular or granular casts, pigments, and crystals can aid in narrowing down the cause of renal dysfunction. For example, patients with ethylene glycol toxicosis may develop calcium oxalate crystalluria within 6–8 hours of exposure; however, absence of oxalate crystals does not rule out ethylene glycol as a potential toxicant, because not all patients will develop detectable crystalluria.

Additional Testing

During the course of patient management, additional testing may be indicated based on the clinical status of the patient or changes in historical information received from clients. Tests such as coagulation profiles, illicit drug screening, other drug or chemical screening, radiography, electrocardiography, and ultrasound can assist in identifying causes and measuring response to therapy.

Coagulation profiles are used to detect changes in the clotting parameters of the blood, especially prolonged prothrombin time (PT) and partial thromboplastin time (aPTT). These profiles (or individual tests) are often performed at the clinic and are helpful in diagnosing coagulopathy from a variety of causes, including anticoagulant rodenticide toxicosis. Anticoagulant rodenticides interfere with recycling of vitamin K in the body, leading to deple-

tion of clotting factors, which results in uncontrolled hemorrhage. Because most animals have a "reserve" of clotting factors, exposure to these rodenticides generally will not result in prolongation of PT or aPTT until 36–48 hours postingestion.

Illicit drug screening has become an invaluable tool used in cases where illicit drug ingestion is suspected. There are several types of these tests available at most pharmacies, designed for home monitoring of drug use. The tests are easy to perform, inexpensive, require only a small amount of urine, and provide results within a matter of minutes. The kits can screen for two to ten substances including amphetamines, barbiturates, benzodiazepines, cocaine, methadone, methamphetamine, nicotine, opiates, phencyclidine, and tricyclic antidepressants. Most of the tests for amphetamines will cross-react with sympathomimetic drugs such as pseudoephedrine or ma huang, so they can sometimes be helpful if ingestion of these legal drugs is suspected. Based on clinical experience, in many kits, the test for marijuana apparently does not give consistent results (i.e., gives false negatives), possibly due to differences in the metabolites excreted between humans and dogs. Other than the issue with marijuana, the kits appear to work very well in a clinical setting. These tests have not been validated in nonhumans, meaning they would not stand up in a court of law, but they have great utility in assisting veterinary staff in diagnosis of suspected drug ingestion. Keep in mind that any positive result based upon the use of a drug screening kit is not considered confirmatory, and false positive or negative results can occur. If someone wishes to pursue a case legally following a positive on an OTC test kit (i.e., suspected malicious poisoning), blood and urine should subsequently be submitted to a validated diagnostic laboratory for analysis that will be acceptable in a court of law. Some clients may be reluctant to have the test performed for fear of police authority involvement. As an animal care provider, it is very important to reassure clients that the only concern is for appropriate therapy for their pet. The cooperation of the client and the ability to provide illicit drug screening allows for a targeted treatment plan that can greatly improve the overall outcome of these patients.

Ethylene glycol testing is used in detecting the presence of high serum concentrations of ethylene glycol. Ethylene glycol (EG) is the major component found in many commercial antifreeze products. This test is most reliable in the first 4 hours after ingestion; however, based on the amount of EG ingested, levels may be detectable in excess of 12 hours postingestion. False negatives and false positives can occur with the existing tests available for in-house use in veterinary clinics. Details of these issues can be found in the discussion on ethylene glycol in Chapter 28.

Human hospital laboratories may be helpful in determining exposure to a variety of toxicants, including EG and acetaminophen. When in-house EG testing is not available, or there is concern that the test result may be a false positive, human hospital laboratories can run an EG test that will give a specific level of EG in the blood. For dogs, the level of concern is 50 mg/dl or greater and for cats the level of concern is 20 mg/dl or greater. Tests run in human hospitals for EG are very sensitive and specific, so the false positives and negatives seen in the in-house veterinary EG tests are not an issue. In many situations, there is concern that a cat or dog may have been exposed to acetaminophen. In these cases, human hospitals can analyze blood for acetaminophen levels, which can tell whether the animal was exposed; unfortunately, nomograms do not exist for dogs and cats to determine subtoxic doses from toxic doses, but these test can help with the question "Did he/she eat it?"

Radiography may be useful in providing evidence of a metallic foreign body. Common radiopaque materials include batteries, screws, galvanized metal, and coins. Some heavy metals are proven to be highly toxic. For example, a patient presenting with acute hemolytic anemia should have radiographs taken to look for coins (pennies minted after 1982) to rule out zinc toxicosis. If radiographs are diagnostic, an endoscopy or a gastrotomy will be required after patient stabilization.

Electrocardiography (ECG) may help detect arrhythmias a patient may be experiencing. Many patients intoxicated with substances such as methylxanthines, amphetamines, cocaine, or albuterol will present with sinus tachycardia or ventricular tachyarrhythmias. Bradycardia and bradyarrhythmias may present in patients exposed to substances such as organophosphorous insecticides, pharmaceuticals (e.g., beta-adrenergic blockers), and alcohol. Bradyarrhythmias can also occur in patients with severe electrolyte abnormalities (e.g., hyperkalemia) secondary to a toxicosis (e.g., digitalis toxicosis). The use of appropriate antiarrhythmic medication will be dictated by the veterinarian based on the type and severity of the abnormal rhythm. Continuous ECG monitoring is recommended when treating these patients.

CONCLUSION

There are a variety of reasons that animals may present to an emergency service, including infectious, inflammatory, metabolic and toxic processes. In many circumstances involving poisoning, the cause of the animal's condition may not be known, particularly in cases where exposure to a toxicant was not witnessed. Having a systematic approach to these patients is paramount to identifying the major health issues present. Patient stabilization is essential to keeping the patient alive while the underlying problem is diagnosed and treated. Evaluation of the patient's clinical status and detailed historical information are often necessary to identify the inciting cause and provide prompt and appropriate treatment.

CHAPTER 6 STUDY QUESTIONS

1. Initial triage of a poisoning patient includes quick assessment of the function of which of the following systems?
   a. Neurologic
   b. Renal
   c. Cardiovascular
   d. Respiratory
   e. All of the above
2. List the four parameters that are used during the assessment of cardiovascular function.
3. Tiffany, a 10-week-old female intact Siamese kitten presents 3 hours after the owner applied a spot-on canine flea control product containing amitraz to the kitten's skin. During the initial assessment, Tiffany is found to be recumbent and drooling. She appears minimally aware of her surroundings but does react to sudden noises (such as the sound of a cage door

closing) or to being touched by lifting her head and jerking slightly. Her level of consciousness is best assessed as
   a. Alert
   b. Depressed
   c. Obtunded
   d. Stuporous
   e. Comatose
4. Tiffany has a heart rate of 70 bpm, capillary refill time of 5 seconds, gray mucous membranes, and thready pulses. Which of the following assessments best match Tiffany's cardiovascular status?
   a. Bradycardic, hypertensive
   b. Bradycardic, hypotensive
   c. Normal heart rate, hypotensive
   d. Tachycardic, hypertensive
   e. Tachycardic, hypotensive

5. Tiffany's body temperature is 96°F and her blood glucose (via quick enzymatic strip test) is >200 mg/dl. Which of the following is the correct assessment for Tiffany?

    a. Hyperthermic, hyperglycemic
    b. Hyperthermic, hypoglycemic
    c. Hypothermic, hyperglycemic
    d. Hypothermic, normoglycemic
    e. Hypothermic, hypoglycemic

6. What is the most appropriate next step to take after Tiffany's initial assessment?

    a. Obtain a detailed history from Tiffany's owner.
    b. Put Tiffany in a cage with a hot water bottle.

    c. Give Tiffany some insulin to drop the blood glucose.
    d. Insert intravenous catheter and initiate IV fluid therapy using warmed fluids.
    e. Bathe the flea product off of Tiffany.

7. Tiffany is stabilized, bathed, and placed in a cage with a heating pad. What parameters should be monitored closely over the next several hours?

    a. Heart rate
    b. Capillary refill time
    c. Fluid ins and outs
    d. Body temperature
    e. All of the above

ANSWERS

1. e. All of these systems must be assessed during patient triage.

2. Determination of mucous membrane color, capillary refill time, heart rate and rhythm, and pulse quality.

3. c. Obtunded animals are minimally responsive to tactile and auditory stimuli.

4. b. A heart rate of <100 bpm in a kitten is bradycardia, and the prolonged capillary refill time, mucous membrane color and poor pulse quality are consistent with hypotension.

5. c. Body temperature <100°F is hypothermia, and blood glucose levels >120 mg/dl indicate hyperglycemia.

6. d. Following assessment, steps should be taken to stabilize the patient. In this case, fluid therapy is indicated to help manage the hypotension. Obtaining a history and bathing the cat should be done after the kitten is stabilized.

7. e. All of these parameters should be monitored closely.

REFERENCES

Plumb, Donald C. 2005. *Plumb's Veterinary Drug Handbook*, 5th ed. Ames, Iowa: Blackwell.

Fitzgerald, Kevin T. 2006. Taking a toxicological history. In *Small Animal Toxicology*, 2nd ed, edited by Michael E. Peterson and Patricia A. Talcot, pp. 38–44. St. Louis: Saunders.

Thrall, Mary A., Connally, Heather E., Grauer, Gregory F., and Hamar, Dwayne. 2006. Zinc phosphide. In *Small Animal Toxicology*, 2nd ed, edited by Michael E. Peterson and Patricia A. Talcot, pp. 38–44. St. Louis: Saunders.

Waddell, Lori S. 2004. Evaluation and Interpretation of Blood Gases. *Proceedings of the Western Veterinary Conference, Reno Nevada*.

Decontamination Procedures

7

Lisa Murphy

SOURCES

Companion animals may need to be decontaminated due to a variety of exposures to potentially harmful substances. The most common scenarios that may require decontamination and follow-up veterinary care are oral, inhalation, dermal, and ocular exposures.

Oral exposures in the animal's environment may include consumption of contaminated food or water, ingesting dropped pills or other items, licking puddles of unknown liquids, grooming, and swallowing particles that are first inhaled then returned to the pharynx from the lower respiratory tract by the mucociliary apparatus (Gwaltney-Brant et al. 2003).

Inhalation exposures can result from exposures to dusts, ash, gases, and toxic fumes (Gwaltney-Brant et al. 2003). Gases and toxic fumes are most dangerous in enclosed spaces, so animals confined indoors may be at the greatest risk for dangerous levels of exposure. Animals can easily inhale dust, ash, and other particulates when displaced by either their own movement or that of people walking through a contaminated area with animals located nearby. Fires are another important source of inhaled smoke, toxic gases, and other hazardous substances.

Dermal exposures can occur in many ways including direct application of sprays, drops, ointments, or other substances by the owner. In addition animals may roll or walk in puddles, spills, or other sources of contamination that they find in their environment, or they may be exposed during intentional uses or accidental releases of various chemicals if the pet is in the vicinity and located down-wind (Murphy et al. 2008). As mentioned previously, dermal exposures can become oral exposures as a result of grooming. It is also important to realize that animals may directly transfer potentially harmful substances from their feet and haircoat to any people, other animals, surfaces, and other objects they come in contact with prior to being decontaminated.

Ocular exposures can occur with liquids, solids, and gases. Liquids can enter the eyes through splashes, immersions, or instillation (accidental or intentional) by the owner. Solid objects and particles that are blown or rubbed into the eyes can cause corneal abrasions and other mechanical trauma. Depending on the compound involved direct chemical effects and even systemic signs may be possible. Irritant gases may come in direct contact with the cornea and surrounding ocular structures and result in a variety of clinical signs.

CLINICAL EFFECTS

Clinical signs caused by toxic compounds will vary depending on the substance(s) involved, the animal's age and health history, the amount the animal comes in contact with, the duration of exposure, and sometimes the route of exposure as well (Poppenga 2004). Table 7.1 shows a variety of local and systemic effects that can result from exposures to hydrocarbons. Common hydrocarbons that companion animals may come in contact with include lighter fluid, furniture polish, kerosene, gasoline, other automotive fluids, and chemical solvents such as mineral spirits. Small exposures of short durations result in mild

Small Animal Toxicology Essentials, First Edition. Edited by Robert H. Poppenga, Sharon Gwaltney-Brant.
© 2011 John Wiley and Sons, Inc. Published 2011 by John Wiley and Sons, Inc.

Table 7.1. Range of clinical effects associated with hydrocarbon exposures

Affected Systems	Possible Syndromes
Skin	Dermatitis, skin eruptions, burns, epidermal necrosis
Eyes	Conjunctivitis, corneal irritation, corneal necrosis
Gastrointestinal tract	Nausea, vomiting, diarrhea, abdominal pain
Respiratory tract	Vascular endothelial damage, petechiation and hemorrhage, atelectasis, dyspnea
Central nervous system	Disorientation, seizures, coma

local irritant effects; larger exposures of longer durations may potentially result in life-threatening systemic signs.

Signs

Animals exposed to toxicants may show no signs, immediate problems, or delayed clinical effects depending on the type and amount of substance involved. Signs may also be either local (e.g., confined to the footpads if an animal walks through a toxic substance) or systemic if significant absorption occurs.

Mild local effects associated with oral exposures to toxicants may be limited to drooling, gagging, and foaming (especially in cats); rubbing and pawing at the mouth; vomiting; and diarrhea. More severe signs, such as deep ulcerations and sloughing of the tongue and mucous membranes can occur with ingestions of alkaline substances such as drain cleaners and electric dishwasher detergents. In severe cases, potential sequelae include scarring or perforations of the esophagus or other structures of the gastrointestinal tract. Severe vomiting and gagging can also put animals at risk of aspiration and subsequent respiratory problems.

Inhalation of particulates and gases can result in immediate coughing, respiratory distress, and damage to the lining of the respiratory tract.

When small quantities of toxic or irritating substances come in contact with the skin, the only signs may be redness, itching, or mild transient hair loss. More extensive or prolonged exposures may result in deep chemical burns, scarring, and permanent hair loss, and

put the animal at risk for infection and thermoregulatory problems.

As shown using the example of hydrocarbons in Table 7.1 ocular exposures may result in signs ranging from mild conjunctivitis, corneal irritation, tearing, and blepharospasm to corneal necrosis, perforation, and permanent blindness.

MANAGEMENT OF EXPOSURES

The goal of decontamination is to minimize exposures to potentially toxic substances. This can be accomplished by preventing or minimizing absorption or enhancing elimination.

Precautions

Proper safety measures should be taken before admitting a patient that is suspected to have been exposed to a toxic substance. Not only are human personnel potentially at risk, but other animals on the premises could also be harmed. The minimum personal protective equipment (PPE) for veterinary personnel performing animal decontamination includes gloves, an apron or other water resistant clothing, and eye protection (Murphy et al. 2008). Specific substances such as pepper spray and other riot control agents also require the use of respiratory protection and adequate ventilation, preferably in an area of the hospital that is isolated from other staff members and patients.

Oral Decontamination

Induction of Vomiting (Emesis)

Induction of vomiting (emesis) is used to remove potentially harmful substances from the stomach. Complete stomach emptying is generally not possible, though the total amount of toxicant available for absorption can be significantly reduced. Emesis in companion animals is typically most useful within 30 to 90 minutes of the ingestion.

There are certain circumstances under which emesis should not be induced (DeClementi 2007). Following ingestions of caustic substances or hydrocarbons an animal could aspirate these substances into its respiratory tract if vomiting occurs. Animals that are already demonstrating clinical signs, such as dyspnea, disorientation, or seizure activity, could also aspirate or develop more severe problems if they are then also made to vomit. Vomiting can also cause an acute worsening of preexisting conditions in patients with a known history of cardiovascular or seizure disorders.

Table 7.2. Hydrogen peroxide dosing recommendations for the induction of vomiting in dogs and cats

Body weight	Volume of 3% hydrogen peroxide
<2.3 kilograms (<5 pounds)	5 ml (1 teaspoon)
2.3–4.5 kilograms (5–10 pounds)	10 ml (2 teaspoons)
4.5–9.1 kilograms (10–20 pounds)	20 ml (1.3 tablespoons)
9.1–13.6 kilograms (20–30 pounds)	30 ml (2 tablespoons)
13.6–18.2 kilograms (30–40 pounds)	40 ml (2.7 tablespoons)
>18.2 kilograms (> 40 pounds)	45 ml (3 tablespoons)

Source: DeClementi 2007.

Hydrogen peroxide (3% USP) can be safely and effectively used to induce vomiting. Acting by local irritation of the stomach, 3% hydrogen peroxide dissociates into nonharmful oxygen and water after it has finished foaming. Table 7.2 outlines general dosing recommendations for dogs and cats. Some clinicians do not recommend using hydrogen peroxide in cats due to the possibility of an increased risk of severe gastritis and reduced efficacy. If no vomiting occurs after 5 to 10 minutes a second oral dose may be administered. Hydrogen peroxide often works most effectively if given after a small soft meal such as bread or canned pet food. Potential adverse effects of the use of hydrogen peroxide include protracted vomiting, hematemesis, and gastritis; these effects are generally the result of overdosing of hydrogen peroxide.

Apomorphine is a centrally acting emetic that is commonly used orally or intravenously, though mild sedation and prolonged vomiting may occur as a side effect. These adverse effects can be minimized by instead instilling apomorphine into the subconjunctival sac and then flushing it out with sterile saline solution when vomiting begins.

Although xylazine will often cause vomiting in cats its effects can be inconsistent and it can result in excessive sedation. The sedation caused by xylazine can be reversed with atipamezole or yohimbine.

Extra precautions should be taken and no unnecessary personnel should be allowed in the treatment area if it is suspected that the animal has ingested something especially noxious, such as zinc phosphide. In these situations the resulting vomitus could lead to dangerous human exposures to the noxious material (e.g., phosphine gas in the case of zinc phosphide). Induction of emesis outdoors or in a well-ventilated area is highly recommended in these cases.

Other substances that are not generally recommended for the induction of emesis include liquid dishwashing detergent, powdered mustard, syrup of ipecac, and salt. Detergents and mustard are not particularly effective in companion animals and can cause significant gastrointestinal irritation. Syrup of ipecac does not consistently induce vomiting in animals and has been associated with adverse cardiovascular effects in people; there is also a significant delay of up to 40 minutes for emesis to occur. Salt is another substance that also often fails to induce emesis after oral administration and if not vomited up can put the animal at risk for potentially life-threatening sodium ion toxicosis.

If vomiting cannot be successfully induced following the ingestion of significant quantities of potentially harmful substances, other decontamination options include diluents, adsorbents, and cathartics.

Diluents

Dilution with fluids such as water works by making ingested compounds less irritating. Other diluents such as milk and liquid antacids can have the added benefit of soothing and coating damaged mucous membrane surfaces. For all diluents, only limited amounts should be offered to reduce the risk of excessive distention of the stomach and subsequent vomiting and possible aspiration. Volumes similar to those recommended for hydrogen peroxide in Table 7.2 based on body weight can be safely offered or administered to otherwise stable and asymptomatic animals.

Activated Charcoal

Activated charcoal is an adsorbent that binds most organic compounds, reducing their absorption and facilitating their elimination in the feces. Available in powder, gel, or liquid formulations the recommended oral dose for all species is 1 to 3 grams per kilogram of body weight. It can be offered to some animals in a dish or administered with a large syringe or stomach tube. Repeated doses may be useful for minimizing the severity and duration of clinical signs associated with ingestions of compounds that undergo enterohepatic recirculation such as barbiturates and ivermectin.

Cathartics

Cathartics enhance elimination of substances, including activated charcoal, by moving them through the gastrointestinal tract more quickly. Bulk cathartics such as psyllium (Metamucil), canned pumpkin, and whole grain breads rely on high fiber content to retain water in the lower gastrointestinal tract and produce bulkier stools. Bulk cathartics can also be useful in facilitating the passage of ingested foreign bodies such as coins, rocks, and glass. Osmotic cathartics pull free body water into the gastrointestinal tract and decrease total gastrointestinal transit time. The most frequently used osmotic cathartic is 70% sorbitol and is often combined with activated charcoal products. Saline cathartics such as sodium sulfate (Glauber's salts) and magnesium sulfate (Epsom salts) work by stimulating gastrointestinal motility and require careful monitoring to avoid harmful electrolyte disturbances. Cathartics should not be administered to animals with preexisting dehydration, electrolyte imbalances, or diarrhea (DeClementi 2007).

Other Gastrointestinal Decontamination Techniques

Enemas, such as warm soapy water or dioctyl sodium sulfosuccinate (DSS), can be useful in eliminating toxicants from the lower gastrointestinal tract. Phosphate enemas should be avoided, particularly in cats.

Gastric lavage requires general anesthesia and the use of a cuffed endotracheal tube, but may be necessary in cases of potentially life-threatening oral exposures. The use of anesthesia also provides an extra measure of safety for animals that may unexpectedly begin to seizure or develop other neurologic signs as a symptom of intoxication. After the lavage has been completed and before the endotracheal tube is removed activated charcoal can be instilled directly into the stomach. Gastric lavage should not be used to remove caustic substances or hydrocarbons due to the risk of aspiration.

General anesthesia is also required for endoscopy, but if available this technique can be extremely useful for the removal of coins, batteries, toys, and other items before they can pass out of the stomach.

Decontamination for Inhalation Exposures

The initial treatment for exposure to inhaled toxicants is removing the patient to fresh air. In the veterinary clinic, symptomatic and supportive care may include administration of supplemental oxygen, intravenous fluid therapy, and pain management if local injury has occurred. Monitoring may consist of blood gas measurements, pulse oximetry, and serial thoracic radiographs. Antidotal treatments and additional diagnostics may be needed for some specific chemical exposures.

Dermal Decontamination

Most dermal exposures are treated by washing the affected area or bathing the entire animal. Liquid dishwashing detergent, used for hand-washing of dishes and distinct from highly alkaline electric dishwasher detergents, is very safe and effective for removing a variety of contaminants, especially greasy or oily substances (DeClementi 2007). It is readily available and relatively nonirritating to skin and mucous membranes. If an animal licks a small amount during bathing, brief drooling or gagging may be expected. Repeated baths may be needed for heavily contaminated animals or if the initial washing needs to be curtailed because the patient begins to shiver or appears stressed. An animal such as a cat that may be particularly fearful of a direct spray of water may be more easily wetted down for washing and subsequent rinsing by gently immersing it up to its neck in a bucket or other suitable container of warm water while carefully supporting its body. After bathing all animals should be carefully monitored in a draft free environment to prevent hypothermia.

Vacuuming or combing is helpful for removing powders and other dry compounds from the haircoats of animals that will tolerate it. This is especially useful for products that would otherwise become sticky or clumped with the addition of water. Shaving or clipping is appropriate for dried paint, tar, and other similar substances.

Oily substances such as mineral oil, vegetable oils, and peanut butter can be used to remove items such as glue traps, asphalt, and tree sap. After applying these to the contaminated skin or hair it can then be gently massaged to work the contaminant into small gummy balls that can then either be combed out or washed away with liquid dishwashing detergent.

Ocular Decontamination

Eyes should be flushed with sterile saline solution or clean room temperature water. Careful irrigation of the nostrils can also facilitate the removal of substances that may have entered the nasolacrimal ducts. Sterile eye wash solutions are available in small handheld bottles. Bagged or bottled intravenous solutions can also be used to flush eyes after removing the needle from the end of the intravenous drip set. Although prolonged or especially dangerous ocular exposures may require the eyes to be flushed as long as 20 to 30 minutes, in many cases it may not be necessary for small splashes involving only mildly irritating chemicals. When more extensive decontamination is needed some animals may tolerate repeated flushings of short durations paired with rest periods in between.

Fluorescein staining should be performed after flushing if the patient history or physical examination suggests a significant ocular exposure or injury. Staining should then be repeated 12 to 24 hours later even if initial staining fails to detect any corneal defects. Instillation of lubricant ointments can then follow the fluorescein staining.

PROGNOSIS

The likelihood of a full recovery for otherwise healthy animals that are promptly decontaminated before significant clinical signs develop is generally excellent. Even animals that display adverse effects may still have a good prognosis if they are closely monitored and receive appropriate symptomatic and supportive care.

CHAPTER 7 STUDY QUESTIONS

1. Barney, a 75-pound, neutered male, 7-year-old golden retriever presents within an hour of his owner finding Barney gobbling down the contents of a 2-pound bag of semisweet chocolate morsels. What is the first step in managing this case?
   a. Assess the patient.
   b. Induce vomiting.
   c. Administer IV fluids.
   d. Radiograph the abdomen.
   e. Administer PO activated charcoal.

2. Barney has melted chocolate smeared on his muzzle, but other than a bad case of "chocolate-breath," he is bright, alert, and responsive. His heart rate is 120, he is panting and his body temperature is 102.5°F. It is determined that it is safe to induce vomiting to try to retrieve some chocolate. Which of the following is/are NOT recommended as an emetic?
   a. 3% hydrogen peroxide
   b. Apomorphine administered PO, IV, or via conjunctival sac
   c. Syrup of ipecac
   d. Salt
   e. c and d

3. Emesis is induced and Barney vomits up a large volume of chocolaty liquid with some clumps of solid chocolate. It is decided to administer activated charcoal because a significant amount of chocolate is still unaccounted for. The rationale behind administering activated charcoal in a toxicity case is to
   a. Cause more vomiting to get more of the toxicant back.
   b. Increase gastrointestinal motility to move the toxicant through the digestive tract faster.
   c. Dilute the toxicant in the digestive tract, making it less toxic.

   d. Adsorb the toxicant to the charcoal in the digestive tract, thereby decreasing absorption of the toxicant.
   e. Adsorb the toxicant to the charcoal in the plasma, preventing the toxicant from reaching its site of action.

4. Which contaminant is correctly matched with the best means of removing it from the hair/skin of a dog or cat?
   a. Motor oil: plain water
   b. Latex paint: mineral oil
   c. Latex paint: paint thinner
   d. Glue-based mouse trap: vegetable oil
   e. Dried tar: soapy water

5. Smurf, a 6-pound, 1-year-old, male Persian cat is boarding at a veterinary clinic. Smurf was being treated with a topical ophthalmic solution for a pre-existing eye condition. By mistake, a staff member accidentally instilled an ear mite medication containing ivermectin into Smurf's eye. The ear mite medication insert indicates that the product may cause mild irritation if ocular exposure occurs. Which of the following is the best course of action?
   a. Flush Smurf's eye with sterile saline for 1–2 minutes and monitor for redness or irritation.
   b. Flush Smurf's eye with soapy water for 1–2 minutes and monitor for redness or irritation.
   c. Flush Smurf's eye with soapy water for 10–20 minutes and then stain with fluorescein.
   d. Flush Smurf's eye with sterile saline for 10–20 minutes and then stain with fluorescein.
   e. Flush Smurf's eye with mineral oil for 10–20 minutes and then stain with fluorescein.

Continued

ANSWERS

1.a. Assess the patient.

2.e. Neither salt nor syrup of ipecac is considered safe or consistently effective emetics for dogs.

3.d. Activated charcoal adsorbs certain compounds, preventing the compounds from being absorbed from the gastrointestinal tract.

4.d. Vegetable oil (or other oily compounds) can help to remove the adhesive properties of glues. Oily compounds are not removed effectively by water-based compounds (and vice versa) unless a detergent is included to break up the oil, so answers a and b are incorrect. Paint thinner and other mineral spirits should never be used on dog or cat skin because chemical burns can develop; this fact and the fact that latex paint is water-based and therefore would not effectively be removed by paint thinner makes answer c incorrect. Dried tar (answer e) will not be removed by soapy water; small amounts may respond to oily compounds, but often tar dried in a hair coat may need to be clipped off.

5.a. Sterile saline is the agent of choice for ocular decontamination. Because the product information indicated that only mild irritation was expected, a short period of flushing and monitoring is acceptable.

REFERENCES

DeClementi, Camille. 2007. Prevention and treatment of poisoning. In *Veterinary Toxicology*, edited by Ramesh C. Gupta, pp. 1139–1158. San Diego: Academic Press-Elsevier.

Gwaltney-Brant, Sharon M., Murphy, Lisa A., Wismer, Tina A., and Albretsen, Jay C. 2003. General toxicologic hazards and risks for search-and-rescue dogs responding to urban disasters. *Journal of the American Veterinary Medical Association*, 222(3):292–295.

Murphy, Lisa A., Slessman, Dawn, Mauck, Bob. 2008. Decontamination of Large Animals. In *Technical Large Animal Emergency Rescue*, edited by Rebecca Gimenez, Tomas Gimenez, and Kimberly Anne May, pp. 293–310. Ames, Iowa: Wiley-Blackwell.

Poppenga, Robert. 2004. Treatment. In *Clinical Veterinary Toxicology*, edited by Konnie H. Plumlee, pp. 13–21. St. Louis: Mosby.

Antidotes

8

Tina Wismer

INTRODUCTION

Antidotes are remedies to counteract poisons. They can prevent, reverse, or decrease the action of a toxicant. While many clients "just want the antidote," there are some very real obstacles to this in many situations (Post and Keller 1999). First, the vast majority of toxicants have no specific antidote, so treatment is symptomatic and supportive. Second, even in situations where an antidote exists, there are often obstacles to its use (cost, availability, etc.). Many manufacturers do not produce antidotes because there is little profit to be made. Third, antidotes themselves can cause intoxication or adverse reactions. Unfortunately, there is no universal antidote and choices must be made depending on the specific situation. Almost all antidotes are off-label use in veterinary patients.

There are three major classifications of antidotes: chemical, pharmacological, and functional (Bateman and Marrs 1999). The chemical antidotes include the chelators, commercial antibodies, and enzyme inhibitors. Chemical antidotes act directly on a toxicant to decrease toxicity or to increase excretion. Pharmacological antidotes antagonize or compete with the toxicant at its receptor site or through other macromolecules. They can bind to the toxicant itself or to the target to prevent the toxicant from binding. Functional antidotes treat the symptoms caused by the toxicant (symptomatic care). Antidotes can be in different classification groups depending on which toxic substance they are treating.

CHEMICAL ANTIDOTES

Chelators

Chelators, from the Greek word for *claw*, bind toxicants (usually metals) in a ring structure to increase their water solubility and excretion (Bateman and Marrs 1999). Chelators decrease levels of free toxicant in the blood, decrease tissue concentrations, and increase elimination. A chelator should be chosen that is resistant to biotransformation, is able to reach sites of toxicant storage, forms nontoxic complexes with toxic substances, has a low affinity for essential metals, and is easily excreted from the body. Unfortunately, no chelators can fulfill all of these requirements.

Calcium Disodium EDTA (Riker, Versenate®)

Calcium disodium EDTA (CaEDTA, sodium calcium edentate, calcium disodium edathamil, calcium disodium edetate, calcium disodium ethylenediaminetetra-acetate, calcium disodium versenate, disodium calcium tetrace-mate) is used to chelate many heavy metals. It is used mostly in the treatment of lead and zinc toxicoses, but it can also chelate cadmium, copper, cobalt, iron, nickel, chromium, manganese, plutonium, thorium, uranium, yttrium, and possibly vanadium (Chisolm 1992). The divalent or trivalent metal displaces the calcium in CaEDTA to form a water-soluble complex that is excreted in the urine.

Small Animal Toxicology Essentials, First Edition. Edited by Robert H. Poppenga, Sharon Gwaltney-Brant.
© 2011 John Wiley and Sons, Inc. Published 2011 by John Wiley and Sons, Inc.

All metal should be removed from the GI tract before administration, because CaEDTa will increase absorption of metal from the GI tract. It is recommended that CaEDTA is given slowly IV, because IM injections are very painful. Calcium disodium EDTA therapy is not benign. It can cause nephrotoxicity (renal tubular necrosis) and GI irritation. Maintaining hydration will help decrease the renal toxicity. Calcium disodium EDTA can also chelate essential metals (e.g., zinc, iron), resulting in deficiency; this is especially problematic when chelation is required for an extended period of time (Plumb 2008). Chronic use of CaEDTA may lead to zinc and iron deficiency and supplementation should be implemented.

Monitor animals closely when starting CaEDTA therapy because initially blood lead levels will increase due to removal from body stores; this may worsen clinical signs or precipitate signs in asymptomatic animals with high body burdens of lead. Calcium disodium EDTA and BAL may be used together in severe cases. Do not use sodium EDTA (edentate disodium); it chelates calcium and can cause severe hypocalcemia (Plumb 2008).

Deferoxamine (Ciba, Desferal®)

Deferoxamine (DFO, desferoxamine mesylate) is a chelating agent approved for use in humans for the treatment of acute and chronic iron poisoning and aluminum overload in patients on chronic dialysis (Westlin 1971). It has also been used to treat doxorubicin, paraquat, aminoglycoside, and acetaminophen poisonings. Deferoxamine has been used off-label to treat iron toxicosis in animals (Plumb 2008).

Deferoxamine chelates free iron, which is then excreted in the urine and bile. Early administration, within the first 24 hours, is most effective. The dose is given IM every 4–8 hours. If using the IV route, the animal should be monitored for development of pulmonary edema and hypotension (Ioannides and Panisello 2000). Pink to orange-red urine ("vin rose") indicates excretion of chelated iron (Plumb 2008). Excretion of deferoxamine can be increased by giving ascorbic acid after the gut has been cleared of iron. Therapy may be stopped if asymptomatic and the urine is clear. Deferoxamine will artificially elevate total iron-binding capacity and depress serum iron levels, so these diagnostic parameters are no longer valid measurements during treatment (Gevirtz and Wasserman 1966).

One advantage of using deferoxamine includes the lack of chelation of other trace metals (except aluminum). Adverse effects include pain at the injection site, vomiting, and diarrhea; chronic high doses can cause hypocalcemia

and thrombocytopenia. Animals treated with deferoxamine are at risk to develop certain infections. Deferoxamine supplies the iron siderophore growth factor needed by both *Yersinia* bacteria and *Rhizopus* fungus to grow (Melby et al. 1982). Humans have reported cataracts, retinal abnormalities, night blindness, and hearing loss after treatment (Levine et al. 1997). Although these effects have not yet been reported in dogs and cats, the potential for their development should be taken into consideration when choosing this compound for use in companion animals.

Dimercaprol (Taylor, BAL in Oil®)

Dimercaprol (BAL, British anti-Lewisite, dimercaptopropanol, dithioglycerol) provides sulfhydryl groups to chelate heavy metals. It was originally developed during WWII as an antidote to the blistering agent Lewisite (Kosnett 2005a). Dimercaprol can be used to chelate lead, arsenic, gold, inorganic mercury, antimony, bismuth, chromium, nickel, copper, zinc, and tungsten (Kosnett 2005a). In veterinary medicine, BAL is most commonly used to treat arsenic toxicosis and occasionally lead, mercury, and gold intoxications. It should not be used with iron, cadmium, and selenium poisoning, because the chelated complex is more toxic than the metal alone.

Dimercaprol can remove lead from the brain and red blood cells and may be the recommended chelator in small animal cases where severe CNS signs are present. Binding to dimercaprol is not irreversible and metals can dissociate in an acidic environment. Alkalinizing the urine will increase excretion and decrease renal toxicity. BAL is nephrotoxic and is extremely painful on injection. Hypertension, hyperpyrexia, tachycardia, vomiting, and seizures can occur with higher dosages (Kosnett 2005a).

Intravenous Lipid Solutions (Intralipid®, Lipsosyn®)

Intravenous lipid solutions (ILS) are intravenous fat emulsions used to provide parenteral nutrition. These emulsions can be used to treat systemic drug toxicoses. Highly fat-soluble drugs will bind to the lipids and be removed from the blood stream similar to chylomicrons (Waitzberg et al. 2006). Intravenous lipid solutions have been used to treat local anesthetics, bupropion, barbiturate, propranolol, verapamil, tricyclic antidepressants, and avermectin toxicoses (Turner-Lawrence and Kerns 2008).

D-penicillamine (Merck, Cuprimine®; Wallace, Depen®)

D-penicillamine (D-3-mercaptovaline, beta,beta-dimethylcysteine) is a hydrolytic product of penicillin, but has no antimicrobial action. It is used to chelate a variety of heavy metals such as copper, cadmium, mercury, iron, and lead (Lyle 1981). D-penicillamine is used most commonly in veterinary medicine to treat copper-storage hepatopathies (dogs), but can also be used in lead poisoning.

D-penicillamine is less effective than other chelating agents (CaEDTA or dimercaprol) for the treatment of severe lead poisoning, but it has the benefit of being given orally. Penicillamine should be given on an empty stomach because food decreases the bioavailability. Vomiting is a common side effect that may be minimized by splitting doses or pretreating with dimenhydrinate (Plumb 2008). Penicillamine should not be given if metal is still present in GI tract because it will increase absorption. Penicillamine will also chelate essential metals, including zinc, cobalt, and manganese. Pyrexia, depression, anorexia, diarrhea, proteinuria, lymphadenopathy, immune-complex glomerulonephropathy, and blood dyscrasias are rare but can be seen.

Protamine sulfate (Various, Generic)

Protamine sulfate combines with acidic glycosaminoglycans and is used in the treatment of heparin overdosage. Protamine and heparin bind to form an inactive stable salt (Plumb 2008). Protamine can also be used in the treatment of low molecular weight heparins (dalteparin, enoxaparin), but it does not completely inhibit their activity (Plumb 2008). Protamine begins to neutralize heparin within 5 minutes after IV administration (Plumb 2008). Protamine should be given over 1–3 minutes because too rapid administration of protamine can cause hypotension, bradycardia, and dyspnea (Plumb 2008).

Succimer (Sanofi-Synthelabs, Chemet®)

Succimer (2,3-dimercaptosuccinic acid, DMSA) is an oral heavy metal chelator used primarily in the treatment of childhood lead poisoning (Kosnett 2005b). It has also been used to treat arsenic and mercury poisoning in humans (Kosnett 2005b). Succimer is used off-label to treat lead poisoning in dogs, cats, other small mammals, and birds (Plumb 2008). It can be given orally or per rectum if the animal is vomiting. Dosing for caged birds is critical because overdoses have caused death in cockatiels (Denver et al. 2000).

The advantages of succimer include less nephrotoxicity than BAL, oral administration, and lower incidence of GI upset, and it is also less likely than the others to induce zinc, iron, calcium, or magnesium deficiency. Unlike other chelators, succimer will not increase the absorption of lead from the GI tract, so it can be used in situations where the GI tract may not be free of metal. Succimer is more expensive than penicillamine or CaEDTA. Succimer can be used alone or following CaEDTA or BAL. Concurrent use with other chelating agents is not recommended. Succimer can cause a sulfurous odor to the breath, saliva, feces, or urine (Kosnett 2005b).

Trientine (Merck, Syprine®)

Trientine (TETA, triethylenetetramine) is an oral copper chelator. It is used in the treatment of copper-associated hepatopathies in dogs (Plumb 2008). Trientine is more expensive than penicillamine and may need to be compounded into smaller dosages, but it has fewer adverse effects (vomiting). It does need to be administered in a capsule since topical exposure to trientine causes dermatitis. Trientine also chelates zinc and iron and so supplementation may be needed during treatment.

Commercial Antibodies

Commercial antibodies include antitoxin-specific serum and monoclonal antibodies. These products decrease the free form of the toxicant, decrease tissue concentration, and increase elimination. Commercial antibodies are dosed depending on plasma concentrations of the agent to be removed, not the patient's body weight. Commercial antibodies also do not penetrate tissue so they need to be given early in the syndrome while there is still circulating toxicant. New technology employing Fab fragments has decreased the antigenicity (allergic reactions) seen with commercial antibodies, but it also increases their excretion. Fab fragment products may require a larger volume due to this short half-life (Sevcik et al. 2007).

Antivenin, Black Widow (Merck, Sharp, and Dohme; Lyovac®)

Black widow antivenin neutralizes *Latrodectus mactans* (black widow spider) venom. Antivenin is used only to treat patients with severe signs because most cases will recover with just supportive care. Antivenin administration is recommended if severe hypertension is present, or if pain is not controlled (Clark et al. 1992). Antivenin will reverse muscle cramping, pain, central nervous system effects, and hypertension (Clark et al. 1992). With most veterinary patients, usually one vial is sufficient. As with any antivenin of equine origin, anaphylactic reactions may occur.

Antivenin, Crotalidae Polyvalent (Equine) (Boehringer Ingelheim)

Antivenin, Crotalidae Polyvalent is approved for use in dogs. It is used to neutralize the venom of crotalids (pit vipers) native to North, Central, and South America. It can be used to treat envenomations from *Crotalus* (diamondback rattlesnake, Cascabel), *Bothrops* (fer-de-lance), *Agkistrodon* (copperhead, cottonmouth), and *Lachesis* (bushmaster). Early use (within 4 hours) is recommended but if clinical signs are present, antivenin therapy should be implemented. The antivenin should be reconstituted in sodium chloride or 5% dextrose and given intravenously. As this product is from equine origin, monitor closely for anaphalytic reactions.

Antivenin, Crotalidae Polyvalent Immune Fab (Ovine) (Protherics, CroFab®)

Antivenin, Crotalidae Polyvalent Immune Fab (Ovine) is approved in humans for the management of North American crotalid snake envenomation (Sevcik et al. 2007), animal use is off-label. The antivenin can be used to treat envenomation by ten different North American crotalid species (see Table 8.1). Early use (within 6 hours of snakebite) is best, but if coagulation abnormalities exist, administration of antivenin can still be beneficial after this time period. Crotalid Fab has good efficacy in dogs although some did require more than 1 vial (average dosing was 1.25 vials) (personal communication, Michael Peterson). However, there are fewer reactions to this product when compared to the IgG antivenin. The biggest drawback to using this antivenin is the cost.

Table 8.1. Cross-reactivity of Crotalidae polyvalent immune Fab

Scientific Name	Common Name
Agkistrodon picivorus	Cottonmouth, water moccasin
Agkistrodon contortrix contortrix	Copperhead
Crotalus adamanteus	Eastern diamondback rattlesnake
Crotalus atrox	Western diamondback rattlesnake
Crotalus horridus atricaudatus	Canebrake rattlesnake
Crotalus horridus horridus	Timber rattlesnake
Crotalus molossus molossus	Northern blacktail rattlesnake
Crotalus scutulatus	Mojave rattlesnake
Crotalus viridis helleri	Southern Pacific rattlesnake
Sistrurus malarius barbouri	Pygmy rattlesnake

Antivenin, North American Coral Snake (Wyeth-Ayrst, Elapid Polyvalent, Horse, Antivenin®)

Antivenin (*Micrurus fulvius*) neutralizes the venom of Eastern (*M. fulvius fulvius*) and Texas (*M. fulvius tenere*) coral snakes, fer-de-lance, and Central and South American rattlesnakes. This antivenin is *NOT* effective for Arizona or Sonoran coral snakes (*M. euryxanthus*) envenomations. There are many factors involved in the potential seriousness of a coral snake bite (size of victim, bite site, number of bites, species of snake, etc.). Bites in which the snake "hangs on" and "chews" result in a higher venom exposure (Kitchens and Van Mierop 1987). Early administration of antivenin is recommended because once clinical signs appear it is not always possible to stop the progression. The antivenin is expensive. Wyeth Pharmaceuticals has recently stopped manufacturing of Elapid Antivenin, and there is currently no alternative FDA-approved supplier of this product.

Digoxin Specific Antibody Fragments (GalaxoSmithKline, Digibind®)

Digoxin-immune Fab will bind directly to digoxin or digitoxin and inactivate it. Antidigitoxin Fab fragments can also be effective against bufotoxins from Bufo toads and against cardiac glycosides from plants (see Table 8.2)

Table 8.2. Cross-reactivity of antidigoxin Fab fragment with plant cardiac glycosides

Scientific Name	Common Name
Acokanthera oblongifolia	
Adenium sp	Desert Rose
Adonis microcarpa	Pheasant's eye
Asclepias sp	Milkweed
Byrophyllum tubiflorum	Mother of millions
Calotropis procera	King's crown
Carissa laxiflora	
Cerbera manghas	Sea mango
Convallaria majalis	Lily of the valley
Crytostegia grandioflora	Rubber vine
Digitalis sp	Foxglove
Helleboros sp	
Nerium oleander	Oleander
Ornithogalum sp	Star of Bethlehem
Scilla hyacinthoides	Scilla hyacinth
Strophanthus sp	Corkscrew Flower
Thevetia neriifolia, T. peruviana	Yellow oleander
Urginea maritima	Squill

(Binder and Lewander 1998). Patients who fail to respond to supportive care should be given antidigitoxin Fab fragments, which are expensive but can be life-saving (Ward et al. 1999). They can reverse severe ventricular arrhythmias (ventricular tachycardia, ventricular fibrillation), progressive bradyarrhythmias (severe sinus bradycardia), and second- or third-degree heart block not responsive to atropine (Megarbane et al. 2005). Monitor potassium closely because reactivation of ATPase may lead to hypokalemia (Megarbane et al. 2005).

Enzyme Inhibitors

Enzyme inhibitors inhibit formation of toxic metabolites by either competitive inhibition or irreversible inhibition. They are used to treat substances that become toxic through in vivo metabolism by decreasing the amount of toxic metabolite. They may increase the time needed for elimination of the parent drug and need to be dosed before excessive toxic metabolites are produced (Dalefield 2004).

Ethanol (Various, Generic)

Ethanol (etoh, ethyl alcohol, grain alcohol) may be used to treat ethylene glycol (EG; antifreeze) toxicosis. Ethanol is a competitive inhibitor of alcohol dehydrogenase. By competing for this enzyme, ethanol delays the breakdown of EG to its more toxic metabolites (Dalefield 2004; Mathews 2006). Ethylene glycol is then excreted in the urine unchanged. Ethanol sources include medical or laboratory grade alcohol or clear commercially available liquors (Everclear®, vodka).

Ethanol is well absorbed orally, but is administered intravenously for management of EG toxicosis. Ethanol can be dosed in boluses or as a constant-rate infusion (Plumb 2008). Ethanol must be given very early after ingestion of EG for it to be effective. In dogs it should be given within the first 6–8 hours, in cats, before 3 hours (Connelly et al. 2002). Ethanol is inexpensive and readily available, but it can worsen metabolic acidosis and CNS depression.

Fomepizole (Paladin Labs, Antizol-vet®)

Fomepizole (4-methylpyrazole, 4-MP) is approved for use in the treatment of EG toxicity in dogs. It is a competitive inhibitor of alcohol dehydrogenase. By inhibiting this enzyme, EG is excreted unchanged in the urine, without being biotransformed into the more toxic metabolites responsible for metabolic acidosis and renal tubular necrosis. The benefits of using fomepizole rather than ethanol are that it does not induce CNS depression, hyperosmolality, or diuresis (Gaddy 2001). While immediate treatment holds the best prognosis, dogs may be treated as late as 8 hours postingestion and can still have a favorable prognosis. Fomepizole slows down the metabolism of EG and so serum EG levels may still be detectable at 72 hours after ingestion. Continue treatment if the EG test is still positive. Fomepizole is expensive, but each vial will treat a 60 lb dog. Fomepizole is not labeled for use in cats but can be used off-label at high doses (Connally et al. 2002). Cats will become ataxic and depressed at these high doses. With EG poisoned cats, therapy must be started within 3 hours or the prognosis is grave.

PHARMACOLOGICAL ANTIDOTES

Atipamezole (Pfizer, Antisedan®)

Atipamezole is an α2-adrenergic antagonist approved for use in dogs as the reversal agent for medetomidine (Domitor®). It can also be used off-label to treat several toxicoses. Atipamezole will reverse other α2-adrenergic agonists (amitraz, xylazine, imidazoline decongestants, bromonidine, clonidine, and tizanidine) (Gwaltney-Brant 2004). Atipamezole quickly reverses the sedation, hypotension, and bradycardia seen in these toxicoses. It can be given IM or IV. Atipamezole reversal lasts about 2–3 hours and may need to be repeated (Plumb 2008).

Atropine (Various, Generic)

Atropine (tropine tropate, *dl*-tropyl tropate, *dl*-hyoscyamine) may be used to treat the muscarinic signs caused by anticholinesterase pesticides (OPs, carbamates) (see Table 8.3), physostigmine excess, antimyasthenic

Table 8.3. Selected organophosphates and carbamates

Aldicarb	Bromophos	Carbaryl	Chlofenvinphos	Chlorpyrifos
Diazinon	Dicrotophos	Dioxathion	Disulfoton	Fensulfothion
Fenthion	Fumarate	Malathion	Methidathion	Methiocarb
Methomyl	Parathion	Paraxon	Profenphos	Propoxur
Terbufos	Tetraethyl pyrophosphate			

agents, nerve gas agents (sarin, soman, tabun, VX), synthetic choline esters, cholinergic agonists, and clitocybe and inocybe mushrooms (Balali-Mood and Balali-Mood 2005). Atropine blocks the effects of accumulated acetylcholine at the synapse. Atropine is also used as an adjunct in treating bradyarrhythmias. Muscarinic (SLUDDE) signs include salivation, lacrimation, urination, defecation, dyspnea, and emesis. Atropine sulfate does not control nicotinic signs (muscle tremors, muscle weakness).

Atropine should be used to treat bradycardia and dry up excess bronchial secretions; patients not experiencing either of these signs do not require atropine. Atropine is not indicated if drooling or miosis are the only clinical signs. Atropine may be given IV, IM, SQ, endotracheally, or intraosseously (Prete et al. 1987). Atropinization may need to be maintained for hours to days, depending on the toxicant. Overdoses of atropine can cause CNS stimulation, seizures, sinus tachycardia, hypertension, and ileus (Plumb 2008).

Atropine can also be used as a diagnostic test for poisoning by cholinesterase inhibitors (e.g., organophosphorus or carbamate insecticides). The heart rate is measured before and after a preanesthetic dose of atropine is given. If the heart rate increases, it is not a cholinesterase inhibitor toxicosis, because it takes about ten times this amount to raise the heart rate in poisoned patients (Fikes 1990).

Calcium Salts (Various, Generic)

Calcium salts (calcium chloride, calcium gluconate, calcium borogluconate, calcium lactate, calcium phosphate) can be used in veterinary toxicology for treating various toxicoses. Calcium salts can be used in treating fluoride, hydrofluoric acid, ethylene glycol, calcium channel blocker (verapamil, diltiazem, etc.), beta blocker, and nondepolarizing neuromuscular blocking agent poisonings (see Table 8.4) (el Saadi et al. 1989; Roder 2004b). They can also be used to reverse hypocalcemia, hyperkalemia, hypermagnesemia, oxalic acid, and oxalate poisoning. Calcium salts can also be helpful in relieving muscular spasm associated with black widow spider bites (Henninger and Horst 1997; Roder 2004a).

Folinic Acid (Lederle, Leucovorin®)

Folinic acid (calcium folinate, citrovorum factor) is the reduced active form of folic acid. It is used to treat methotrexate, trimethoprim, pyrimethamine, and *Gyromitra esculenta* mushroom ingestions (Lambie and Johnson 1985; Leathem and Dorran 2007). These toxins stop conversion of folic acid to folinic acid (active form) by block-

Table 8.4. Nondepolarizing neuromuscular blocking agents

Atracurium
Curare
Gallamine
Metocurine
Pancuronium bromide
Tubocurarine
Vecuronium

ing the enzymes needed for this reaction. By administering the active form, these enzyme blockades are bypassed. Folinic acid should be given as soon as possible for the best results.

Flumazenil (Roche, Romazicon®)

Flumazenil (flumazepil) is a competitive blocker of benzodiazepines and reverses sedation and respiratory depression within 1–2 minutes (Gwaltney-Brant 2002). The dose may need to be repeated because the half-life for flumazenil is about 1 hour. Flumazenil is usually limited to animals at risk of respiratory depression. Flumazenil is contraindicated in animals with tricyclic antidepressant overdoses because it can cause seizures (Plumb 2008).

Glucagon (Bedford, GlucaGen®)

Glucagon (HGF) is a hormone with glycemic and inotropic actions. It is used in beta adrenergic blockers, calcium channel blockers, and tricyclic antidepressant overdoses that produce severe bradycardia, AV block, or hypotension (Love and Howell 1997). Glucagon can also be used to treat hypoglycemia from insulin and oral hypoglycemic agents (sulfonylureas, etc.) because it stimulates hepatic glycogenolysis. Glucagon is administered as an IV bolus, followed by a CRI. Patients should be monitored for hyperglycemia with secondary hypokalemia (Plumb 2008).

Hydroxocobalamin (EMD, Cyanokit®)

Hydroxocobalamin (vitamin B12a, alpha-cobione) is a vitamin B12 precursor. It is used to treat cyanide toxicosis. Hydroxocobalamin combines with cyanide to form cyanocobalamin (vitamin B12) (Hall and Rumack 1998). Cyanocobalamin is eliminated through the urine. Cyanide poisoning can be seen secondary to nitroprusside, acetonitrile, cyanogenic glycoside plant (see Table 8.5) ingestion, and hydrogen sulfide inhalation. Hydroxocobalamin does not produce either methemoglobinemia or hypoten-

Table 8.5. Cyanide-containing plants

Scientific Name	Common Name
Acacia	Acacia
Alocasia	Elephant's Ear
Amelanchier	Serviceberry, Shadebush, Juneberry
Canavalia	Wonder Bean
Cercocarpus	Mountain Mahogany
Chenopodium	Goosefoot, Wormseed
Contoneaster	Contoneaster
Cynodon	Stargrass, Bermudagrass
Drosera	Sundew
Eucalyptus	Eucalyptus
Glyceria	Mannagrass
Heteromeles	Christmas Berry, California Holly
Hydrangea	Hydrangea
Juncus	Rushes
Lotus	Bird's-foot Trefoil, Nevada Deer Vetch
Manihot	Cassava
Nandina	Bamboo
Panicum	Switchgrass, Kleingrass, Millet
Phalaris	Canarygrass
Prunus	Apricot, Cherry, Plum, Chokecherry, Peach, Almond, Mock Orange
Pyracantha	Firethorn
Ranunculus	Buttercup
Rhodotypos	Jetbead
Sambucus	Elderberry
Sorghum	Sorghum, Sudangrass
Sorghastrum	Indiangrass
Spirea	Spirea, Bridal Wreath
Suckleya	Suckleya
Stillingia	Stillingia
Trifolium	Clovers
Triglochin	Arrowgrass

sion, as sodium nitrite does. Administration of hydroxocobalamin can interfere with AST, total bilirubin, creatinine, magnesium, and iron measurements (Curry 1992).

Hyperbaric Oxygen

Hyperbaric oxygen (HBO) therapy can be used in the treatment of carbon monoxide, methylene chloride, carbon tetrachloride, cyanide, and hydrogen sulfide toxicosis to reverse methemoglobinemia (Tomaszewski and Thom 1994). By delivering 100% oxygen at pressures greater than 1 atmosphere, it displaces CO and increases the elimi-

nation of other toxicants. Hyperbaric chambers may be available at larger veterinary referral centers.

Methylene Blue (Various, Generic)

Methylene blue (tetramethylthionine chloride trihydrate) is an oxidation-reduction agent that helps convert methemoglobin (Fe^{3+}) to hemoglobin (Fe^{2+}) (Plumb 2008). Methylene blue is used in small animal medicine to treat methemoglobinemia from aniline dyes, nitrites, nitrates, naphthalene, and local anesthetics (benzocaine, etc.) (Plumb 2008). Methylene blue should not be given unless methemoglobinemia is evident, especially in cats, because methylene blue can induce methemoglobinemia in normal animals. The new methylene blue found in laboratory dyes can *NOT* be substituted for methylene blue, because new methylene blue can be toxic if injected.

N-acetylcysteine (Apothecon, Mucomyst®; Cumberland Pharmaceuticals, Acetadote®)

N-acetylcysteine (NAC, mercapturic acid) is a mucolytic that can also reduce the extent of liver injury and methemoglobinemia after ingestion of acetaminophen. NAC is a precursor of glutathione, provides organic sulfate needed for the sulfation pathway and directly binds with acetaminophen metabolites to enhance elimination (Plumb 2008). N-acetylcysteine has been used in high doses to treat *Amanita phalloides* (death cap mushroom) poisoned people. It was effective in preventing permanent hepatic injury in 10 of 11 people (Montanini et al. 1999). NAC can also be used to treat white/yellow phosphorus, cyclophosphamide, and carbon tetrachloride toxicoses. NAC may be given orally (use a taste masking agent) or slow IV. Oral administration can cause vomiting. When treating acetaminophen toxicosis, especially in cats, it is recommended that acetylcysteine be dosed before the activated charcoal.

Naloxone (DuPont, Narcan®)

Naloxone (N-allylnoroxymorphone hydrochloride) is an opioid antagonist that competes with and displaces narcotics from their receptor sites (mu, kappa, and sigma) (Plumb 2008). Naloxone is most commonly used to reverse opiates (buprenorphine, butorphanol, codeine, fentanyl, hydrocodone, hydromorphone, methadone, morphine, oxycodone, oxymorphone, tramadol, etc.). It can also be used to reverse CNS depression associated with dextromethorphan, benzodiazepines, ACE inhibitors, alpha2-agonists, imidazoline decongestant overdoses, and ethanol (Jefferys and Volans 1983). Naloxone may be administered IV, IM, SQ, intraosseous, and even sublingual. Naloxone acts within minutes and has a duration of action from 45–90 minutes (Plumb 2008). When treating long-acting substances, naloxone may need to be repeated.

Pralidoxime (Wyeth-Ayerst, Protopam®)

Pralidoxime (2-PAM, 2-pyridine aldoxime methylchloride, 2-formyl-1-methylpyridinium chloride oxime) is an oxime used to control the nicotinic signs (muscle and diaphragmatic weakness, fasciculations, muscle cramps, etc.) seen in organophosphate toxicoses (Fikes 1990). 2-PAM is a cholinesterase reactivator, which displaces the acetylcholinesterase enzyme from its receptor site. It binds with the insecticide and is excreted in the urine. 2-PAM works best if administered as soon as possible; however, this can vary with some compounds (Vale 2005). Once the organophosphate receptor bond "ages," oximes are no longer effective. Since "aging" varies with the compound, oximes may be effective even hours to days after exposure (Vale 2005). Oximes are generally not recommended for use in carbamate poisoning, due to the lack of "aging" in these compounds (Vale 2005).

Pyridostigmine (ICN, Mestinon®; Various, Generic)

Pyridostigmine is an anticholinesterase. Pyridostigmine competes with acetylcholine for binding to acetylcholinesterase so acetylcholine accumulates in the synapse. It is used to treat nondepolarizing neuromuscular blocking agents (see Table 8.4) and botulism. It may also be used in the treatment of atropine, avermectin, Coral (*Micrurus*) and Cobra (*Naja*) snake bites, tetrodotoxins (Porcupine fish [*Diodon*]), and anticholinergic alkaloid plants poisonings (see Table 8.6) (Martinez and Mealey 2001). Other drugs in this group (neostigmine, edrophonium, physostig-

mine, etc.) can also be used to treat these toxicoses, but they have a much shorter duration of action.

Pyridoxine (Various, Generic)

Pyridoxine (vitamin B6) is used in the management of coma and seizures associated with overdoses of isoniazid or hydrazines, seizures due to *Gyromitra* mushroom (false morel) poisoning, penicillamine-induced seizures, and as an adjunct therapy for EG toxicosis (Dyer and Shannon 2005).

Silymarin (Various, Generic)

Silymarin (milk thistle) is a nutraceutical that can be used as a hepatoprotectant agent. It has been shown to be effective as an adjunct in the treatment of cyclopeptide mushroom (*Amanita*) and acetaminophen toxicoses (Jahn et al. 1980; Fakurazi et al. 2008).

Silymarin should be started within the first 48 hours and continued for several weeks. Oral silymarin can cause vomiting but is otherwise well tolerated. Because silymarin is considered a nutritional supplement by the FDA, quality and content can vary between different formulations. Choose a product that states the concentration (usually 70%–80%) of silymarin contained in the product.

Yohimbine (Lloyd, Yobine ®)

Yohimbine (aphrodine hydrochloride) is an α2-adrenergic antagonist approved as a reversal agent for xylazine in dogs, but it can also be used to treat other α2-adrenergic agonist toxicoses (amitraz, clonidine, etc). The onset of action is within minutes, and yohimbine has a short half-life (1.5 to 2 hours), so repeated dosing may be required (Jernigan et al. 1988). Dogs receiving five times the recommended dose developed muscle tremors and seizures (Plumb 2008).

FUNCTIONAL ANTIDOTES

Acepromazine (Ft. Dodge, PromAce®; Vetus, Aceproject®)

Acepromazine (ace, acetazine, acetopromazine, acetylpromazine) is a neuroleptic phenothiazine. It is approved for use in dogs and cats (Plumb 2008). Acepromazine is used to decrease the CNS stimulation associated with amphetamine, methamphetamine, serotonergic drugs, 4-methylimidazole, and metaldehyde toxicosis (Andrews and Humphries 1982). Intravenous injection will have the quickest onset, but acepromazine can be given IM, SQ, or orally. Acepromazine can cause hypotension at high

Table 8.6. Anticholinergic alkaloid plants

Scientific Name	Common Name
Atropa	Belladonna
Cestrum	Jasmine
Datura	Jimsonweed
Hyoscyamus	Henbane
Lycium	Boxthorn
Lycopersicon	Tomato
Mandragora	Mandrake
Physalis	Ground Cherry
Solanum	Nightshade, Bittersweet
	Various mushrooms

doses, and blood pressure should be monitored after administration.

Bicarbonate, Sodium (Various, Generic)

Sodium bicarbonate (sodium hydrogen carbonate, monosodium carbonate, sodium acid carbonate, baking soda) has many uses in veterinary toxicology. It is a systemic alkalinizer, which can be used to correct metabolic acidosis, QRS prolongation, and rhabdomyolysis and to alkalinize urine in poisonings (Kolecki and Curry 1997). Administration of sodium bicarbonate to a serum pH of 7.45–7.55 will help decrease the cardiac toxicity of tricyclic antidepressants (amitriptyline, doxepin, imipramine, nortriptyline, etc.) and type 1 antidysrrhythmics (quinidine) (Kolecki and Curry 1997).

Urinary alkalinization with sodium bicarbonate traps weak acids and enhances the elimination of salicylates, phenobarbital, chlorpropamide, and chlorophenoxy herbicides (Wax 2011). Oral sodium bicarbonate may decrease the absorption of anticholinergics, histamine 2 blockers (cimetidine, ranitidine, etc.), iron, ketoconazole, and tetracyclines, but increase the amount of naproxen absorbed and reduce the efficacy of sucralfate (Plumb 2008). Urinary alkalinization will decrease excretion of some drugs (e.g., quinidine, amphetamines, ephedrine).

Chlorpromazine (SmithKlineGlaxo, Thorazine®; Various, Generic)

Chlorpromazine (aminazine) is a phenothiazine used in the treatment of monamine oxidase inhibitor, amphetamine, and metaldehyde toxicoses (Grantham et al. 1964; Kisseberth and Trammel 1990). It is used to decrease the stimulatory signs. Chlorpromazine is less potent than acepromazine, but has a longer duration of action. Chlorpromazine can be given orally, IV or IM. Do not administer IM in rabbits because it causes severe muscle pain and swelling (Plumb 2008). Do not use chlorpromazine with physostigmine or paraquat toxicoses because it may increase the toxicity (Plumb 2008).

Cyproheptadine (Merck, Periactin®; Various, Generic)

Cyproheptadine has been used traditionally in veterinary medicine for its antihistaminic and appetite-stimulant effects (cats) but is now being used to help treat serotonin syndrome (Gwaltney-Brant 2002). Serotonin syndrome is caused by excess serotonin within the CNS and can be characterized by tremors, seizures, hyperthermia, ataxia, vomiting, diarrhea, abdominal pain,

excitation or depression, and hyperesthesia. Serotonin syndrome is seen secondary to the ingestion of drugs that increase brain serotonin levels (selective serotonin reuptake inhibitors, amphetamines, tricyclic antidepressants, 5-hydroxytryptophan, etc.) (Gwaltney-Brant 2002). The dose may be given PO or per rectum (if vomiting or activated charcoal already given). Discontinue if no effect after the second dose (Gwaltney-Brant et al. 2000).

Dantrolene (Procter and Gamble, Dantrium®)

Dantrolene is used in veterinary toxicology to treat the malignant hyperthermia-like syndrome seen in dogs after ingestion of hops (*Humulus lupulus*) (Duncan et al. 1997). It is a direct acting muscle relaxant that reverses muscle rigidity and associated hyperthermia. Dantrolene can be given orally or IV (injectable is expensive). Hepatotoxicity has been seen in humans with high dose chronic therapy (Plumb 2008). It is unknown if this occurs in animals.

Dapsone (Wyeth-Ayerst, Avlosulson®; Jacobus, Dapsone®)

Dapsone (diaminodiphenylsulfone, diphenylsulfone) decreases neutrophil chemotaxis, complement activation, lysosomal enzyme synthesis, and antibody production (Plumb 2008). Because of these leukocyte inhibitory effects, dapsone is used for adjunctive treatment of Brown recluse spider (*Loxosceles* sp.), Wolf spider (*Lycosidae* sp.), and Funnel Web spider (*Dipluidae* sp.) bites (Hansen and Russell 1984). It is thought to decrease the tissue necrosis seen after these envenomations. Dapsone should be used cautiously in cats due to the possibility of neurotoxicity and hemolytic anemia. All patients should be monitored for hepatotoxicity, anemia, thrombocytopenia, neutropenia, gastrointestinal effects, neuropathies, and cutaneous drug eruptions (photosensitivity) (Plumb 2008).

Dextrose (Various, Generic)

Dextrose is used in the treatment of hypoglycemia, which may result directly from toxicants (alpha lipoic acid, biguanides, insulin, sulfonylureas, xylitol) or indirectly (clonidine, ethanol, salicylates, organophosphates, Ackee [*Blighia*], Sneezeweed [*Helenium*], Desert Marigold *Baileya*], Paperflowers [*Psilostrophe*], Sartwellia *Sartwellia*], Periwinkle [*Catharanthus*], Balsam Apple and Pear [*Momordica*], Castor Bean [*Ricinus*], Bitterweed and Rubberweed [*Asteraceae*]) (Browning et al. 1990). Multiple bolus doses or a CRI may be required.

Methocarbamol (Fort Dodge, Robaxin®, Robaxin®V)

Methocarbamol (guaiphenesin carbamate) is approved in animals as a centrally acting skeletal muscle relaxant. It is used in toxicology to treat tremors associated with permethrin, metaldehyde, strychnine, tetanus (*Clostridium*), White Snakeroot (*Eupatorium*), ergot alkaloids (*Claviceps*), *Penicillium,* and other tremorgenic mycotoxins (Richardson 2000; Richardson et al. 2003; Gwaltney-Brant 2002; Schell 2000). Methocarbamol depresses pathways in the spinal cord without interfering with muscle function. It may be given intravenously, orally, or rectally (crush tablets in saline).

Nitroprusside (Various, Generic)

Nitroprusside—(OC-6-22)-pentakis(cyano-C)nitrosylferrate dihydrate, sodium nitroferricyanide dehydrate—is used for treatment of severe hypertension secondary to poisonings (phenylpropanolamine, etc.). It causes peripheral arterial and venous vasodilation. Nitroprusside has an immediate onset and short duration of action, which allows accurate titration of blood pressure (Plumb 2008). Blood pressure should be monitored closely because it will return to pretreatment levels within 1–10 minutes once the CRI is stopped. Prolonged use may lead to potential cyanide toxicosis, especially in patients with hepatic or renal insufficiency. Metabolic acidosis and delirium are early signs of cyanogen toxicosis (Plumb 2008).

Norepinephrine (Sanofi-Sybthelabo, Levophed®)

Norepinephrine (noradrenalin) is an alpha-adrenergic agonist used to reverse hypotension by increasing systolic and diastolic blood pressure through vasoconstriction. It is used to treat alpha adrenergic blockers (see Table 8.7) and other toxicants that cause acute hypotension (Amanita mushrooms [*Amantia*], beta blockers, calcium channel blockers, ergot alkaloids, lily of the valley [*Convallaria*], periwinkle [*Vinca*], phenothiazines, quinine sulfate, tetrodotoxins, tricyclic antidepressants, Yew [*Taxus*]) (Brent et al. 2005). Norepinephrine must be given IV because extravasation causes severe necrosis.

Pamidronate (Novartis, Aredia®; Various, Generic)

Pamidronate (ADP sodium) is a synthetic bisphosphonate that binds to the hydroxyapatite found in bone. It inhibits osteoclastic bone resorption and is used in veterinary toxicology to treat hypercalcemia secondary to vitamin D and its analogs (cholecalciferol, calcipotriene, calcitriol) (Pesillo et al. 2002). Pamidronate is administered as a slow IV infusion over 2–4 hours. It has an advantage over salmon calcitonin in that it has long-lasting effects (may need to repeat once in 5–7 days). Do not use in combination with calcitonin, because it increases mortality (Rumbeiha et al. 1997). Pamidronate can cause hypomagnesemia, renal toxicity, and arrhythmias (Kadar et al. 2004).

Salmon Calcitonin (Sandoz, Calcitonin Micalcin®; Lennod, Salmonine®)

Calcitonin is a hormone used to control hypercalcemia. It inhibits osteoclastic bone resorption and reduces tubular reabsorption of calcium (Plumb 2008). Calcitonin is used to treat vitamin D analog toxicoses (see pamidronate). Calcitonin's use is limited by expense, availability, frequent dosing schedule, pain at injection site, and development of resistance to its effects after several days. Bisphosphonates are frequently used instead.

SAMe (Nutramax, Denosyl®; Vetoquinol, Zentonil®)

SAMe (S-Adenosyl-Methionine, ademetionine) is a nutraceutical used as a treatment for acetaminophen toxicity in small animals (Plumb 2008; Wallace et al. 2002). It has also been used for liver support in chronic hepatitis, hepatic lipidosis, cholangiohepatitis, feline triad disease, and osteoarthritis. SAMe is formed from the amino acid methionine and ATP. It plays an essential role in major biochemical pathways (transmethylation, transsulfuration, and aminopropylation). Through these pathways SAMe provides compounds (sulfur, glutathione) important in liver support (Plumb 2008).

SAMe should be given on an empty stomach, because food will greatly reduce the amount of drug absorbed. SAMe is well tolerated and adverse effects are rare. Because SAMe is considered a nutritional supplement by the FDA, there are no standards for potency, purity, safety, or efficacy. Due to this lack of oversight, a well-known brand name should be used.

Table 8.7. Alpha-adrenergic blockers

Generic Name	Trade Name
Atipamezole	Antisedan®
Doxazosin	Cardura®
Phenoxybenzamine	Dibenzyline®
Phentolamine	
Prazosin	Minipress®
Tamsulosin	Flomax®
Terazosin	Hytrin®
Tolazoline	Tolazine®
Yohimbine	Yobine®

Vitamin K1 (Merck, Mephyton®; Various, Generic)

Vitamin K1 (phytonadione, phylloquinone, phytomenadione) is used to treat anticoagulant rodenticides, coumarin, and sulfaquinoxaline toxicoses (Plumb 2008). Vitamin K1 is needed for the regeneration of blood clotting factors II, VII, IX, and X. After administration it takes about 6–12 hours for new clotting factors to be synthesized. Vitamin K1 can be given PO, IM, or SQ. IV use is not recommended due to a high incidence of anaphylactoid reactions. Giving vitamin K1 with a fatty meal will increase bioavailability (Plumb 2008). Because vitamin K1 does not accumulate in the liver and it may take several weeks to eliminate some of the anticoagulant rodenticides from the body, the drug must be dosed daily.

CHAPTER 8 STUDY QUESTIONS

1. Functional antidotes differ from chemical or pharmacological antidotes in that
   a. They increase the excretion of toxicant from the body.
   b. They decrease the absorption of the toxicant from the gastrointestinal tract.
   c. They treat the clinical signs caused by the toxicant.
   d. They increase the metabolism of the toxicant.
   e. They decrease the metabolism of the toxicant.
2. Which of the following best describes the mechanism of action of chelators?
   a. They bind to target-organ receptors to prevent the toxicant from binding.
   b. They bind to a toxicant to increase the toxicant's water solubility and enhance excretion.
   c. They enhance excretion of a toxicant by increasing toxicant metabolism.
   d. They bind to a toxicant to decrease absorption of the toxicant from the gastrointestinal tract.
   e. They bind to a toxicant and cause the toxicant to be sequestered with a specific organ (e.g., spleen).
3. When using chelators to treat heavy metal toxicoses, it is necessary that the gastrointestinal tract be free of any metal or the chelator will actually increase the further absorption of metal from the gastrointestinal tract into the bloodstream. This statement is true for all chelators and metals with which exception?
   a. Use of calcium disodium EDTA to treat lead poisoning
   b. Use of deferoxamine to treat iron poisoning
   c. Use of dimercaprol to treat lead poisoning
   d. Use of d-penicillamine to treat lead poisoning
   e. Use of succimer to treat lead poisoning
4. Antibodies have been developed to treat intoxication from all of the following except
   a. Rattlesnake venom
   b. Digitalis
   c. Coral snake venom
   d. Fire ant venom
   e. Black widow spider venom
5. When treating ethylene glycol toxicosis, fomepizole has all of the following advantages over ethanol except that
   a. Fomepizole does not cause significant CNS depression.
   b. Fomepizole does not cause hyperosmolality and diuresis.
   c. Fomepizole is less expensive than ethanol.
   d. Fomepizole administration and monitoring are less labor-intensive than ethanol.
   e. Fomepizole is FDA-approved for use in dogs.

ANSWERS

1.c. Functional antidotes help manage clinical signs caused by the toxicant but have no impact on the level of toxicant in the body.
2.b. Chelators bind toxicants to increase water solubility and enhance excretion.
3.c. Succimer does not enhance the absorption of lead from the gastrointestinal tract.
4.d. No antivenom exists to treat envenomation from fire ants.
5.c. Fomepizole is more expensive than ethanol to obtain; however, because ethanol requires more monitoring and constant administration of IV fluids, the cost of nursing care for ethanol may make the difference in cost much less significant.

REFERENCES

Anthony H. Andrews, David J. Humphreys. 1982. *Poisoning in Veterinary Practice*, 2nd ed. pp. 76–77, 112. Middlesex: National Office of Animal Health Ltd.

Kia Balali-Mood, Mahdi Balali-Mood. 2005. Atropine. In *Critical Care Toxicology Diagnosis and Management of the Critically Poisoned Patient*, edited by Jeffrey Brent, Kevin L. Wallace, Keith K. Burkhart, Scott D. Phillips, J. Ward Donovan, pp. 1517–1521. Philadelphia: Mosby.

Nicholas Bateman, Timothy Marrs. 1999. Antidotal studies. In *General and Applied Toxicology*, vol. 1, 2nd ed., edited by Bryan Ballantyne, Timothy C. Marrs, Tore Syversen, pp. 425–435. New York: Nature Publishing Group.

W.D. Binder, William J. Lewander. 1998. Digoxin. In *Emergency toxicology*, 2nd ed., edited by Peter Vicellio, Tod Bania, pp. 707–722. Philadelphia: Lippincott-Raven.

Jeffrey Brent, Kevin L. Wallace, Keith K. Burkhart, Scott D. Phillips, J. Ward Donovan. 2005. *Critical Care Toxicology Diagnosis and Management of the Critically Poisoned Patient*. pp. 35, 410, 421, 1258. Philadelphia: Mosby.

Randall G. Browning, David W. Olson, Harlan A. Stueven, James R. Mateer. 1990. 50% Dextrose: Antidote or toxin? *Ann Emerg Med* 19(6):683–687.

J. Julian Chisolm Jr. 1992. BAL, EDTA, DMSA, and DMPS in the treatment of lead poisoning in children. *Clin Toxicol* 30:493–504.

R.F. Clark, S. Wethern-Kestner, M.V. Vance, R. Gerkin. 1992. Clinical presentation and treatment of black widow spider envenomation: A review of 163 cases. *Ann Emerg Med* Jul;21(7):782–787.

Heather E. Connally, Dwayne W. Hamar, Mary Anna Thrall. 2002. Safety and efficacy of high dose fomepizole as therapy for EG intoxication in cats (Abstract). 8th IVECCS, San Antonio, TX. *J Vet Emerg Crit Care* 12:191.

Steven C. Curry. 1992. Hydrogen cyanide and inorganic salts. In *Hazardous Material Toxicology: Clinical Principles of Environmental Health*, edited by John B. Sullivan, Gary R. Krieger, pp. 698–709. Baltimore: Williams and Wilkins.

Rosalind Dalefield. 2004. Ethylene glycol. In *Clinical Veterinary Toxicology*, edited by Konnie H. Plumlee, pp. 150–154. St. Louis: Mosby.

M. Denver, Lisa A. Tell, Frank D. Galey, J.G. Trupkiewicz, Philip H. Kass. 2000. Comparison of two heavy metal chelators for treatment of lead toxicosis in cockatiels. *Am J Vet Res* 61:935–940.

Karen L. Duncan, William R. Hare, William B. Buck. 1997. Malignant hyperthermia-like reaction secondary to ingestion of hops in five dogs. *J Am Vet Med Assoc* Jan1; 210(1):51–54.

K. Sophia Dyer, Michael Shannon. 2005. Pyridoxine. In *Critical Care Toxicology Diagnosis and Management of the Critically Poisoned Patient*, edited by Jeffrey Brent, Kevin L. Wallace, Keith K. Burkhart, Scott D. Phillips, J. Ward Donovan, pp. 1537–1538. Philadelphia: Mosby.

Magdi S. el Saadi, Alan H. Hall, Priscilla K. Hall, Betty S. Riggs, W. Lynn Augenstein, Barry H. Rumack. 1989. Hydrofluoric acid dermal exposure. *Vet Hum Toxicol* Jun;31(3):243–247.

Sharida Fakurazi, Ithnin Hairuszah, U. Nanthini. 2008. Moringa oleifera Lam prevents acetaminophen induced liver injury through restoration of glutathione level. *Food Chem Toxicol* Aug;46(8):2611–2615.

James D. Fikes. 1990. Organophosphorus and carbamate insecticides. *Vet Clin North Am Small Anim Pract* 20: 353–367.

Jonathan Gaddy. 2001. Pharm profile fomepizole. *Compend Contin Educ Pract Vet X* 1073–1074.

Norman R. Gevirtz, Louis R. Wasserman. 1966. The measurement of iron and iron-binding capacity in plasma containing deferoxamine. *J Pediatr* 68:802–804.

Julie Grantham, W. Neel, R.W. Brown. 1964. Toxicity reversed: Reversal of imipramine-monamine oxidase inhibitor induced toxicity by chlorpromazine. *J Kans Med Soc* 65:279–280.

Sharon Gwaltney-Brant. 2004. Amitraz. In *Clinical Veterinary Toxicology*, edited by Konnie H. Plumlee, pp. 177–178. St. Louis: Mosby.

Sharon Gwaltney-Brant, Jay Albretsen, Safdar Khan. 2000. 5-hydroxytryptophan toxicosis in dogs: 21 cases (1989–1999). *JAVMA* 216:1937–1940.

Sharon Gwaltney-Brant, Wilson Rumbeiha. 2002. Newer antidotal therapies. In *The Veterinary Clinics of North America Small Animal Practice*, edited by Robert H. Poppenga, Petra A. Volmer, pp. 323–339. Philadelphia: Saunders.

Alan H. Hall, Barry H. Rumack. 1998. Cyanide and related compounds. In *Clinical Management of Poisoning and Drug Overdose*, 3rd ed., edited by Lester M. Haddad, Michael W. Shannon, James F. Winchester, pp. 899–905. Philadelphia: Saunders.

Ronald C. Hansen, Findlay E. Russell. 1984. Dapsone use for *Loxosceles* envenomation treatment. *Vet Hum Toxicol* 26:260.

Richard W. Henninger, J. Horst. 1997. Magnesium toxicosis in two horses. *J Am Vet Med Assoc* Jul1;211(1):82–85.

Adonis S. Ioannides, Jose M. Panisello. 2000. Acute respiratory distress syndrome in children with acute iron poisoning: The role of intravenous desferrioxamine. *Eur J Pediatr* 159:158–159.

Wolfgang Jahn, Heinz Faulstich, Thomas Wieland. 1980. Pharmacokinetics of (3H)-methyl-dihydroxymethyl-amanitin in the isolated perfused rat liver, and the influence of several drugs. In *Amanita Toxins and Poisoning*, edited by Heinz Faulstich, Burkhard Kommerell, Thomas Wieland, pp. 80–85. Baden-Baden, Germany: Witzstrock.

David B. Jefferys, Glyn N. Volans. 1983. An investigation of the role of the specific opioid antagonist naloxone in clinical toxicology. *Hum Toxicol* Apr;2(2):227–231.

Antoinette D. Jernigan, Robert C. Wilson, Nicholas H. Booth, Roger C. Hatch, Ali Akbari. 1988. Comparative pharmacokinetics of yohimbine in steers, horses and dogs. *Can J Vet Res* Apr;52(2):172–176.

Elissa Kadar, John E. Rush, Lois Wetmore, Daniel L. Chan. 2004. Electrolyte disturbances and cardiac arrhythmias in a dog following pamidronate, calcitonin, and furosemide administration for hypercalcemia of malignancy. *J Am Anim Hosp Assoc* Jan–Feb;40(1):75–81.

Willam C. Kisseberth, Harold L. Trammel. 1990. Illicit and abused drugs. In *The Veterinary Clinics of North America Small Animal Practice*, edited by Val R. Beasley, pp. 405–418. Philadelphia: Saunders.

Craig S. Kitchens, Lodewyk H.S. Van Mierop. 1987. Envenomation by the Eastern coral snake (Micrurus fulvius fulvius). A study of 39 victims. *JAMA* Sep25;258(12):1615–1818.

Paul Francis Kolecki, Steven C. Curry. 1997. Poisoning by sodium channel blocking agents. *Crit Care Clin* Oct;13(4):829–848.

Michael J. Kosnett. 2005a. Dimercaprol (BAL). In *Critical Care Toxicology Diagnosis and Management of the Critically Poisoned Patient*, edited by Jeffrey Brent, Kevin L. Wallace, Keith K. Burkhart, Scott D. Phillips, J. Ward Donovan, pp. 1499–1501. Philadelphia: Mosby.

———. 2005b. Succimer (DMSA). In *Critical Care Toxicology Diagnosis and Management of the Critically Poisoned Patient*, edited by Jeffrey Brent, Kevin L. Wallace, Keith K. Burkhart, Scott D. Phillips, J. Ward Donovan, pp. 1505–1507. Philadelphia: Mosby.

D.G. Lambie, R.H. Johnson. 1985. *J Rheumatol Suppl* Jan–Feb;7:96–99.

Anne M. Leathem, Thomas J. Dorran. 2007. Poisoning due to raw Gyromitra esculenta (false morels) west of the Rockies. *CJEM* Mar;9(2):127–130.

Jon E. Levine, Aaron Cohen, M. MacQueen, M. Martin, Patricia J. Giardina. 1997. Sensorimotor neurotoxicity associated with high-dose deferoxamine treatment. *J Pediatr Hematol Oncol* Mar–Apr;19(2):139–141.

Jeffrey N. Love, John M. Howell. 1997. Glucagon therapy in the treatment of symptomatic bradycardia. *Ann Emerg Med* Jan;29(1):181–183.

W.H. Lyle. 1981. Penicillamine in metal poisoning. *J Rheumatol Suppl* Jan–Feb;7:96–99.

Elizabeth A. Martinez, Katrina A. Mealey. 2001. Muscle relaxants. In *Small Animal Clinical Pharmacology and Therapeutics*, edited by Dawn Merton Boothe, pp. 473–481. Philadelphia: Saunders.

Karol A. Mathews. 2006. Ethylene Gycol Intoxication. In *Veterinary Emergency and Critical Care Manual*, edited by Karol A. Mathews, pp. 655–659. Guelph, Ontario: Lifelearn Inc.

Bruno Megarbane, Stephen W. Borron, Frederic J. Baud. 2005. Anti-Digitalis fab Fragments. In *Critical Care Toxicology Diagnosis and Management of the Critically Poisoned Patient*, edited by Jeffrey Brent, Kevin L. Wallace, Keith K. Burkhart, Scott D. Phillips, J. Ward Donovan, pp. 1575–1579. Philadelphia: Mosby.

Kjetil Melby, Sofie Slordahl, Tore Jarl Gutteberg, Svein Arne Nordbo. 1982. Septicemia due to Yersinia enterocolitica after oral overdoses of iron. *Br Med J* 285:467–468.

S. Montanini, D. Sinardi, C. Praticò, A.U. Sinardi, G. Trimarchi. 1999. Use of acetylcysteine as the live-saving antidote in *Amanita phalloides* (death cap) poisoning. Case report on 11 patients. *Arzneimittelforschung* 49:1044–1047.

S.A. Pesillo, Safdar A. Khan, Elizabeth A. Rozanski, John E. Rush. 2002. Calcipotriene toxicosis in a dog successfully treated with pamidronate disodium. *J Vet Emerg Crit Care* 12:177–181.

Donald C. Plumb. 2008. *Plumb's Veterinary Drug Handbook*, Sixth Edition. pp. 3–5, 10–12, 79–80, 83–86, 121–122, 186–187, 240–241, 250–253, 256–257, 334–335, 365–366, 396, 425–426, 597–599, 641–642, 659–661, 734–736, 783–784, 809–810, 822–824, 839–840, 868–870, 906–907, 938–939. Ames, Iowa: Blackwell.

Lynn O. Post, W.C. Keller. 1999. An update of antidote availability in veterinary medicine. *Vet Hum Toxicol* 41:258–261.

M.R. Prete, C.J. Hannan, F.M. Bunce. 1987. Plasma atropine concentrations via intravenous, endotracheal, and intraosseous administration. *Am J Emerg Med* 5:101–104.

Jill A. Richardson. 2000. Permethrin spot-on toxicoses in cats. *J Vet Emerg Crit Care* 10:103–106.

Jill A. Richardson, Sharon M. Gwaltney-Brant, Joel D. Huffman, Marcy E. Rosendale, Sharon L. Welch. 2003. Metaldehyde toxidoses in dogs. *Compend Contin Educ Pract Vet* 25:376–379.

Joseph D. Roder. 2004a. Black Widow. In *Clinical Veterinary Toxicology*, edited by Konnie H. Plumlee, pp. 111–112. St. Louis: Mosby.

———. 2004b. Calcium Channel Blocking Agents. In *Clinical Veterinary Toxicology*, edited by Konnie H. Plumlee, pp. 308–309. St. Louis: Mosby.

Wilson K. Rumbeiha, J. Kruger, S. Fitzgerald, J. Render, R. Nachreiner, J. Kaneene, R. Vrable, M. Richter, C. Chiapuzio. 1997. The use of pamidronate disodium for treatment of vitamin D₃ toxicosis in dogs. *Proceedings 40th Annual Meeting AAVLD*, Louisville, Kentucky. pp. 71.

Mary M. Schell. 2000. Tremorgenic mycotoxin intoxication. *Vet Med* 95:283–286.

Carlos Sevcik, Victor Salazar, Patricia Díaz, Gina D'Suze. Initial volume of a drug before it reaches the volume of distribution: Pharmacokinetics of F(ab')2 antivenoms and other drugs. *Toxicon* 2007 Oct;50(5):653–665.

Christian A. Tomaszewski, S.T. Thom. 1994. Use of hyperbaric oxygen in toxicology. *Emerg Med Clin North Am* 12(2):437–459.

D.E. Turner-Lawrence, Ii W. Kerns. 2008. Intravenous fat emulsion: A potential novel antidote. *J Med Tox* 4(2):109–114.

J. Allister Vale. 2005. Oximes. In *Critical Care Toxicology Diagnosis and Management of the Critically Poisoned Patient*, edited by Jeffrey Brent, Kevin L. Wallace, Keith K. Burkhart, Scott D. Phillips, J. Ward Donovan, pp. 1523–1530. Philadelphia: Mosby.

Dan L. Waitzberg, Raquel Susana Torrinhas, Thiago Manzoni Jacintho. 2006. New parenteral lipid emulsions for clinical use. *J Parenter Enteral Nutr* 30:351–367.

Kevin P. Wallace, Sharon A. Center, Fiona H. Hickford, Karen L. Warner, Scott Smith. 2002. S-adenosyl-L-methionine (SAMe) for the treatment of acetaminophen toxicity in a dog. *J Am Anim Hosp Assoc* May–Jun;38(3):246–254.

Daniel L. Ward, S. Dru Forrester, T.C. DeFrancesco, Gregory C. Troy. 1999. Treatment of severe chronic digoxin toxicosis in a dog with severe cardiac disease, using ovine digoxin-specific immunoglobulin G Fab fragments. *JAVMA* 215(12):1808–1812.

Paul M. Wax. 2011. Sodium bicarbonate. In *Goldfrank's Toxicologic Emergencies*, edited by Lewis S. Nelson et al., PP. 520–527. China: McGraw-Hill.

W.F. Westlin. 1971. Deferoxamine as a chelating agent. *Clin Toxicol* 4:597–602.

Investigating Fatal Suspected Poisonings

9

Safdar A. Khan

INTRODUCTION

Veterinary staff may encounter situations where they are asked to investigate cause of death of a companion animal that was apparently healthy when observed last but was later found dead by the owner. In many such situations, the animal may have had clinical signs that went unnoticed by the owner, or the animal may not have been observed during the time of illness. Investigating sudden death in dogs and cats in the absence of clinical signs can be quite challenging. The definition of sudden death in terms of time may vary from person to person. For the purpose of this discussion, sudden, unattended, or unexplained death is defined as death occurring in an apparently healthy animal within a 12- to 24-hour period with no premonitory clinical signs or with minimal clinical signs (Casteel and Turk 2002). The purpose of this chapter is to outline the approach to take in the investigation of sudden death and to provide some common toxicologic rule-outs that should be included for investigating sudden acute unattended death in dogs and cats (Table 9.1).

CAUSES OF SUDDEN DEATH

A list of common causes of acute sudden death is available for large animals. However, for small animals, limited information is available on this topic. Animal poisoning (accidental or malicious) in dogs, according to one 10-year retrospective study, is the second most cause of sudden death in dogs after heart diseases (Table 9.2) (Olsen and Allen 2000).

In cats, however, poisoning has not been listed as a cause of acute sudden death (Table 9.3) (Olsen and Allen 2001).

Investigation of sudden death in a dog or a cat is no different than investigation of any other disease condition. Nontoxicologic rule-outs including infectious, metabolic, nutritional, physical, and miscellaneous causes must be considered along with poisoning when investigating sudden death in a pet.

It is important to realize that the effects of a toxicant on the body are dose-dependent. Many of the toxicants listed in the rule-out list from Table 9.1 may not be expected to cause acute sudden death with small exposures. However, the list includes the most common/likely toxicants that possess the potential to cause acute sudden death with the right amount (dose) of exposure. The reader is encouraged to review more detail about a particular topic or agent listed in this text once a reasonable cause of death has been narrowed down.

DIAGNOSTIC APPROACH

History

The investigation of acute sudden death involves close cooperation between client, veterinary staff, and diagnostic laboratory personnel. A complete and thorough case history is essential for such investigations. A good case history can help expedite the process of putting together all the pieces and eliminate several unnecessary steps early. Obtaining a recent case history from the client may

Small Animal Toxicology Essentials, First Edition. Edited by Robert H. Poppenga, Sharon Gwaltney-Brant.
© 2011 John Wiley and Sons, Inc. Published 2011 by John Wiley and Sons, Inc.

Table 9.1. Common toxicants that can cause sudden death in dogs and cats

Agent	Comments
5-Flurouracil	Topically used anticancer medication; seizures, vomiting, cardiac arrhythmias; acute death possible with large ingestion
5-hydroxytryptophan (5-HTP)	Used as OTC sleep aid and antidepressant; seizures, hyperthermia; acute death with large ingestions possible
Acetaminophen	Death due to methemoglobinemia within hours with large ingestion; cats more sensitive
Albuterol	Prescription bronchodilator for asthma; acute death with large ingestion possible; cardiac arrhythmias, hypokalemia
Amphetamines	Recreational or human prescription; hyperthermia, hyperactivity, circling, hypertension, tachyarrhythmias; acute death with large ingestion possible
Anticoagulant rodenticides	Internal bleeding 3–5 days postingestion; acute death due to pulmonary hemorrhage possible
Antidepressants	Common human prescription medications; acute death possible with large ingestion; CNS and cardiac effects
Arsenic	Toxicosis uncommon; watery diarrhea, abdominal pain, shock, acute death possible
Baclofen	Prescription drug; coma, hypothermia, respiratory depression; death with large ingestion
Barbiturates	Common anticonvulsant, accidental ingestion of large doses; farm dogs eating flesh/carcass of animals euthanized by barbiturates; coma, hypothermia, and death
Blue-green algae	History of drinking from a lake/pond; algae on the muzzle; collapse, shock, seizures, liver failure, death
Botulism	Acute death rare; ingestion of preformed toxins from eating a carcass; progressive weakness, paralysis, death
Brunfelsia spp ingestion	Strychnine-like signs (seizures, rigidity); dogs attracted to fruit/seed pods/flowers; acute death possible with large ingestion
Bufo toad	Common in Florida and other Southern states; acute collapse, salivation, cardiac arrhythmias, seizures, death
Caffeine	Ingestion of chocolate or caffeine pills; acute death with large ingestion possible; vomiting, CNS signs, cardiac arrhythmias
Carbon monoxide	Uncommon; bright red mucous membranes
Cardiac glycosides-containing plants	Acute death uncommon; evidence of plant ingestion
Castor beans	Acute death unlikely; only possible if several seeds have been ingested
Cocaine	Recreational drug; acute death possible
Ethylene glycol	Acute death with large ingestions possible; cats more sensitive
Garbage poisoning	History of eating garbage; acute death possible with some Salmonella, E. coli toxins; vomiting, progressive shock and death
Hepatotoxic mushrooms	Vomiting, diarrhea, abdominal pain, shock, liver failure, death
Hops (used for beer flavoring)	Malignant hyperthermia-like syndrome in dogs; acute death possible
Ionophores (e.g., monensin, lasalocid)	Eating cattle feed; farm dog; acute death with large ingestion (premix) possible
Iron	Multivitamins; large ingestions, acute death uncommon, vomiting, shock, liver damage
Isoniazid ingestion	Antituberculosis drug; seizures, acute death possible

Table 9.1. *Continued*

Agent	Comments
Lidocaine and other local anesthetics	Uncommon toxicosis; CNS, and cardiovascular effects
Metaldehyde	Used mostly as slug bait; seizures, hyperthermia, acute death with large ingestion possible
Moldy food ingestion (tremorgenic mycotoxins)	History of ingestion of moldy food; seizures, hyperthermia, vomiting, acute death possible
Nicotine	Acute death with large ingestion possible; GI, CNS and cardiac effects
Organochlorine type pesticides	Lindane, eldrin, dieldrin; use not common anymore; cats more sensitive; seizures, tremors, and acute death
Organophosphates/Carbamate insecticides	Some highly toxic OPs/carbamates like methomyl, aldicarb (tres pasitos), disulfoton; usually SLUD signs present; acute rapid death possible
Paint ball ingestion (glycols)	Ingestion of large amounts; acute death not common, seizures due to hypernatremia possible
Pseudoephedrine	OTC decongestant; amphetamine-like signs; acute death with large overdose possible
Pyrethrins/pyrethroids (permethrin in cats)	Cats more sensitive to concentrated products; tremors, seizures, death
Sago palm	Acute death unlikely; only possible if several seeds have been ingested; seizures, liver failure
Salt (sodium chloride)	Homemade play-dough ingestion; some use for inducing emesis; seizures, hypernatremia, death possible
Smoke inhalation	History of pet trapped in the house during fire
Snake bite	Mohave rattle snake, eastern rattle snake; acute death possible
Strychnine	Used as a rodenticide bait; rapid onset, seizures, hyperthermia, rigidity, death, rapid onset rigor mortis
Tetrodotoxins	Acute death rare; ingestion of dried puffer fish, pet salamander; paresis, respiratory failure, death
Water intoxication	History of being on the beach/swimming; hyponateremia, hypochloremia, polydipsia
Xylitol ingestion	Acute death due to severe hypoglycemia possible; acute liver failure possible 1–3 days after ingestion
Zinc phosphide	Available as gopher bait; vomiting, CNS effects; acute death with large ingestion possible

sometimes be difficult, especially in situations where the animal was unsupervised immediately prior to death. Clients may be too distraught to have good recollection of recent events, and it is not uncommon for them to focus on one particular event (e.g., herbicide recently applied to lawn) as the potential cause of death. Patient and tactful questioning is paramount to getting a history that is as accurate as possible.

Important historical questions must include animal signalment (breed, sex, weight, and age); previous medical history, vaccination history, and any medications the pet was taking; information regarding other animals present in the household; timeline of death (i.e., when the pet was last seen alive, where and when the pet was found dead); where pet had been in the hours/days prior to death (e.g., traveling, beach, park, neighbors, pet sitter, party); evidence of clinical signs (e.g., vomiting, diarrhea, seizure); number of affected animals (i.e., any other sick animals in the household); information about the animal's environment (indoor vs. outdoor, free-roaming vs. fenced), location (urban vs. rural), time of the year (summer vs. winter); recent renovations, construction or updates; availability of recreational drugs (amphetamines, cocaine) or human medications in the animal's environment (antidepressants,

Table 9.2. Underlying causes of sudden and unexpected deaths in 151 dogs as reported in the literature

General Cause of Death	Number of Cases	% of Total
Heart disease	33	21.9
Toxicosis	25	16.6
Gastrointestinal disease	20	13.2
Trauma	19	12.6
Hemorrhage not associated with trauma	10	6.6
Malnutrition or dehydration	8	5.5
Respiratory disease	6	4.0
Urogenital disease	5	3.3
Central nervous system disease	2	1.3
Peritonitis	2	1.3
Pancreatic disease	2	1.3
Undetermined	19	12.6
Total	151	100

Source: Olsen and Allen 2000.

Table 9.3. Underlying causes of sudden and unexpected deaths in 79 cats as reported in the literature

General Cause of Death	Number of Cases	% of Total
Trauma	31	39.2
Heart disease	16	20.3
Intestinal disease	6	7.6
Respiratory disease	5	6.3
Urinary tract disease	4	5.1
Feline leukemia virus–related disease	3	3.8
Menengioencephlitis	1	1.3
Hepatic necrosis	1	1.3
Sepsis	1	1.3
Hemorrhage not associated with trauma	1	1.3
Undetermined	10	12.7
Total	79	100.2[a]

Source: Olsen and Allen 2001.
[a]Exceeds 100 due to rounding.

painkillers, stimulants, nutritional supplements, overnight visitors taking prescription medications); the presence of insecticides, flea/tick control products, herbicides, or rodenticides in the house or yard; recent visits by pest control or lawn care companies; and information about presence of indoor or outdoor plants and lawn/garden fertilizers or chemicals) (Cote and Khan 2005). Information about disputes involving the neighbors, coworkers, family members, or others may help determine if the death could be malicious.

Sample Collection

The best way to investigate acute sudden death is by having a complete necropsy (gross and histopathologic examination) performed, preferably by a board certified veterinary pathologist (Volmer and Meerdink 2002). After obtaining an initial history, multiple digital pictures of the dead animal with any lesions (hemorrhage, mucous membrane color, broken skin/bones etc.) along with incriminating agent (if any) and surrounding environment (plants, chewed-up container, bait, feed, water etc.) should be taken. Stringent written documentation and chain of custody protocols should be followed for all potential medicolegal cases; if necessary, contact local animal control or law enforcement for details on securing potential legal evidence. For shipment to a diagnostic laboratory, triple-bag the dead animal and ship it to a diagnostic

laboratory on ice or dry ice through an express mail. Inform the diagnostic laboratory about the shipment before shipping. Avoid shipping over the weekends or holidays. Talk to the shipping carrier before shipping the animal to discuss packaging and labeling requirements.

Unfortunately, in many situations the options for a complete necropsy may not be feasible due to economics, animal size, or shipment constraints. In such circumstances, appropriate postmortem samples should be obtained from the animal and the environment. Collection of inappropriate type or amount of samples, and inadequate preservation techniques are some of the most common errors that hinder investigation by diagnostic laboratories. To avoid cross-contamination, all samples should be collected in separate containers, properly labeled with the patient's and owner's name, and dated. For histopathologic examination, a full set of tissues from all major organ systems should be cut 4–5 mm thick and placed in 10% formalin.

Most toxicologic analyses require frozen or refrigerated samples. Important samples for toxicologic investigations include liver, kidney, stomach contents, urine, abdominal fat, brain, heart clot blood and serum, hair, feed, water, or suspected bait (if available). The preferred anticoagulant for storage of whole blood is EDTA, although heparin is also acceptable in some case. Whole blood, serum, or urine samples should be refrigerated or chilled until analyzed. The amount of samples should be reasonable. Generally, the larger the amount, the better it may be. You can always discard the excessive amount or extra samples later if not needed. Larger amounts can allow the toxicologist to repeat an analysis, test for additional potential toxicants, and confirm the results with a different method if necessary. An entire set of samples must be collected for toxicologic analysis even when the diagnosis may be obvious or apparent (Casteel and Turk 2002; Volmer and Meerdink 2002).

Sample Submission

A concise history of events should be submitted to the diagnostic laboratory along with your request for analyses. For a completed necropsy or toxicologic analysis an accredited diagnostic laboratory should be utilized whenever possible. Most laboratories now have websites that detail sample submission requirements. Discuss cost, turnaround time, limitations of analytical methods if any, and interpretations of results with the diagnostic toxicologist if needed. The latter is especially important, because with modern analytical equipment it is possible to detect a wide variety of compounds at levels far below those that would have clinical significance. The toxicologist can assist in determining whether the levels found are consistent with a toxicosis.

CONCLUSION

The sudden death of a companion animal can be an emotionally challenging time for animal owners and veterinary staff. It is important that the veterinary staff understand the steps that need to be taken to investigate the cause of death so that the right questions can be answered and the appropriate samples are collected.

CHAPTER 9 STUDY QUESTIONS

1. A client brings a dead adult male cat into the hospital. What is the first step in dealing with this case?
   a. Collect samples for toxicology.
   b. Perform a necropsy.
   c. Obtain a history.
   d. Take radiographs.
   e. Draw some blood for a chemistry profile.

2. The client says that the cat was a stray that she and several neighbors had been feeding for several months. One neighbor had taken the cat to be neutered and vaccinated 2 months ago, and the cat appeared generally healthy. The client had fed the cat last night and he seemed fine; this morning he was lying dead on her porch. The client called the neighbors who were helping to feed the cat; no one saw anything out of the ordinary in the past 24 hours, and none had administered medication or flea control to the cat within the past week. The client is suspicious that the cat has been maliciously poisoned and wants to know why the cat died. A cursory external exam of the shows no lesions or evidence of why the cat may have died. What is the next step?
   a. Collect samples for toxicology.
   b. Perform a necropsy.
   c. Take radiographs.
   d. Draw some blood for a chemistry profile.

3. A necropsy is performed and samples are taken for histopathology. Additional samples are collected for toxicology, but are kept at the clinic pending the results of the necropsy and histopathology. What is the preferred means of storage of these samples until they are ready to be submitted to the toxicology laboratory?
   a. Frozen
   b. Refrigerated
   c. Fixed in 10% buffered formalin solution
   d. a and b
   e. a, b, and c

4. The necropsy and histopathology on the cat were highly suggestive of ethylene glycol (antifreeze) toxicosis. What is the next step?
   a. Call the diagnostic laboratory to determine which sample(s) to submit for ethylene glycol.
   b. Call animal control to report a malicious poisoning.
   c. Call the neighbors to see whether they suspect anyone of poisoning the cat.

5. The toxicologic analysis of the submitted samples confirmed the presence of ethylene glycol in the cat's stomach contents, fat, and kidney. Is this proof that the cat was maliciously poisoned? Why or why not?

Continued

ANSWERS

1.c. Obtain a history to determine the most appropriate course of investigation.

2.b. A necropsy holds the best chance of determining why the cat died.

3.d. Samples for toxicology can be stored either refrigerated or frozen prior to submitting to the laboratory.

4.a. Determine which samples to submit and have them analyzed by the diagnostic laboratory.

5. No. Without a witnessed exposure it is not possible to say for sure whether the exposure was malicious or accidental.

REFERENCES

Casteel S.W., Turk J.R. 2002. Collapse/sudden death. In *Large Animal Internal Medicine*, 3rd edition, edited by B.P. Smith, pp. 246–253. St. Louis: Mosby-Elsevier.

Cote E., Khan S.A. 2005. Intoxication versus acute, non-toxicologic illness: Differentiating the two. *Ettinger and Feldman's Text Book of Veterinary Internal Medicine*, 6th edition, pp. 242–245. St. Louis: Elsevier-Saunders.

Olsen T.F., Allen A.L. 2000. Causes of sudden and unexpected death in dogs: A 10-year retrospective study. *Canadian Veterinary Journal* 41:873–875.

————. 2001. Causes of sudden and unexpected death in cats: A 10-year retrospective study. *Canadian Veterinary Journal* 42:61–62.

Volmer P.A., Meerdink G.L. 2002. Diagnostic toxicology for the small animal practitioner. *Veterinary Clinics of North America Small Animal* 32:357–365.

Toxicologic Testing and Using Diagnostic Laboratories

10

Lisa Murphy

SOURCES

Toxicologic testing may be available at many levels: in the veterinary clinic (for example, ethylene glycol testing), at a local or regional commercial veterinary diagnostic laboratory, or at a veterinary diagnostic laboratory associated with a veterinary school or state department of agriculture. When selecting a diagnostic laboratory the following criteria should be considered: cost, turnaround time, experience with the sample type, available detection limits for the toxicant of concern, quality assurance and quality control programs, and assistance in the interpretation of results (Galey 2004).

The use of specialized instruments and highly trained personnel will often make toxicologic testing quite expensive compared to other diagnostic tests routinely performed for small animal patients. Many laboratories also charge additional fees for samples that are sent from another state, so be sure to ask about any additional fees that may apply.

Turnaround time refers to how long it will generally take to receive test results once samples arrive at the laboratory. Since some toxicologic tests may take several days or sometimes more than a week to complete, it will still be necessary to stabilize, decontaminate, and begin to treat the patient while waiting for results. Since some analyses can be completed more quickly, especially if the laboratory receives prior notice, it is important to contact the laboratory directly before submitting samples for critically ill patients.

Common sample types submitted for toxicologic testing in veterinary medicine include blood, urine, stomach contents, tissues, food, baits, water, and plant material. Each distinct sample type may require its own specific type of processing and analysis to detect the same toxic substance. Not all sample types may be appropriate for obtaining reliable results for all toxicologic tests. Diagnostic laboratories should be able to recommend which sample types are best or preferred for specific toxicologic tests.

Detection limits refer to the minimum amount of a toxic substance that must be present to reliably produce a positive test result. Detection limits will often be listed on a diagnostic report as the MDL, the minimum detection limit or method detection limit. When a toxic substance is either not found in a sample or appears to be present at a very low level below the MDL that is not confirmable, the result may be reported as either "none detected" or less than the MDL. If a specific level of detection of a toxicant is needed for either diagnostic or treatment purposes it is probably worthwhile to contact the veterinary toxicology laboratory ahead of time to be sure that its method is able to adequately provide the desired information.

Quality assurance and quality control are the practices laboratories use to ensure that the results they report are consistent and accurate. This reliability is typically accomplished by the use of standard reference materials, standard data curves, spiked samples, regular use of check samples, and participation in multilaboratory proficiency tests. When using an unfamiliar laboratory for the first time, it may be prudent to inquire about its quality assurance and quality control program.

Once a test has been completed, interpretation of the results by a trained professional such as a veterinary

Small Animal Toxicology Essentials, First Edition. Edited by Robert H. Poppenga, Sharon Gwaltney-Brant.
© 2011 John Wiley and Sons, Inc. Published 2011 by John Wiley and Sons, Inc.

Table 10.1. Environmental sample types and amounts for toxicologic testing

Sample Type	Amount	Collection/Storage Method
Human or animal foods	500 grams (approximately 2 cups)	Refrigerate or freeze in a well-sealed plastic bag or container.
Baits	Entire amount present up to 500 grams (approximately 2 cups)	Refrigerate or freeze in a well-sealed plastic bag or container.
Plants	Whole green plant including the roots; a fresh tree, or shrub branch with leaves (and flowers if present); entire nut, fruit, berry, or other characteristic part of the plant	Press or wrap in newspaper, place in a sealed plastic bag, and then send to the diagnostic laboratory either fresh or frozen.
Mushrooms	Whole mushroom or as much as possible if the only remaining source is from the animal's vomitus or stomach contents	Keep relatively cold and dry in a paper bag to reduce moisture accumulation and subsequent spoilage.
Water	0.5–1 L (approximately 2–4 cups)	Ideally, collect into a new, unused, clean, and dry glass container that is free of any detergent, chemical, food, or beverage residues.
Other unidentified substances or medications	Representative amount of what is present up to 500 grams (approximately 2 cups)	Refrigerate or freeze in a well-sealed plastic bag or container.

toxicologist, can be critical in determining its significance to the case as a whole and may be used to direct additional patient care or diagnostic testing. To determine whether a patient's result is abnormal or diagnostically significant, something should be known about what "normal" results are expected to be for an animal of a particular species, age, or gender. As an example anticoagulant rodenticides would not be expected to be present in the blood of an unexposed animal, while a low level of lead in the same animal's blood could be considered normal and not expected to be associated with signs of lead toxicity.

An experienced veterinary toxicology laboratory will be able to provide reliable, accurate, and useful results in a timely matter.

DIAGNOSTICS

The appropriate selection of diagnostic tests in cases of suspected intoxications will rely heavily on obtaining a good case history. Based on the historical information provided, a veterinary toxicology laboratory's professional staff should be able to assist veterinary clinics with questions about which tests should be selected for a given case, the best and appropriate sample types to submit, and the desirable sample quantities needed to run the requested analyses.

Environmental Samples

Many toxicants cannot be successfully detected in animal tissues or bodily fluids, so the collection and submission of environmental samples may be critical to identifying an animal's access to a potentially toxic substance. Common environmental samples that could represent sources of intoxication to small animals include foods, baits, plants, mushrooms, water, and other unidentified substances or medications. For a description of typical sample amounts and how they should be collected, stored, and submitted for toxicologic testing, see Table 10.1.

Antemortem

Common sample types that can be obtained from a live patient for toxicology testing include whole blood, serum, urine, vomitus, stomach contents, feces, biopsy specimens, and hair. Samples should be obtained preferably at the earliest feasible opportunity after the animal arrives at the clinic. If specimens cannot be collected before extensive medical treatments are instituted, any drugs administered or treatments given should be noted as part of the case history when submitting toxicology samples for testing. Suggested sample amounts and how they should be stored and transported are described in Table 10.2. The sample size that can be safely collected from tiny patients

Table 10.2. Suggested antemortem samples for toxicologic testing

Sample Type	Amount	Collection/Storage Method
Whole blood	2–4 ml	Refrigerate in calcium EDTA or heparin tube.
Serum	2–4 ml	Spin and refrigerate or freeze the serum in a plain glass or plastic blood tube to separate from the red blood cells. Use a special all-plastic royal blue top for accurate zinc levels.
Urine	At least 10–20 ml	Refrigerate or freeze in a clean, tightly sealed plastic container.
Vomitus or stomach contents	At least 10–20 ml	Refrigerate or freeze in a clean, tightly sealed plastic bag or container.
Feces	At least 100 grams	Refrigerate or freeze in a clean, tightly sealed plastic bag or container.
Biopsy specimens	At least 2–5 grams	Refrigerate or freeze in a clean, tightly sealed plastic bag or container.
Hair	5–10 grams	Place in a clean, tightly sealed plastic bag or container.

Table 10.3. Postmortem samples for toxicologic testing

Sample Type	Amount	Storage Method
Stomach contents	At least 10–20 ml	Refrigerate or freeze in a clean, tightly sealed plastic bag or container.
Liver	At least 5–10 grams	Refrigerate or freeze in a clean, tightly sealed plastic bag or container.
Kidney	At least 5–10 grams	Refrigerate or freeze in a clean, tightly sealed plastic bag or container.
Brain	Half of the brain	Cut in half sagittally, leaving the other half and the midline intact for histopathology. Refrigerate or freeze in a clean, tightly sealed plastic bag or container.
Body fat	At least 5–10 grams	Refrigerate or freeze in a clean, tightly sealed plastic bag or container.
Eye	One globe	Refrigerate or freeze in a clean, tightly sealed plastic bag or container; allows testing of either ocular fluid or retina
Injection site	Surrounding tissue	Refrigerate or freeze in a clean, tightly sealed plastic bag or container.

such as neonates and exotic species may be limited. Some form of toxicologic testing can still be performed in most cases, though the number and types of tests along with the ability to verify any positive results may be severely limited.

Postmortem

When patients have died as a result of a suspected toxicosis it may be beneficial to refrigerate or freeze samples for potential toxicologic testing while awaiting results of other diagnostic tests such as complete blood counts, serum chemistries, gross necropsies, and histopathology. These results may provide valuable information about possible cause(s) of death and subsequently what specific toxicologic analyses should be pursued. One exception may be if other animals in the same household or neighborhood are sick or at risk. In these cases toxicologic testing may be pursued more quickly when the history and clinical signs observed are strongly supportive of or suspicious for

poisoning. Common postmortem sample types are described in Table 10.3. Rarely, collection of other postmortem sample types may be necessary for the detection of some compounds, such as lung tissue for paraquat. This kind of special testing information can be obtained by consulting with the toxicology laboratory.

MANAGEMENT OF EXPOSURES

Diagnostic testing should not be substituted for general patient care and case management. All patients should be evaluated as individuals and life-threatening signs such as respiratory distress, cardiovascular compromise, and central nervous system abnormalities such as seizures should be addressed first. Once the patient has been stabilized, diagnostic tests can be performed and specific care can be provided. Even in the event that diagnostic toxicologic testing is not readily available, most intoxicated animals can recover if close monitoring, symptomatic treatment, and good nursing care are provided.

CHAPTER 10 STUDY QUESTIONS

1. Manny, a 6-year-old, intact male, 65-pound German shepherd dog, presents to the veterinary hospital with a history of vomiting and muscle tremors that began about 2 hours ago. Prior to development of signs, Manny had been roaming free on the owner's farm. The owners are concerned that Manny may have gotten into the shed that houses the farm pesticides. They also noted that Manny was seen digging in the compost pile in the pasture. Besides blood or serum, list two other samples from Manny that might be helpful to aid in diagnosis.

2. For each of the two samples selected in Question 1, indicate the amount to collect and the best method of storage/handling of the sample for submission to a diagnostic laboratory.

3. Which of the following is not correct regarding diagnostic toxicology samples?
   a. Freezing or refrigeration is an acceptable means of preserving samples prior to submission to the diagnostic laboratory.
   b. Veterinary diagnostic laboratory personnel can assist the veterinary technician in determining the best test and sample for a particular suspected toxicology case.
   c. When determining whether a laboratory result is clinically significant, the diagnostic toxicologist will compare the result with a range of "normal" values.
   d. Toxicology testing should always be the first step in attempting to diagnose the cause of death in a suspected poisoning case.
   e. Environmental samples that may be submitted in a suspected toxicology case include animal foods, plants, mushrooms, and water.

4. Which of the following is true regarding the MDL (minimum detection limit)?
   a. Refers to the minimum amount of toxicant in an animal that will cause a toxicosis
   b. Refers to the highest amount of toxicant that the diagnostic test can detect in a sample

   c. Refers to the minimum amount of a toxic substance that must be present to reliably produce a positive test result
   d. Refers to the lowest level of toxicant that will be toxic to a particular animal
   e. Refers to the smallest amount of a nontoxicant (i.e., contaminant) that will give a false positive result

5. The appropriate selection of diagnostic tests in cases of suspected intoxications will rely heavily on the diagnostic laboratory obtaining _____.
   a. An adequate blood sample
   b. A good case history
   c. A freshly dead animal
   d. Frequent calls from the veterinary clinic asking for results
   e. Payment in advance

ANSWERS

1. Urine, vomitus (stomach content), feces.
2. Urine, collect at least 10–20 ml and submit refrigerated or frozen in a clean, tightly sealed plastic container. Vomitus (stomach contents), collect at least 10–20 ml or g and submit refrigerated or frozen in a clean, tightly sealed plastic container. Feces, submit at least 100 g and submit refrigerated or frozen in a clean, tightly sealed plastic container.
3. d. In most cases toxicology testing should be performed after other testing (necropsy, histopathology, clinical pathology) results are obtained in order to help narrow down the potential toxicants to analyze for.
4. c.
5. b. A good case history is essential in knowing what kind of testing would be most appropriate for a particular case.

REFERENCE

Galey, Frank D. 2004. Diagnostic Toxicology. In *Clinical Veterinary Toxicology*, edited by Konnie H. Plumlee, pp. 22–27. St. Louis: Mosby.

Section 2

A Systems-Affected Approach to Toxicology

Nervous System

11

Tina Wismer

INTRODUCTION

The nervous system is a target for an extremely large number of toxic agents including drugs, environmental and industrial chemicals, and "natural" products such as bacterial toxins and animal venoms (Tables 11.1–11.4). Many of these agents are able to bypass the nervous system's protective blood-brain barrier and cause neurologic dysfunction. Many agents that affect the nervous system, especially psychotropic drugs, exert their effects through biochemical mechanisms that do not leave any telltale clinical pathologic changes or anatomic lesions to aid in diagnosis in animals experiencing a toxicosis. Because the nervous system has a limited number of responses to injury, the clinical effects of toxicoses affecting nervous system function will resemble effects from other causes of neurologic dysfunction such as infectious, metabolic, traumatic, and neoplastic injury. Definitive diagnosis of nervous system toxicosis can therefore be quite challenging.

ANATOMY AND PHYSIOLOGY

The nervous system encompasses both the central nervous system (CNS) and the peripheral nervous system (PNS). The CNS coordinates the activity of all parts of the body and consists of the brain and spinal cord. The PNS connects the CNS with the limbs and organs.

The basic functional unit of the nervous system is the neuron. Neurons initiate and conduct nerve stimuli. The basic structure of a neuron contains the body (soma), dendrites, and axons. The dendrites are short branches off the body that receive stimuli from other neurons and transmit it to the soma. The axon carries impulses away from the soma, and is often covered by myelin, a fatlike substance that increases the speed of impulse conduction (Spencer 2000). Nervous impulses cross the synapses between neurons by the release of chemicals termed neurotransmitters (Anthony et al. 2001). Neurotransmitters include acetylcholine, catecholamines (dopamine, norepinephrine, epinephrine), amino acid derivatives (serotonin, gamma amino butyric acid or GABA, glycine, histamine, aspartic acid, glutamic acid), and various other neuropeptides (substance P, orexins, endorphins, vasopressin, thyroid-releasing hormone) (Beasley 1999; Spencer 2000).

Neurotransmitters can be excitatory and/or inhibitory. Excitatory neurotransmitters stimulate postsynaptic membranes, and inhibitory neurotransmitters decrease (or make less likely) the transmission of an impulse. Acetylcholine is both excitatory and inhibitory. It has inhibitory effects on the heart but stimulatory effects on other organs. The catecholamines are hormones that are released by the adrenal glands in reaction to stress. Epinephrine and norepinephrine are associated with the sympathetic nervous system (fight or flight response). Dopamine is found in the brain and affects muscle control and autonomic functions. GABA is the main inhibitory neurotransmitter. GABA regulates neuronal excitability throughout the nervous system. Glycine is also an inhibitory neurotransmitter found in the spinal cord, brainstem, and retina.

The major protective mechanism in the CNS is the blood-brain barrier. The blood-brain barrier forms a "wall" between capillaries in the brain and the nervous tissue. The tight junctions allow small molecules and lipid soluble molecules to enter easily, but keep other substances out of

Small Animal Toxicology Essentials, First Edition. Edited by Robert H. Poppenga, Sharon Gwaltney-Brant.
© 2011 John Wiley and Sons, Inc. Published 2011 by John Wiley and Sons, Inc.

Table 11.1. Pesticides

Toxicant	Possible Effect on the Nervous System
4-aminopyridine (Avitrol®)	Stimulation, tremors, seizures
Amitraz	Depressant
Anticholinesterase insecticides (organophosphates, carbamates)	Seizures
Avermectins (ivermectin, moxidectin)	Weakness, ataxia, tremors, seizures, coma
Bromethalin	Stimulant at high doses; depressant at low doses
3-chloro-*p*-toluidine hydrochloride (Starlicide®)	Depressant, weakness, paralysis
DEET (diethyltoluamide)	Seizures
Metaldehyde	Seizures, tremors
Organochlorine insecticides (lindane, DDT)	Seizures
Pyrethrins	Tremors
Sodium fluoroactate (1080)	Intermittent seizures, stimulation
Strychnine	Seizures
Zinc phosphide	Ataxia, seizures

Table 11.2. Biologic agents

Toxicant	Possible Effect on the Nervous System
Asclepias spp. (Milkweed)	Weakness, tremors, seizures
Atropa belladonna (Deadly nightshade, Belladonna)	Tremors, paralysis, hallucinations
Black widow spider envenomation	Flaccid paralysis
Blue-green algae (anatoxin-a, anatoxin-a[s])	Tremors, seizures
Botulism	Flaccid paralysis
Brunfelsia spp. (Yesterday, Today, and Tomorrow)	Tremors (can last for weeks), seizures
Calycanthus spp. (Bubby bush)	Seizures
Cannabis sativa (Marijuana)	Depressant, ataxia, coma; possible agitation
Cicuta spp. (Water hemlock)	Seizures
Conium spp. (Poison hemlock)	Initial stimulation, followed by depressive signs
Coral snake envenomation	Ataxia, tremors, paralysis
Datura spp. (Jimsonweed, Angel's trumpet)	Tremors, paralysis, hallucinations
Essential oils	Depressant, ataxia, weakness, tremors; seizures with large doses
Eupatorium rugosum (White snakeroot)	Tremors, ataxia, stiff gait, weakness
Ipomoea spp. (Morning glory)	Stimulation, hallucinations
Lobelia spp. (Lobelia)	Initial stimulation, followed by depressive signs
Lupinus spp. (Lupine)	Initial stimulation, followed by depressive signs
Macadamia nuts	Weakness, tremors (dogs only)
Mushrooms, isoxazole	Alternating CNS stimulation and depression
Mushrooms, monomethylhydrazines	Tremors, seizures, coma
Mushrooms, psychedelic	Ataxia, tremors, hallucinations
Nerium oleander (Oleander)	Tremors, seizures
Nicotine (cigarettes, *Nicotiana* spp.)	Initial stimulation, followed by depressive signs
Tetanus	Muscle rigidity
Tick paralysis	Weakness, paralysis
Tremorgenic mycotoxins (Penitrem A, roquefortine)	Tremors, seizures

Table 11.3. Pharmaceuticals

Toxicant	Possible Effect on the Nervous System
Amphetamines (Ritalin®, Adderall®, crack, methamphetamine, MDMA)	Stimulation
Antihistamines (diphenhydramine, hydroxyzine, loratadine)	Stimulant at high doses; depressant at low doses
Atropine	Seizures with high doses
Barbiturates (phenobarbital)	Depressant
Benzodiazepines (diazepam, alprazolam)	Depressant, ataxia; rarely agitation
Bromide	Depressant, weakness, ataxia
Bupropion (Wellbutrin®)	Stimulant at high doses; depressant at low doses
Buspirone	Stimulant at high doses; depressant at low doses
Cocaine	Stimulation
Cyproheptadine	Stimulant at high doses; depressant at low doses
Decongestants (pseudoephedrine, phenylephrine, Ma huang, ephedra)	Stimulation
5-fluorouracil (Efudex®)	Seizures
General anesthetics (isoflurane, halothane, propofol)	Depressant
Ibuprofen	Seizures, coma with high doses
Isoniazid	Seizures
Lithium	Seizures
Local anesthetics (lidocaine, benzocaine)	Seizures with high doses
LSD	Stimulation, hallucinations
MAO inhibitors (Anipryl®)	Stimulant at high doses; depressant at low doses
Methylxanthines (caffeine, theobromine, theophylline)	Stimulation
Mirtazepine (Remeron®)	Stimulant at high doses; depressant at low doses
Nefazadone, trazodone	Stimulant at high doses; depressant at low doses
Opiates (hydrocodone, morphine, codeine, butorphanol, tramadol)	Depressant; rarely agitation and seizures
Phenothiazines (acepromazine, chlorpromazine)	Depressant
Piperazine	Ataxia, tremors
Salicylates	Seizures with high doses
Serotonergic drugs (Prozac®, Paxil®, 5-hydroxytryptophan, Effexor®)	Stimulant at high doses; depressant at low doses
Tricyclic antidepressants (amitriptyline, clomipramine)	Stimulant at high doses; depressant at low doses

Table 11.4. Nonmedicinal agents

Toxicant	Possible Effect on the Nervous System
Alcohol	Depressant
Carbon monoxide	Depressant, weakness, ataxia
Ethylene glycol	Depressant effect, ataxia, tremors, seizures
Lead	Intermittent stimulation and depression
Liver toxicants	Secondary to hepatic encephalopathy
Organic alkyl mercury	Blindness, ataxia, paralysis, coma
Phenol	Tremors, seizures with large doses
Propylene glycol	Depressant effects, ataxia, seizures
Sodium	Tremors, seizures
Thiaminase (raw fish)	Depression, ataxia, paresis
Thallium	Tremors, weakness, seizures
Turpentine	Depressant, weakness, ataxia, coma

the brain. The PNS is not protected by the blood-brain barrier, leaving it exposed to toxicants.

MECHANISMS OF TOXICOLOGIC INJURY

In small animal toxicology, most toxicants work directly on the neurons or affect the release and/or binding of neurotransmitters. Toxicant-induced alteration of neurotransmitters can result in stimulation or inhibition of postsynaptic neurons, resulting in excitatory or depressive clinical effects depending on the type of neurotransmitter affected, type of postsynaptic neuron, and amount of neurotransmitter and receptors involved. For instance, CNS stimulation (manifested as hyperactivity, agitation and/or seizures) may be caused by increasing the synaptic levels of an excitatory neurotransmitter (e.g., stimulation of acetylcholine release by organophosphorus insecticides) or by decreasing the synaptic levels of an inhibitory neurotransmitter (e.g., strychnine-induced decrease in glycine neurotransmission).

The brain is very susceptible to injury because it requires a continual high level of oxygen. It has a high percentage of blood flow for an organ of relatively small mass. Hypoxia is a common cause of neuronal injury. It may be secondary to systemic hypotension, cerebral infarction, vascular injury, or oxygen deprivation. Respiratory compromise leading to hypoxia is the primary life-threatening issue in many toxic exposures causing alterations of consciousness (Anthony et al. 2001). Brain damage can also occur secondary to hypoglycemia. During periods of low blood sugar, neuronal damage to dentate and granule cells occurs. Hypoglycemia can result in either cerebral cortex or brainstem deficits. Other mechanisms of toxicologic injury to the nervous system include ion balance disruption (excessive intracellular accumulation of calcium), cytoskeleton damage, decreased protein synthesis (loss of rough endoplasmic reticulum), and glial cell damage (Anthony et al. 2001).

Disruption or dysfunction of the blood-brain barrier may result in normally excluded compounds entering the CNS, resulting in neurologic injury and/or dysfunction.

PATTERNS OF TOXICOLOGIC INJURY

Toxicological insults to the nervous system produce a wide range of clinical signs when compared to other organ systems. Toxicants can affect multiple areas of the nervous system depending on the dose, route of exposure, and species of animal. To make diagnosis more difficult, toxicants can cause a progression of clinical signs (e.g., initial CNS depression, followed by CNS stimulation).

Many neurotoxicants effect neurotransmission and leave no obvious lesions. Functional neurotoxicants can affect the CNS, PNS, and autonomic nervous system (ANS). They act by preventing synthesis, storage, release, binding, reuptake, or degradation of neurotransmitters. Functional neurotoxicants may also interfere with axonal transmission via sodium, potassium, chloride or calcium channels, and alter action potentials (Spencer 2000).

There are a few structural changes caused by neurotoxicants. These include neuronopathy, anoxopathy, and myelinopathy. In neuronopathy, neurotoxicants directly target the cell body, causing cell death and secondary axonal degeneration. The response to the loss of neurons is gliosis, proliferation of astrocytes, and/or microglial cells (Anthony et al. 2001). Neuronopathies can be selective or diffuse.

In axonopathy, in contrast to neuronopathy, the neuronal cell body remains intact, but the portion of the axon distal to the lesion degenerates (Wallerian degeneration) (Mandella 2002). Histologic changes can be seen in the Nissl substance. These changes include chromatolysis (dissolution of the Nissl substance) as well as movement of the nucleus to the periphery of the cell body. Neurons with axons of the greatest length are most susceptible to axonal damage.

Myelinopathy occurs when toxicants cause a loss of myelin (demyelination) or edema in the myelin sheath and subsequent separation of myelin layers. This slows down nerve transmission.

HEALING AND REPAIR

Damage to the nervous system is frequently irreversible because the adult neuron does not divide. With peripheral neuronopathies the prognosis for at least partial regeneration is good. However, this is not true in the CNS. Central neuronopathies, with few exceptions, are not reversible.

In axonopathies, glial cells debride the area. The cell body undergoes central chromatolysis which may lead to cell death. If the cell body does not die, axonal regrowth may occur slowly (approximately 1 mm per day). Secondary demyelination can be seen with axonal injury (Mandella 2002). Remyelination can occur in some cases, more often in the PNS than in the CNS.

CHAPTER 11 STUDY QUESTIONS

1. Many psychotropic drugs alter nervous system function by changing the brain biochemistry through alterations of
   a. Hormones
   b. Neurotransmitters
   c. Cytokines
   d. Tight junctions
   e. Glial cells

2. The functional unit of the nervous system is the _____, composed of _____ that receive stimuli from other cells, _____ that carry impulses away from the cell body, and the cell body, also known as the _____.
   a. Soma, dendrites, axons, neuron
   b. Dendrites, soma, axons, neuron
   c. Neuron, axons, dendrites, soma
   d. Neuron, dendrites, axons, soma
   e. Soma, axons, dendrites, neuron

3. GABA is an inhibitory neurotransmitter within the CNS. The most significant effect of inhibition of the action of GABA would be expected to be
   a. CNS depression and coma
   b. CNS stimulation and seizures
   c. Fight or flight response
   d. Corticosteroid release
   e. Immunosuppression

4. The blood-brain barrier
   a. Keeps all foreign compounds out of the CNS regardless of size
   b. Protects the CNS and PNS from entry of potentially damaging compounds

   c. Repels negatively charged compounds, keeping them from entering the nervous system
   d. Is readily traversed by inflammatory cells
   e. Is composed of tight junctions that allow the passage of small molecules and lipid-soluble compounds but prevent passage of other substances

5. Which of the following is not a potential cause of brain injury?
   a. Hypoglycemia
   b. Hypoxia
   c. Blood-brain barrier disruption
   d. Disruption of ion balance
   e. All of the above are potential causes of brain injury.

ANSWERS

1. b. Neurotransmitters
2. d. The neuron is composed of dendrites that receive stimuli, axons that transmit impulses, and the soma, or cell body.
3. b. Inhibition of CNS inhibitory neurotransmitters such as GABA and glycine commonly cause CNS stimulation and, potentially, seizures.
4. e.
5. e.

REFERENCES

Douglas C. Anthony, Thomas J. Montine, William M. Valentine, Doyle G. Graham. 2001. Toxic responses of the nervous system." In *Casarett & Doull's Toxicology: The Basic Science of Poisons*, 6th ed., edited by Curtis D. Klassen, pp. 535–563. New York: McGraw-Hill.

Val R. Beasley. 1999. *Veterinary Toxicology*. International Veterinary Information Service. www.ivis.org/advances/Beasley/toc.asp.

Rosemary C. Mandella. 2002. Applied neurotoxicology. In *Handbook of Toxicology*, 2nd ed., edited by Michael J. Derelanko, Mannfred A. Hollinger, pp. 371–399. Boca Raton: CRC Press.

Peter S. Spencer. 2000. Biological principles of chemical neurotoxicity. In *Experimental and Clinical Neurotoxicology*, 2nd edition, edited by Peter S. Spencer, Herbert H. Schaumburg, pp. 3–54. New York: Oxford University Press.

Cardiovascular System

12

Karla R. Smith

INTRODUCTION

Cardiovascular toxicity can be broadly defined as adverse effects on the heart and blood vessels following exposure to toxic agents. These toxicants can produce direct or indirect effects on the heart and/or vascular system. Agents that affect the heart may increase the force of contraction (*cardiotonic or positive inotropic effect*), may increase the rate of contraction (*positive chronotropic effect*), or may have cardiac depressant effects (*negative inotropic or chronotropic effects*).

ANATOMY AND PHYSIOLOGY

The cardiovascular system can be divided into two categories: the heart and the blood vessels. The heart is made up of two large pumps; the right and left ventricle, which work in concert to pump blood through the blood vessels.

The right ventricle pumps blood through the lungs where it is oxygenated. The left ventricle pumps blood through the systemic circulation. The smaller pumps, the right and left atria, move blood into their associated ventricles. The right atrium houses the sinoatrial (SA) node, which is responsible for initiating cardiac impulses.

Electrical impulses begin in the SA node and are transmitted throughout the atria, causing them to contract and force blood into the ventricles. When the electrical impulse reaches the atrioventricular (AV) node, there is a slight delay in conduction, which allows complete filling of the ventricles before the impulse is transmitted throughout the ventricles via the AV bundle and Purkinje fibers (Fox et al. 1999).

The cardiac muscle (myocardium) does the work of the heart. The myocardium is a type of involuntary striated muscle found only in the walls of the heart. It shares some similarities with skeletal muscle but is unique in many ways. The striations observed in cardiac muscle are due to alternating thick (myosin) and thin (actin) protein filaments. It is the sliding of actin filaments past myosin filaments that causes contraction of the myocardium. This action requires both ATP and an adequate concentration of sodium and calcium (Kittleson and Kienle 1998).

The blood vessels make up the circulatory system, which transports blood throughout the body. The arteries transport blood away from the heart, the capillaries are small vessels that allow the exchange of oxygen and nutrients and connect the arterial and venous sides of the vascular system, and the veins transport blood back toward the heart. The blood vessels have limited ability to contribute to forward blood flow. Arteries can regulate their inner diameter by contraction or relaxation of the vascular smooth muscle layer. This vasoconstriction or vasodilation can be an important mechanism in cardiovascular toxicity, contributing to hypertension or hypotension. All blood vessels are lined with endothelial cells that interface between circulating blood and the vessel wall. The endothelial cells have multiple functions, including helping to control blood pressure and forming specialized barriers, such as the blood brain barrier.

Small Animal Toxicology Essentials, First Edition. Edited by Robert H. Poppenga, Sharon Gwaltney-Brant.
© 2011 John Wiley and Sons, Inc. Published 2011 by John Wiley and Sons, Inc.

MECHANISMS OF TOXIC INJURY TO THE HEART

Toxicologic injury to the cardiovascular system may develop by either direct or indirect means. Direct means include those that have a primary effect on the functional or biomechanical properties of the heart and vascular system. An example would be the tricyclic antidepressant clomipramine, which inhibits myocardial sodium channels, leading to cardiac dysrhythmias. Indirect toxicity arises when the cardiovascular system is secondarily affected by toxicosis to another body system. For example, ingestion of bromodialone, an anticoagulant rodenticide, can cause significant blood loss leading to hypovolemic shock. The fall in blood volume causes a drop in systemic blood pressure. Reflex vasoconstriction causes splenic contraction in an effort to increase the circulating blood volume, and the heart rate elevates as the heart attempts to move the remaining blood through the circulatory system more rapidly.

PATTERNS OF TOXIC INJURY TO THE HEART

Direct Myocardial Injury

Some toxicants can cause degeneration and necrosis of the myocardium, either by direct injury to the myocardial cells or by hemodynamic alterations resulting in ischemic injury. Depending on the toxicant, the pattern of injury on the heart can vary from small areas of necrosis to massive necrosis of the myocardium, resulting in congestive heart failure (CHF), cardiomyopathy, conduction disturbances, or death. Areas of myocardial necrosis will appear as pale spots or streaks in the heart muscle; older lesions may be more pronounced due to fibrosis or mineralization. Agents that can cause this type of myocardial injury in dogs and cats include doxorubicin, thallium, sodium fluoroacetate (a pesticide also known as 1080), and minoxidil (DeClementi et al. 2004).

Conduction Disturbances

It is important to recognize when specific cardiac arrhythmias and ECG findings may be related to exposure to a cardiotoxic agent. Three mechanisms contribute to production and maintenance of arrhythmias: (1) abnormal impulse initiation, (2) abnormal triggered rhythms, and (3) abnormal impulse conduction. Toxicants causing myocardial conduction disturbances leave few to no lesions in the heart unless significant cardiac ischemia occurs during the toxicosis, in which case areas of myocardial necrosis may be identifiable.

Abnormal impulse initiation may occur when there is increased automaticity of the atrial or ventricular myocardial cells unassociated with the SA or AV nodes. This area is generally referred to as an *ectopic focus*. If the firing rate of the ectopic focus is greater than the SA node, the ectopic focus will become the predominant pacemaker of the heart. The drugs digitoxin and digoxin are digitalis glycosides, which are used in both human and veterinary medicine to treat congestive heart failure and atrial fibrillation. They act by depressing the rate of cardiac impulses initiated by the SA node, and increasing intracellular calcium, leading to slower and more forceful cardiac contraction. While they are effective drugs used in treating atrial fibrillation commonly seen with dilated cardiomyopathy, they have a narrow margin of safety, with both acute and chronic toxicity being observed. Toxic doses cause marked slowing of conduction through the AV node, potentially allowing an ectopic focus to take over as the prominent pacemaker of the heart. Increased intracellular calcium can also cause cardiac arrhythmias to develop. Clinical signs typically include ventricular tachycardia and preventricular contractions.

Abnormal triggered rhythms occur from either potassium channel blockade or intracellular calcium overload. Barium salts, which are used to create green colors in fireworks, cause intracellular trapping of potassium along with cardiac dysrhythmias, including preventricular contractions, ventricular tachycardia, or bradycardia.

Abnormal impulse conduction occurs when electrical impulses traveling through the myocardium reach an area that, due to ischemia, disease, or toxicant exposure is not appropriately able to conduct these impulses. When these impulses are completely blocked, bradyarrhythmias may occur. Slow conduction may trigger a reentry circuit, causing either supraventricular or ventricular tachycardia. The sympathomimetic drug phenylpropanolamine has been shown to cause myocardial necrosis when ingested at toxic doses. This myocardial necrosis may be partially responsible for arrhythmias seen following toxicity (Pentel et al. 1987).

CARDIOTOXIC AGENTS

Many substances cause cardiac toxic responses directly or indirectly. However, the next section will focus on drugs that have primary cardiac toxicity.

Calcium Channel Blockers

There are several classes of calcium channel blocking drugs that are currently in use in both human and veterinary medicine. The formulations most likely to be encountered in a clinical veterinary medicine setting are verapamil, amlodipine, nifedipine, and diltiazem. These drugs are used to treat angina, supraventricular arrhythmias, and myocardial infarction in humans and supraventricular arrhythmias, hypertension, and hypertrophic cardiomyopathy in domestic pets. The calcium channel blockers affect both the myocardium and cardiac pacemaker cells. Ultimately there is slowing of impulse initiation by the SA node, conduction through the AV node, and decreased cardiac contractility. Clinical signs of overdose may include hypotension, bradycardia or tachycardia, heart block or other arrhythmias, electrolyte imbalances, vomiting, and lethargy.

Beta-adrenergic Blocking Agents

The beta-blocking drugs act by inhibiting catecholamine binding to beta receptors in the heart, kidneys, and vascular smooth muscle. They are common drugs, used to treat hypertension, tachycardia, congestive heart failure, and glaucoma. Formulations include atenolol, esmolol, metoprolol, and propranolol. Overdose of a beta-blocking agent is most likely to cause hypotension, bradycardia and metabolic acidosis.

Angiotensin-Converting Enzyme Inhibitors (ACE Inhibitors)

The ACE inhibitor enalapril is often one of the first drugs administered to dogs suffering from CHF, hypertension, or valvular disease. The ACE inhibitors work by blocking angiotensin II. Angiotensin II is a potent vasoconstrictor and mediator of sodium reabsorption in the kidneys. Ultimately this leads to increased blood volume and blood pressure. By blocking angiotensin II the ACE inhibitors lower blood pressure. In an overdose situation the primary concern is for hypotension.

Angiotensin II Antagonists

The angiotenisn II antagonists are very similar to the ACE inhibitors but are not used in veterinary medicine. They are used to treat hypertension by blocking the vasoconstricting effects of angiotensin II. Clinical signs in small animal patients are not expected to be severe, but they may include hypotension and reflex tachycardia. The angiotensin II antagonists will also act synergistically with ACE inhibitors, calcium channel blockers, and beta blockers to cause hypotension.

Cardiac Glycosides

Digoxin and digitoxin are used in veterinary medicine to treat CHF, atrial fibrillation, and supraventricular tachycardias. The glycosides act by increasing intracellular calcium concentrations, leading to increased myocardial contractility. They also decrease conduction through the AV node, slowing the heart rate and allowing for more complete filling of the ventricles. Digoxin and digitoxin have narrow therapeutic indices, meaning that the therapeutic dose and toxic dose are very close together. In a clinical setting patients may be seen with either chronic or acute toxicity from these agents. Clinical signs may include those related to the cardiovascular system, such as heart block, tachycardia, or preventricular contractions. Other clinical signs may include gastrointestinal upset, depression, and electrolyte changes.

Pimobendan

Pimobendan is a selective phosphodiesterase (PDE) III inhibitor currently approved only to manage CHF in dogs. It has positive inotropic and vasodilator effects, leading to increased cardiac output and reduction in systemic vascular resistance. Pimobendan appears to have a wide margin of safety, with tachycardia, lethargy, and hypotension being the most common clinical signs associated with overdose.

Sympathomimetics

The sympathomimetics have been available as a drug class since the 1st century AD when Pliny used ephedrine to treat bleeding. Sympathomimetics currently used in veterinary medicine include phenylpropanolamine (PPA), albuterol, dopamine, ketamine, and terbutaline. Pet owners may have sympathomimetics in their houses either legally in the form of methylphenidate (Ritalin®), dextroamphetamine (Adderall®), pseudoephedrine and phenylephrine or illegally in the form of cocaine or methamphetamine.

Sympathomimetics are defined as catecholamine-like substances that have physiologic actions similar to those observed with activation of the sympathetic nervous system. They have an overall excitatory effect on the heart, and those formulations that cross the blood brain barrier cause CNS stimulation. In general signs of overdose include mydriasis, tachycardia, hypertension, and agitation.

In large overdoses, phenylpropanolamine may cause such significant hypertension that a reflex bradycardia may develop rather than the expected tachycardia (Hoffman and Nelson 2005). Phenylpropanolamine has also been shown to cause focal cardiac necrosis when administered to rats at doses greater than 4 mg/kg (Pentel et al. 1987).

Methylxanthines

Theophylline, caffeine, and theobromine are naturally occurring plant alkaloids. They are found in food (chocolate) and drinks (colas) for human consumption, over- the-counter medications that promote wakefulness, and as therapeutic agents to treat asthma. Clinical signs of methylxanthine overdose may include tachycardia, premature ventricular contractions, and hypotension. Ingestion of medications containing both caffeine and ephedrine (a sympathomimetic) can cause hemorrhagic myocardial necrosis (Nyska et al. 2005).

MECHANISMS OF TOXIC INJURY TO THE VASCULAR SYSTEM

The potential for toxic injury to the vascular system may be underestimated in veterinary medicine when it is considered that all toxicants, following absorption, contact the vascular system. The vascular endothelial cells are frequently the immediate target of toxic agents, followed by the vascular smooth muscle cells. Both of these cells types are metabolically active, and systems present in these cells may bioactivate some toxicants. Oxygen-derived free radicals formed during bioactivation may injure endothelial cells, leading to changes in permeability. Toxicants can also cause alterations in the structure of the vessels. Hypertonic intravenous solutions can cause the endothelial cells to shrink, leading to increased permeability (Weddle and Morgan 2004).

Cholecalciferol

Cholecalciferol or vitamin D_3 is the most common agent seen in veterinary medicine that does significant, lasting damage to the vascular system. Cholecalciferol (or its analogues) can be found in rodenticides, vitamins, and prescription creams for the treatment of psoriasis. Cholecalciferol overdose causes an increase in serum calcium and phosphorus levels due to increased renal tubular reabsorption of calcium, increased intestinal absorption of calcium, and increased release of calcium from bone. This excess calcium and phosphorus in the blood causes deposition of these minerals within the vascular wall. The vessel then becomes hard and rigid, and sudden death may result (Weddle and Morgan 2004).

Carbon Monoxide

Small animal patients may be exposed to carbon monoxide due to accidental exposures to automobile exhaust or household fires. Short-term exposure to carbon monoxide can cause direct damage to vascular endothelial cells and smooth muscle cells. Carbon monoxide also causes a direct vasodilatory response on coronary circulation. The primary toxic effect of carbon monoxide is due to its reversible interaction with hemoglobin. It binds preferentially to hemoglobin, impairing oxygen delivery, which leads to cellular hypoxia (Ramos et al. 2001). Clinical signs in the pet may include tachycardia, dyspnea, lethargy. and coma.

CONCLUSION

Ultimately any toxic exposure may cause some effect on the cardiovascular system, and an important aspect of managing toxicosis is providing support to the cardiovascular system. This typically includes intravenous fluid therapy and appropriate drugs to regulate heart rate and blood pressure.

CHAPTER 12 STUDY QUESTIONS

1. A cardiac drug that increases the rate of heart contraction and decreases the strength of heart contraction would be classified as
   a. Negative chronotrope, positive inotrope
   b. Negative chronotrope, negative inotrope
   c. Positive chronotrope, positive inotrope
   d. Positive chronotrope, negative inotrope
   e. Cardiotonic
2. Cardiac electrical impulses stimulate the coordinated contraction of myocardial cells. These impulses are initiated by the
   a. Interventricular node
   b. Sinoatrial node

   c. Submandibular node
   d. Atrioventricular node
   e. Popliteal node
3. Missy, a 12-pound, 2-year-old, spayed female Maltese presents with lethargy, vomiting, and weakness. Her body temperature is 98°F, her heart rate is 65, and her mean arterial blood pressure (MAP) is 55 mmHg. Missy's condition is best described as
   a. Hypothermic, bradycardic, hypotensive
   b. Hyperthermic, bradycardic, hypertensive
   c. Hypothermic, tachycardic, hypotensive
   d. Hyperthermic, tachycardic, hypertensive
   e. Hypothermic, tachycardic, normotensive

4. Missy's owner is concerned that the dog may have ingested one of the husband's heart medications. She is able to tell you the general class of drugs that her husband takes. Which of the following is LEAST likely to be responsible for Missy's condition.
   a. Beta blocker
   b. Calcium channel blocker
   c. Cardiac glycoside
   d. Sympathomimetic
   e. ACE inhibitor
5. Cholecalciferol rodenticides affect the cardiovascular system by
   a. Causing massive blood loss through disruption of normal blood coagulation.
   b. Causing direct myocardial necrosis and fibrosis.
   c. Causing mineralization within the walls of blood vessels.
   d. Causing necrosis of pulmonary endothelial cells, resulting in pulmonary edema.
   e. Causing dilation of peripheral vessels, resulting in hypotension.

ANSWERS

1. d. Chronotropy refers to heart rate and inotropy refers to force of contraction. Cardiotonic drugs increase the force of contraction (i.e., positive inotropes).
2. b. The sinoatrial (SA) node is responsible for initiation of myocardial contraction.
3. a. Missy's body temperature, blood pressure, and her heart rate are all below normal.
4. d. Sympathomimetics are cardiovascular stimulants, so they would be expected to cause hypertension and tachycardia.
5. c.

REFERENCES

Camille DeClementi, Keith L. Bailey, S.C. Goldstein, and M.S. Orser. 2004. Suspected toxicosis after topical administration of minoxidil in 2 cats. *Journal of Veterinary Emergency and Critical Care* 14(4):287–292.

Philip R. Fox, David Sisson, and N. Sydney Moise. 1999. *Textbook of Canine and Feline Cardiology Principles and Clinical Practice*, 2nd ed. Philadelphia: W.B. Saunders Company.

Robert J. Hoffman and Lewis S. Nelson. 2005. Sympathomimetic agents. In *Critical Care Toxicology Diagnosis and Management of the Critically Poisoned Patient*, edited by Jeffrey Brent et al. pp. 465–473. Philadelphia: Elsevier Mosby.

Mark Kittleson and Richard D. Kienle. 1998. *Small Animal Cardiovascular Medicine*. St. Louis: Mosby.

Abraham Nyska et al. 2005. Acute hemorrhagic myocardial necrosis and sudden death of rats exposed to a combination of ephedrine and caffeine. *Toxicological Sciences* 83(2):388–396.

Paul R. Pentel, Jeffrey Jentzen, and Jenny Siever. 1987. Myocardial necrosis due to intraperitoneal administration of phenylpropanolamine in rats. *Fundamental and Applied Toxicology* 9:167–172.

Kenneth S. Ramos, J. Kevin Kerzee, Napoleon F. Alejandro, and Kim P. Lu. 2001. Vascular toxicity: A cellular and molecular perspective. In *Cardiovascular Toxicology*, edited by Daniel Acosta Jr. pp. 479–524. London: Taylor and Francis.

Diann L. Weddle and Sherry J. Morgan. 2004. Cardiovascular System. In *Clinical Veterinary Toxicology*, edited by Konnie H. Plumlee. pp. 48–54 St. Louis: Mosby.

Pulmonary System

13

John A. Pickrell, Kiran Dhakal, and Sharon Gwaltney-Brant

INTRODUCTION

Inhalation toxicology refers to the pulmonary route of exposure; *pulmonary toxicity* refers to toxicity to the lung. Lung toxicity is most commonly caused by inhaling airborne poisons, but some toxicants can locate primarily in the lung from other exposure routes (e.g., paraquat from oral exposure) and cause lung toxicity. In addition to the lung, inhaled toxicants can cause injury in other areas of the respiratory tract such as the nasal cavity or conducting airways.

ANATOMY AND PHYSIOLOGY

Anatomy of the Respiratory Tract

The nares are the external openings into the nasal cavity. The nares lead to the nasal cavity, which is largely filled with the nasal turbinates, which moisten and warm inhaled air as well as filter out larger particulates. The nasal cavity is lined by ciliated and olfactory epithelium. Air passes through the nasal cavity into the nasopharynx. The nasopharynx is lined by pseudostratified columnar ciliated epithelium with goblet cells (Dungworth 1993). The eustachian tubes extend from the middle ear to the nasal cavity (Dungworth 1993). Many animals, especially horses and small laboratory rodents, are obligate nose breathers. Other animals, such as dogs and cats, can breathe with either their nose or mouth. Brachycephalic dog breeds have a variety of upper respiratory abnormalities that can result in respiratory compromise, including stenotic nares, elongated soft palate, and hyperplastic tongue (Dupre 2009).

Conducting airways consist of trachea, bronchi, and progressively smaller generations of bronchioles as the airways extend deeper into the lung. Animals performing for speed have progressively larger diameter airways to accommodate additional needed airflow. Some toy and brachycephalic dogs may have hypoplastic and/or collapsing tracheas that limit airflow and contribute to respiratory compromise (Dupre 2009). Terminal bronchioles lead to alveoli, where gas exchange with blood occurs. All of the airways but the alveoli are lined with ciliated and nonciliated pseudostratified columnar epithelial cells with a few goblet cells interspersed (Dungworth 1993). Mucus secreted by these cells traps inhaled particulates, and ciliary action propels the mucus and particulates upward toward the pharynx, where they are coughed up or swallowed. The most important of the alveolar epithelia are type II epithelial cells, which make the surfactant that forms a single layer and keeps the alveoli open and functioning. Release of significant serum protein will flood the alveoli (edema), reduce surfactant function, and allow the alveoli to stick together (atelectasis).

Deposition of Inhaled Particulates

Inhaled particulates that are >5 micrometers in diameter deposit in the nasopharyngeal region and larger conducting airways (Witschi et al. 2008). Smaller particles are transported to the deeper airways and alveoli; those deposited in bronchioles are phagocytized by bronchiolar macrophages, which travel via the mucociliary escalator to the pharynx, whereas those entering the alveoli are removed

Small Animal Toxicology Essentials, First Edition. Edited by Robert H. Poppenga, Sharon Gwaltney-Brant.
© 2011 John Wiley and Sons, Inc. Published 2011 by John Wiley and Sons, Inc.

by pulmonary macrophages and isolated in the interstitium or local lymph nodes.

MECHANISMS AND PATTERNS OF RESPIRATORY TRACT INJURY

Respiratory toxicants can exert their adverse effects to the respiratory tract in a variety of ways (Woods and Wilson 2004). Displacement asphyxia results when gases such as methane, carbon dioxide, and nitrogen displace oxygen in the immediate environment, resulting in hypoxia and hypoxemia. Gases that interfere with oxygen transport in the blood or oxygen release to tissues, such as cyanide or carbon monoxide, cause asphyxia in the presence of adequate environmental oxygen. Many inhaled toxicants exert their effect through irritation of the respiratory mucosa, resulting in damage to respiratory epithelium. Inhalation of respiratory irritants can result in loss of mucosal cells and breakdown of the protective barriers (e.g., mucociliary escalator) within the airways. Respiratory irritants that reach the alveoli can damage alveolar epithelium, resulting in loss of surfactant and atelectasis; in severe cases, necrosis of alveolar cells can result in leakage of serum or blood into alveoli and lower airways. Loss of alveolar surface area results in decreased oxygen exchange and hypoxia. Some toxicants enter the lung via the blood and may cause damage to the alveolar capillaries, resulting in noncardiogenic pulmonary edema. Other bloodborne toxicants cause damage to alveolar epithelial cells. Damage to alveolar epithelium or alveolar capillary endothelium may not manifest until several hours after the toxic insult, resulting in a delay in the onset of pulmonary edema of up to 24 hours following exposure to the toxicant (Smith 2005). Table 13.1 lists some respiratory toxicants and their action on the respiratory tract.

HEALING AND REPAIR

Epithelial Hyperplasia

Healing by epithelial hyperplasia (primary intent) is quite frequently the normal course of events following lung microinjury. In the smallest of these injuries, epithelial rearrangement is so successful that the tissue seems entirely normal. Function is normal and no veterinary intervention is needed.

Fibrosis

Healing by secondary intent, often called "pulmonary fibrosis," may be either reversible or irreversible depending on the degree of injury to the lung. When lung injury is too high, or intense or persists too long to heal spon-

Table 13.1. Respiratory toxicants

Mechanism	Toxicant
Displacement asphyxiation	Carbon dioxide
	Methane
	Natural gas
	Nitrogen gas
Oxygen transport asphyxiation	Carbon monoxide
	Cyanide
Airway irritation	Ammonia
	Chlorine
	Phosphine (zinc/aluminum phosphide)
Increased bronchial secretions	Anticholinesterase insecticides
	Muscarinic mushrooms (*Clitocybe, Inocybe*)
Pneumonia, aspiration	Hydrocarbons
	Iatrogenic (e.g., barium, activated charcoal)
Pulmonary edema	Chlorine
	Cisplatin (cats)
	Paraquat
	Phosphine (zinc/aluminum phosphide)
	Pine oil
	Sulfluryl fluoride (Vikane®)
Pulmonary fibrosis	Paraquat

taneously (e.g., with high levels of paraquat), fibroblasts will attempt to fill the void caused by death of the alveolar epithelial cells. Fibroblast proliferation impairs gas exchange, making a portion of the lung volume less functional than normal. If minimal to moderate alterations in pulmonary architecture are present the lung will spontaneously resolve (Pickrell et al. 1983). If greater alterations have been made to pulmonary architecture in response to high levels of alveolar damage, the interstitial fibrosis may become irreversible and form dense fibrous scars (Pickrell et al. 1983). The clinical implication of this change depends on the amount of lung tissue that is lost. In the case of paraquat, for example, the pulmonary injury tends to be progressive and ultimately the patient dies of asphyxia as fibrous connective tissue replaces functional lung tissue.

Emphysema

Emphysema has been defined as enlarged air space with tissue destruction (Pickrell 2007; Witschi et al. 2008). Loss of gas exchange membrane, specifically alveolar capillary membrane, causes a reduction in the gas exchange area; as the alveoli collapse, air spaces become distended and irregular, and the possibility of trapping air increases. This makes it difficult to get enough air to exchange (sometimes called "air hunger"). Minimal to no air exchange takes place in these alveoli. It is even more difficult to expel the air once it is in the distended alveoli. Clinically, dyspnea with forced expirations will be present. Emphysema is usually a progressive, ultimately terminal, condition as the airways continue to deteriorate over time.

LUNG CANCER

In humans, it has been estimated that 80%–90% of all lung tumors are caused by inhaling cigarette smoke (Witschi

et al. 2008). Dogs are companion animals that live with their owners over long periods of time. The most frequent tumors in dogs are mammary tumors, which may metastasize to the lung. Spontaneous lung tumors in companion animals such as dogs are much less frequent. Although infrequent, some dogs have developed either nasal or lung tumors after being exposed to their owner's second-hand cigarette smoke (Reif et al. 1992). These tumors were carcinomas, which are epithelial in origin and malignant. Dogs with long noses (dolichocephalic breeds) deposit the tumor-causing (carcinogenic) particles in the nasal cavity and develop nasal carcinomas. Dogs with shorter noses (brachycephalic breeds) allow the cigarette smoke particles to deposit in the upper airways and develop bronchogenic carcinomas (Reif et al. 1992).

CHAPTER 13 STUDY QUESTIONS

1. The function of the mucociliary escalator of the respiratory tree is to
   a. Filter out particulates to prevent them from entering deeper into the lung.
   b. Move trapped particulates up the respiratory tree to the pharyngeal area where they are coughed up or swallowed.
   c. Move particulate matter deeper into the bronchi, where the particulates are engulfed by bronchiolar macrophages.
   d. Move particulates to the rostral nasal area, where they are sneezed out.
   e. Prevent aspiration pneumonia by moving inhaled ingesta out of the lungs.

2. Small particulates entering the pulmonary alveoli undergo which fate?
   a. The particulates are moved up the respiratory tree via the mucociliary escalator.
   b. The particulates cross the alveolar wall and enter the bloodstream.
   c. The particulates are translocated to the alveolar interstitium, where they reside for the life of the animal.
   d. The particulates are coughed up out of the lung to the pharyngeal area where they are swallowed.
   e. The particulates are engulfed by pulmonary macrophages.

3. Direct injury to the respiratory tissues can result in all of the following except
   a. Loss of alveolar surfactant
   b. Noncardiogenic pulmonary edema

   c. Dysfunction of mucociliatory escalator
   d. Displacement asphyxia
   e. Atelectasis

4. Alterations to the respiratory system following injury may be reversible or permanent. Which of the following is a reversible change?
   a. Nasal carcinoma
   b. Epithelial hyperplasia
   c. Pulmonary fibrosis
   d. Emphysema
   e. Tracheal stricture

ANSWERS

1.b.

2.e. Particulates that manage to reach the alveoli are removed by pulmonary intraalveolar macrophages.

3.d. Displacement asphyxia occurs when a gas such as methane displaces oxygen, resulting in a hypoxic environment.

4.b. Hyperplasia is an increase in cell numbers caused by irritation or inflammation and is a reversible change. Fibrosis (pulmonary fibrosis or tracheal stricture), emphysema, and nasal carcinoma are permanent changes.

REFERENCES

Dungworth, D. 1993. The respiratory system. In *Pathology of Domestic Animals*, 4th ed., edited by K.V.F. Jubb, P.C. Kennedy, and N. Palmer, pp. 539–699. New York: Academic Press.

Dupre, G.P. 2009. Brachycephalic obstructive syndrome: diagnosis and underlying pathology. *Proceedings of the British Small Animal Veterinary Congress. Vienna, Austria.*

Pickrell, J.A. 2007. Respiratory toxicity. In *Veterinary Toxicology, Basic and Clinical Principles*, edited by Ramesh C. Gupta, pp. 193–205. New York: Elsevier.

Pickrell, John A., Diel, J.H., Slauson, D.O., Halliwell, W.H., and Mauderly, J.L. 1983. Radiation-induced pulmonary fibrosis resolves spontaneously if dense scars are not formed. *Experimental and Molecular Pathology* 38(1): 22–32.

Reif, J.S., Dunn, K., Ogilvie, G.K., and Harris, C.K. 1992. Passive smoking and canine lung cancer risk. *American Journal of Epidemiology* 135(3):234–239.

Smith, Dorsett D. 2005. Irritant and toxic respiratory injuries. In *Critical Care Toxicology*, edited by Jeffrey Brent et al., pp. 1011–1028. Philidelphia: Mosby-Elsevier.

Witschi, HansPeter, Pinkerton, Kent E., Van Winkle, Laura S., and Last, Jerold A. 2008. Toxic responses of the respiratory system. In *Casarett and Doull's Toxicology, the Basic Science of Poisons*, 6th ed., edited by Curtis D. Klaasen, pp. 609–630. New York: McGraw-Hill Medical.

Woods, Leslie W. and Wilson, Dennis W. 2004. Respiratory System. In *Clinical Veterinary Toxicology*, edited by Konnie H. Plumlee, pp. 80–88. St. Louis: Mosby.

Hepatobiliary System

14

Sharon Gwaltney-Brant

ANATOMY AND PHYSIOLOGY

The liver is situated in the proximal-most area of the peritoneal cavity immediately distal to the diaphragm and is divided into grossly distinguishable lobes. Closely associated with the ventral aspect of the liver in the dog and cat is the gall bladder. The liver plays a critical role in a variety of functions including nutrient homeostasis, filtration of particulates, protein synthesis, bioactivation, and detoxification, formation of bile and biliary secretion (Jaeschke 2008). Hepatic injury due to chemicals and drugs is the most common cause of acute liver failure in humans in the United States and is the leading cause of regulatory action against drugs (Watkins and Seef 2006). Epidemiologic studies into the incidence of drug- and chemical-induced liver injury in animals is lacking, but as the number of pharmaceuticals, neutraceuticals, and "natural" remedies for our companion animals increases, it is likely that the incidence of drug-induced liver injuries in companion animals will also increase.

Understanding the toxicologic changes that can occur in the liver requires understanding of its structural and functional anatomy. When viewed microscopically, the liver appears to be composed of hexagonal *lobules* surrounding a central blood vessel (*central vein*) and bordered by six *portal triads* at the outer edge of each lobule; each portal triad consists of a branch from each of the *hepatic artery*, *portal vein*, and *bile duct* (Figure 14.1). Between the portal triads and central vein are single-cell–wide cords of *hepatocytes* arranged radially around the central vein. Between the hepatocellular cords, *sinusoids* carry blood from the portal triads to the central vein. In this *lobule* model of the liver, the lobule is divided into three areas: the *centrilobular* region surrounding the central vein, the *periportal* region at the periphery of the lobule that incorporates the portal triads, and the *midzonal* region between the centrilobular and periportal regions. Pathology reports on liver histology frequently use these terms associated with the lobular model of the liver.

From a functional point of view, the hepatic lobule can be divided differently based on the flow of blood as it passes through the liver. Blood enters the liver lobule through branches of the hepatic artery (carrying oxygen) and the portal vein (carrying nutrients and other absorbed compounds, including toxicants, from the gastrointestinal tract) of the portal triads. The blood then filters within the sinusoids along the cords of hepatocytes until emptying into the central vein, giving up oxygen and picking up wastes as it passes from triad to central vein. Using the *acinar* model of the liver, the *acinus* is centered on a line from portal triad to portal triad. The area immediately around this line is termed *Zone 1* and is equivalent to the periportal region. *Zone 2* is equivalent to the midzonal region and *Zone 3* is equivalent to the centrilobular region. Zone 1 receives blood with the highest oxygen and nutrient content, and Zone 3 is relatively oxygen and nutrient depleted. For instance, blood in Zone 1 contains approximately 9%–13% oxygen compared to 4%–5% in Zone 3 (Bischoff and Ramaiah 2007).

From a toxicological perspective, the acinar model tends to be more relevant because it can help predict where in the liver toxicant-induced damage may occur (Table 14.1). Toxicants that are directly injurious to cells (e.g.,

Small Animal Toxicology Essentials, First Edition. Edited by Robert H. Poppenga, Sharon Gwaltney-Brant.

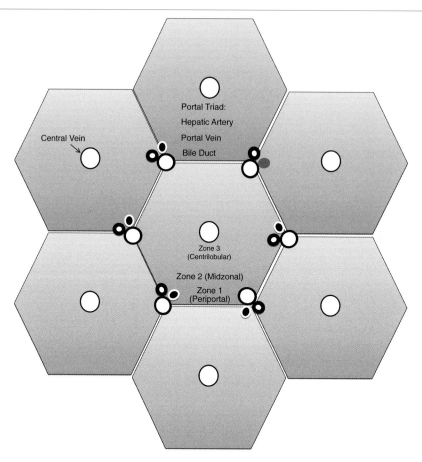

Figure 14.1. Schematic illustration of the microanatomy of the liver. Each hexagon represents a hepatic lobule centered around a central vein with portal triads at the periphery. The portal triads are each composed of a portal vein, hepatic artery, and bile duct. The central lobule is divided into the three anatomic and functional zones: Zone 1 or periportal region, Zone 2 or midzonal region, and Zone 3 or centrilobular region.

iron salts, white phosphorus) will cause damage to the first hepatocytes they encounter, thus injury from these types of toxicants appears primarily in Zone 1 (periportal). Zone 3 contains a higher level of cytochrome P450 metabolic enzymes, making this area most prone to injury from compounds that are bioactivated by these enzymes (e.g., acetaminophen). Some toxicants can produce hepatocellular injury so severe that zonal patterns are lost as the entire lobule undergoes *massive necrosis*, with necrosis extending from portal triads to central veins.

In contrast to blood flow through the hepatic acinus, *bile* flows from the *canaliculi* between hepatocytes into channels that empty into the bile ducts within the portal triad; these bile ducts in turn empty into the gall bladder, which stores and concentrates bile prior to emptying the bile into the duodenum (Bischoff and Ramaiah 2007). Bile is a complex mixture of bile acids, phospholipids, proteins, and other compounds that is important in the uptake of lipids from the small intestine, protection of the small intestine from oxidative injury, and the excretion of endogenous and xenobiotic compounds (Jaeschke 2008). Biliary excretion is an important route of elimination for certain xenobiotics (e.g., ivermectin, naproxen in dogs) that are poorly excreted through the urine. Compounds excreted through the bile may undergo *enterohepatic recirculation* whereby the compound that is excreted into the duodenum from the bile duct is then reabsorbed and reenters the portal and systemic circulations. Compounds that undergo enterohepatic recirculation tend to have half-lives that are measured in days rather than hours. For example, naproxen in humans is eliminated primarily through the kidneys and has a half-life of about 6 hours. In dogs, naproxen is elimi-

Table 14.1. Patterns of hepatotoxicity

Causes of Nonzonal Hepatic Injury
NSAIDs
Cyclophosphamide
Phenobarbital
Phenytoin
Sulfonamides
Ketoconazole

Causes of Zone 1 (Periportal) Hepatic Injury
Aflatoxin
Iron salts
Organic arsenic
White phosphorus

Causes of Zone 2 (Midzonal) Hepatic Injury
Cisplatin
Hexachlorophene (cats)

Causes of Zone 3 (Centrilobular) Hepatic Injury
Acetaminophen
Aflatoxin
Blue-green algae
Castor bean (*Ricinus*)
Chloroform
Cycad palms (*Cycas, Zamia*)
Diazepam (cats)
Hepatotoxic mushrooms (e.g., Amanita phalloides*)*
Naphthaene
NSAIDs (e.g., carprofen, ibuprofen)
Phenols
Xylitol

Causes of Massive Hepatic Necrosis
Acetaminophen
Cisplatin
Cycad palms (*Cycas, Zamia*)
Diazepam (cats)
Iron
Mebendazole (dogs)
Microcystin LR (*Microcystis aeruginosa*)

Sources: Bischoff and Ramaiah 2007, Haschek et al. 2007.

nated through the bile, undergoes enterohepatic recycling and has a half-life of 74 hours (Frey and Rieh 1981; Talcott 2006).

MECHANISMS OF TOXICOLOGIC INJURY

The mechanisms behind hepatic injury can be divided into two categories: intrinsic and idiosyncratic. Intrinsic liver injury is a dose-dependent, predictable reaction to a toxicant and it is the most common type of liver injury in animals (Bischoff and Ramaiah 2007). There is frequently a predictable latent period between exposure to the toxicant and the development of clinical signs of liver insufficiency. Intrinsic liver injury is often caused by highly reactive by-products of xenobiotic metabolism, especially free radicals and electrophiles. Idiosyncratic liver injury is an unpredictable response to a xenobiotic. Idiosyncratic reactions are rare and non–dose-dependent and may be associated with extrahepatic lesions. Idiosyncratic reactions frequently occur following unremarkable initial exposure (sensitization) and manifest upon reexposure to the xenobiotic. With idiosyncratic drug reactions, it is not uncommon for there to be a delay of a few weeks to several months between the time of initial exposure and development of liver injury. Extrahepatic changes may include fever and dermal erythema or rash.

Free Radical–Induced Injury

The generation of free radicals within hepatocytes can occur during xenobiotic biotransformation, normal metabolic processes involving oxidation/reduction reactions, inflammatory states (mediated by nitric oxide (NO)), and exposure to ionizing radiation (Bischoff and Ramaiah 2007). Free radicals have unpaired electrons, which make them highly susceptible to binding to other macromolecules, including lipoproteins of cell membranes, enzymatic proteins, and DNA. Binding of free radicals to cellular macromolecules generates even more free radical production, resulting in an escalating effect. Normally cells have scavenger molecules (e.g., glutathione) to react with and detoxify free radicals, but excessive free radical production can result in depletion of scavenger stores, resulting in increased binding of free radicals to vital cellular structures. Free radical damage can cause alterations of cell membrane permeability, inactivation of membrane-associated proteins, and loss of polarity to mitochondrial membranes. Inactivation of enzymatic proteins can interfere with normal cellular metabolism, leading to cellular degeneration or necrosis. Free radical-induced DNA damage can result in interference with transcription or translation, resulting in decreased protein synthesis.

Calcium Homeostasis Disruption

Within the cell, calcium is sequestered within organelles such as mitochondria and endoplasmic reticulum, which maintain a relatively low level of calcium within the cytosol. Xenobiotics that interfere with the pumps that maintain calcium balance can result in increased release of calcium into the cytosol. The released calcium ions impede normal cytoskeletal function and activate a variety of cytosolic enzymes including ATPases, phospholipases and proteases. Subsequently, mitochondrial membrane permeability increases, which causes induction of necrosis and apoptosis (programmed cell death) (Bischoff and Ramaiah 2007).

Mitochondrial Injury

Mitochondria are the source of energy production within the cell, and toxicants that disrupt mitochondrial function can result in cell death. Toxicants induce mitochondrial injury by altering mitochondrial DNA, interfering with oxidative phosphorylation, damaging mitochondrial membranes, or inactivating mitochondrial enzymes.

Cytoskeletal Disruption

The cytoskeleton of the cell is vital to maintaining normal shape and position of hepatocytes. Agents that damage cytoskeletal structure result in cellular deformation and detachment. The blue-green algae toxin microcystin-LR, produced by *Microcystis aeruginosa* causes hepatocellular cytoskeletal injury and severe liver damage (Haschek et al. 2007).

Cholestasis

Toxicants that interfere with bile transport can result in cholestasis, leading to injury to biliary ducts and hepatocytes. Bile duct hyperplasia and biliary fibrosis may result. Cholestasis can also occur secondary to hepatocellular swelling due to degeneration or lipidosis. Clinically, cholestatic disorders can result in dermal photosensitization, whereby areas of skin exposed to the sun develop burns similar to sunburn. Epidermal and dermal burns from photosensitization are rapid in onset and occur following exposure to wavelengths of light that would cause no injury in normal animals. Animals with white areas on their haircoats and upigmented skin are most susceptible to photosensitization. In veterinary medicine, photosensitization is more commonly seen in large animals grazing plants that cause bile stasis, but it has occasionally been reported in dogs with hepatic injury.

Idiosyncratic Reactions

Many idiosyncratic drug reactions are considered to be immune-mediated, triggered by the formation of adducts of reactive drug metabolites with cellular macromolecules. These adducts are identified by the immune system as foreign, and an immune response is mounted, leading to death of individual hepatocytes ("piecemeal necrosis").

This mechanism has been postulated, but not proven, as the mechanism by which the nonsteroidal anti-inflammatory drug carprofen causes idiosyncratic liver injury in dogs (McPhail et al. 1998). The exact mechanisms of other types of idiosyncratic liver injury await further study to be elucidated.

PATTERNS OF TOXICOLOGIC INJURY

Toxic hepatic injury can manifest as hepatocellular degeneration, hepatocellular necrosis, immune-mediated injury, biliary disorders, and sinusoidal disorders.

Hepatocellular Degeneration

Hepatocellular degeneration is a common, nonspecific response of the liver to toxic insult. Hepatocellular degeneration represents a sublethal insult to the liver that can often resolve if the inciting cause is removed. Although some cellular processes may be altered, the degenerative hepatocyte still retains some degree of functional integrity. Degenerating hepatocytes are generally swollen and may accumulate various compounds, including metals, pigments, water, and lipids. It is important to realize that in most situations the accumulation of these compounds is a *result* of some form of hepatocellular dysfunction rather than the primary *cause* of hepatocellular degeneration.

Hepatic Lipidosis

Hepatic lipidosis (steatosis, fatty liver) is a form of hepatocellular degeneration characterized by accumulation of lipid within the hepatocyte cytosol. Lipidosis can be the result of transient disruptions in lipid metabolism, or it can reflect a more serious metabolic condition. Severe lipid accumulation can result in sufficient hepatocellular swelling to cause cholestasis.

Hepatocellular Necrosis or Apoptosis

Both hepatocellular necrosis and apoptosis represent death of hepatocytes with the difference being that apoptosis is a controlled, orderly "shutdown" of cellular processes leading to death of the cell. Necrosis occurs when cells are subject to insurmountable insults resulting in loss of cellular membrane integrity and disruption of cellular machinery. What follows is cellular swelling, leakage of cellular contents into the adjacent environment, disintegration of nuclear material and an influx of inflammatory cells to remove cellular debris (Jaeschke 2008). Because the necrotizing insult is generally locally intense, whole groups of hepatocytes, as well as support structures, may be affected. In contrast, apoptosis results when enzymes termed *caspases* trigger the activation of various cytosolic and nuclear enzymes that compartmentalize cellular structures and proceed to shut down cellular activity. Apoptotic cells are shrunken, with condensed cytosol and fragmented nuclei that pinch off along with the cell membrane (which has remained intact) to form *apoptotic bodies*. Apoptotic bodies are then phagocytized by hepatic macrophages (Kuppfer cells) or are taken up into adjacent hepatocytes without inciting an inflammatory response. Apoptosis is the means by which normal tissues eliminate unneeded or senescent cells, and it generally affects single cells. Apoptosis can be triggered by a variety of external stimuli, including ionizing radiation, drugs (NSAIDs, corticosteroids), and physiologic conditions such as stress.

HEALING AND REPAIR

The liver has a tremendous capacity for regeneration—so much so that human liver transplants can be done from liver lobes donated by living donors. Following successful transplant, both recipient and donor will eventually regenerate sufficient hepatic parenchyma to have normal liver function. As with most organs that have regenerative ability, the capacity to regenerate is dependent upon the retention of the basic tissue scaffold. Conditions that result in loss of this scaffold can result in hepatic healing via fibrosis instead. Fibrosis occurs most commonly along the terminal plates at the edges of the hepatic lobule and surrounding the central vein. Fibrous tissue that bridges between portal triad and central vein can result in loss of functional integrity of the acinus. Regenerative nodules of hepatocytes within bands of fibrous tissue are often disconnected from access to central veins and are minimally functional. *Cirrhosis* is the term in human medicine for the end-stage form of liver injury, with irregular patches of fibrous tissue surrounding rounded nodules of hepatocytes.

Although the liver has a high regenerative capacity, massive acute loss of hepatocytes can result in death from liver failure if insufficient hepatocytes remain to allow the patient to survive long enough for regenerated hepatocytes to begin to function.

CHAPTER 14 STUDY QUESTIONS

1. Milo, a 2-year-old, 135-pound, neutered male St. Bernard dog has been successfully treated for acute hepatic insufficiency. A liver biopsy had been taken and the pathology report indicated that there was substantial centrilobular necrosis. All of the following toxicants are potential causes for Milo's liver injury except
   a. Iron
   b. Blue-green algae
   c. Acetaminophen
   d. Hepatotoxic mushrooms
   e. Xylitol

2. In what way does enterohepatic recirculation alter the kinetics of a xenobiotic?
   a. Increases elimination
   b. Increases absorption
   c. Shortens the half-life
   d. Lengthens the half-life
   e. Enhances metabolism

3. Intrinsic liver injury is characterized by all of the following except
   a. Dose-dependent
   b. Predictable latent period
   c. Rare in animals
   d. Often caused by free radicals and electrophiles
   e. Predictable clinical course

4. Blue-green algae induce liver injury by which of the following mechanisms?
   a. Free radical formation
   b. Disruption of calcium homeostasis
   c. Cytoskeletal damage
   d. Immune-mediated mechanisms
   e. Cholestasis

ANSWERS

1.a. Iron causes primarily periportal or Zone 1 injury in the liver.

2.d. Enterohepatic recirculation increases the half-life of a xenobiotic.

3.c. Intrinsic liver injury is the most common type of liver injury identified in animals.

4.c. Blue-green algae disrupt the structural support of hepatocytes resulting in cytoskeletal failure.

REFERENCES

Bischoff, Karen and Ramaiah, Sashi K. 2007. Liver toxicity. In *Veterinary Toxicology: Basic and Clinical Principles*, edited by Ramesh C. Gupta, pp. 145–160. New York: Elsevier.

Frey, H.H. and Rieh, B. 1981. Pharmacokinetics of naproxen in the dog. *American Journal of Veterinary Research* 42(9):1615–1617.

Haschek, Wanda M., Rousseaux, Colin G., and Wallig, Matthew A. 2007. The liver. In *Fundamentals of Toxicologic Pathology*, 2nd ed., pp. 197–235. San Diego: Academic Press-Elsevier.

Jaeschke, Hartmut. 2008. Toxic responses of the liver. In *Casarett and Doull's Toxicology, the Basic Science of Poisons*, 6th ed., edited by Curtis D. Klaasen, pp. 557–582. New York: McGraw-Hill Medical.

McPhail, C.M., Lappin, M.R., Meyer, D.J., Smith, S.G., Webster, C.R., and Armstrong, P.J. 1998. Hepatocellular toxicosis associated with administration of carprofen in 21 dogs. *Journal of the American Veterinary Medical Association* 212(12):1895–1901.

Moeller, Robert B. 2004. Hepatobiliary system: Toxic response of the hepatobiliary system. In *Veterinary Clinical Toxicology*, edited by Konnie H. Plumlee, pp. 61–68. St. Louis: Mosby.

Plumlee, Konnie H. 2004. Hepatobiliary system: differential diagnosis. In *Veterinary Clinical Toxicology*, edited by Konnie H. Plumlee, p. 61. St. Louis: Mosby.

Talcott, Patricia A. 2006. Nonsteroidal antiinflammatories. In *Small Animal Toxicology*, 2nd ed., edited by Michael E. Peterson and Patricia A. Talcott, pp. 902–933. St. Louis: Saunders.

Watkins, P.B., Seef, L.B. 2006. Drug-induced liver injury: summary of a single topic clinical research conference. *Hepatology* 43:618–631.

Urinary System

15

Erin Freed

INTRODUCTION

This chapter focuses on the basic anatomy and physiology of the urinary system, the mechanisms and patterns of toxicological injury including common toxic substances that affect the urinary system, and the healing and repair after toxicological damage.

ANATOMY AND PHYSIOLOGY

The urinary system of dogs and cats consists of the kidneys, ureters, bladder, and the urethra. The function of the urinary system is to filter blood, reabsorb important nutrients, and eliminate wastes in the form of urine. The kidneys regulate the amount of water reabsorbed and excreted, maintain the pH of the blood, and control the concentration of electrolytes (Na, K, Ca, and Cl), proteins, and hormones in the blood. Additionally, the kidneys secrete hormones that regulate blood pressure, water balance, red blood cell production, and calcium homeostasis (Haschek et al. 2007).

The kidneys receive approximately 25% of the cardiac output and can be divided into three main parts: the outer cortex, which receives 90% of the renal blood flow; the medulla, which receives 6%–10% of blood flow; and renal papilla, which receives 1%–2% of the total renal blood flow.

The functional unit of the kidney is the nephron, which is composed of a glomerulus, proximal convoluted tubule, loop of Henle, distal tubule, and collecting duct. The glomerulus is composed of an anastomosing tuft of fenestrated endothelial cells that form a filter for the blood, with the initial filtrate flowing into Bowman's space surrounding the glomerulus and progressing into the proximal tubule. The renal tubules reabsorb 60%–80% of the filtered solute, including water, electrolytes, glucose, amino acids, small peptides, and organic acids. In the medulla, the loops of Henle play a major role in the concentration of urine and maintenance of the blood's electrolyte balance. The filtrate then passes into collecting ducts, which control the excretion rates of electrolytes and urea as well as further maintain acid/ base and water balances. The renal papilla empties the urine through the renal pelvis into the ureters. From the ureters the urine passes into the bladder where it is stored until it is excreted through the urethra.

Renal function is largely measured clinically by the serum renal markers blood urea nitrogen (BUN) and creatinine; due to reserve capacity of the kidney, approximately 50%–75% of nephrons must be damaged before these values become significantly elevated. *Azotemia*, the term for elevations of serum BUN and creatinine, can occur due to prerenal, renal, and postrenal causes. Prerenal azotemia is most commonly the result of dehydration and occurs without renal insufficiency. Renal azotemia is caused by kidney dysfunction, generally due to injury by infectious, metabolic, toxic, or neoplastic processes. Postrenal azotemia is usually associated with obstruction of urine outflow (e.g., bladder "stones"), resulting in a back pressure of urine within the kidney that decreases glomerular filtration. Determination of whether azotemia is prerenal, renal, or postrenal is essential to aid in diagnosis and therapeutic management of the patient. When

Small Animal Toxicology Essentials, First Edition. Edited by Robert H. Poppenga, Sharon Gwaltney-Brant.
© 2011 John Wiley and Sons, Inc. Published 2011 by John Wiley and Sons, Inc.

azotemia is present along with the clinical signs associated with renal failure (vomiting, gastrointestinal bleeding, gastritis, oliguria/anuria/polyuria), the condition is termed *uremia*.

MECHANISMS OF TOXICOLOGICAL INJURY

Renal tubular injury is the most common form of nephrotoxic insult in animals (Haschek et al. 2007). Tubular damage may result from direct injury to the epithelial cells by the toxicant or its metabolites, from mechanical obstruction of the tubules, from mineralization of the basement membrane, or from ischemia due to vasoconstriction of renal blood vessels. Toxicants such as lead, arsenic, aminoglycoside antibiotics, and many anticancer drugs cause direct injury to the tubular epithelium. Renal epithelium, particularly in the proximal tubules, contains high levels of metabolic enzymes that can detoxify some compounds present in the filtrate. However, other compounds (e.g., diquat, acetaminophen) can be bioactivated into toxic metabolites by these same enzymes and result in injury to the epithelial cells. Pigments such as hemoglobin (e.g., due to intravascular hemolysis from zinc toxicosis) or myoglobin (e.g., due to muscle damage from monensin toxicosis in dogs) are also directly injurious to renal tubular epithelium.

Some toxicants will result in the precipitation of crystals into the urine as the tubular filtrate becomes more concentrated. Overdoses of drugs such as penicillins, cephalosporins, and acyclovir may result in transient crystalluria, and the crystals can cause mild epithelial damage, which is usually reversible. Tubular obstruction by calcium oxalate crystals is a major cause of renal injury in ethylene glycol intoxication; however, direct tubular epithelial injury due to acidosis also contributes to lesions seen in ethylene glycol toxicosis. Mineralization (deposition of calcium) of renal tubules can result from hypercalcemia associated with some toxicoses (e.g., cholecalciferol rodenticide toxicosis) and can also occur as a sequel of uremia. Mineralization along the tubular basement membrane, within epithelial cells, and within renal blood vessels (impeding blood flow) results in degeneration and necrosis of tubular epithelial cells, cell sloughing, and decreased tubular regenerative ability.

Agents that cause vasoconstriction can impede glomerular filtration as well as cause ischemic damage to the renal tubules. The renal papilla is especially susceptible to ischemic injury because it normally receives only 1% of total renal blood flow, but any portion of the nephron may be affected. Nonsteroidal anti-inflammatory drugs (NSAIDs; e.g., ibuprofen, aspirin, phenylbutazone) decrease prostaglandin levels within the kidney, decreasing prostaglandin-mediated vasodilation and resulting in vessel constriction (Sebastian et al. 2007). Other agents (e.g., the antifungal amphotericin B) induce vasoconstriction by direct interaction with renal arterioles (Sawaya et al. 1995).

Injury to renal tubules impairs water and solute reabsorption, resulting in dilute urine (isosthenuria) due to loss of concentrating ability, as well as spillage of amino acids, glucose, small peptides, and other solutes into the urine. Polyuria will occur unless the tubules become obstructed by swollen tubular epithelium, crystals, sloughed epithelial cells, pigments, or other debris; in these instances oliguria or anuria can occur. When blockages occur, increased tubular pressure counteracts the capillary hydrostatic pressure in the glomerulus, resulting in further decrease in glomerular filtration. A nephron that has damaged tubules can leak filtrate into the systemic circulation, contributing to azotemia as BUN and creatinine are reintroduced into the bloodstream from the damaged tubules.

PATTERNS OF TOXICOLOGICAL INJURY

Nephrotoxic agents can cause renal insufficiency that may progress to acute renal failure (ARF) or chronic renal failure (CRF) depending on the toxicant involved, dose, and duration of exposure. ARF often results from exposure to a relatively high dose of a nephrotoxic agent, causing sudden loss of kidney function, whereas CRF tends to occur more insidiously and may be the result of repeated insults to the kidney (e.g., from repeated exposures to nephrotoxins over time) or it may reflect progression of acute disease. An individual may be more or less susceptible to toxic renal damage due to genetic factors, age, prior renal disease, general overall health, or concurrent medication administration. Patients with CRF oftentimes adapt to their renal disease and may maintain a relatively normal clinical appearance for quite some time in spite of fairly high elevations of serum BUN and creatinine (compensated CRF). Generally, these patients display polyuric renal failure and are able to maintain themselves, provided they have access to adequate fresh water in order to compensate for the increased fluid losses. However, with progression of the renal disease or sudden change in hydration status, these patients may suddenly decompensate and present with clinical signs similar to an ARF patient.

Because of its high blood flow, high metabolic activity and concentration of wastes, the kidney is especially susceptible to toxic injury. While the glomeruli and proximal tubules are exposed to large amounts of bloodborne toxicants, the more distal aspects of the nephron and lower urinary tract are exposed to higher concentrations of toxicants for a greater period of time as a result of accumulation of toxicants within tubular lumens.

Renal toxicants may cause glomerular damage, resulting in a decrease in glomerular filtration and resulting in azotemia, or increasing the "pore" size of the glomerular filter resulting in the leakage of proteins into the urine. Renal toxicants affecting glomeruli are rare in animals, although some rattlesnake venoms have been associated with glomerular injury (Fitzgerald and Rumbeiha 2004).

Their relatively high metabolic activity, high content of metabolic enzymes, and closer proximity to glomerular filtrate make the proximal tubules more susceptible to a wider range of toxicants than the rest of the nephron (Sebastian et al. 2007). In domestic animals, the proximal renal tubules are most commonly affected by nephrotoxicants, although the distribution of tubular lesions can vary depending on the toxicant involved. For example, tubular injury from melamine:cyanuric acid crystals, the lesion seen in kidneys of animals affected by melamine-contaminated pet foods in the U.S. in 2007, tends to occur in the distal tubules and collecting ducts, whereas calcium oxalate crystals from ethylene glycol metabolism tend to affect primarily the proximal tubules (Puschner et al. 2007). In nephrons undergoing degeneration necrosis, affected tubular cells will swell (degeneration) and then shrink and slough. Cellular debris from damaged tubules manifests as granular casts in the urine sediment.

Damage to the renal papilla can disrupt loops of Henle, resulting in loss of urine-concentrating ability as well as electrolyte imbalances.

Toxic damage to the distal areas of the urinary tract—renal pelvis, ureters, urethra, and bladder—is relatively uncommon. The rapid flushing of urine through the pelvis, ureters, and urethra may explain their relative resistance to toxicologic injury. The urinary bladder, because it stores urine, has occasionally been associated with syndromes arising from toxicants (e.g., cyclophosphamide-induced cystitis).

HEALING AND REPAIR OF THE URINARY SYSTEM

Because much of the nephron is comprised of epithelial cells there is potential for cellular regeneration following toxic injury, provided the tubular basement membrane has remained intact and adequate residual epithelial cells are present. Regeneration of tubular epithelium is usually visible microscopically within 3 days of insult, but it can take up to 3 weeks for the tubules to return to normal structure (Haschek et al. 2007) and up to several more weeks for return to full renal function. The glomerulus tends to be less forgiving, and glomeruli damaged by toxic insults may be permanently dysfunctional (Table 15.1).

Table 15.1. Nephrotoxicants

Lesion	Toxicant	Species
Nephrosis (renal tubular degeneration and necrosis)	Metals (lead, mercury, arsenic, cadmium)	Dogs, cats
	Nonsteroidal anti-inflammatory drugs (e.g., ibuprofen, aspirin, phenylbutazone, carprofen, deracoxib)	Dogs, cats
	Lilies (*Lilium* or *Hemerocallis*)	Cats only
	Grapes/raisins/Zante currants/Sultanas (*Vitis* spp.)	Dogs, (cats anecdotal only)
	Antineoplastics (e.g., cisplatin)	Dogs, cats
	Diquat/paraquat	Dogs, cats
	Ethylene glycol	Dogs, cats
	Zinc phosphide	Dogs, cats
	Melamine	Dogs, cats
	Amphotericin B	Dogs, cats
Mineralization	Cholecalciferol and analogues (vitamin D_3, cholecalciferol rodenticides, calcitriol, calcipotriene)	Dogs, cats
Glomerular injury	Rattlesnake venom	Dogs, cats
Bladder injury	Cyclophosphamide	Dogs, cats

CHAPTER 15 STUDY QUESTIONS

1. The most common form of renal injury in animals is
   a. Glomerular injury
   b. Renal tubular injury
   c. Interstitial injury
   d. Tubulointerstitial injury
   e. Papillary necrosis

2. In renal tubular injury, the most common manifestation is _____ except when massive necrosis of tubular epithelial cells results in occlusion of the lumens of renal tubules, in which case _____ or _____ may occur.
   a. Anuria, polyuria, oliguria
   b. Oliguria, polyuria, anuria
   c. Oliguria, anuria, polyuria
   d. Polyuria, oliguria, anuria
   e. Anuria, oliguria, polyuria

3. Cellular debris from damaged renal tubules can be seen in the urinary sediment in the form of
   a. Hyaline casts
   b. Oxalate crystals
   c. Granular casts
   d. Struvites
   e. Dhole bodies

4. The ability of renal tubular epithelium to regenerate depends on the presence of sufficient residual cells and on the integrity of the
   a. Renal papilla
   b. Interstitium
   c. Glomerular mesangium
   d. Renal tubular basement membrane
   e. Vascular endothelium

ANSWERS

1.b. Tubular injury is the most common form of renal injury in animals.

2.d. Polyuric renal insufficiency is the most common manifestation of renal tubular injury.

3.c. Granular casts.

4.d. The integrity of the tubular basement membrane is considered an essential factor in whether tubular epithelium can regenerate following an injury.

REFERENCES

Fitzgerald, S.D. and Rumbeiha, W.K. 2004. Urinary system. In *Clinical Veterinary Toxicology*, edited by Konnie H. Plumlee, pp. 91–96. St. Louis: Mosby.

Haschek, Wanda M., Rousseaux, Colin G., and Wallig, Matthew A. 2007. Kidney and lower urinary tract. In *Fundamentals of Toxicologic Pathology*, 2nd ed., pp. 261–371. San Diego: Academic Press.

Puschner, Birgit, Poppenga, Robert H., Lowenstine, L.J., Filigenzi, M.S., and Pesavento, P.A. 2007. Assessment of melamine and cyanuric acid toxicity in cats. *Journal of Veterinary Diagnostic Investigation* 19(6):616–624.

Sawaya, B.P., Briggs, J.P., and Schnemann, J. 1995. Amphotericin B nephrotoxicity: The adverse consequences of altered membrane properties. *Journal of the American Society of Nephrology* 6(2):154–164.

Sebastian, M.M., Baskin, S.I., Czerwinski, S.E. 2007. Renal toxicity. In *Veterinary Toxicology: Basic and Clinical Principles*, edited by Ramesh C. Gupta, pp. 161–176. San Diego: Elsevier.

Other Systems

16

Sharon Gwaltney-Brant DVM, PhD

ALIMENTARY TRACT

Making a diagnosis of alimentary tract toxicosis is difficult because, in dogs and cats, there are numerous conditions that can cause gastrointestinal signs (nausea, hypersalivation, vomiting, abdominal discomfort, and diarrhea) that are not toxic in nature. When presented with a patient displaying gastrointestinal signs, the list of potential differential diagnoses is quite long and not easily shortened; one must avoid the temptation to decide "it must be toxic" just because an obvious answer is not immediately forthcoming. Patients presenting with gastrointestinal signs should be worked up thoroughly to rule out other potential etiologies. Infectious, inflammatory, metabolic, nutritional, neoplastic, and mechanical (e.g., foreign body) diseases need to be considered in addition to toxic agents. Table 16.1 lists toxicants that have a primary effect on the gastrointestinal tract.

Many agents that damage the alimentary tract do so by causing erosion or ulceration to the tissues (Haschek et al. 2007). *Erosion* is the loss of integrity of the superficial mucosal (epithelial) layer of the alimentary tract. *Ulceration* occurs when the lesions extend deeper into the tissues, penetrating into the blood vessels and tissues of the submucosa. *Perforation* is a full thickness defect in the wall of the gastrointestinal tract leading to leakage of ingesta into the pleural (esophageal perforation) or peritoneal cavity.

Oral Cavity

The most common toxicological injuries to the oral cavity are direct irritation or corrosion. Irritants (e.g., insoluble calcium oxalate crystals) cause discomfort and possibly mild erythema but do not compromise the integrity of the oral mucosa. Corrosive agents (acids, alkalis, cationic detergents) cause chemical burns to the tissues of the oral cavity which can result in severe pain, extensive tissue damage and, potentially, sloughing of oral tissues (e.g., tongue). In severe cases, damage to pharyngeal and/or esophageal tissues may also occur.

Gastrointestinal Tract

Toxic injury to the gastrointestinal tract can occur through several mechanisms (Haschek et al. 2007). Mild gastrointestinal irritation can occur from agents such as hydrocarbons, household detergents, and insoluble calcium oxalate containing plants. These agents will cause local irritation, leading to nausea (often manifested by hypersalivation), vomiting, and/or diarrhea, but they are not appreciably absorbed and are not expected to cause any systemic signs (note: volatile hydrocarbons such as gasoline have a high risk of aspiration if vomiting occurs, which can result in aspiration pneumonia; see Chapter 28, "Household and Industrial Toxicants"). Intense vomiting caused by these agents may result in rupture of gastric blood vessels, leading to blood-tinged vomitus. Corrosive injury resulting in erosion, ulceration, and/or perforation of the gastrointestinal tract can occur through ingestion of corrosive agents such as acids or alkalis (e.g., leaking alkaline batteries), resulting in gastrointestinal hemorrhage. Agents that alter blood supply to the gastrointestinal mucosa (e.g., nonsteroidal anti-inflammatory drugs, arsenic) can cause injury due to hypoxia, resulting in

Table 16.1. Toxicants affecting the gastrointestinal tract

Mechanism (Clinical Effects)	Toxicant	Comment
Irritation (hypersalivation, nausea, vomiting, diarrhea, abdominal discomfort)	Bleach	Household bleaches are irritants; industrial/commercial strength may be corrosive
	Boric acid	Ant baits, borax powder
	Cycad palms	Primary concern is liver injury
	Detergents	Household cleaners, shampoos, and soaps
	Fertilizers	Other ingredients (e.g., insecticides, herbicides) may pose other risks
	Hydrocarbons/petroleum products	Risk of aspiration of volatile hydrocarbons
	Ice melts	See corrosive injury
	Insoluble calcium oxalate-containing plants	*Aglaonema, Alocasia, Colocasia, Anthurium, Arisaema, Arum, Caladium, Calla, Dieffenbachia, Epipremnum, Monstera, Philodendron, Scindapsius, Spathiphyllum, Symplocarpus, Syngonium, Xanthosoma, Zantedeschia* and others
	Ornamental bulb plants	*Amaryllus, Crocus, Hyacinthus, Iris, Narcissus, Tulipa*, and others
	Zinc	U.S. pennies minted after 1983 (also cause hemolysis), zinc oxide ointments
Corrosive injury (similar to irritants but more severe; can see oral, pharyngeal, or esophageal burns; gastric ulceration, hematemesis, melena, or hematochezia)	Acids	Car/boat batteries, drain openers, oven cleaners, etching compounds, gun barrel cleaners, pool sanitizers, rust removers
	Alkalis	Anhydrous lime, cement, drain openers, fabric softeners, industrial strength bleaches, liquid dishwasher detergents, low phosphate laundry detergents, pool chemicals
	Batteries	Car/boat batteries contain acid; alkaline and disk batteries contain alkali
	Calcium chloride ice melts	Corrosive to GI tract and skin
	Cationic detergents	Disinfectants, sanitizers, pool algicides
	Essential oils	Concentrated forms can be corrosive
	Phenols	Concentrations <5% are corrosive; lower concentrations are found in household cleaners, sore-throat lozenges, gargles, ointments, mouthwashes
Altered mucosal blood flow (leads to gastrointestinal hemorrhage)	Arsenic	Damages endothelium of gastrointestinal mucosa causing submucosal hemorrhage
	Cadmium	Inhibition of prostaglandin formation, resulting in decreased blood flow
	NSAIDs	Inhibition of prostaglandin formation, resulting in decreased blood flow

Table 16.1. *Continued*

Mechanism (Clinical Effects)	Toxicant	Comment
Epithelial cell necrosis (hemorrhagic gastroenteritis, ±mucosal shreds)	5-Fluorouracil	Topical treatments for skin cancers, dermatosis
	Abrus precatoris (precatory pea, rosary pea)	Damage to seed coat (e.g., chewing) allows toxin release
	Colchicine	Pharmaceutical, autumn crocus (*Colchicum*), glory lily (*Gloriosa*)
	Corrosives	See above.
	Iron salts	Vitamins, fertilizers, hand warmers
	Methotrexate	Rheumatoid arthritis medications, anticancer therapy
	Quercus spp. (Oak)	Tannins are toxic principle precipitate proteins
	Ricinus communis (Castor bean)	Damage to seed coat (e.g., chewing) allows toxin release
Impeded nutrient or water absorption	Cadmium	Inhibits calcium absorption, alters fat and protein metabolism
(weight loss, dehydration)	Ethanol	Reduces absorption of B vitamins and carbohydrates
	Laxatives	Increases gastrointestinal transit time resulting in decreased time for nutrient absorption; osmotic laxatives can decrease free body water stores
Altered motility		
Hypomotility (constipation, obstipation, ileus)	Opioids	Decreases gastric emptying and gut contractility through local and central effects
Hypermotility (watery diarrhea, ±blood)	Organophosphorus or carbamate insecticides	Overstimulation of cholinergic receptors enhances GI smooth muscle contraction

necrosis, ulceration, and/or perforation. Toxicants that damage the rapidly dividing cells of the mucosal crypts (e.g., colchicine, 5-fluorouracil) can result in villous atrophy and loss of absorptive capacity of the gastrointestinal tract; this type of injury is sometimes termed *radiomimetic* because the lesion resembles that seen following exposure to ionizing radiation. Some gastrointestinal toxicants alter the absorption of water or nutrients without causing significant physical derangement of gastrointestinal tissues. For example, cadmium can alter the absorption of calcium from the gastrointestinal tract (Haschek et al. 2007), while compounds having a laxative effect (e.g., high viscosity hydrocarbons) can result in decreased nutrient absorption due to rapid gastrointestinal transit time as well as increased water loss due to diarrhea. Other toxicants can reduce (e.g., opioids) or increase (e.g., organophosphorous insecticides) motility by altering the neuromuscular activity of the gastrointestinal tract.

HEMATOPOIETIC

Alteration in the number, structure, or function of hematic cells (red blood cells, white blood cells, platelets) can occur from a variety of toxicants (Haschek et al. 2007a). Some agents (e.g., estrogen, 5-fluorouracil) can result in suppression of bone marrow with decreased red and/or white blood cell production. Other agents (e.g., lead) can cause anemia by inhibition of enzymes that allow normal red blood cell maturation. Certain oxidative compounds (e.g., acetaminophen metabolites, garlic) can denature hemoglobin to form methemoglobin within red blood cells. Other oxidants (e.g., zinc, naphthalene) cause non–immune-mediated hemolytic anemia. Platelet function can

Table 16.2. Toxicants affecting the hematopoietic system

Mechanism	Toxicant	Comments
Hemolytic anemia	*Allium* spp.	Onions, garlic, etc.; powdered, concentrated forms more toxic
	Crotalid snake venom	Direct RBC membrane damage
	Naphthalene	Mothballs, urinal disks, toilet bowl blocks
	Propylene glycol	Heinz body anemia in cats
	Zinc	U.S. pennies minted after 1983; other zinc-containing hardware; zinc oxide ointments
Methemoglobinemia	Acetaminophen	Primarily cats; dogs with high doses
	Benzocaine/lidocaine	Primarily cats
	Chlorates	Matches, fireworks, gunpowder
	Phenols	Primarily cats
Decreased formation of RBC, WBC, and/or platelets	5-fluorouracil	Bone marrow suppression; primarily WBC ± RBC
	Estrogen	Suppresses bone marrow formation of RBC and platelets
	Methotrexate	Bone marrow suppression
	Lead	Interferes with RBC maturation
Coagulopathy	Anticoagulant rodenticides; Warfarin	Prevents vitamin K recycling resulting in clotting factor deficiency
	Aspirin	Inhibits platelet function
	Crotalid snake venom	Contains platelet aggregation inhibitors and inhibitors of fibrin formation
Asphyxiants	Carbon dioxide	Displacement of oxygen
	Carbon monoxide	Interference with oxygen delivery to tissues
	Cyanide	Uncoupling of cellular respiratory chain
	Hydrogen Sulfide	Paralysis of respiratory center in CNS
	Methane	Displacement of oxygen

be altered by toxicants such as aspirin, and platelet numbers can be reduced through the action of toxicants such as estrogen. Alteration of coagulation factors can result in uncontrolled hemorrhage, such as that seen with anticoagulant rodenticides Anticoagulant rodenticides inhibit vitamin K epoxide reductase, preventing the recycling of vitamin K and the formation of vitamin K–dependent clotting factors. When existing clotting factor stores are depleted, hemorrhage occurs. Some toxicants inhibit the ability of the blood to carry oxygen or to deliver oxygen to tissues (e.g., carbon monoxide, cyanide). Table 16.2 lists some common hematopoietic toxicants.

The sensitivity of the feline red blood cell to oxidative injury is well known, and it is no surprise that cats are more sensitive to oxidant-induced hemoglobin damage. A large part of this sensitivity is due to the fact that cats have 8 sulfhydryl groups on each hemoglobin molecule, compared to 4 in dogs and 2 in humans (Bischoff 2007). These

sulfhydryl groups are highly reactive areas of the molecule and interact with oxidants such as the acetaminophen metabolite para-aminophenol, which denatures the hemoglobin molecule to form methemoglobin (McConkey et al. 2009). Additionally, compared to other species, cat red blood cells are relatively deficient in methemoglobin reductase, resulting in a diminished ability to convert methemoglobin back to hemoglobin (Bischoff 2007).

INTEGUMENTARY

The skin is the largest organ in the body and acts as a barrier against exogenous injury and excessive water loss (Haschek et al. 2007b). The skin has an outer *epidermis* composed of an outer *stratum corneum* that consists of keratinized epithelium and an inner basal layer of proliferating epithelial cells that replenish the stratum corneum as they mature into keratinocytes. The thickness of the epidermis varies significantly between species and is rela-

Table 16.3. Toxicants affecting the skin

Mechanism	Toxicant	Comments
Direct injury (irritation, erosion or ulceration of skin)	Acids	Car/boat batteries, drain openers, oven cleaners, etching compounds, gun barrel cleaners, pool sanitizers, rust removers
	Alkalis	Anhydrous lime, cement, drain openers, fabric softeners, industrial strength bleaches, liquid dishwasher detergents, low phosphate laundry detergents, pool chemicals
	Cationic detergents	Disinfectants, sanitizers, pool algicides
	Essential oils	Concentrated d-limonene, tea tree oil, eugenol
	Hydrocarbons (e.g. motor oil, mineral spirits)	Volatile hydrocarbons (e.g., kerosene, mineral spirits) very damaging to canine and feline skin
Immune-mediated	Essential oils	D-limonene
	Medications	Idiosyncratic; penicillins, cephalosporins, levamisole, thrimethoprim-sulfa, others

tively thin in dogs and cats compared to many other species. The *dermis* is the tissue immediately under the epidermis and is composed of fibrous connective tissue, blood vessels, and adnexal structures such as hair follicles and sebaceous glands. Beneath the dermis is the subcutaneous adipose tissue.

Toxicants that are lipophilic can more readily penetrate the outer layers of the epidermis to reach the more metabolically active cells in the lower epidermis (Haschek et al. 2007b). These cells have the ability to metabolically deactivate many potential toxicants, preventing them from reaching the dermis. Compounds reaching the dermis may be removed through the blood or lymphatics. In this way, the skin serves as an effective barrier against a large number of potential toxicants. Some highly lipophilic organic solvents (e.g., dimethyl sulfoxide) have the ability to penetrate these layers and can be used as "carriers" to aid other molecules in passing through the integument.

There are three basic mechanisms of toxic skin injury: (1) direct injury to the skin, (2) immune-mediated injury, and (3) phototoxic injury (Haschek et al. 2007b). Direct injury from a topically applied agent results in irritation that can range from mild dermatitis to severe corrosive injury depending on the toxicant and degree of exposure. Immune-mediated skin injury results from stimulation of the immune system by exposure to a compound that is ingested, inhaled, or injected; only rarely is this reaction seen due to topical exposure. As with any other reaction involving the immune system, immune-mediated skin injury requires prior sensitization before an immune reaction will occur. Phototoxic injury is a direct immediate interaction between light and photosensitizing compound within the dermis. The photosensitizing compound may be a toxicant or its metabolite, and it interacts with certain wavelengths of light to produce free radicals in the skin, resulting in damage to cellular structures. The net effect resembles a severe sunburn. Phototoxicity is less commonly seen in dogs and cats than humans or grazing animals due to their protective hair coats and lack of exposure to the types of compounds (plant toxins, some pharmaceuticals) that cause photosensitization. Table 16.3 lists toxicants that affect the skin.

MUSCULOSKELETAL SYSTEM

The musculoskeletal system is composed of bones, joints, and skeletal muscle (Plumlee 2004). Bones and joints are relatively spared from the effects of acute toxic insults and most toxic changes are due to chronic exposure to toxicants. Toxicants affecting bone or cartilage can alter their formation or remodeling. Skeletal muscle is similar to cardiac muscle in structure and function, and many toxicants that affect the myocardium will also affect skeletal muscle cells. Skeletal muscle toxicants can alter neuromuscular action, interfere with myofiber biochemical processes, or cause direct myofiber degeneration or necrosis. Table 16.4 contains a listing of musculoskeletal toxicants.

Table 16.4. Toxicants affecting the musculoskeletal system

Mechanism	Toxicant	Comments
Alteration of cartilage formation	Fluoroquinalones (e.g., enrofloxacin)	Growing animals
Muscle weakness, paralysis	Ionophores (e.g., monensin)	Dogs
	Macadamia nuts	Dogs
Muscle tremors, fasciculations	Tremorgenic mycotoxins	Dogs most commonly affected
	Pyrethroids	Concentrated pyrethroids, especially in cats

REFERENCES

Bischoff, Karen. 2007. Toxicity of over-the-counter drugs. In *Veterinary Toxicology: Basic and Clinical Principles*, edited by Ramesh C. Gupta, pp. 363–390. San Diego: Elsevier.

Haschek, Wanda M., Rousseaux, Colin G., and Wallig, Matthew A. 2007. Gastrointestinal tract. In *Fundamentals of Toxicologic Pathology*, 2nd ed., pp.163–196. San Diego: Academic Press-Elsevier.

———. 2007a. Hematopoietic system. In *Fundamentals of Toxicologic Pathology*, 2nd ed., pp.491–512. San Diego: Academic Press-Elsevier.

———. 2007b. Skin and oral mucosa. In *Fundamentals of Toxicologic Pathology*, 2nd ed., pp. 135–162. San Diego: Academic Press-Elsevier.

McConkey, S.E., Grant, D.M., and Cribb, A.E. 2009. The role of para-aminophenol in acetaminophen-induced methemoglobinemia in dogs and cats. *Journal of Veterinary Pharmacology and Therapeutics*, 32(6):585–595.

Plumlee, Konnie H. 2004. Musculoskeletal system. In *Clinical Veterinary Toxicology*, edited by Konnie H. Plumlee, p. 69. St. Louis: Mosby.

Section 3

Specific Toxicants

Rodenticides

17

Eric Dunayer

INTRODUCTION

Rodenticides are pesticides that are intended to kill rodents and other small mammals. Frequently, however, dogs, cats, pet rodents, and other "nontarget" animals ingest the agent either unintentionally or due to malicious poisoning. At the ASPCA Animal Poison Control Center (APCC), rodenticides were the fourth most common ingestion in dogs (Meadows and Gwaltney-Brant 2006) while anticoagulant rodenticides (AR) were the ninth most common exposure reported in cats (Merola and Dunayer 2006).

There are several different rodenticides currently available. They come in various forms including pellets, blocks, dust, and place packs (paper packages left out for the rodents to chew open). Some rodenticides are mixed with seeds or grain to attract the rodents. Many rodenticides are dyed green or blue, but other colors such as red, tan, and white are also common. Rodenticides cannot be identified by their color or form; they can be identified only by locating their active ingredient or the Environmental Protection Agency (EPA) registration number (EPA Reg. no.) on the packaging. Properly identifying the agent is necessary for determining the appropriate treatment for the ingestion. However, even if the agent cannot be identified, treatment should not be delayed while trying to obtain the information.

ANTICOAGULANT RODENTICIDES

Sources/Formulations

Anticoagulant rodenticides (AR) were originally derived from studying the effects of moldy clover on cattle. Mold infecting sweet clover (*Melilotus officinalis* and *M. alba*)

converted the harmless chemical coumarin into the toxic metabolite dicoumarol. Chronic ingestion of the infected hay led to coagulopathy and death in cattle (Knight and Walter 2001). Warfarin, the first commercially available anticoagulant rodenticide, was developed in the 1940s as a derivative of dicoumarol; it was named for the Wisconsin Alumni Research Foundation (WARF), the organization that uncovered the link between dicoumarol and coagulopathy (Merola 2002; Murphy 2007). Warfarin is also used therapeutically as an anticoagulant in human and veterinary medicine.

While warfarin was the original anticoagulant rodenticide, others were soon synthesized. Warfarin requires many days of ingestion to cause signs. Also, rodents developed resistance to warfarin's effects. To overcome these drawbacks, second-generation anticoagulant rodenticides were developed. These are capable of being lethal with a single feeding (Murphy 2007). The various compounds are listed in Table 17.1.

AR are sold in various forms (as discussed in the introduction) and under dozens of trade names. Warfarin baits generally contain 0.025% of active ingredient or 7 mg of warfarin per ounce of bait. Second-generation anticoagulant rodenticides come as a 0.005% bait (1.4 mg of active ingredient per ounce of bait) with the exception of difethialone, which is 0.0025% (0.7 mg of difethialone per ounce of bait).

Due to the unintended poisoning of children, pets, and wildlife by rodenticides, the EPA in 2008 announced a regulation to ban the over-the-counter sale of second-generation anticoagulant rodenticides directly to consumers. The use of AR will be restricted to licensed Pest

Small Animal Toxicology Essentials, First Edition. Edited by Robert H. Poppenga, Sharon Gwaltney-Brant.
© 2011 John Wiley and Sons, Inc. Published 2011 by John Wiley and Sons, Inc.

Table 17.1. Anticoagulant rodenticides

First-Generation	Second-Generation
Warfarin	Brodifacoum
Chlorophacinone	Bromadiolone
Diphacinone	Difenacoum
Pindone	Difethialone

Control Operators, and the rodenticide must be in a tamperproof bait station. Other rodenticides will still be available for direct purchase by consumers, but they can only be sold in a bait station; loose pellet baits are banned (USEPA 2008).

Kinetics

Most AR are well absorbed after ingestion. Once absorbed, a large percentage is bound to plasma proteins. Ingestion of other highly protein-bound drugs (such as NSAIDs, thyroid supplements, and corticosteroids) can increase the toxicity of the anticoagulant by displacing it from the protein. The half-lives of the agents vary but, in general, first-generation agents have a much shorter half-lives (14 hours) than second-generation products (up to 6 days) (Merola 2002).

Mechanism of Action

AR interfere with the ability of the liver to recycle vitamin K, which is necessary for the production of the active forms of clotting factors II, VII, IX, and X. Without continuous production of new factors, the animal depletes those that are present in the blood. When the factors are depleted (generally 3 to 7 days or more after ingestion), spontaneous hemorrhage begins (Merola 2002).

Toxicity

The toxicity of these products varies greatly by compound and by form (Murphy and Talcott 2006). Often, when the chemical is incorporated into bait, its toxicity is greatly increased. Warfarin requires a much higher single dose to cause toxicosis compared to repeated daily ingestions. Because of the wide variation in toxic doses in the literature, the APCC recommends using 0.02 mg/kg as a dosage of concern for all second-generation agents.

Clinical Effects

Signs

The initial signs of AR toxicosis are generally vague and include anorexia, weakness, and lethargy. Once bleeding begins, signs depend on where the hemorrhage has occurred. For instance, hemorrhage into the chest can lead to signs of dyspnea. Heavier dogs, due to pressure on their joints, might bleed into joint spaces and subsequently develop lameness. Hemorrhage under the skin can cause swelling of limbs. Bleeding into the brain and spinal cord can cause a sudden onset of paralysis and seizures. Most commonly, hemorrhage occurs into body "spaces" such as pleural or peritoneal cavities. Some dogs die suddenly without any obvious signs. Bleeding generally will not start until 3–7 days after the exposure due to the requirement that existing vitamin-K–dependent clotting factors be consumed. Younger animals, which have less of a reserve of coagulation factors, potentially start to develop coagulopathy sooner. Also, animals with preexisting liver disease are also more susceptible to intoxication (Merola 2002).

Laboratory

Depending on the length of time bleeding has occurred, the animal might be anemic with a decreased hematocrit. Platelet counts are often slightly decreased as platelets are consumed to try to stop the bleeding. Increases in the coagulation parameters prothrombin time (PT) and partial thromboplastin time (PTT) are the most consistent findings. Factor VII (critical for the extrinsic coagulation pathway) has the shortest half-life in dogs (6.2 hours) and as it is depleted, the PT (which assesses both the extrinsic and common coagulation pathways) will become abnormal first, generally by 48–72 hours (Murphy 2007). A second test known as PIVKA (proteins induced by vitamin K_1 antagonism) can be used instead of the PT to monitor the patient but it may not be as readily available.

Differential Diagnoses

Differential diagnoses include naturally occurring bleeding defects such as hemophilia, von Willebrand disease, and other inherited or acquired clotting disorders. Because the liver produces the clotting factors, liver failure can lead to spontaneous bleeding. Finally, bleeding due to trauma should be ruled out.

Diagnostics

Antemortem

A diagnosis of AR toxicosis is based on history and results of coagulation testing. In some cases, particularly where there is no history of exposure, analysis of whole blood or serum for the presence of a specific AR can confirm exposure (Murphy 2007).

Postmortem

Typically, no microscopic lesions are noted. The animal will have widespread hemorrhage into body cavities, joints, skin, CNS, or other tissues. AR can be detected, most typically in liver tissue, to confirm exposure (Murphy 2007).

Management of Exposures

In animals with recent exposures (<4 hours), emesis should be performed. This can be followed with a single dose of activated charcoal; multiple doses of activated charcoal have not been shown to be beneficial. Next, one of two courses should be followed (Merola 2002). Vitamin K_1 can be started at a dose of 3–5 mg/kg divided twice a day. The length of treatment depends on the agent ingested. For warfarin, a minimum of 14 days is recommended; for bromadiolone, the recommended treatment period is 21 days; and for all other first and second-generation agents, at least 30 days of treatment should be done. Injections of vitamin K_1 should not be used if possible as this increases the risk of allergic or anaphylactic reactions. Oral vitamin K_1 should be given with a small, fatty meal, such as canned dog or cat food, because this enhances absorption. For rodents and small puppies or kittens, the injectable vitamin K_1 solution can be given orally if appropriately sized tablets are not available. Approximately 48 and 72 hours after stopping the vitamin K_1, a PT should be run to see if additional treatment is necessary (Merola 2002).

Alternatively, instead of starting vitamin K_1 immediately, the patient's PT can be monitored. A baseline PT level should be obtained and then rechecked at 48 and 72 hours after the exposure. If the PT becomes prolonged, vitamin K_1 therapy, as indicated above, should be instituted (Merola 2002). As mentioned above, the PIVKA test, if available, can be used instead of the PT to monitor the patient.

A study done at the University of Pennsylvania showed that over 90% of dogs decontaminated with emesis and/or activated charcoal after anticoagulant ingestion did not need treatment with vitamin K_1 when their PT was monitored; none of the animals developed signs during the period that the PT was being run (Pachtinger et al. 2008). Therefore, waiting to monitor PTs rather than immediately starting vitamin K_1 is an acceptable treatment plan.

In patients that are actively bleeding, emesis should not be performed as exposure likely occurred several days before presentation. The animal should be stabilized for shock with fluids. If the anemia is severe, a blood transfusion should be performed (Merola 2002). Vitamin K_1 therapy should be started as soon as possible. However, since vitamin K_1 takes 6–12 hours before new clotting factors can be produced, the patient should receive a fresh frozen plasma an/or whole blood transfusions to supply clotting factors until the body manufactures a sufficient quantity on its own (Murphy and Talcott 2006). Strict cage rest should be enforced. For animals that are dyspneic due to bleeding into the pleural cavity, the chest can be carefully tapped to relieve pressure (Merola 2002). Blood from a thoracocentesis can be autotransfused back to the patient especially if anemia is present.

Prognosis

For asymptomatic animals, vitamin K_1 therapy is effective and should prevent signs from developing. If bleeding has begun, the prognosis is more guarded, depending on extent and location of the hemorrhage. However, most symptomatic animals can recover with appropriate therapeutic intervention.

BROMETHALIN

Sources/Formulations

Bromethalin was developed to kill AR-resistant rodents. Despite its name being similar to some of the AR (bromadiolone, brodifacoum), it is not an anticoagulant; it is neurotoxic. As with AR, bromethalin is sold in various forms and under many different brand names. It generally comes as a 0.01% concentration (2.84 mg bromethalin per oz of bait) (Dunayer 2003). For mole control, it is also sold in the form of a "worm" bait. In these products, the bromethalin concentration is 0.025%.

Kinetics

Bromethalin is rapidly absorbed after ingestion and plasma levels peak in about 4 hours. In the liver, bromethalin is converted to a toxic metabolite desmethylbromethalin. Bromethalin is excreted in the bile and undergoes enterohepatic recirculation. The half-life of bromethalin is about 6 days in rats (Dunayer 2003; Gupta 2007).

Mechanism of Action

Bromethalin and its metabolite desmethylbromethalin uncouple oxidative phosphorylation. This leads to decreased production of energy in cells so levels of ATP fall. Without ATP, Na-K ATPase pumps in the cell membrane are unable to pump sodium out of the cell. Because sodium builds up inside the cell, water is pulled in and the cell swells. Nerves cells are the most sensitive tissue and so signs of neurotoxicity are seen. In the CNS, myelin sheaths that surround nerve cells swell and vacuoles form

Table 17.2. Toxicity of bromethalin in various species

Species	Oral LD_{50} (mg/kg)
Rat	2.0
Mouse	5.3
Rabbit	13.0
Guinea pig	<1000
Dog	4.7
Cat	1.8

Source: Van Lier and Cherry 1988.

within the nerve cell. As the cells and the myelin sheaths swell with fluid, internal pressure increases; there is also an increase in cerebrospinal fluid pressure. Together, these changes cause nerve dysfunction (Dunayer 2003, Gupta 2007).

Toxicity

For most species, the toxicity of bromethalin is very similar (see Table 17.2). However, cats are much more sensitive to the effects of bromethalin than dogs. Guinea pigs are relatively insensitive to bromethalin as they are unable to produce the toxic metabolite desmethylbromethalin (Dunayer 2003). Interestingly, if guinea pigs are fed desmethylbromethalin, the toxic dose is similar to bromethalin (Van Lier and Cherry 1988). Based on cases reported to the APCC, dogs have died at dosages of 0.95 mg/kg and cats have developed signs at 0.24 mg/kg (Dunayer 2003).

Clinical Effects

Signs

In dogs, the onset of signs depends on the dose ingested. At lower doses, the onset is slow, taking from 24–86 hours to be seen. Initial signs include hindlimb weakness, which can progress to paresis and paralysis. CNS depression also develops. Once signs develop, they may last for days to weeks before they resolve (Dorman et al. 1990b). In dogs ingesting doses at or above the LD_{50}, the onset of signs is more rapid, from 4–36 hours. In these dogs, hyperexcitability develops followed by tremors, seizures, and death (Dorman et al. 1990b).

In cats, the most common sign is ataxia. Other signs include focal motor seizures, recumbency, abdominal distension, decreased conscious proprioception, and a decerebrate posture. Onset of signs occurs from 3–7 days after exposure. As noted with dogs, higher ingested doses generally lead to earlier onset of signs (Dorman et al. 1990a).

Laboratory

There are no significant laboratory changes expected with bromethalin toxicosis. (Dorman et al. 1990b).

Differential Diagnoses

For the paralytic form of bromethalin toxicosis, toxic differentials include botulism, ivermectin toxicosis, and ionophore toxicosis. In seizing patients, differentials include metaldehyde (snail bait), strychnine, zinc phosphide, and sodium fluoroacetate (Compound 1080) intoxications.

Diagnostics

Antemortem

Antemortem diagnosis relies on a history of exposure and occurrence of compatible clinical signs. Although blood can be tested for the presence of bromethalin, this is not a standard test and results are typically not available prior to the need to institute treatment.

Postmortem

Bromethalin can be detected in various organs including the brain and liver. Histopathology of the CNS shows spongy degeneration of the white matter with an accumulation of fluid within the myelin sheaths (Dunayer 2003).

Management of Exposures

There is no antidote for bromethalin, so the management of exposure is focused on decontamination. Decontamination recommendations vary depending on the species, dosage, and time since ingestion. Tables 17.3a and b summarize the APCC's recommendations for decontamination (Dunayer 2003). Since bromethalin is not an anticoagulant, vitamin K_1 is not indicated as a treatment.

Once signs begin, treatment is supportive and symptomatic. Recumbent animals should be well padded to prevent pressure sores. Seizures should be controlled as needed. Mannitol, furosemide, and corticosteroids have been suggested to treat the cerebral edema. Although these might slow progression of signs, they do not prevent their occurrence. In addition, when the treatment is stopped, the animal may deteriorate rapidly (Dunayer 2003).

Prognosis

Prompt decontamination can often prevent signs from occurring. In mild cases, recovery is possible but full recovery can take weeks. Animals who are paralyzed or having seizures have a guarded prognosis, although even these animals can recover with intensive care.

Table 17.3a. Decontamination recommendations for bromethalin ingestion: Recommendations for dogs

Time since Exposure	Dosage Ingested (mg/kg)	Action
<4 hours	0.1–0.49	Emesis or one dose of activated charcoal
>4 hours	0.1–0.49	One dose of activated charcoal
<4 hours	0.5–0.75	Emesis and three doses of activated charcoal over 24 hours
>4 hours	0.5–0.75	Three doses of activated charcoal over 24 hours
<4 hours	>0.75	Emesis and three doses of activated charcoal a day for 48 hours
>4 hours	>0.75	Three doses of activated charcoal a day for 48 hours

Table 17.3b. Decontamination recommendations for bromethalin ingestion: Recommendations for cats

Time since Exposure	Dosage Ingested (mg/kg)	Action
<4 hours	0.05–0.1	Emesis or one dose of activated charcoal
>4 hours	0.05–0.1	One dose of activated charcoal
<4 hours	0.1–0.3	Emesis and three doses of activated charcoal over 24 hours
>4 hours	0.1–0.3	Three doses of activated charcoal over 24 hours
<4 hours	>0.3	Emesis and three doses of activated charcoal a day for 48 hours
>4 hours	>0.3	Three doses of activated charcoal a day for 48 hours

Source: Dunayer 2003.

CHOLECALCIFEROL

Sources/Formulations

Cholecalciferol is a form of vitamin D_3. It is generally found in a 0.075% bait (21.3 mg cholecalciferol per oz of bait). As with other rodenticides, it is available in different forms and from different manufacturers (Morrow 2001). Vitamin D toxicosis can also occur due to chronic overdosing with vitamin D supplements or as a result of improperly formulated dog or cat foods. Although over-the-counter daily multivitamins contain vitamin D, it is generally present in such low concentrations (<1000 IU per capsule) that vitamin D toxicosis from acute overdoses of these products is rare. However, prescription products containing between 5,000 and 50,000 IU per capsule may result in toxicosis if sufficient numbers are ingested. Additionally, certain medications that contain vitamin D analogs such as calcipotriene, a topical cream for treating psoriasis, can cause toxicosis similar to cholecalciferol (Rumbeiha 2006).

Kinetics

Cholecalciferol is rapidly absorbed after ingestion. It is mainly excreted by the liver and undergoes enterohepatic recirculation (Morrow 2001). Vitamin D_3 is highly fat-soluble so it can be stored in body fat. After absorption, cholecalciferol is transported to the liver on vitamin D–binding proteins. In the liver, cholecalciferol is metabolized to 25-hydroxycholecalciferol, also known as calcifediol. Calcifediol circulates in the blood and, in the kidneys, is further metabolized to 1,25-dihdroxycholcalcerifol or cacitriol, which is the most active form of vitamin D (Morrow 2001; Rumbeiha 2006).

Mechanism of Action

Calcitriol increases blood calcium and phosphorus levels via various mechanisms: increased gastrointestinal absorption of calcium, increased calcium reabsorption by the kidneys, and increased bone resorption and release of phosphorus and calcium into the blood (Morrow 2001; Rumbeiha 2006). The overall effect is to increase blood phosphorus and calcium levels. When the calcium × phosphorus product exceeds 60, soft tissue mineralization may occur. Mineralization of the kidneys can lead to acute renal failure although any tissue can be affected. (Morrow 2001).

Toxicity

In dogs dosages of 10 mg/kg have been fatal (Gupta 2007). Based on experience at the APCC, dosages of 0.5 mg/kg can cause signs (Morrow 2001). Therefore, the APCC recommends that decontamination and monitoring for signs be performed on dogs ingesting more than 0.1 mg/kg.

Clinical Effects

Signs

Onset of signs is usually within 12 to 36 hours of ingestion. Initial signs include vomiting and diarrhea (possibly bloody). The animal will then show depression, polyuria, and polydipsia. Acute renal failure can occur in as little as 24 hours (Morrow 2001).

Laboratory

After ingestion, serum phosphorus usually increases first, generally around 12 hours. The serum calcium increases by about 24 hours. Increases in BUN and creatinine consistent with renal failure can begin shortly after the phosphorus and calcium product exceeds 60 (Morrow 2001).

Differential Diagnoses

Any condition that increases serum calcium levels should be considered as a differential. This includes primary hyperparathyroidism in which the parathyroid gland produces excessive levels of parathormone (PTH), usually due to a tumor of the gland. In addition, certain tumors, such as lymphoma and anal gland carcinomas can secrete a protein that acts like PTH. In these syndromes, unlike cholecalciferol toxicity, phosphorus levels are usually normal (Rumbeiha 2006).

Diagnostics

Antemortem

In addition to measuring serum calcium, phosphorus, and assessing renal function, vitamin D_3 and calcitriol levels can be measured in blood. In cholecalciferol toxicosis, these are markedly elevated. In addition, PTH levels should be determined since they will be reduced (Rumbeiha 2006).

Postmortem

Lesions on postmortem examination include mineralization of soft tissues, especially the kidneys. However, this can occur with any condition that causes hypercalcemia. The bile and kidneys can be tested for calcifediol levels to confirm toxicity (Rumbeiha 2006).

Management of Exposures

If ingestion is within 6–8 hours, emesis can be performed. Since cholecalciferol undergoes enterohepatic recirculation, multiple doses of activated charcoal (every 6–8 hours) might increase clearance. Baseline levels of calcium, phosphorus, BUN, and creatinine should be obtained and monitored daily for at least 4 days (Morrow 2001).

In patients with elevated calcium and phosphorus concentrations, intensive therapy is indicated to prevent renal failure and other signs. The animal should receive 0.9% saline IV at twice maintenance rates; sodium competes for reabsorption with calcium in the kidney and increases calcium loss. Furosemide should be administered as it increases calcium excretion by the kidneys. Corticosteroids such as prednisone will decrease bone resorption and decrease intestinal absorption while increasing renal excretion of calcium. In addition, a low calcium/phosphorus diet should be fed and phosphate binders, such as aluminum or magnesium hydroxide, can be given (Morrow 2001; Rumbeiha 2006).

If these measures are not successful in reducing calcium levels, other treatments should be initiated. Salmon calcitonin is a hormone that lowers calcium levels. However, it must be given several times a day and some animals develop a tolerance to it. The preferred treatment is pamidronate, a bisphosphonate used to lower serum calcium in people with hypercalcemia due to malignancy. Pamidronate is given in normal saline by slow IV infusion over 2 to 4 hours. Its effects can last up to a week. It can be repeated as needed. Other bisphosphonates such as clodronate also appear to be effective (Ulutas et al. 2006). Calcitonin and pamidronate (or other bisphosphonates) should not be used together (Morrow 2001).

Treatment should be continued until the calcium × phosphorus product is less than 60. At that point, treatments can be slowly reduced while the calcium and phosphorus values are watched closely for signs of recurrence over the course of several weeks (Morrow 2001).

Prognosis

The prognosis is good with prompt decontamination and if no signs develop. The prognosis is guarded once signs develop because mineralization is poorly reversible. Chronic renal failure can be a permanent sequela. Sudden deaths have occurred weeks later, probably due to cardiac arrhythmias from calcified heart muscle or the rupture of a major artery like the aorta (Morrow 2001).

STRYCHNINE

Sources/Formulations

Strychnine is an alkaloid obtained from the seeds and bark of the strychnine tree (*Strychnos nux-vomica* and *S.*

ignatti). These trees grow in Southeast Asia and Australia (Gupta 2007). Strychnine is one of the oldest rodenticides; it was first used in the 16th century (Talcott 2006). Strychnine is sold in various formulations, usually mixed with grain. It is often dyed red or green. Formulations contain 0.5%–3% strychnine. It is intended for killing rodents as well as porcupines, rabbits, and pigeons (Talcott 2004). Strychnine is labeled for use underground in animal burrows (Talcott 2004).

Kinetics

Strychnine is rapidly absorbed from the small intestine (Gupta 2007). It is metabolized in the liver, but up to 20% of the dose may be excreted in the urine unchanged (Talcott 2004). It rapidly distributes to many different tissues and has a half-life of about 6 hours (Gupta 2007).

Mechanism of Action

Strychnine competitively blocks the effects of the amino acid glycine, an inhibitory neurotransmitter in the spinal cord. Normally, glycine prevents repetitive nerve activity that stimulates muscle contractions. Without this inhibition, the nerve continues to fire rapidly and leads to muscle spasms. Eventually, the animal develops muscle rigidity (tetanic spasms) (Talcott 2004; Gupta 2007). Because extensor muscles are stronger than flexor muscles in the limbs and neck, an extensor rigidity develops.

Toxicity

Strychnine is considered extremely toxic. In dogs, the minimum lethal dosage is about 0.75 mg/kg (Gupta 2007); this is about 0.15 g/kg of a 0.5% bait or about 0.5 teaspoon in a 35 lb (16 kg) dog. In cats, the LD_{50} is about 2 mg/kg (Talcott 2004).

Clinical Effects
Signs

Signs can occur from 10 minutes to 2 hours after ingestion depending on when the stomach empties since strychnine is better absorbed in the intestines (Talcott 2004). Vomiting is uncommon (Gupta 2007). Initially, the animal may be anxious, tachypneic, and salivating heavily. Signs then progress to ataxia followed by collapse with violent muscular seizures. The legs will be extended and rigid and the neck may be arched. Stimulation by noise or lights typically causes signs to worsen. The animal can be hyperthermic due to extreme muscle activity. Death is likely due to respiratory arrest from paralysis of the diaphragm (Talcott 2004; Gupta 2007).

Laboratory

There are no specific changes associated with strychnine toxicosis (Talcott 2004).

Differential Diagnoses

Many toxicants and conditions can cause severe tremors similar to strychnine. These include metaldehyde, bromethalin, tremorgenic mycotoxins, zinc phosphide, tetanus, organochlorine insecticides, anticholinesterase insecticides, and *Brunfelsia* spp. (Talcott 2006).

Diagnostics
Antemortem

Strychnine can be detected in urine and stomach contents from gastric lavage (Gupta 2007; Talcott 2004). However, some animals die so quickly that strychnine can't be detected in their urine (Beasley et al. 1999). In addition, the results of the tests are not likely to be available before the patient has either died or recovered.

Postmortem

There are no specific lesions associated with strychnine toxicosis. Strychnine can be detected in stomach contents, urine, bile, liver, and kidney to confirm exposure (Talcott 2004).

Management of Exposures

Emesis can be induced before the animal is symptomatic; however, due to rapid onset of signs in most cases, this may not be practical. Activated charcoal may be useful but care should be taken to avoid aspiration (Talcott 2004). In general, treatment is aimed at controlling the tremors and seizures. Barbiturates, methocarbamol, propofol, and gas anesthesia may be used to control signs. In severe cases, the patient may need to be kept under anesthesia for 24–48 hours. IV fluids to support hydration should be administered. Sensory stimulation should be kept to a minimum to prevent worsening of the signs. Treatment should be continued until signs have resolved, which may take 24–72 hours (Talcott 2004; Gupta 2007).

Prognosis

Prognosis is guarded once signs have begun.

ZINC PHOSPHIDE

Sources/Formulations

Zinc phosphide is an inorganic rodenticide that has been available for over 70 years (Albretson 2004). It is sold as a 2% bait (566 mg zinc phosphide per oz of bait). Zinc phosphide can be found in several different forms such as in pellets, in place packs, and mixed with grains. In addition to mice and rats, it is also used to kill voles, moles, rabbits, and other rodents (Gupta 2007).

Kinetics

After ingestion, zinc phosphide reacts with acids in the stomach to produce phosphine gas, which can be absorbed from the stomach or may be inhaled as it escapes the stomach (Albretson 2004). Intact zinc phosphide may be absorbed as well from the gastrointestinal tract.

Mechanism of Action

The exact mechanism of zinc phosphate and phosphine gas intoxication is not known. It is thought that phosphine gas blocks the enzyme cytochrome oxidase, which decreases energy production by cells. Without energy, cells are unable to maintain normal function and cell death occurs (Albretson 2004; Gupta 2007). Phosphine gas is also thought to be directly irritating, especially to the lungs (Albretson 2004).

In addition to its immediate effects, zinc phosphide can cause delayed liver and kidney failure. It is not known whether this is due to phosphine gas or the absorption of intact zinc phosphide.

Toxicity

The LD_{50} of zinc phosphide is about 40 mg/kg in dogs and cats. The LD_{50} in rats is 12 mg/kg. Because zinc phosphide is a strong emetic, dogs and cats are less sensitive to zinc phosphide than rodents because they can vomit and partially decontaminate themselves after ingestion (Albretson 2004).

Clinical Effects

Signs

The onset of signs varies from 15 minutes to 4 hours. Rapidity of onset appears to be influenced by whether or not the animal has food in its stomach. The presence of food increases the production of hydrochloric acid, which in turn increases the production of phosphine gas (Albretson 2004). Vomiting, often bloody, is common. The animal's breath or its vomitus can have a garlicky or rotten fish smell from the phosphine gas (Knight 2006). Severe gastrointestinal pain can develop. CNS signs include anxiety, initial depression progressing to increased activity, tremors, and seizures. Increased respiratory sounds and rate are common (Knight 2006).

Laboratory

There are no specific clinical laboratory changes noted (Albretson 2004).

Differential Diagnoses

The differential diagnoses are similar to those for strychnine. These include metaldehyde, bromethalin, tremorgenic mycotoxins, zinc phosphide, tetanus, organochlorine insecticides, anticholinesterase insecticides, and *Brunfelsia* spp.

Diagnostics

Antemortem

Diagnosis is based on history and the presence of the characteristic smell of phosphine gas. Stomach contents samples can be tested for the presence of phosphine.

Postmortem

Diagnosis can be made by the detection of phosphine in stomach contents.

Management of Exposures

If exposure was recent, the patient should be given oral liquid antacids to neutralize stomach acid and reduce the production of phosphine gas. Emesis can be performed early but a centrally active emetic such as apomorphine should be used rather than hydrogen peroxide, which could increase the production of phosphine gas (Albretson 2004). Emetics are not indicated in animals that have already vomited. In patients who are seizuring, gastric lavage can be considered. Activated charcoal has been recommended, but there is no proof of efficacy (Knight 2006). In vomiting animals, activated charcoal may increase the risk of aspiration and it may delay healing of gastric erosions.

There are no antidotes for zinc phosphide toxicosis. Treatment should be directed to providing support and controlling signs such as fluids for shock, seizure control, and correcting acid-base imbalances. Liver protectants such as n-acetylcysteine, B-vitamins, SAMe, and dextrose may be useful but proof of efficacy is lacking (Albretson 2004; Knight 2006).

When presented with a poisoned animal, there is a real risk to attending medical staff. Phosphine gas coming from the patient's stomach or vomitus can affect human personnel in the room. The odor of phosphine gas can be detected by the human nose at about 2 ppm. However, levels of 1 ppm or less, depending on the length of exposure, can be toxic (Knight 2006). If possible, induction of emesis should be performed outdoors or in a well-ventilated room. Vomitus or gastric lavage material should be cleaned up rapidly and placed in an airtight bag. If the smell of phosphine gas is detected, personnel should be evacuated and the room aired out thoroughly.

Prognosis

In asymptomatic animals, the prognosis is good. If signs do develop, the prognosis is guarded especially for the first 48 hours. Even those animals that survive the initial period may develop acute renal and hepatic failure over the next 2 weeks.

REFERENCES

Albretson, Jay C. 2004. Zinc phosphide. In *Clinical Veterinary Toxicology*, edited by Konnie H. Plumlee, pp. 456–458. St. Louis: Mosby.

Beasley, Val R., Dorman, David C., Fikes, James D., Diana, Stephen G., and Woshner, Victoria. 1999. *A Systems Affected Approach to Veterinary Toxicology*. St Louis: Mosby.

Dorman, David C., Parker, Alan J., Dye, Janice A., and Buck, William B. 1990a. Bromethalin neurotoxicosis in the cat. *Progress in Veterinary Neurology* 1(2):189–196.

Dorman, David C., Parker, Alan J., and Buck, William B. 1990b. Bromethalin toxicosis in the dog: Part I: Clinical effects. *Journal of the American Animal Hospital Association* 26:589–594.

Dunayer, Eric. 2003. Bromethalin: The other rodenticide. *Veterinary Medicine* 98(9):732–736.

Gupta, Ramesh C. 2007. Non-anticoagulant rodenticides. In *Veterinary Toxicology: Basics and Clinical Principles*, edited by Ramesh C. Gupta, pp. 548–563. New York: Elsevier.

Knight, Anthony P. and Walter, Richard G. 2001. *A Guide to Plant Poisoning of Animals in North America*. Jackson, Wyoming: Teton New Media.

Knight, Michael W. 2006. Zinc Phosphide. In *Small Animal Toxicology, Second Edition*, edited by Michael E. Peterson and Patricia A. Talcott, pp. 1101–1118. St. Louis: Elsevier Saunders.

Meadows, Irina and Gwaltney-Brant, Sharon. 2006. The 10 most common toxicoses in dogs. *Veterinary Medicine* 101 (3):142–148.

Merola, Valentina. 2002. Anticoagulant rodenticides: Deadly to pests, dangerous to pets. *Veterinary Medicine*. 101(6): 339–342.

Merola, Valentina and Dunayer, Eric. 2006. The 10 most common toxicoses in cats. *Veterinary Medicine* 101 (10):905–911.

Morrow, Carla. 2001. Cholecalciferol poisoning. *Veterinary Medicine* 96(12):905–911.

Murphy, Michael. 2007. Anticoagulant rodenticides. In *Veterinary Toxicology: Basics and Clinical Principles*, edited by Ramesh C. Gupta, pp. 525–547. New York: Elsevier.

Murphy, Michael J. and Talcott, Patricia A. 2006. Anticoagulant Rodenticides. In *Small Animal Toxicology*, 2nd ed., edited by Michael E. Peterson and Patricia A. Talcott, pp. 563–577. St. Louis: Elsevier Saunders.

Pachtinger, Garret E., Otto, Cynthia M., and Syring, Rebecca S. 2008. Incidence of prolonged prothrombin time in dogs following gastrointestinal decontamination for acute anticoagulant rodenticide ingestion. *Journal of Veterinary Emergency and Critical Care* 18(3):285–291.

Rumbeiha, Wilson K. 2006. Cholecalciferol. In *Small Animal Toxicology*, 2nd ed., edited by Michael E. Peterson and Patricia A. Talcott, pp. 629–642. St. Louis: Elsevier Saunders.

Talcott, Patricia A. 2004. Strychnine. In *Clinical Veterinary Toxicology*, edited by Konnie H. Plumlee, pp. 454–456. St. Louis: Mosby.

———. 2006. Strychnine. In *Small Animal Toxicology*, 2nd ed., edited by Michael E. Peterson and Patricia A. Talcott, pp. 1076–1082. St. Louis: Elsevier Saunders.

Ulutas, B., Voyvoda, H., Pasa, S. and Alingan, M.K. 2006. Clodronate treatment of vitamin D-induced hypercalcemia in dogs. *Journal of Veterinary Emergency and Critical Care* 16(2):141–145.

USEPA (U.S. Environmental Protection Agency). 2008. Final Risk Mitigation Decision for Ten Rodenticides. Accessed at http://www.epa.gov/pesticides/reregistration/ rodenticides/finalriskdecision.htm#proposed on December 20, 2008.

Van Lier, Robert B.L., Cherry, Linda D. 1988. The toxicity and mechanism of action of bromethalin: A new single-feeding rodenticide. *Fundamental and Applied Toxicology* 11:664–672.

Insecticides

18

Petra A. Volmer

AMITRAZ

Sources/Formulations

Amitraz is a formamidine acaricide with activity against ticks, mites, and lice. It is used in veterinary medicine for the control and eradication of demodex mites and for the prevention of tick infestations. For small animals amitraz is commercially available under the trade names Mitaban® dip (19.9% for dilution), Preventic® collar (9.0%), and ProMeris® topical solution (15%). It is also available as an emulsifiable concentrate (12.5% for dilution) for use on pigs and cattle.

Kinetics

Amitraz is rapidly absorbed following oral administration of technical material. Clinical signs can be seen by 1 hour of ingestion and peak plasma concentrations occur by 5 hours. The elimination half-life is approximately 23.4 hours (Hugnet et al. 1996). Absorption and duration of effects following ingestion of amitraz-impregnated collars tend to be prolonged due to slow release of the active ingredient from the collar. Although dermal absorption is low, intoxication has been reported following topical application in dogs (Paradis 1999).

Mechanism of Action

The alpha-2 adrenergic agonist characteristics of amitraz account for its sedative and hyperglycemic effects. The effects on blood glucose are thought to be due to alpha-2– mediated inhibition of insulin release (Plumb 2005).

Toxicity

Amitraz is classified by the EPA as slightly toxic to mammals if ingested orally. The oral LD_{50} for amitraz in rats is 523–800 mg/kg and for mice is greater than 1600 mg/kg. The dermal LD_{50} for rats and rabbits is greater than 1600 mg/kg and greater than 200 mg/kg, respectively (Extoxnet 1995). Cats tend to be more sensitive than dogs to the effects of amitraz.

Clinical Effects

Signs

Signs of amitraz toxicosis can begin within 1 to 4 hours, but can be delayed as long as 12 hours. Intoxicated dogs and cats exhibit vomiting, depression, somnolence, ataxia, disorientation, ileus, bradycardia, hypertension, or hypotension, coma, hypothermia, and seizures. Some of the neurological signs might be attributed to the xylene carrier found in dip formulations. Equids may display similar neurological signs and are at risk of developing life-threatening ileus and impaction.

Laboratory

Biochemical changes include hyperglycemia and elevated hepatic enzymes.

Differential Diagnosis

Toxicants causing central nervous system depression should be considered. These include ethanol, methanol, isopropanol, the avermectins, marijuana, ethylene glycol,

Small Animal Toxicology Essentials, First Edition. Edited by Robert H. Poppenga, Sharon Gwaltney-Brant.
© 2011 John Wiley and Sons, Inc. Published 2011 by John Wiley and Sons, Inc.

barbiturates, benzodiazepines, opioids, and antidepressants. Other differentials include CNS trauma and primary CNS disease.

Diagnostics

Antemortem

Amitraz can be detected in stomach contents, urine, feces, and skin, although laboratories performing the analysis are limited.

Postmortem

No specific gross or histopathological lesions are expected on necropsy. Tissue analysis for the presence of the compound can confirm exposure.

Management of Exposures

The most common routes of exposure are dermal and oral. In either case, patients should be stabilized if necessary, clinical signs treated, and further exposure prevented.

For dermal exposures, the animal should be stabilized according to clinical signs and then bathed in a liquid dish detergent to remove any product remaining on the skin. Care should be taken to prevent the development of hypothermia subsequent to bathing. Mild signs following label use often do not require treatment and resolve in 24–72 hours. For more severe signs, yohimbine and atipamizole are alpha-2 adrenergic antagonists that effectively reverse bradycardia, CNS depression, hyperglycemia, and ileus (Plumb 2005). Atipamezole is thought to have fewer cardiorespiratory effects than yohimbine (Andrade and Sakate 2003). Atropine should not be used in the treatment of amitraz-induced bradycardia, because it can potentiate hypertension and ileus (Hsu et al. 1986). Seizures can be treated with diazepam or a barbiturate. Animals should be closely monitored for severe CNS depression following use of these drugs. In all cases exhibiting clinical signs, symptomatic and supportive care including IV fluids and thermoregulation is indicated.

Oral exposures are usually the result of ingestion of either spot-on or concentrated dip formulations containing volatile hydrocarbons, or from ingestion of an amitraz-containing collar. The induction of emesis should be avoided or done with care for products containing solvents due to the risk of aspiration and subsequent chemical pneumonitis. Emesis is recommended for asymptomatic animals that have ingested a collar. Activated charcoal binds amitraz; however, administration may also aggravate an already upset stomach and cause vomiting and possible aspiration. Activated charcoal is more suitable for cases in which a collar has been ingested. However, if surgery is required to remove collar pieces, activated charcoal can obscure the surgical field. Yohimbine and atipamezole might hasten passage of collar fragments from the gastrointestinal tract by reversing depressed GI motility. Saline cathartics can also enhance elimination.

Prognosis

Animals receiving prompt, aggressive treatment have a good prognosis. Animals exhibiting severe signs such as coma or seizures, have a guarded to poor prognosis.

ORGANOCHLORINES

Sources/Formulations

The organochlorine insecticides (OCs) (also referred to as "chlorinated hydrocarbons") reached the height of their popularity as insecticides from approximately the 1950s to the 1970s. They were prized because of their effectiveness as insecticides and relatively low acute mammalian toxicity (compared to the organophosphorus and carbamate compounds at the time). Additionally they were lipophilic and slow to degrade, requiring fewer applications. These characteristics, however, also contributed to their environmental persistence and biomagnification through the food chain. Because of this, the OCs have been replaced by newer and safer insecticides. However, old containers may resurface from storage in sheds, barns, and other structures, thus posing a hazard.

There are three main categories of OCs based on chemical structure. The diphenyl aliphatic compounds include agents such as DDT, methoxychlor, perthane, and dicofol. The aryl hydrocarbons include lindane, mirex, kepone, and paradichlorobenzene. The cyclodiene insecticides include aldrin, dieldrin, endrin, chlordane, heptachlor, and toxaphene. Although DDT and most of the other OCs have been banned from use in the United States, lindane topical products are still available as "second line" treatments for scabies and head lice in humans if "first line" treatments are not effective. Lindane-based dips for dogs, though not popular, continue to be available.

Kinetics

The OCs are well absorbed through most exposure routes. Blood concentrations initially increase following absorption, but then they decline rapidly as distribution takes place to liver, kidney, brain, and lipid-rich tissues such as adipose where OCs are stored. Body fat may serve as a source of OC poisoning if weight loss occurs and stored OCs are released into the general circulation. Because of their lipophilicity, OCs will be secreted into milk and eliminated from the body via this route. Some OCs are excreted through the bile and reabsorbed (enterohepatic recirculation), contributing to persistence in the body.

Mechanism of Action

The OCs exert their effects through two main mechanisms. In general, the diphenyl aliphatics interfere with sodium channel kinetics, resulting in partial depolarization. The aryl hydrocarbons and cyclodienes act to inhibit the binding of GABA (an inhibitory neurotransmitter) to GABA receptors. For both of these mechanisms, clinical signs reflect nervous stimulation. DDT metabolites also cause selective necrosis of the adrenal gland zona fasciulata and zona reticularis. The OCs have demonstrated potent estrogenic and enzyme-inducing properties, which interfere with fertility and reproduction in wildlife and laboratory animals.

Toxicity

The acutely toxic dose varies depending upon the OC, but in general the group is less toxic than the organophosphorus or carbamate insecticides. The one exception is endrin with a rat acute oral LD_{50} of 3 mg/kg (Buck et al. 1976).

Clinical Effects

Signs

Signs can occur anywhere from minutes to days following exposure. Initial signs include salivation, nausea, vomiting, followed by agitation, apprehension, hyperexcitability, incoordination, nervousness, and tremors. These can progress to clonic-tonic seizures, opisthotonus, paddling, and clamping of the jaw. Seizure activity can persist for 2–3 days (due to lipophilicity and enterohepatic recirculation). Coma and death are possible.

Laboratory

No diagnostic or suggestive changes occur. Although performing CBC and chemistry profiles will not rule in or out a diagnosis of an OC toxicosis, they are recommended to determine the overall health of the poisoned patient.

Differential Diagnosis

Any agent or disease process causing neurological stimulation should be included in the differential diagnosis list. Such conditions include infectious encephalitis, lead poisoning, rabies, eclampsia, canine distemper, strychnine, metaldehyde, 4-aminopyridine, methylxanthines, and other toxicants causing seizures.

Diagnostics

Confirmation of an OC poisoning is based on history of exposure and appropriate clinical signs along with detection of the compound in tissues. Samples for OC analysis should be collected and submitted in clean glass containers or wrapped in aluminum foil (dull side toward sample) to prevent contamination from plasticizers which can interfere with analysis.

Antemortem

Blood, milk, or adipose tissue (from a biopsy), or suspect feed or product can be analyzed. However, finding OC residues is not alone diagnostic because of the widespread persistence of these compounds in the environment.

Postmortem

Liver, brain, adipose tissue, and ingesta collected during necropsy can be analyzed.

Management of Exposures

Treatment is aimed at controlling neurological signs and preventing further exposure. No specific antidote exists, so therapy is largely symptomatic and supportive. Neurological stimulation can be addressed with antiseizure medications (e.g., diazepam, barbiturates, gas anesthetics, propofol, etc.) but may be difficult to control. For dermal exposures animals should be bathed with a liquid dish detergent. Activated charcoal is recommended for oral exposures. Personnel should use protective measures to prevent self-exposure.

Prognosis

The prognosis is dependent upon the OC involved, the dose, and how quickly treatment is initiated. Those animals with few or mild signs and that receive prompt treatment have a good prognosis. Animals with prolonged or severe signs, or for which treatment has been delayed have a guarded prognosis.

ORGANOPHOSPHORUS AND CARBAMATE INSECTICIDES

Sources/Formulations

This group of compounds is characterized by their ability to inhibit the enzyme acetylcholinesterase. There are a number of organophosphorus (OP) and carbamate insecticides developed for use on animals and crops, as well as around buildings or in structures such as ships and airplanes. The development of newer and safer insecticides has limited the use of this class of compounds to some extent, but many of these products are still available and in use. Older formulations can turn up from storage in old outbuildings such as sheds and barns. Most OP and carbamate insecticides are applied topically to the animal or plant, but some are designed to be absorbed and act systemically. The OPs and carbamates can be found in various formulations including dusts, wettable powders, and emulsifiable concentrates. They have been used in dips, sprays, flea collars, shampoos, flea foggers, and ant and roach baits.

The organophosphorus insecticides are aliphatic carbon, cyclic, or heterocyclic phosphate esters. They can be identified by the presence of the terms *phosphate*, *phosphorothioate*, *phosphoramidate*, *phosphonate*, *phosphoryl*, or *phosphorothiolate* somewhere in their long chemical name. Carbamates are derivatives of carbamic acid and generally have the terms *carbamate*, or *carbamoyl*, somewhere in their long chemical name. Tables 18.1 and 18.2 provide common and chemical names of some representative OPs and carbamates, and their acute oral LD_{50}.

Kinetics

Ultimately, absorption is dependent upon lipid solubility and carrier formulation, but in general, the cholinesterase inhibitors tend to be well absorbed from any exposure route. They are rapidly distributed to tissues throughout the body.

The cholinesterase inhibitors are metabolized primarily in the liver. In most cases the metabolic process detoxifies the compound but some organophosphorus insecticides may be activated or have an increase in activity following metabolism. In particular, phosphorothioates and phosphorodithioates (sulfur-containing compounds) undergo oxidative desulfuration reactions to form the oxon derivatives that have increased potency. General oxidation and hydrolysis reactions, in particular the cleavage of the ester linkage, markedly reduce toxicity (Taylor 2001). Most OPs and carbamates are excreted as degradation products in the urine.

Mechanism of Action

The OP and carbamate insecticides inhibit the enzyme acetylcholinesterase (AChE). AChE functions to break down the neurotransmitter acetylcholine (ACh) into acetate and choline, which are then recycled to form more acetylcholine. Acetylcholine is the neurotransmitter found between preganglionic and postganglionic neurons of the autonomic nervous system; at the junction of postganglionic parasympathetic neurons in smooth muscle, cardiac muscle, or exocrine glands; at neuromuscular junctions of the somatic nervous system; and at cholinergic synapses in the CNS. AChE is also found on the surface of red blood cells, although its function there is uncertain. Inhibition of AChE results in excess ACh at the postsynaptic receptor,

Table 18.1. Common organophosphorus compounds

Compound	Chemical Name	Acute Oral LD_{50} (mg/kg; rat)
Chlorpyrifos	O,O-diethyl O-(3,5,6-trichloro-2-pyridyl) **phosphorothioate**	135
Diazinon	O,O-diethyl O-(2-isopropyl-4-methyl-6-pyrimidyl) **phosphorothioate**	300
Dichlorvos	2,2-dichloro-vinyl dimethyl **phosphate**	25
Disulfoton (aka Disyston)	O,O-diethyl S-2-[(ethylthio) ethyl] **phosphorodithioate**	2
Phosmet	O,O-dimethyl S-phthalimidomethyl **phosphorodithioate**	147
Terbufos	S[(tert-butylthiomethyl] O,O-diethyl**phosphorodithioate**	1.6
Trichlorfon	Dimethyl (2,2,2-trichloro-1-hydroxyethyl) **phosphonate**	630

Table 18.2. Common carbamate compounds

Compound	Chemical Name	Acute Oral LD_{50} (mg/kg; rat)
Aldicarb	2-methyl-2-(methylthio)propionaldehyde-O-(**methylcarbomoyl**)oxime	0.9
Carbaryl	1-naphthyl **methylcarbamate**	307
Carbofuran	2,3-dihydro-2,2-dimethyl-7-benzofuranyl **methylcarbamate**	8
Methomyl	S-methyl N-(**methylcarbamoyloxy**) thioacetimidate	17
Propoxur	O-isopropoxyphenyl **methylcarbamate**	95

and thus exaggerated stimulation. Normally, depolarization and transmission of the action potential occurs with temporary binding of acetylcholine and ends upon degradation. When AChE is phosphorylated (due to binding of OPs) or carbamylated (due to binding of carbamates) ACh binds to the postsynaptic membrane but is not broken down. Continued stimulation and depolarization of the postsynaptic membranes may progress to paralysis because repolarization cannot occur.

The OPs and carbamates occupy the anionic and esteratic sites of AChE. The binding of OPs to AChE is considered "irreversible" since the phosphorus atom of the OP attached to the esteratic site of AChE is a fairly strong bond with a half-life of hours or days. The binding of the carbonyl structure of carbamates to the esteratic site is considered a "reversible" bond because of its relatively shorter half-life of 30 to 40 minutes. The phenomenon of "aging" can occur with some OPs but not with carbamates. Aging occurs when the phosphorus atom attached to the esteratic site is demethylated or deethylated, resulting in a stable, unbreakable bond. (Sultatos 1994; Fukuto 1990) The rate at which aging occurs varies with the OP. Once aging has occurred, the enzyme will no longer be active and the body must synthesize new enzyme over days to weeks. Reexposure to a cholinesterase-inhibiting compound during this time will cause further depression of already compromised AChE activity with potentially devastating results.

Toxicity

The acute oral toxicity of this class of compounds varies widely, from highly toxic (<1 mg/kg) to practically nontoxic (>5 gm/kg) depending upon formulation, route, and species. Cats and fish tend to be very sensitive to the cholinesterase inhibitors. The minimum oral lethal dose of chlorpyrifos in cats is 10–40 mg/kg (Fikes 1992). Information on toxicities of specific insecticides can be found on MSDSs, other product data literature, and reputable websites. In most cases, acute toxicosis is the most likely problem encountered. Tables 18.1 and 18.2 provide acute oral LD_{50} for some commonly encountered OPs and carbamates.

Clinical Effects

Signs

Clinical signs can be related to either muscarinic or nicotinic effects, and the predominance of a particular sign as well as the rate of its progression can vary with the OP and species involved. Muscarinic signs are the classic cholinergic or SLUDDE signs (salivation, lacrimation, urina-

tion, diarrhea, dyspnea, and emesis). In addition, animals can exhibit miosis and/or bradycardia. Alternatively, due to sympathetic override, mydriasis or tachycardia can be seen. Dyspnea is the result of excess bronchial secretions. Nicotinic signs are related to effects at the neuromuscular junction and can manifest as muscle fasciculations or tremors, generalized tetany, and paralysis. CNS signs, though less common, can include depression or hyperstimulation, and seizures.

A delayed neuropathy syndrome (Organophosphorus Induced Delayed Neuropathy, OPIDN) was described in humans during prohibition following ingestion of Jamaican Ginger tainted with triorthocresylphosphate ("Ginger Jake paralysis"), with signs starting 1 week to 1 month later and resulting in permanent disability. A similar syndrome (intermediate syndrome) has been reported in cats exposed to chlorpyrifos, with signs accompanied by persistently depressed blood cholinesterase activity, starting within days of exposure.

Laboratory

No diagnostic changes are noted on routine CBC or chemistry evaluations. Although performing CBC and chemistry profiles will not rule in or out a diagnosis of OP or carbamate toxicosis, they are recommended to determine the overall health of the poisoned patient.

Differential Diagnosis

Differential diagnoses include agents causing neuromuscular effects as well as those producing muscarinic-type signs including tremorgenic mycotoxins, amitraz, pyrethrins/pyrethroids, pancreatitis, and garbage intoxication.

Diagnostics

Confirmation of an OP or carbamate poisoning is based on history of exposure and appropriate clinical signs, detection of the compound in tissues, and suppression of cholinesterase activity. Samples for cholinesterase determination should be chilled, not frozen.

Antemortem

A test dose of atropine can be used to help differentiate an OP/carbamate toxicosis from another cause of signs. Administration of a preanesthetic dose of atropine (0.02 mg/kg IV) will not produce signs of atropinization in these cases. A much higher dose is required (see below in treatment).

Appropriate samples for chemical detection are ingesta, bait, urine, and hair (if dermal exposure is suspected).

Whole blood should be collected in the clinical patient for determination of cholinesterase activity. Whole blood should be refrigerated, not frozen. Depression of cholinesterase activity of 50% to 80% of normal is typical and is consistent with exposure and intoxication.

Postmortem

Liver, ingesta, hair, urine, and any suspect bait should be collected on necropsy for chemical identification. In addition, collect retina (collect entire globe of eye), and brain (entire brain or hemisphere) for cholinesterase determination. Retina and brain should be chilled, not frozen.

Management of Exposures

The clinical course of many OP and carbamate intoxications progresses rapidly and requires immediate and intensive therapy. The goals of treatment are to correct and support respiratory and cardiovascular function, control nervous stimulation, and eliminate further exposure through decontamination.

Respiratory compromise is the most common cause of death from this class of compounds due to bronchoconstriction, increased bronchial secretions, and bradycardia. Oxygen therapy should be instituted. Atropine is indicated for life-threatening muscarinic signs (Mensching and Volmer 2008). Give to effect, but do so cautiously, because atropine toxicosis can occur with overzealous administration. Atropine is not effective against nicotinic signs.

Pralidoxime chloride (2-PAM; Protopam chloride), a cholinesterase reactivator, at 10–15 mg/kg IM or SC twice daily is indicated for the treatment of neuromuscular (nicotinic) signs (Plumb 2005). Pralidoxime binds to the OP-AChE complex, liberating the enzyme. It is not effective for treatment of muscarinic signs, or if aging has occurred. However, because the aging process varies with the OP, administration of 2-PAM is worthwhile. If no improvement is seen after 3 consecutive doses, 2-PAM should be discontinued, because at high doses (150 mg/kg) it can also inhibit AChE. Diazepam or another anticonvulsant medication is indicated for seizures.

The goal of decontamination is to prevent further absorption. Care should be taken to protect personnel from exposure. Animals exposed dermally should be bathed in a liquid dish detergent. Care should be taken to maintain normal body temperature. Insecticide collars should be removed. Clipping may be necessary for animals with long or matted hair.

Because clinical signs can develop rapidly with some agents, and the carriers for some products may be hydrocarbon-based, induction of vomiting should be done with caution following oral exposures (see Chapter 7, "Decontamination Procedures"). Gastric lavage might be preferable in some cases. Activated charcoal is effective in binding OP and carbamate insecticides.

In all cases of exposure, animals should be monitored and provided with appropriate supportive therapy if necessary.

Prognosis

The prognosis is dependent upon the OP or carbamate involved, the dose and time of exposure, formulation, and species. The more potent AChE agents can produce clinical signs and death within minutes to hours. For these cases, the prognosis is guarded even with prompt and aggressive intervention.

PYRETHRINS AND PYRETHROIDS

Sources/Formulations

Because of concern for toxicity and environmental persistence of the organochlorine and organophosphorus insecticides, there was a shift toward greater use of pyrethrins and pyrethroids in the 1970s. Recent estimates state that pyrethrins and pyrethroids currently make up more than 25% of the world insecticide market (Vais et al. 2001). This class of insecticides is effective against a number of insect pests and products are marketed as sprays, dusts, dips, shampoos, spot-ons, gels, foggers, ear tags, pour-ons, back rubbers, and face rubbers.

Pyrethrum is a mixture of six active insecticidal compounds termed pyrethrins: pyrethrin I and II, cinerin I and II, jasmolin I and II. Pyrethrum occurs naturally in the flowers of *Chrysanthemum* species. Chemically, pyrethrins are esters of alcohols and acids. Synthetic modification of the basic pyrethrin structure has resulted in a series of "pyrethroids," which tend to have greater insecticidal potency and are more environmentally stable than the pyrethrins. Potency is enhanced with the addition of a cyano group, leading to the classification of the type I (lacking a cyano group) and type II (containing a cyano group) pyrethroids.

Kinetics

The pyrethrins and pyrethroids tend to have poor dermal absorption (>2% in humans) (Woollen et al. 1992). However, the grooming behavior of animals results in oral exposure even when products are applied dermally. Carriers and solvents can also influence absorption. Pyrethrins and pyrethroids are incompletely absorbed following oral exposure, with approximately 40%–60% of an oral dose absorbed (ATSDR 2001). Once absorbed they are rapidly distributed and because of their lipophilicity will accumulate in nervous tissue (Anadon 2009). Pyrethrins and pyrethroids are hydrolyzed in the GI tract and metabolized by a variety of tissue types throughout the body. Metabolites and parent compounds are eliminated via bile and urine.

Mechanism of Action

The primary mode of action of the pyrethrins and pyrethroids is through disruption of normal sodium channel function, resulting in a prolongation of sodium channel opening, a less polarized membrane, and ultimate repetitive firing of action potentials. Differences in type I and type II mechanisms have been identified with type II pyrethroids more likely to cause depolarization, but this has little significance in either the occurrence of clinical signs or the treatment of the poisoned patient. Pyrethrins also act on GABA receptors at high doses, but this mechanism also appears to be of little clinical significance (Anadon 2009).

Toxicity

Toxicity varies widely and is dependent upon the individual pyrethrin or pyrethroid, species of animal, formulation, and route of exposure. In general, the pyrethroids are considered less acutely toxic than the OP and carbamate insecticides. Adverse effects are often the result of extralabel use, but can also occur from individual hypersensitivity reactions and genetic-based idiosyncratic reactions (Hansen 2006). Animals that are weak or debilitated from a large flea burden or from other causes are at increased risk. Fish are highly sensitive to this class of compounds. Care should be taken to avoid contamination of water bodies when using these compounds outdoors. Indoor aquaria should be protected when using foggers or sprays in the home. The air pump intake should be turned off and the tank and intake covered during application. The home must be well ventilated before returning to use (Volmer 2004). Cats are exquisitely sensitive to concentrated permethrin products, likely because of their reduced ability to metabolize permethrin.

Clinical Effects

Signs

Because the pyrethrins and pyrethroids are applied via the dermal route, most signs are attributed to skin sensitivity. Cats sprayed with a pyrethrin-based spray might exhibit paw shaking, ear twitching, flicking of the tail, and twitching of the skin on their backs. Some cats hide or are reluctant to move or walk, holding a leg out to the side.

Signs generally begin within minutes to hours postapplication, and resolve with minimal treatment by 24–48 hours (Volmer 2004). Hypersalivation can occur from grooming soon after application. This might be due to the unpleasant taste or to a tingling sensation on the tongue and mouth. Dermal reactions might also be due to a tingling sensation (paresthesia) produced by the product.

Cats mistreated with concentrated permethrin spot-on products (36%–65% permethrin) intended for dogs can develop life-threatening seizures. Cats can also develop a toxicosis following grooming of freshly treated dogs before the product has dried. Signs develop within 12–18 hours and include initial apprehension and agitation, hypersalivation, and vocalization, progressing to tremors and seizures by 18–24 hours. Convulsions are severe and can be difficult to control. Death can occur in untreated cats (Volmer 2004).

Dogs can also develop signs associated with dermal hypersensitivity. They act uncomfortable, lick or chew at their skin, roll on the floor, or rub their backs. Occasionally an episode of vomiting or diarrhea occurs, and is not considered a true toxic effect but a nonspecific stress effect.

Laboratory

No specific clinical pathological alterations are associated with exposure to the pyrethrins and pyrethroids. However, for animals with severe signs, a CBC and chemistry is recommended to assess the overall health of the poisoned patient.

Differential Diagnosis

The differential diagnosis list should include any toxic agents or other conditions that cause nervous stimulation. Toxic agents include strychnine, metaldehyde, methylxanthines, illicit drugs (cocaine, amphetamines), and organophosphorus or carbamate insecticides.

Diagnostics

Diagnosis is based on history of exposure and appropriate clinical signs.

Antemortem

Analysis for pyrethrins and pyrethroids is limited to a few laboratories. Preferred samples include whole blood, serum, and urine. Unfortunately, concentrations are not well correlated to clinical signs. Hair samples can be analyzed for permethrin to verify exposure in cats suspected of receiving an inappropriate application. A spot-on application should be considered if a greasy or oily area is noted on the animal's fur.

Postmortem

Hair, brain, and liver can be used for chemical analysis. Because analyses for pyrethrins and pyrethroids are not widely available, consultation with a diagnostic laboratory is recommended prior to submission. No pathognomonic lesions are expected on gross necropsy or histopathology.

Management of Exposures

Treatment is aimed at controlling excess neurological stimulation and preventing further exposure. For mild effects such as hypersalivation, ear twitching, and paw shaking that are often associated with use of a pyrethrin spray, no treatment is usually required. Offering a tasty treat such as milk or tuna juice can alleviate hypersalivation. If mild signs persist the animal can be bathed in a liquid dish detergent and kept warm. Rinsing alone will not remove most topical products. Clinical signs usually resolve rapidly following bathing. Animals with moderate to severe discomfort may require treatment with an antihistamine. In addition, vitamin E oil applied to the application site might help to alleviate the irritation.

Cats mistreated with a permethrin product intended for dogs should be considered a medical emergency. If the exposure was recent and the animal is not exhibiting clinical signs, the cat should be thoroughly bathed in a liquid dish detergent, dried well, and kept warm. The animal should be monitored for the next 12–18 hours for the development of clinical signs. If the cat is already exhibiting tremors or seizures, hospitalization is required. Methocarbamol, a centrally acting skeletal muscle relaxant, is effective in controlling the tremors and seizures. One-third to one-half of the dose is administered as a bolus (not exceeding 2 ml/min). As the cat begins to relax the administration is paused, and the remainder is given to effect. Methocarbamol can be repeated as needed to a maximum daily dose of 330 mg/kg. Complete termination of the tremors might not occur and is not necessary (Volmer 1998a,b) Diazepam alone is ineffective in controlling severe signs. Barbiturates, gas anesthetics, and propofol have also been used with varying results to control the signs.

Once stabilized the cat should be bathed in liquid dish detergent to remove any residual permethrin, dried well, and kept warm. Activated charcoal is not indicated unless the permethrin product was administered orally to the cat. General supportive care should be instituted including IV fluids, blood glucose monitoring and correction, and thermoregulation. For most cats receiving appropriate treatment, recovery is achieved by 24 to 72 hours, and permanent sequelae are not expected. Fine muscle tremors may linger for several days. However, this should not preclude releasing the patient to the owners as long as the animal is able to eat, drink, and use the litter box. Atropine is not indicated.

Prognosis

Most animals experiencing a pyrethrin or pyrethroid toxicosis are expected to have an excellent prognosis. Cats exposed to concentrated permethrin products have a good prognosis if timely and intensive treatment is initiated. Cats exhibiting severe or prolonged signs, or for which timely treatment is denied, have a guarded prognosis.

NEONICOTINOIDS

Sources/Formulations

Neonicotinoids, the only major new class of insecticides developed in the past 3 decades, have been synthesized for use against insect pests on crops and companion animals. Worldwide annual sales of neonicotinoids account for 11%–15% of the total insecticide market (Tomizawa 2005). Of the 7 neonicotinoids in use today, only 3 are of primary significance to companion animals: imidacloprid (Advantage®), nitenpyram (Capstar®), and dinotefuran (Vectra®). Imidacloprid and dinotefuran are used in topical formulations, and nitenpyram is the active ingredient in an oral product. Imidacloprid and nitenpyram are chloronicotinyl compounds developed based on the structure of nicotine. Dinotefuran is a furanicotinyl compound developed using acetylcholine as the lead compound. The chloronicotinyl compounds are considered first generation neonicotinoids, and the furanicotinyl compounds are third generation. The second generation neonicotinoids are thianicotinyl compounds and are used primarily for crop protection (Wakita 2003).

Kinetics

The neonicotinoids tend to be rapidly absorbed following oral exposure. There are a number of pathways for metabolism depending upon the specific neonicotinoid and species. Elimination is primarily via urine with some fecal excretion. The neonicotinoids tend to have short half-lives in the body and thus pose little risk for bioaccumulation.

Mechanism of Action

The neonicotinoids are considered neurotoxins that bind to the nicotinic acetylcholine receptor (nAChR). They have a much higher binding affinity to the nAChR of insects than mammals (Tomizawa and Casida 2005).

Table 18.3. Toxicological profiles of neonicotinoid insecticides

| | Rat | | Bird |
| | Acute Oral | NOAEL | Acute Oral |
Compound	LD_{50} (mg/kg)	(mg/kg/day)	LD_{50} (mg/kg)
Imidacloprid	450	5.7	31
Nitenpyram	1628	—	>2250
Dinotefuran	2400	127	>2000

Source: Tomizawa 2005.

Dinotefuran is thought to bind to a unique location on the receptor compared to imidacloprid and nitenpyram (Wakita et al. 2005). In normal nerve tissue, the neurotransmitter acetylcholine is rapidly broken down by AChE to end the synaptic transmission and return the membrane to its normal resting state. The neonicotinoids bind at or near the site where nicotine binds, producing unregulated stimulation and ultimately death of the insect.

Toxicity

Because of their low affinity for mammalian nicotinic receptors and rapid metabolism, the neonicotinoids in general have a wide margin of safety. Table 18.3 lists some toxicity values of the 3 common neonicotinoids.

Clinical Effects

Signs

Because of their wide margin of safety, toxic effects from imidacloprid, nitenpyram, and dinotefuran are rare and are likely due to other components of the formulation. Oral exposures can result in self-limiting vomiting. Dermal exposures can result in erythema, pruritus, and alopecia.

Laboratory

No clinical laboratory changes are expected from the neonicotinoids.

Diagnostics

Antemortem

There are no routine diagnostic tests for the neonicotinoids in tissues. Consultation with a diagnostic laboratory is recommended prior to submission.

Postmortem

No lesions are expected on gross necropsy or histopathology.

Management of Exposure

For most clinical cases the signs are transient and require no treatment. Bathing and administration of an antihistamine may be required for some cases of dermal discomfort. Oral exposures can be treated by diluting with milk or water. If vomiting occurs, food and water should be removed for a brief period (1–2 hours) to allow the GI tract to settle down.

Prognosis

Because of their exceptional safety profiles, rapid metabolism, and their availability only in limited quantities for companion animals, exposures carry an excellent prognosis.

REFERENCES

Anadon, A., Martinez-Larranaga, M.R., and Martinez, M.A. 2009. Use and abuse of pyrethrins and synthetic pyrethroids in veterinary medicine. *The Veterinary Journal* 182:7–20.

Andrade, S.F. and Sakate, M. 2003. The comparative efficacy of yohimbine and atipamezole to treat amitraz intoxication in dogs, *Veterinary and Human Toxicology* 45(3): 124–127.

ATSDR (Agency for Toxic Substances and Disease Registry). 2001. Toxicological profile for pyrethrins and pyrethroids: draft for public comment, Washington, D.C., U.S. Department of Health and Human Services, Public Health Service.

Buck, William B., Osweiler, Gary D., Van, Gelder, and Gary, A. 1976. Organochlorine insecticides. In *Clinical and Diagnostic Veterinary Toxicology*, 2nd edition, edited by Gary A. Van Gelder, pp. 191–204. Dubuque: Kendall Hunt.

EXTOXNET. Pesticide information profile for amitraz, 1995, Oregon State University, http://extoxnet.orst.edu/pips/amitraz.htm

Fikes, J.D. 1992. Feline chlorpyrifos toxicosis. In *Current Veterinary Therapy XI: Small Animal Practice*, edited by Robert W Kirk and John D Bonagura. p. 188. Philadelphia: W.B. Saunders.

Fukuto, T.R. 1990. Mechanism of action of organophosphorus and carbamate insecticides. *Environmental Health Perspectives* 87:245–254.

Hansen, Steve R. 2006. Pyrethrins and pyrethroids. In *Small Animal Toxicology*, edited by Michael E. Peterson and Patricia A. Talcott, pp. 1002–1010. St. Louis: Saunders.

Hsu, W.H., Lu, Z.X., and Hembrough, F.B. 1986. Effect of amitraz on heart rate and aortic blood pressure in conscious dogs: Influence of atropine, prazosin, tolazoline, and yohimbine. *Toxicology and Applied Pharmacology* 84(2): 418–422.

Hugnet, C., Buronrosse, F., Pineau, X., Cadore, J.L., Lorque, G., and Berny, P.J. 1996. Toxicity and kinetics of amitraz in dogs, *American Journal of Veterinary Research* 57(10): 1506–1510.

Mensching, Donna, Volmer, Petra A. 2008. Insecticides and Molluscicides. *In Handbook of Small Animal Practice*, edited by Rhea V. Morgan, pp. 1197–1204. St. Louis: Saunders Elsevier.

Paradis, M. 1999. New approaches to the treatment of canine demodicosis. *Veterinary Clinics of North America Small Animal Practice* 29(6):1425–1436.

Plumb, D.C. 2005. *Veterinary Drug Handbook*, 3d ed. Ames, Iowa: Blackwell Publishing.

Sultatos, LG. 1994. Mammalian toxicology of organophosphorus pesticides. *Journal of Toxicology and Environmental Health* 43(3):271–289.

Taylor, Palmer. 2001. Anticholinesterase agents. In *Goodman and Gilman's the Pharmacological Basis of Therapeutics*, 10th edition, edited by Joel G. Hardman, Lee E. Limbird, and Alfred G. Gilman, pp. 175–192. New York: McGraw-Hill.

Tomizawa, Motohiro, Casida, John E. 2005. Neonicotinoid insecticide toxicology: Mechanisms of selective action. *Annual Review of Pharmacology and Toxicology* 45: 247–268.

Vais, H., Williamson, M.S., Devonshire, A.L., Usherwood, P.N. 2001. The molecular interactions of pyrethroid insecticides with insect and mammalian sodium channels. *Pest Management Science* 57(10):877–888.

Volmer, P.A., Kahn, S.A., Knight, M.W., and Hansen, S.R. 1998a. Warning against use of some permethrin products in cats. *Journal of the American Veterinary Medical Association* 213(6):800–801.

———. 1998b. Permethrin spot-on products can be toxic in cats. *Veterinary Medicine* 93(12):1039.

Volmer, Petra A. 2004. Pyrethrins and pyrethroids. In *Clinical Veterinary Toxicology*. edited by Konnie H. Plumlee, pp. 188–190. St. Louis: Mosby.

Wakita T., Kinoshita, K., Yamada, E., Yasui, N., Kawahara, N., Naoi, A., Nakaya, M., Ebihara, K., Matsuno, H., and Kodaka, K. 2003. The discovery of dinotefuran: A novel neonicotinoid. *Pest Management Science* 59(9):1016–1022.

Wakita, T., Yasui, N., Yamada, E., Kishi, D. 2005. Development of a novel insecticide, dinotefuran. *Journal of Pesticide Science* 30(2)122–123.

Woollen, B.H., Marsh, J.R., Laird, W.J., Lesser, J.E. 1992. The metabolism of cypermethrin in man: Differences in urinary metabolite profiles following oral and dermal administration. *Xenobiotica* 22(8):983–991.

Other Pesticides

19

Robert H. Poppenga

INTRODUCTION

A pesticide is defined as any substance or mixture of substances intended for preventing, destroying, repelling, or mitigating any pest. A pesticide may be a chemical substance, a biological agent (such as a virus or bacterium), an antimicrobial, a disinfectant, or a device used against any pest. Pests include insects, plant pathogens, weeds, molluscs, birds, mammals, fish, parasites, and microbes that destroy property, spread disease, or are a vector for disease or cause a nuisance. Pesticides can be categorized based upon the type of pest they are intended to control (i.e., insecticides, rodenticides, herbicides, fungicides, avicides, etc.). There are literally hundreds of different chemicals used as pesticides with diverse chemical structures, formulations, and toxicities. Although there are obvious benefits to the use of pesticides, there are also potential risks such as potential toxicity to humans and other animals.

Insecticides and rodenticides are commonly involved in animal intoxications and are discussed in separate chapters. This chapter is intended to discuss several other diverse pesticides that have been associated with pet intoxication; it is not intended to be comprehensive in its scope. Interested readers are referred to an excellent website under the auspices of the National Pesticide Information Center (NPIC) that has a wealth of information on various pesticides: http://npic.orst.edu/index.html. This website has numerous pesticide fact sheets and toxicity information and a section specifically addressing pesticide use on or around animals. The USEPA-sponsored publication entitled *Recognition and Management of Pesticide Poi-*sonings, 5th edition, is a valuable source of information regarding the toxicology and general treatment approaches for a large number of pesticides typically not discussed in veterinary textbooks (Riegart and Roberts 1999). The entire manual is available from http://npic.orst.edu/ rmpp.htm. It is important to keep in mind that there is limited species-specific toxicity data for many pesticides and that for the majority of pesticides discussed below, treatment of poisoned animals involves appropriate and timely decontamination along with symptomatic and supportive care; specific antidotes are typically not available.

MISCELLANEOUS INSECTICIDES AND REPELLANTS

Boric Acid and Borates

Sources and Formulations

Boric acid is formulated as tablets and powders to kill insect larvae in livestock confinement areas and cockroaches, ants, and other insects in residences. Powders and tablets scattered on floors present a hazard for pets; cats can be exposed by grooming paws after contact with powders spread on floors.

Kinetics and Toxicity

Absorption of boric acid from the GI tract is rapid (Welch 2004). Following absorption it is found at highest concentrations in the brain, liver, and kidneys. It is eliminated unchanged by the kidneys with a half-life of 5 to 21 hours. The acute oral LD_{50} reported for rats range from 2 to approximately 5 g/kg. Thus, it is considered slightly toxic.

Small Animal Toxicology Essentials, First Edition. Edited by Robert H. Poppenga, Sharon Gwaltney-Brant.
© 2011 John Wiley and Sons, Inc. Published 2011 by John Wiley and Sons, Inc.

However, chronic exposure to lower doses is a potential problem.

Mechanism of Action

The mechanism of action of boric acid is unknown, but it is considered to be cytotoxic.

Clinical Effects

The GI tract, vascular system, brain, and kidneys are primary target organs. In acute, single-dose, oral exposures, signs include hypersalivation, vomiting, depression, anorexia, diarrhea, and abdominal pain. Depending on the dose ingested, weakness, ataxia, tremors, focal or generalized seizures, oliguria or anuria, renal tubular nephrosis, and liver damage may occur, although the latter is uncommon (Welch 2004). Seizures can be followed by metabolic acidosis, depression, coma, and death. Chronic, toxic exposures cause anorexia, weight loss, vomiting, loose stools, rashes, alopecia, anemia, and death.

Diagnostics

Antemortem

A history of exposure, occurrence of compatible clinical signs, and possibly the detection of elevated levels of boron in blood, plasma, or urine support a diagnosis.

Postmortem

Significant lesions can be found in target organs such as the GI tract, kidneys, brain, liver, and skin. No lesions are unique to boric acid, but a constellation of lesions might support a diagnosis. Measurement of boron in kidneys and liver might also be helpful to confirm exposure.

Management of Exposures

Standard decontamination procedures should be followed with suspected exposures. Exposed hair and skin should be washed with mild soap or shampoo and water followed by thorough rinsing. Emetics or cathartics might not be indicated if an animal has already vomited or exhibited diarrhea. Activated charcoal is generally not administered due to poor adsorption of boric acid. Symptomatic and supportive care is often needed. Intravenous balanced electrolyte solutions and glucose are administered as needed. GI protectants and antiemetics might be indicated. Maintaining urine flow is important to prevent or correct kidney damage. Although dialysis (hemo- or peritoneal dialysis) might be indicated if renal failure occurs, it does not appear to increase borate clearance. Benzodiazepines can be given to control seizures.

Prognosis

Most exposures result in rather mild GI signs; in such cases the prognosis is good. With large acute ingestions or chronic exposures, the prognosis is more guarded.

Diethyltoluamide (DEET)
Sources and Formulations

DEET is a widely used liquid insect repellant suitable for application to skin or fabrics. Products contain a range of concentrations from 5% to 100%.

Kinetics and Toxicity

DEET is well absorbed following dermal or oral exposures (Dorman 2004). The amount absorbed increases with increasing concentrations, and the solvents used in many products enhance absorption as well (Riegart and Roberts 1999). The clearance of absorbed DEET is rapid with a half-life measured in hours. It is primarily eliminated via the urine. The toxicity of DEET is low with rat oral LD_{50} ranging from 1.8 to 2.7 g/kg body weight. Dermal toxicity is also low based on studies in rabbits where single applications of 2 to 4 g/kg did not cause any clinical signs.

Mechanism of Action

The mechanism of toxic action of DEET is unknown.

Signs

Repeated topical exposures can cause dermal and ocular irritation. Clinical signs observed in dogs and cats with suspected acute DEET intoxication include vomiting, tremors, excitation, ataxia, and seizures (Dorman 1990). There are no characteristic laboratory findings associated with DEET intoxication.

Diagnostics

Antemortem

An antemortem diagnosis relies on a history of exposure (perhaps noticing a residue on skin or hair). Testing for DEET is not widely available, although contacting a veterinary diagnostic laboratory might be helpful; detection of residues on hair or in biological specimens only confirms exposure and not necessarily intoxication.

Postmortem

There are no characteristic postmortem findings.

Management of Exposures

Treatment involves standard dermal, ocular, and GI decontamination procedures including induction of emesis if early after an oral ingestion, washing skin and hair with mild soap and water followed by a thorough rinse, and flushing eyes following an ocular exposure. Initially, seizures should be treated with a benzodiazepine such as diazepam. Other symptomatic and supportive care is provided as needed.

Prognosis

Most animals with mild DEET intoxication recover uneventfully in several days.

Macrocyclic Lactone Parasiticides

Sources and Formulations

Macrocyclic lactone parasiticides (also known as *macrolides*) are compounds used to treat or prevent a variety of parasitic diseases in domestic animals and humans. These products are derived from fermentation products of *Streptomyces avermitilis* and *S. cyaneogriseus*. They are often referred to as *endectocides* due to their ability to kill both internal (*endo*) and external (*ecto*) parasites (Lanusse et al. 2009). Macrolides include ivermectin, abamectin, doramectin, eprinomectin, milbemycin oxime, moxidectin, and selamectin. These products are used for prevention of heartworms in dogs and cats, treatment of feline ear mites, prevention of internal nematode infestation, and management of a variety of other parasitic diseases such as scabies and infestations of lice (Mealey 2006). Several macrolides are used in food animals and horses for the prevention and treatment of internal and external parasites. Abamectin b_1 is a macrocyclic lactone that is present in some household insecticides, in ant and roach bait stations, and in agricultural insecticides. Products containing macrolides include tablets, chewable tablets, spot-on products, gels, pour-on liquids, injectable solutions, otic solutions, premixes, and granules.

Kinetics and Toxicity

In general, macrolides are well absorbed orally and some (e.g., selamectin) are also well absorbed dermally (Mealey 2006). Many of these compounds are lipophilic, with moxidectin being the most lipophilic of the group (Lanusse et al. 2009). The macrolides have relatively long half-lives due to their wide tissue distribution, lipophilicity (fat storage), extensive biliary, and intestinal secretion and enterohepatic recycling (Lanusse et al. 2009).

The macrolides have a wide margin of safety in mammals due to the fact that they do not cross the blood-brain barrier under normal circumstances (Lanusse et al. 2009). Animals with blood-brain barrier defects are at increased risk for toxicosis from doses of macrolides that would not affect animals with intact blood-brain barriers.

Table 19.1. Breeds known to carry the MDR1 P-glycoprotein genetic polymorphism

Collie	Wäller
Longhaired whippet	White Swiss shepherd
Shetland sheepdog	Old English sheepdog
Miniature Australian shepherd	Border collie
Australian shepherd	German shepherd dog

A genetic polymorphism in some breeds of dogs causes a defect in the P-glycoprotein of a multidrug resistant pump (coded for by the MDR1, or ABCB1, gene) in the blood-brain barrier. As a consequence of this defect, the blood-brain barriers of affected dogs do not exclude certain xenobiotics (including the macrolides) from the brain. Additionally, the same P-glycoprotein acts within the intestine to limit absorption of macrolides, so dogs with the MDR1 defect may absorb more drug after ingestion and attain higher blood concentrations of macrolides (Lanusse et al. 2009). Higher blood and CNS concentrations of macrolide put MDR-1 defective dogs at risk for toxicosis at dosages of macrolides that are well tolerated by dogs without this genetic polymorphism. However, the doses of macrolides commonly used for heartworm preventative are well below the levels expected to cause clinical signs in MDR-1 defective dogs, and no problems are expected with the monthly heartworm treatments even in affected dogs. Table 19.1 lists the dog breeds that to date have had the MDR1 defect confirmed through genetic testing. Because this defect is an autosomal recessive trait, only a fraction of dogs within these breeds would be expected to be affected.

The minimum toxic dose of ivermectin in MDR1-defective dogs is 100 mcg/kg, which is approximately 16 times higher than the monthly heartworm preventive dose; moxidectin toxicosis has been reported in a collie at 90 mcg/kg (30 times the monthly heartworm preventive dose); milbemycin toxicosis has been reported in MDR1-defective collies at 5 mg/kg (10 times the monthly heartworm preventive dose); and selamectin caused ataxia when administered orally to MDR1-defective collies at 2.5 times the therapeutic dose. In contrast, dogs without the MDR1 defect can generally tolerate ivermectin dosages up to 600 mcg/kg and milbemycin dosages up to 1.6 mg/kg for treatment of ectoparasites (Mealey 2006). Based on results in laboratory dogs, the minimum toxic dosage of ivermectin had been reported to be 2.5 mg/kg. A recent review of ivermectin toxicosis in dogs revealed that some individuals are intolerant of dosages as low as 0.2 mg/kg in spite of them belonging to breeds not associated with the MDR1 defect (Merola et al, 2009), so the potential for individual sensitivity to macrolides needs to be considered whenever treatment with higher doses is contemplated.

Mechanism of Action

The macrolides cause death of parasites by paralyzing nematodes and arthropods through actions on chloride channels of the pharyngeal pump and somatic musculature of the parasites. As a result, the parasite loses the ability to obtain nutrients and its muscular movements are inhibited. Macrolides also may stimulate some parasite GABA receptors.

Mammals are largely protected from the actions of macrolides on the nervous system, as the target receptors exist only within the central nervous system in mammals, and the macrolides are excluded from the CNS by the P-glycoprotein pump of the blood-brain barrier (Gramer 2010). Animals with defects in the blood-brain barrier due to inflammation, anatomic anomaly or trauma can be at increased risk of macrolide toxicosis. Additionally, the MDR1 pump can be overwhelmed in cases of macrolide overdose, allowing excessive amounts of macrolide into the CNS and resulting in toxicosis. Once in the CNS, the macrolides alter chloride channels and GABA activity, resulting in CNS depression.

Clinical Effects

Clinical signs associated with macrolide toxicosis include mydriasis, ataxia, CNS depression, hypersalivation, vomiting, clinical blindness, coma, tremors and seizures (Roder 2004). Hypothermia may develop secondarily in recumbent animals. Signs generally occur soon after an overdose, but in animals being treated with daily doses signs may not develop until several days of treatment have passed. Additionally, dogs being treated with injectable macrolides may have a delay in onset and delay in peak effect as the macrolide is slowly absorbed from the subcutaneous injection site.

Diagnostics

Macrolides can be detected in various body tissues, but the utility of such analysis in aiding in diagnosis of emergent cases is minimal. Diagnosis is based on history of exposure and consistent clinical signs. There are no expected consistent postmortem lesions in animals succumbing to macrolide toxicosis.

A DNA test is available to detect dogs with MDR1 polymorphisms. The test uses cheek swabs and can be helpful in identifying dogs that are at increased risk for macrolide toxicosis.

Management of Exposures

The goals of managing exposures to macrolides are patient stabilization, decontamination, and supportive care for recumbent animals. In recent ingestions with no serious clinical signs, induction of emesis should be considered. Because of the rapid absorption of macrolides from liquids and gels, if more than 30 to 60 minutes have elapsed from ingestion, it may be more beneficial to administer activated charcoal. Repeated doses of activated charcoal should be administered to all animals showing more than mild signs in order to try to reduce the half-lives of the macrolides. Animals that become comatose will need intensive nursing care to prevent hypothermia, decubital ulcers, and aspiration. Recently, intravenous lipid solution infusions (ILS) have been used to successfully manage severe macrolide toxicosis (Crandell 2009), although anecdotally not all animals appear to respond to this treatment modality.

Prognosis

The prognosis depends on the dosage ingested, the MDR1 status of a dog, and the availability of good nursing care to manage comatose animals. Comatose animals surviving more than 24 hours have a reasonable chance of recovery if adequate nursing care is provided.

FUNGICIDES

Fungicides constitute a chemically diverse group of pesticides. The risk of intoxication from fungicides is low given use restrictions, available formulations, and low bioavailability of these compounds (Osweiler, 1996; Riegart and Roberts 1999). Many fungicides are formulated as suspensions of wettable powders or granules, which prevent rapid and efficient absorption from sites of exposure. Most pets are likely to be exposed to fungicides as a result of their application to lawns. The reader is referred to several sources for additional information (Gerken 1995; Osweiler 1996; Riegart and Roberts 1999; and Yeary 2000; the NPIC website).

Toxicity

Fungicides vary in terms of their acute toxicity. Many are almost nontoxic with rodent LD_{50} greater than 0.5 g/kg body weight (Osweiler 1996). However, some have relatively low rodent oral LD_{50} (e.g., cyclohexamide with a rat LD_{50} of 2 mg/kg). The four fungicides listed by Yeary (2000) for lawn use—flutolonil, iprodione, propiconazole and thiophanate-methyl—have rat oral LD_{50} of >5000 mg/kg, >2000 mg/kg, 1517 mg/kg, and 6640 mg/kg, respectively.

Clinical Effects

Clinical signs are most often nonspecific and include anorexia, depression, weakness, and diarrhea (Osweiler 1996). Many fungicides are irritating to skin, eyes, and mucous membranes. There are no characteristic laboratory findings.

Diagnostics

A diagnosis of intoxication primarily relies on a history of exposure. Testing for specific fungicides in biological samples is typically not available.

Management of Exposures

Treatment involves standard decontamination procedures. For known exposures to fungicides that have low toxicity, GI decontamination is probably not necessary due to the unlikely occurrence of clinical signs. There are no antidotes, so in the unlikely event of intoxication, symptomatic and supportive care is indicated.

HERBICIDES

Herbicides are widely used around farms and homes and constitute a diverse group of chemicals. They come in a variety of formulations that are designed to prevent plants from growing (preemergent herbicides) or kill plants that are already growing(postemergent herbicides). Preemergent herbicides are typically incorporated into soil to prevent germination, and postemergent herbicides are applied directly to the growing plant. Several major categories of herbicides include chlorophenoxy herbicides (e.g., 2,4-D), nitrophenolic and nitrocresolic herbicides (e.g., dinitrocresol, dinitrophenol, dinocap, and dinoseb, among others), triazine herbicides (e.g., atrazine and simazine), and bipyridyls (e.g., paraquat and diquat). An extensive list of other herbicides with associated toxicity information can be found in Riegart and Roberts (1999). Only chlorophenoxy and dipyridyls are discussed below.

Chlorophenoxy Herbicides

Sources and Formulations

These compounds are used alone or mixed into commercial fertilizers to control broadleaf weeds. There are numerous commercial products that contain chlorophenoxy herbicides; 2,4-D is one of the most commonly used herbicides around the home. 2,4-D is available in several chemical forms including salts, esters, and an acid form;

toxicity is dependent on the chemical form. Also, products containing 2,4-D can be in liquid, dust, or granular formulations.

Kinetics and Toxicity

Following ingestion, 2,4-D is rapidly absorbed; the degree of dermal absorption varies with the formulation of 2,4-D and species (Yeary 2006). Absorbed 2,4-D is widely distributed throughout the body, but it does not accumulate in fat. Elimination is via the renal anion transport system of the kidney; this system is not as efficient in dogs as other species, making dogs more susceptible to exposures to 2,4-D. In dogs, oral dosages of 2,4-D exceeding 175 mg/kg resulted in toxicosis, characterized primarily by myotonia. Although dosages this high are possible if dogs were exposed to very concentrated solutions, at the concentrations used in residential areas (<1%) exposure of dogs to toxic levels of 2,4-D is extremely unlikely. A NOAEL of 1 mg/kg/day has been established for dogs in a chronic study (Yeary 2006).

Clinical Effects

Signs

Chlorophenoxy herbicides are moderately irritating to skin and mucous membranes. Inhalation of sprays can cause a burning sensation in the nasopharynx and chest and result in coughing. Manifestations of systemic toxicity of these herbicides are known mainly from deliberate, suicidal exposures in people (Riegart and Roberts 1999). Most reports of fatal outcomes involve acidosis, electrolyte imbalances, renal failure, and multiple organ failure. Early signs following exposure include vomiting, diarrhea, confusion, behavioral changes, and tachycardia. Muscle weakness, moderate increases in body temperature, hyperventilation, and seizures can also occur, but they are less common. Laboratory changes include low arterial pH and bicarbonate, elevated serum CPK concentrations due to muscle damage, elevated BUN and creatinine, and electrolyte disturbances (hyperkalemia and hypocalcemia). Mild leukocytosis and liver enzyme elevations have also been noted.

Clinical signs of 2,4-D toxicosis in dogs include vomiting, anorexia, reluctance to move, muscle rigidity, ataxia, CNS depression, and muscle weakness (Yeary 2006). Spastic movements or clonic spasms may occur in severe cases.

Diagnostics

A diagnosis relies on a history of recent exposure. Depending on the nature of the exposure, a peculiar odor might be noted on the hair or breath of an exposed animal. Although antemortem or postmortem analysis of biological specimens is possible, such testing is not widely available.

Management of Exposures

Initial management should include consideration of standard skin and gastrointestinal decontamination procedures. Significant vomiting prior to presentation would make induction of emesis contraindicated. Other treatment is largely symptomatic and supportive. Antiemetics should be used as needed to control vomiting. Dogs presenting with myotonia may benefit from the use of muscle relaxants such as methocarbamol. Intravenous fluid administration to induce diuresis is warranted. Forced alkaline diuresis has been used successfully in the management of attempted suicides in people (Riegart and Roberts 1999). Alkalinizing the urine with sodium bicarbonate dramatically accelerates excretion of 2,4-D.

Prognosis

The prognosis is typically good. However, in people, myotonia and muscle weakness can persist for months after acute poisonings.

Dipyridyl Herbicides

Paraquat

Sources and Exposure

Paraquat is widely used as an herbicide for weed and grass control. In the U.S., paraquat is available primarily as a liquid in various strengths. It is classified as "restricted use," which means that it can be used only by people who are licensed applicators.

Paraquat is one of the more common agents used in suicidal attempts. Because paraquat is highly poisonous, the form marketed in the U.S. has a blue dye to keep it from being confused with beverages such as coffee, a sharp odor to serve as a warning, and an added agent to cause vomiting if ingested. Paraquat has also been used to maliciously poison pets (Bischoff et al. 1998; Cope et al. 2004).

Kinetics and Toxicity

Paraquat is poorly absorbed from the GI tract (only 5 to 10%), although it can persist in the GI tract for many hours (Oehme and Pickrell 2004). It is primarily excreted via the kidneys. Paraquat has a unique affinity for lung tissue and accumulates in alveolar epithelial cells. In animals, paraquat has oral LD_{50} ranging from 22 to 262 mg/kg. Clinical experience in humans provides a rough dose-response scale associated with the severity of intoxication. Dosages of <20 mg/kg body weight are associated with mild GI signs and likely recovery. Dosages of 20 to 40 mg/kg are associated with pulmonary fibrosis and death within 2 to 3 weeks postexposure. Dosages >40 mg/kg are associated with multiple organ damage with mortality within 1 to 7 days (before the delayed pulmonary damage occurs) (Riegart and Roberts 1999).

Mechanism of Action

Paraquat forms free radicals that can damage cell membranes. In the lung, one of the major target tissues, paraquat undergoes repeated redox cycling that increases production of reactive oxygen species such as superoxide ions (O_2^-) while decreasing important intracelluar reducing species such as NADPH (Oehme and Pickrell 2004). Superoxide radicals are converted to hydrogen peroxide by superoxide dismutase. Both superoxide radicals and hydrogen peroxide damage epithelial cell membranes and cause pulmonary damage. Paraquat is also an irritant and vesicant and can cause significant localized damage upon contact with skin, eyes, or mucous membranes.

CLINICAL EFFECTS

SIGNS

Dermal contact can result in erythema and blistering. Eye contact results in significant corneal damage. Systemic signs following exposure typically occur in three phases. Phase one reflects the corrosive action of paraquat and the development of gastrointestinal signs including vomiting, dysphagia, and abdominal pain. The second phase is manifested by renal and liver damage; this occurs 2 to 3 days after exposure. The third phase is characterized by development of pulmonary fibrosis, which is ultimately responsible for most fatalities.

LABORATORY

There are no specific laboratory findings noted with paraquat poisoning. Radiographic evidence of pulmonary edema or other pulmonary abnormalities is present if the animal survives for a sufficient length of time for lesions to develop.

Diagnosis

ANTEMORTEM

Antemortem diagnosis relies on a history of exposure and occurrence of compatible clinical signs. Detection of paraquat in serum/plasma or urine samples is possible.

POSTMORTEM

Postmortem detection of paraquat in tissues or urine is possible. Because paraquat accumulates in the lungs, samples of this tissue are often positive for paraquat when other tissues are negative. Pathologic changes in the lungs are also rather unique.

Management of Exposures

There are no antidotes for paraquat intoxication. If an animal is known to have just ingested paraquat, the goal is removal from the stomach of as much of the toxicant as possible as quickly as possible to prevent absorption. Emesis should be induced or gastric lavage should be performed. The administration of activated charcoal or Fuller's earth should be started immediately and continued every 4–6 hours for 3–7 days following ingestion. Intravenous fluids and furosemide should be administered to create a forced diuresis, increasing the rate of excretion of paraquat via the kidneys (Cope et al. 2004). Diuresis is most useful in the first 72 hours after ingestion. Hemodialysis is another useful modality in the treatment of paraquat ingestion, but it also must be performed within the first 72 hours to improve outcomes. The lack of availability of hemodialysis to most veterinarians makes this treatment option more theoretical than practical.

Once an animal presents with clinical signs of respiratory distress, treatment is limited to supportive care. Interestingly, oxygen therapy is not recommended as part of the initial stabilization or treatment of paraquat ingestion. This is because oxygen increases the amount of O_2^- formed and O_2^- formation is one of the main causes of pulmonary damage.

Prognosis

The prognosis, as mentioned earlier, is dependent on the degree of exposure. The prognosis is good if only gastrointestinal signs occur. However, the prognosis is poor in patients developing multiple organ failure or pulmonary impairment.

Herbicide Exposure and Cancer

The association between pesticide exposure and the occurrence of various human cancers has long been debated and studied. Studies linking the occurrence of malignant lymphoma in dogs with the owner's use of 2,4-D and of seminomas in military working dogs in Vietnam to pesticide exposure raised the issue of an association in veterinary medicine (Hayes et al. 1990, 1991). A review of the malignant lymphoma study refuted an association with the use of 2,4-D because of numerous limitations to the original study design (Carlo et al. 1992). An epidemiologic study of household dogs reported an increased risk of bladder cancer with topical insecticide use (Glickman et al. 1989). Studies have also associated an increase in transitional cell carcinomas in Scottish terriers with the use of topical spot-on flea control products and exposure of lawns to herbicides (Glickman et al. 2004; Raghavan et al. 2004). Unfortunately, there are not enough data to draw any firm conclusions concerning pesticide exposure and cancer or other chronic disease processes in animals.

Molluscicides

Metaldehyde

Sources and Formulations

Metaldehyde is found in a number of snail and slug baits that are commonly used in and around gardens. Baits are available in liquid, powder, pellet, and granular formulations. The concentration of metaldehyde in these products ranges from 2% to 4%. Some states require that certain formulations be designed so that they are unattractive to nontarget species such as dogs (Talcott 2004).

Kinetics and Toxicity

In the stomach, metaldehyde undergoes acid hydrolysis to acetaldehyde, which is rapidly absorbed (Richardson et al. 2003). Metaldehyde is also absorbed from the stomach intact. Metaldehyde is rapidly metabolized in the liver by cytochrome P450. Acetaldehyde is also rapidly metabolized to carbon dioxide. Less than 10% of absorbed metaldehyde is eliminated in the urine as parent compound. The half-life of metaldehyde is unknown for dogs and cats, but is approximately 27 hours in people.

Mechanism of Action

The mechanism of toxic action is unknown, but likely involves alterations of neurotransmitters such as GABA, serotonin, and norepinephrine in the brain (Richardson et al. 2003).

Clinical Effects

SIGNS

A common presentation of intoxicated animals is termed "shake and bake." Signs can commence as soon as 30 minutes postexposure. The most common clinical signs in dogs include tachycardia, nystagmus, hyperpnea, ataxia, seizures, acidosis, cyanosis, diarrhea, dehydration, and hyperthermia (Richardson et al. 2003). Uncontrolled hyperthermia can lead to DIC and multiple organ failure. Temporary blindness has been reported in dogs (Talcott 2004). Heightened sensitivity to noise, light, and touch is also commonly noted. Signs are similar in other intoxicated species.

LABORATORY

There are no characteristic laboratory changes. Hemoconcentration, alterations of renal and liver function (possibly secondary to uncontrolled hyperthermia), and mild metabolic acidosis have been reported.

Diagnosis

ANTEMORTEM

A diagnosis relies on a history of exposure and occurrence of compatible clinical signs. Laboratory detection of metaldehyde in stomach contents, serum/plasma and urine can confirm exposure; such tests are commonly available in areas where metaldehyde-containing products are frequently used.

POSTMORTEM

There are no characteristic lesions noted. Analysis of GI contents or urine can confirm exposure.

Management of Exposures

Treatment is directed toward decontamination, controlling muscle tremors and seizures, correcting hyperthermia, and providing adequate cardiovascular and respiratory support (Talcott 2004).

Standard decontamination protocols are recommended. In asymptomatic animals, emetics can be used. In symptomatic animals they are not recommended due to the risk of aspiration. Alternatively, gastric lavage might be considered, particularly if the animal is anesthetized to control muscle tremors or seizures. Activated charcoal with or without a cathartic is indicated.

A variety of drugs are used to control muscle tremors or seizures including benzodiazepines, barbiturates, gas anesthetics, propofol, and methocarbamol. Methocarbamol is likely to be effective and should be tried first (Richardson et al. 2003). Hyperthermia usually resolves one muscle tremors are controlled. If not, evaporative cooling, cool water baths, or cool water enemas might be indicated. Other treatment is symptomatic and supportive. Regular monitoring of blood gas concentrations, anion gap, and urine pH is recommended to identify metabolic acidosis if present. Metabolic acidosis also tends to resolve once muscle tremors are controlled.

Prognosis

The overall prognosis is good with appropriate decontamination and control of muscle tremors and seizures.

AVICIDES

4-aminopyridine

Sources and Formulations

4-aminopyridine (4-AP) is registered as Avitrol® by the EPA for use against red- winged blackbirds, grackles, and blackbirds in agricultural fields, pigeons, and sparrows in public buildings, and various birds around livestock feeding pens. It is usually formulated as a grain (e.g., corn) bait with 0.5 to 3% active ingredient; it is also available as a powder. It is a restricted use pesticide that can be used only by certified applicators. 4-AP repels birds by poisoning a few individual members of a flock of birds, causing them to become hyperactive and to utter distress calls, which signal other birds to leave the site. Only a small number of birds need to be affected to cause alarm in the rest of the flock. After one alarming exposure, birds will usually not return to treated areas.

Kinetics and Toxicity

The chemical is rapidly absorbed from the GI tract. It is rapidly metabolized by the liver and metabolites are excreted via the kidneys (Schell 2004). 4-AP is highly toxic for mammals and birds with LD_{50}s ranging from 3.7 mg/kg for dogs to 20 mg/kg for rodents. Horses have been intoxicated with as little as 3 mg/kg.

Mechanism of Action

4-AP blocks potassium ion channels, which causes an increased release of acetylcholine within synapses and enhanced nerve transmission.

Clinical Effects

Reported clinical signs include salivation, hyperexcitability, tremors, incoordination, tonic-clonic seizures, and cardiac arrhthymias. Signs can begin within 15 minutes of exposure, reflecting rapid absorption of the chemical from the gastrointestinal tract. Laboratory changes are nonspecific and include alterations consistent with metabolic acidosis and possibly mild liver dysfunction.

Diagnosis

An antemortem or postmortem diagnosis relies on a history of exposure and the occurrence of compatible clinical signs and detection of 4-AP in suspect bait samples, GI contents, liver, kidney, or urine.

Management of Exposures

Treatment involves minimizing absorption and controlling CNS signs, along with other necessary symptomatic and supportive care. Standard and timely decontamination procedures are indicated. Benzodiazepines or barbiturates are recommended to control seizures. Monitoring of acid-base status and ECGs are recommended. Tachyarrhythmias are controlled with β-blockers such as propanolol.

Prognosis

Animals surviving beyond 4 hours postexposure reportedly have a good prognosis.

LARGE PREDATOR CONTROL

Sodium Fluoroacetate (Compound 1080)

Sources

Sodium fluoroacetate is a naturally occurring compound found in several plant species in Africa, Australia, and South America. In the U.S., it has been used for predator control (particularly coyotes) under strict guidelines. Its use is limited to inclusion in livestock protection collars (LPCs) primarily used on sheep and goats in several states registered with the EPA (an EPA-approved certification and training program is required) (Parton 2004). LPCs used on sheep and goats contain 30 ml of 1% sodium fluoroacetate (300 mg of active ingredient).

Kinetics and Toxicity

Fluoroacetate is readily absorbed from the GI tract, lungs, and mucous membranes. The parent compound is considered to be nontoxic, but it is metabolized to monofluoroacetic acid by hydrolysis. The monofluoroacetic acid reacts with coenzyme A (CoA) to form fluoroacetyl CoA. Parent compound and metabolites are eliminated primarily via the kidneys.

Fluoroacetate is highly toxic. Oral lethal dosages have been determined for a number of animal species and range from 0.06 to 0.2 mg/kg for dogs to 10 to 30 mg/kg for birds (Parton 2004).

Mechanism of Action

Fluoroacetyl CoA combines with oxaloacetate in the tricarboxylic acid cycle (TCA) and is converted to fluorocitrate. Fluorocitrate inhibits the enzyme aconitase and the oxidation of citric acid, resulting in blockage of the cycle. This results in cellular energy depletion, increases in citrate and lactate concentrations and a decrease in blood pH.

Clinical Effects

Signs

Signs appear rapidly in intoxicated animals (as soon as 30 minutes after exposure). Signs are primarily related to CNS stimulation: anxiety, frenzied behavior, hyperesthesia, and seizures. Vomiting, salivation, urination, defecation, tenesmus, and hyperthermia also can occur. Seizures are tonic-clonic in nature and seizure episodes are interspersed with periods of relative normalcy. Anoxia associated with continuous seizing leads to respiratory failure, coma, and death. Cardiac arrhythmias are reported in cats. Animals exposed to sublethal doses of fluoroacetate exhibit severe depression, anorexia, listlessness, teeth grinding, and weakness.

Laboratory

Consistent clinical pathologic changes include hyperglycemia, hypocalcemia (ionized), acidosis, and elevations of citrate. Cardiac arrhthymias in cats might be secondary to hypocalcemia.

Differentials

Diseases associated with seizures and CNS stimulation should be strongly considered as differentials. These include numerous intoxications: strychnine, chlorinated hydrocarbon insecticides, bromethalin, lead, metaldehyde, methylxanthines, prescription and illicit drugs (e.g., amphetamines, cocaine), cyanide, and tremorgenic mycotoxins.

Diagnosis

A diagnosis is based upon a history of exposure to the compound, compatible clinical signs, and detection of the toxicant in source material or vomitus. Analysis of tissues is possible, but the parent compound is typically present at very low levels and few laboratories offer sufficiently sensitive tests. Postmortem findings are nonspecific although rapid onset of rigor mortis is reported (Parton 2004).

Management of Exposures

The rapidity of onset of clinical signs often precludes institution of decontamination procedures. Administration of activated charcoal is recommended, but this might require control of seizures first.

Perhaps the most critical intervention is the IV administration of sodium bicarbonate (Parton 2004). Although sodium bicarbonate administration might worsen hypocalcemia and cause hyperkalemia, the benefits outweigh the risks. Frequent monitoring of electrolytes is warranted.

Prognosis

The prognosis is typically poor.

REFERENCES

Bischoff, K., Brizzee-Buxton, B., Gatto, N. et al. 1998. Malicious paraquat poisoning in Oklahoma dogs. *Vet Hum Toxicol* 40(3):151–153.

Carlo, G.L., Cole, P., Miller, A.B., Munro, I.C., Soloman, K.R., and Squire, R.A. 1992. Review of a study reporting an association between 2,4-dichlorophenoxyacetic acid and canine malignant lymphoma: report of an expert panel. *Regul Toxicol Pharmacol* 16:245–252.

Cope, R.B., Bildfell, R.J., Valentine, B.A. et al. 2004. Fatal paraquat poisoning in seven Portland, OR dogs. *Vet Hum Toxicol* 46(5):258–264.

Crandell, D.E., Weinberg, G.L. 2009. Moxidectin toxicosis in a puppy successfully treated with intravenous lipids. *J Vet Emerg Crit Car* 19(2):181–186.

Dorman, D.C. 1990. Diethyltoluamide (DEET) insect repellant toxicosis. *Vet Clin North Am Small Anim Pract* 20:387–392.

———. 2004. Diethyltoluamide. In Plumlee, K.H., ed. *Clinical Veterinary Toxicology*, pp. 180–182. St. Louis: Mosby.

Gerken, D.F. 1995. Lawn care products. In Bonagura, J.D., ed. *Kirk's Current Veterinary Therapy XII: Small Animal Practice*, pp. 248–249. Philadelphia: W.B. Saunders.

Glickman, L.T., Raghavan, M., Knapp, D.W., Bonney, P.L., and Dawson, M.H. 2004. Herbicide exposure and the risk of transitional cell carcinoma in Scottish Terriers. *J Am Vet Med Assoc* 224:1290–1297.

Glickman, L.T., Schofer, F.S., McKee, L.J., Reif, J.S., and Goldschmidt, M.H. 1989. Epidemiologic study of insecticide exposures, obesity, and risk of bladder cancer in household dogs. *J Toxicol Environ Health* 28:407–414.

Gramer, I., Leidolf, R., Döring, B., Klintzsch, S., Krämer, E.M., Yalcin, E., Petzinger, E., and Geyer, J. 2010. Breed distribution of the nt230(del4) MDR1 mutation in dogs. *Veterinary Journal*, in press.

Hayes, H.M., Tarone, R.E., Cantor, D.M., Jessen, C.R., McCurnin, D.M., and Richardson, R.C. 1991. Case-control study of canine malignant lymphoma: Positive association with dog owner's use of 2,4-dichlorophenyoxyacetic acid herbicides. *J Natl Cancer Inst* 83:1226–1231.

Hayes, H.M., Tarone, R.E., Casey, H.W., and Huxsoll, D.L. 1990. Excess of seminomas observed in Vietnam service U.S. military working dogs. *J Natl Cancer Inst* 82:1042–1046.

Lanusse, Carlos E., Lifschitz, Adrian L., Imperiale, and Fernanda A. 2009. Macrocyclic lactones: Endectocide compounds. In *Veterinary Pharmacology and Therapeutics*, 9th ed., edited by Jim E. Riviere and Mark G. Papich, pp. 1119–1144. Ames, Iowa: Wiley-Blackwell.

McCurnin, D.M. and Richardson, R.C. 1991. Case-control study of canine malignant lymphoma: positive association with dog owner's use of 2,4-dichlorophenyoxyacetic acid herbicides. *J Natl Cancer Inst* 83:1226–1231.

Mealey, Katrina L. 2006. Ivermectin: Macrolide antiparasitic agents. In *Small Animal Toxicology*, 2nd ed., edited by Michael E. Peterson and Patricia A. Talcott, pp. 785–794. St. Louis: Saunders.

Merola, Valentina M., Khan Safdar A., and Gwaltney-Brant, Sharon M. 2009. Ivermectin toxicosis in dogs: A retrospective study. *Journal of the American Animal Hospital Association* 45(3):106–111.

Oehme, F. and Pickrell, J.A. 2004. Dipyridyl herbicides. In Plumlee, K.H., ed. *Clinical Veterinary Toxicology*, pp. 146–148. St. Louis: Mosby.

Osweiler, G.D. 1996. *Toxicology: The National Veterinary Medical Series*, Philadelphia: Williams and Wilkins.

Parton, K.H. 2004. Sodium fluoroacetate. In Plumlee, K.H., ed. *Clinical Veterinary Toxicology*, pp. 451–454. St. Louis: Mosby.

Raghavan, M., Knapp, D., Dawson, M.H., Bonney, P.L., and Glickman, L.T. 2004. Topical flea and tick pesticides and the risk of transitional cell carcinoma of the urinary bladder in Scottish terriers. *J Am Vet Med Assoc* 225: 389–394.

Richardson, J.A., Welch, S.L., Gwaltney-Brant, S.M. et al. 2003. Metaldehyde toxicosis in dogs. *Compend Contin Edu Vet* 25(5):376–380.

Riegart, J.R. and Roberts, J.R. 1999. *Recognition and Management of Pesticide Poisonings*, EPA 735-R-98-003.

Roder, Joseph D. 2004. Antiparasiticals. In *Veterinary Clinical Toxicology*, edited by Konnie H. Plumlee, pp. 302–305. St. Louis: Mosby.

Schell, M.M. 2004. 4-aminopyridine. In Plumlee, K.H., ed. *Clinical Veterinary Toxicology*, pp. 443–442. St. Louis, Mosby.

Talcott, P.A. 2004. Metaldehyde. In Plumlee, K.H., ed. *Clinical Veterinary Toxicology*, pp. 182–183. St. Louis, Mosby.

Welch, S. 2004. Boric acid. In Plumlee, K.H., ed. *Clinical Veterinary Toxicology*, pp. 143–145. St. Louis, Mosby.

Yeary, R.A. 2000. Lawn care products. In Bonagura, J.D., ed. *Kirk's Current Veterinary Therapy XIII: Small Animal Practice*, pp. 221–222. Philadelphia: W.B. Saunders.

Yeary, Roger A. 2006. Miscellaneous herbicides, fungicides, and nematocides. In *Small Animal Toxicology*, 2nd ed., edited by Michael E. Peterson and Patricia A. Talcott, pp. 732–743. St. Louis: Saunders.

Plants

20

Joanna Delaporte and Charlotte Means

INTRODUCTION

This chapter covers common household and yard plants that might cause household pet intoxication. There are a few details to keep in mind when managing a plant exposure. First, the plant must be positively identified. Potential sources of identification include local plant nurseries, garden stores, university extension offices, or veterinary diagnostic laboratories. If the whole plant cannot be transported, a small branch with leaves, fruit, flowers, or nuts should be obtained. Ideally, the scientific name of the plant rather than the common name should be sought, because common names can be shared among totally unrelated plants. Next, it is important to keep in mind that even nontoxic plants can cause signs of digestive upset such as vomiting, diarrhea, and mild nausea or drooling if they are ingested. Also, the toxicity of plant material can vary tremendously depending on growing conditions. Finally, in cases where signs have already developed, decontamination by induction of emesis may be contraindicated.

There are several plant-related intoxications that are discussed in Chapter 24, "Food-Associated Intoxications," including *Allium* spp. (onions, garlic), *Persea americana* (avocado), grapes and raisins, and macadamia nuts. Additional plant-related intoxications are discussed in Chapter 21, "Dietary Supplements and Herbs."

DIGESTIVE SYSTEM

Aloe spp.

Aloe vera (Figure 20.1) is also known as *A. barbadensis*. This plant is different from American aloe. *Aloe* contains anthraquinone glycosides, which are potent purgatives concentrated in the latex of the leaves. Chewing on *Aloe vera* leaves can result in severe diarrhea. Fluid and electrolyte imbalances may need to be managed if dehydration develops.

Asparagus spp.

Also called asparagus fern, these plants contain steroidal saponins, with the highest concentration being present in the berries. These plants are considered a contact allergen and can cause irritation after dermal contact. After ingestion, signs such as salivation, vomiting, and diarrhea can occur. Symptomatic treatment for gastrointestinal signs may be needed.

Begonia spp.

In contrast to plants that contain only insoluble calcium oxalate, *Begonia* (Figure 20.2) contains both insoluble calcium oxalates and soluble oxalates (soluble salts of oxalic acid such as sodium, potassium, ammonium, and acid potassium oxalates). The oxalate crystals are especially concentrated in the tubers and stems. Insoluble calcium oxalate crystals may cause dermal and mucous membrane irritation. Signs that develop can include salivation and vomiting.

Soluble oxalate intoxication is poorly documented in pets or people due to the large quantity of plant material required to induce toxicosis; livestock poisonings are more commonly reported. In animals, nausea, rapid respiration, and stupor occur early followed by vomiting, bloody diarrhea, coma, and tetany due to hypocalcemia. Oliguria,

Small Animal Toxicology Essentials, First Edition. Edited by Robert H. Poppenga, Sharon Gwaltney-Brant.
© 2011 John Wiley and Sons, Inc. Published 2011 by John Wiley and Sons, Inc.

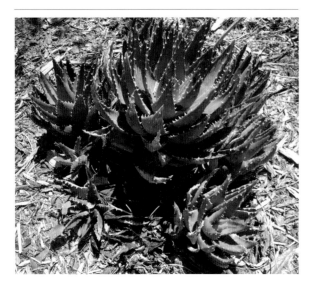

Figure 20.1. Aloe (*Aloe vera*).

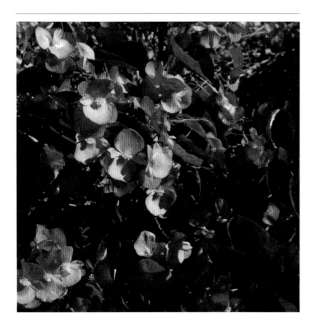

Figure 20.2. Begonia (*Begonia* sp.) (photo courtesy TD Brant).

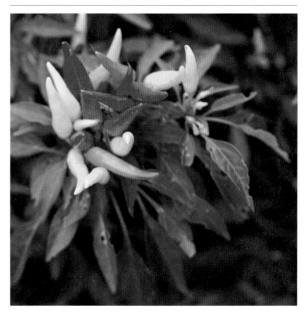

Figure 20.3. Ornamental Pepper (*Capsicum* sp.) (photo courtesy TD Brant).

Capsicum spp.

Capsicum spp. (Figure 20.3) includes chili peppers and other pepper plants that are usually grown in gardens for food or as ornamental plants. The toxin in pepper plants is capsaicin. The highest concentration is found in the fruits, especially in the seeds. Hot peppers are irritating, causing a burning sensation and possibly oral blisters when ingested. Large exposures can cause vomiting and diarrhea. In experiments using rats, very high doses have caused convulsions. Effects of capsaicin are transient and may be relieved by dilution with water or milk or flushing the mouth with water. Demulcents and pain control might also be indicated.

Chrysanthemum spp.

Chrysanthemum plants (Figure 20.4) contain a toxin called arteglasin A, a sesquiterpene lactone. Plant ingestion is associated with hypersensitivity and allergic contact dermatitis.

Clematis spp.

Clematis is also known as virgin's bower and traveler's joy. These plants cause intense GI irritation, vomiting, and diarrhea. Protoanemonin, which is related to the blister beetle vesicant cantharidin, is the toxin. Protoanemonin is

oxaluria, albuminuria, or hematuria can occur due to formation of calcium oxalate crystals in the kidney. Treatment of suspected intoxications has included administration of parenteral calcium salts to correct hypocalcemia as well as intravenous fluid support. These plants are rarely associated with poisonings in companion animals.

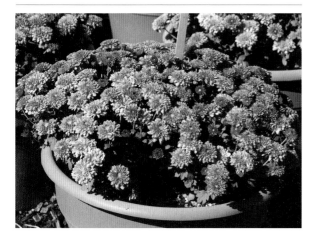

Figure 20.4. Chrysanthemum (*Chrysanthemum* sp.) (photo courtesy TD Brant).

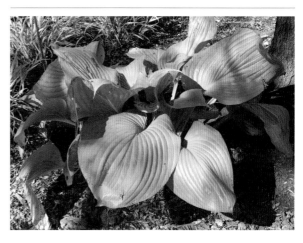

Figure 20.5. Hosta (*Hosta* sp.) (photo courtesy TD Brant).

a subepidermal vesicant, so plants can cause profound dermal irritation on contact. When ingested, plants are bitter and irritating. Excessive salivation, vomiting, and diarrhea are expected signs. Dried plant material contains a polymerized form of protoanemonin, called anemonin, which is not considered to be toxic. Thus, dried plants are considered nontoxic. Treatment includes gastrointestinal protectants, antiemetics, and other symptomatic and supportive care.

Cyclamen spp.

Cyclamen species are native to the Mediterranean and may be known as Persian violet or sow's bread. The toxin contained in *Cyclamen* is a triterpenoid saponin. The saponin is found mainly in the roots, with a small amount in leaves. Ingestion of this plant may lead to nausea, vomiting, and diarrhea. If larger quantities are ingested, the saponin may be absorbed, causing convulsions, seizures, cardiac dysrhythmias, and paralysis. Supportive treatment is typically all that is needed to ensure recovery.

Euphorbia pulcherrima

Euphorbia pulcherrima is commonly known as poinsettia. The toxicity of poinsettia has been greatly exaggerated. In one study using rats, ingestions of up to 15 g/kg for 1 week did not cause behavior changes, clinical signs, or postmortem lesions. However, one group of rats in the study showed a significant increase in thyroid weight. As an estimate of toxicity, human poison experts have calculated that a 50-pound child would need to ingest about 1.25 lb,

or 500–600 leaves, to surpass levels that have been toxic in animal experiments.

Poinsettia plants do contain an irritating milky sap. Pets that chew on the plants develop hypersalivation, vomiting, anorexia, and depression. Signs are usually self-limiting and require minimal treatment. Further GI irritation may be reduced by limiting food and water intake for 1 to 2 hours.

Gypsophilia paniculata

Gypsophilia paniculata is commonly known as Baby's breath, and is often used in floral arrangements. *Gypsophilia* exposures can case dermal irritation due to contact allergen. Ingestion of the plant may lead to vomiting and diarrhea.

Hosta spp.

Members of the *Hosta* genus are also known as hosta lily or August lily (Figure 20.5). Some species contain saponins, which can cause vomiting, diarrhea, depression, and anorexia. They are likely to cause a problem only if consumed in quantity.

Ilex spp.

Holly (Figure 20.6) grows as a small shrub outdoors or can be brought indoors for holiday decoration. A variety of biologically active compounds have been identified in *Ilex* spp. including tannins, caffeine, theobromine, triterpenes, and a hemolytic saponin, among others. With small ingestions vomiting and diarrhea can occur. Anorexia,

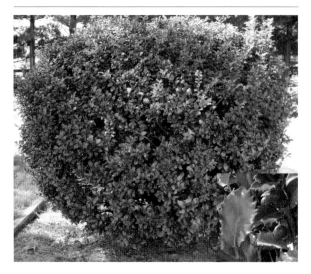

Figure 20.6. American Holly (*Ilex opaca*); i*nsert: Closer view of leaves and berries* (photo courtesy TD Brant).

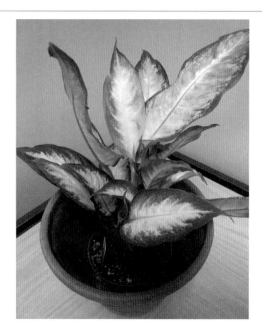

Figure 20.7. Dieffenbachia (*Dieffenbachia* sp.).

head shaking, and lip smacking can also occur. Flushing the oral cavity with water will reduce mucosal irritation.

Insoluble Calcium Oxalate-containing Plants

A number of plants including *Dieffenbachia* spp. (Figure 20.7), *Zantedeschia* spp., *Epipremnun aureum*, *Philodendron* spp., and *Spathiphyllum* spp. (Figure 20.8) contain insoluble calcium oxalate crystals (Spoerke and Smolinske 1990). Chewing on calcium-oxalate containing plants causes mechanical irritation to mucous membranes of the GI tract. As the plant cells are crushed or broken open, needlelike crystals called *raphides* are released and surrounding tissues are penetrated by the crystals. The reaction may be rapid, causing oral pain and swelling of the lips and tongue. The irritation may extend to the esophagus and stomach. However, since the plant cells must be broken open, effects beyond the oral cavity are unlikely with small ingestions. The animal may be inappetent for several days following exposure due to oral discomfort. Vomiting and diarrhea occur rarely. Treatment for insoluble calcium oxalate crystal ingestion is often not needed. Dairy products have been recommended to ease the oral discomfort (Means 2004). In rare severe cases, a soft diet, pain control, NSAIDs, or sedation may be useful.

Ornamental Bulbs

Ornamental bulb plants include tulips (*Tulipa* spp., Figure 20.9), daffodils (*Narcissus* spp.), hyacinth (*Hyacinthus*

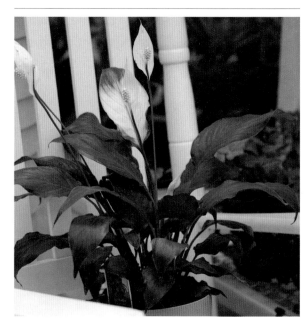

Figure 20.8. Peace Lily (*Spathiphyllum* sp.) (photo courtesy TD Brant).

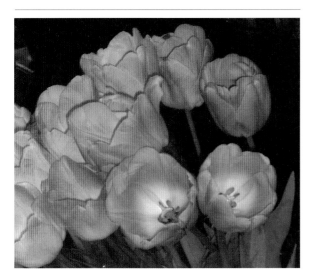

Figure 20.9. Tulip (*Tulipa* sp.).

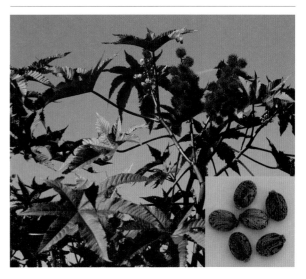

Figure 20.10. Castor Bean plant (*Ricinus communis*); insert: *Castor beans* (photo courtesy TD Brant).

orientalis), spring-blooming crocus (*Crocus* spp., not to be confused with autumn-blooming crocus, *Colchicum*, see below), and iris (*Iris* spp.). All parts of the bulb, especially the roots, flesh, and seed capsules contain pentacyclic terpenoids, which are irritating and cause gastroenteritis. Clinical signs include salivation, abdominal pain, profuse diarrhea with or without blood, and oral lesions. Signs may last hours to days. Treatment includes correction of fluid and electrolyte imbalances and possibly gastrointestinal protectants.

Ricinus communis

Ricinus communis (Figure 20.10) is also known as castor bean or castor oil plant. The principal toxins are ricinine (or ricin) and toxalbumin. The seeds, when well-chewed and ingested in amounts as low as 0.01% of body weight, can cause severe intoxication (Albretson et al. 2000). Intact seeds are expected to pass through the gastrointestinal tract with no negative effects. Leaves or pericarps of fruits require about 2% of body weight (ricin) ingested to cause intoxication. Ricin is water-soluble and is not found in castor oil (Mouser et al. 2007). Heat and aging reduce its toxicity. When ingested, ricin is poorly absorbed and its main site of action is the digestive epithelium. Ricinine appears to have some action on neuroreceptors, since seizures and muscular weakness have been seen in some animals that have chewed and swallowed castor beans (Albretson et al. 2000). The toxins cause edema and necro-

sis of mucosa of stomach and small intestine. However, castor bean intoxication is associated with multiple organ effects: heart, stomach, lungs, liver, kidneys, and pancreas can be affected.

If the seeds are chewed and swallowed, the most common sign is severe diarrhea within about 6 hours (Albretson et al. 2000). The diarrhea may be hemorrhagic. Other signs include hypotension, depression, weakness, trembling, sweating, vomiting, abdominal pain, anorexia, hyperthermia, ataxia, hypersalivation, recumbency, and tachycardia. Signs can be delayed as long as 24 to 48 hours after exposure. Death is attributed to hypovolemic shock.

Treatment involves early decontamination in animals not exhibiting clinical signs. Symptomatic animals need to be stabilized first. Diazepam may be used to control seizures. Intravenous fluid therapy, such as Ringer's lactate solution, is recommended to prevent or treat hypovolemia and to maintain hydration and electrolyte balance. Gastrointestinal protectants such as sucralfate, famotidine, and kaolin-pectin might be indicated to protect and promote healing of the gastrointestinal tract. Antiemetics and pain management might also be needed. Frequent CBC, serum chemistry, and electrolytes monitoring is recommended to assess the extent of organ damage.

Schlumbergera spp.

These plants are commonly called Christmas cactus. Ingestion may result in mild gastrointestinal upset although they are considered to be nontoxic for cats and dogs. If mild gastrointestinal signs occur, withholding food and water for 1 or 2 hours should be sufficient.

CARDIOVASCULAR SYSTEM

Cardiac Glycosides

Several plants contain cardiac glycosides. Cardiac glycoside inhibit cell membrane sodium-potassium ATPase, resulting in decreased electrical conductivity. This can result in the occurrence of a variety of cardiac arrhythmias, both tachy- and bradyarrhythmias, along with abdominal pain and diarrhea. Death can be rapid or delayed for up to 2 days. In general, standard decontamination protocols should be followed when possible and appropriate. Treatment of cardiac arrhythmias varies depending on the specific arrhythmia noted. The electrolytes status of affected animals should be monitored and fluids and electrolytes administered as needed. Treatment with digoxin immune Fab (Digibind®) might be helpful but should be administered as soon as possible after exposure for maximum efficacy. Further information on the effects of cardiac glycosides can be found in Chapter 12, "Cardiovascular System," and Chapter 27, "Prescription Drugs."

Adenium obesum

This plant is known as desert rose and mock azalea. About 30 cardiac glycosides have been isolated from this plant. The plant has been a source for an arrow poison in Africa. There have been no reported cases of animal intoxications. However, the plant is toxic enough to warrant caution if exposure occurs. If sufficient amounts of the plant are ingested, cardiac arrhythmias, heart block, and death may develop. Treatment would be similar to other cardiac glycoside intoxications.

Convallaria majalis

Lily-of-the-valley is the common name for *Convallaria majalis* (Figure 20.11), which contains approximately 38 cardenolides and various saponins. All parts of the plant are toxic, with the greatest toxin concentration in the rhizomes. Signs are as one would expect from cardiac glycosides: vomiting, diarrhea, cardiac arrhythmias, and death. Treatment considerations are as outlined above.

Digitalis purpurea

Foxglove is the common name for *Digitalis purpurea* (Figure 20.12). The plant contains the cardenolides digoxin and digitoxin. All plant parts are toxic, especially the seeds. The dried plant is also toxic. Even water from vases

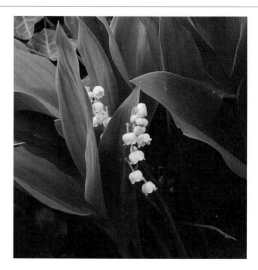

Figure 20.11. Lily-of-the-Valley flowers (*Convallaria majalis*).

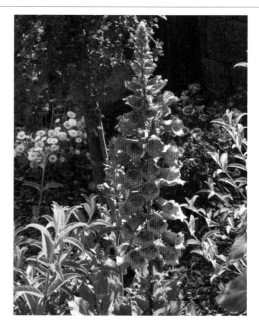

Figure 20.12. Foxglove (*Digitalis* sp.).

where the flowers are kept can be a risk if ingested. The earliest signs of intoxication include marked weakness, stupor, and diarrhea with or without blood. The heartbeat at first may be loud and strong, but then later become faint and barely perceptible, eventually regressing to ventricular fibrillation. Vomiting, increased salivation, and more fre-

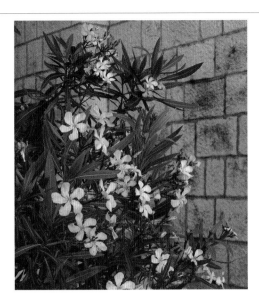

Figure 20.13. Oleander (*Nerium oleander*).

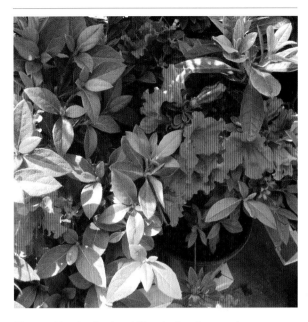

Figure 20.14. Azalea (*Rhododendron* sp.).

quent urination can occur. Treatment is as for other cardiac glycoside-containing plants.

Nerium oleander

Nerium oleander (Figure 20.13) is a shrub that is used as a landscaping plant in warmer parts of the United States, such as California. Oleander is extremely toxic; ingestion of as little as 0.005% body weight can be fatal. Oleander is highly poisonous to birds. Both fresh and dried plant are toxic.

Oleander contains the cardenolides oleandrin, which is concentrated in the leaves, flowers, and seeds. The plant also contains terpenoids. The terpenoids may be responsible for the gastrointestinal irritation seen. Weakness, depression, anorexia, vomiting, abdominal pain, hypersalivation, and diarrhea are likely in cats and dogs. Patients might exhibit signs for many hours and then recover. However, patients can die suddenly from cardiac arrest with few preliminary signs. Patients should be monitored closely with particular attention paid to heart rate and rhythm and electrolyte concentrations. Hyperkalemia and hypocalcemia may develop. Treatment considerations are as outlined above. Intravenous fluids and electrolytes are provided as needed.

Grayanotoxins

Several plants contain cardiotoxins called grayanotoxins. These include *Rhododendron* (azalea, Figure 20.14; moun-

tain rosebay; red laurel; and great laurel, among others), *Kalmia* spp. (mountain laurel), and *Pieris japonica* (Japanese pieris). These plants contain diterpenoid grayanotoxins, which are present in all parts of the plant, although their concentrations vary between plants. Grayanotoxins increase sodium channel permeability, which opens cells to sodium instead of calcium. The channels are slow to close and the cell remains depolarized. Significant effects occur in the heart, skeletal muscles, and CNS. Increased reflexes, increased vagal tone, hypotension, and cardiac arrhythmias occur. Signs include profuse salivation, anorexia, repeated swallowing, persistent retching or vomiting (possibly projectile), severe abdominal pain, and bloat. Severe cases may exhibit weakness and inability or reluctance to stand. Less frequent cardiac effects include bradycardia and AV block. Acute effects last about 24 hours. Weakness and other neurologic effects can last 2 to 3 days. Treatment includes appropriate and timely decontamination and symptomatic and supportive care.

Kalanchoe spp.

Kalanchoe (Figure 20.15) may also be called by another scientific name, *Bryophyllum*. Mother-of-millions is one common name. The significant toxin in *Kalanchoe* is lanceotoxin A, which is a bufadienolide cardiotoxin. These cardiotoxins are similar to the cardiac glycosides

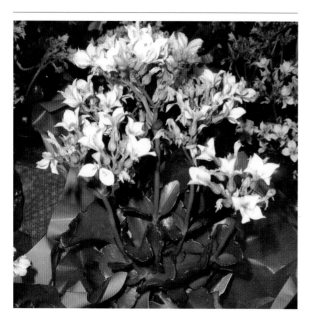

Figure 20.15. Kalanchoe (*Kalanchoe* sp.) (photo courtesy SM Gwaltney-Brant).

found in foxglove, oleander, and lily-of-the-valley. Ingestion of as little as 1% body weight can cause intoxication. The flowers are especially toxic. Natural poisonings are most commonly reported during the plants' flowering season. Known intoxications have occurred in dogs and rabbits.

Signs include vomiting, diarrhea, ataxia, trembling, and sudden death due to cardiac failure. Other signs that have been reported include tachycardia, hypertension, dilated pupils, nystagmus, delirium, weakness, tetany, mild seizures, depression, anorexia, hypersalivation, and mucoid to bloody diarrhea. The diarrhea may persist several days without other signs. Cardiac effects typically require a larger ingestion and signs include increased or decreased heart rate, labored respiration or grunting, arrhythmias, heart block, severe weakness. Serum chemistry abnormalities include increased BUN, creatinine, and glucose concentrations.

Treatment of *Kalanchoe* exposures includes appropriate and timely decontamination and symptomatic and supportive care. Digibind® has not been evaluated for treatment of *Kalanchoe* intoxications. Atropine or propranolol can be used to increase the heart rate and reverse heart block.

Melia azedarach

This plant is known by many common names, including chinaberry, Persian lilac, Texas umbrella tree, among others. The plant is native to Asia, but has become widespread as a landscape plant across the southern United States. Several meliatoxins are present in all parts of the plant, but especially in the fruit. Only the berries have been known to cause intoxication; toxicity of the berries varies by location and species of plant. The toxic dosage is approximately 0.2–0.3 % body weight (Hare et al. 1997). Five to six fruits were lethal to a young dog within 48 hours (Barr 2006). Clinical signs are variable and include hyperthermia, hypothermia, tachycardia, bradycardia, dyspnea, stranguria, muscle rigidity, mydriasis, and miosis. Early signs include hypersalivation, vomiting, anorexia, and diarrhea. If large enough quantities of berries have been ingested, muscle weakness, ataxia, seizures, and paralysis develop. Excitement occurs early, with paralysis developing later. It is possible for sudden death to occur as the only clinical sign. For a recent exposure where signs have not yet developed, emesis helps to remove berries from the stomach followed by activated charcoal administration. Treatment is symptomatic and supportive, because no antidote exists. In severe cases, sedatives and fluid-electrolyte therapy should be used. Animals that recover usually do so within 24–48 hours.

Taxus spp.

Members of *Taxus* spp. (Figure 20.16), also called yews, are shrubs found throughout the United States. Bark, leaves, and seeds are toxic, but not the red flesh of the fruit. The principal toxins are taxines, which cause cardiac conduction disturbances due to interference to the ion channels of cardiac muscle. All domestic animals and birds are at risk for intoxication.

The plant seems to be more toxic in winter. Ingestion of as little as 1 ounce of leaves can be lethal to a dog (Barr 2006). Both fresh and dried leaves are dangerous. Signs exhibited by intoxicated dogs include vomiting, muscle tremors, seizures, panting, dilated pupils, and significant tachycardia. Stressing the patient can cause sudden collapse and death. Sudden death can occur even days after ingestion. Once signs develop it is usually too late for effective treatment due to the peracute nature of the intoxication. However, early decontamination and administration of atropine to reverse bradycardia and heart block should be considered. Syrup of ipecac should not be used to induce emesis due to the potential for vagal nerve stimulation to exacerbate the cardiac effects of yew.

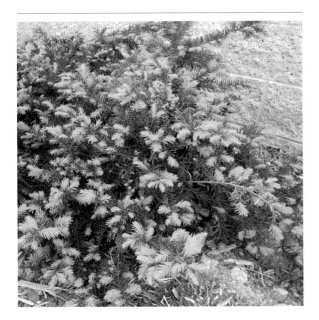

Figure 20.16. Japanese yew (*Taxus* sp.).

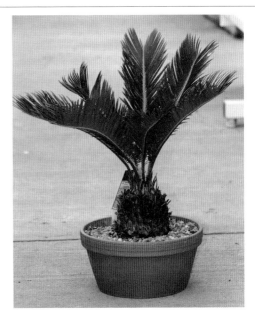

Figure 20.17. Sago Palm (*Cycas revoluta*) (photo courtesy TD Brant).

LIVER

Cycas spp. and *Zamia* spp.

Members of *Cycas* and *Zamia* are referred to as cycad palms, which include common names such as sago palm (Figure 20.17), false sago palm, and fern palm. There are two types of toxins present in cycads: cycasin and macrozamin. The seeds, leaves, and pulp of the cones are primarily hepatotoxic, but the digestive and neuromuscular systems can also be affected. Prolonged consumption of the seeds can cause neurologic signs and lesions. The fruits and seeds of some species remain toxic even after being cooked. The fruits seem to be especially enticing to dogs. In some reported intoxications, parts of the plant have been inappropriately used as an alternative medicine.

Signs that develop after cycad ingestion include persistent vomiting, hypersalivation, excessive water consumption, anorexia, diarrhea or constipation, icterus, thrombocytopenia, hyperbilirubinemia, increase of liver enzymes, elevations of BUN and creatinine, and coagulopathy. Hepatic necrosis and subsequent fibrosis can develop. Treatment primarily involves appropriate and timely decontamination and symptomatic and supportive care. The latter might include the use of hepatoprotectants such as N-acetylcysteine, silimaryin or SAMe, although the efficacy of such therapy is unknown.

Lantana spp.

Members of *Lantana* (Figure 20.18) are also known as shrub verbena, yellow/red/wild sage, and bunchberry. The toxins are triterpenes. There are some varieties much less toxic than others because their triterpene structure is different. All parts of the plants, especially the unripe berries, are toxic, but not all species are toxic. Fully ripe fruits are not toxic, but partially ripe berries can be. All animal species are at risk with ingestions of as little as 1% body weight causing intoxication. Signs associated with intoxication include GI irritation, vomiting, diarrhea, weakness, ataxia, depression, cholestasis, hyperbilirubinemia, hepatic damage, lethargy, cyanosis, labored breathing, depressed tendon reflexes, photophobia, coma, and death.

Triterpenoids cause damage to the bile canaliculi with subsequent development of obstructive cholangitis. They also irritate the GI mucosa and cause diarrhea or constipation. Subacute or chronic exposures are associated with photosensitization. The second or third day after exposure,

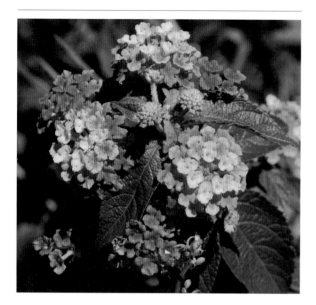

Figure 20.18. Lantana (*Lantana* sp.) (photo courtesy TD Brant).

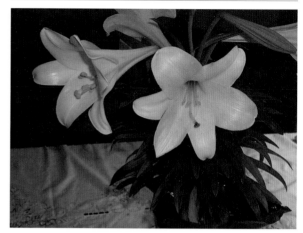

Figure 20.19. Easter Lily (*Lilium longiflorum*).

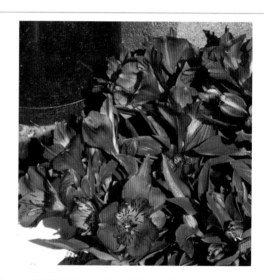

Figure 20.20. Tiger Lily (*Lilium tigrinum*).

icterus and photosensitization may be noticed as well as diarrhea with or without blood. Deaths from *Lantana* toxicoses are mainly due to hepatic and renal failure. Treatment includes appropriate and timely decontamination, fluids, and glucose and electrolyte administration. Symptomatic and supportive might include the use of hepatoprotectants such as N-acetylcysteine, silimaryin, or SAMe although the efficacy of such therapy is unknown. Once signs of liver damage are present, treatment of animals is usually not successful.

URINARY SYSTEM

Lilium spp.

Lilium species including *L. pardalinum, L. candidum, L. speciosum, L. lancifolium* (rubrum or Japanese showy lilies), *L. longiflorum* (Easter lily, Figure 20.19), *L. tigrinum* (Tiger lily, Figure 20.20), and *Hemerocallis* (day lilies, Figure 20.21) are nephrotoxic to cats. Peace lily (*Spathiphyllum,* Figure 20.8) and calla lily (*Zantedeschia*) are not true lilies and are not associated with renal issues, although they do contain insoluble calcium oxalate crystals (see earlier discussion). All true lily plant parts are toxic to cats, and cats are the only species known to be sensitive to lily ingestion. Ingestion of less than one leaf can cause severe toxicosis. Clinical signs include early vomiting, anorexia, and depression; these signs can begin

within 2 hours of exposure (Langston 2002). Vomiting may resolve, but anorexia and depression continue as BUN, creatinine, potassium, and phosphorus concentrations rise 24 to 72 hours after exposure. Epithelial casts and glucose may be detected in the urine within 18 hours. Renal failure is due to an unknown mechanism causing renal tubular necrosis. Fortunately, in cats surviving the acute crisis, affected renal tubular epithelial cells can regenerate since the basement membrane remains intact. Treatment involves early decontamination. Fluid diuresis using LRS at twice maintenance rates (approximately

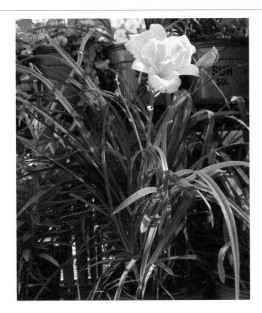

Figure 20.21. Day Lily (*Hemerocallis* sp.) (photo courtesy SM Gwaltney-Brant).

30 ml/kg/day) should be started as soon as possible and continued for at least 48 hours. Baseline BUN and creatinine should be obtained and rechecked daily. Creatinine levels are often disproportionately high when compared to BUN. As long as BUN and creatinine are high, fluid diuresis is continued. If treatment is delayed, there is an increased risk for renal failure and death. Anuric cats have a grave prognosis, but renal function has been restored after peritoneal or hemodialysis dialysis in some cases (Langston 2002).

Soluble Oxalate-Containing Plants

Rhubarb (*Rheum rhabarbarum*, Figure 20.22) contains anthraquinones and soluble oxalates in small quantities (about 0.28% dry weight of leaf material) (Peterson 2006). *Oxalis* spp. (sorrel, wood sorrel, shamrock, soursob, Bermuda buttercup, and Irish shamrock) can contain up to 16% of dry matter as soluble oxalates.

Most of the signs associated with rhubarb leaf ingestion can be attributed to the cathartic action of anthraquinones. In theory, the soluble oxalates can precipitate within the renal tubules causing kidney damage. However, renal oxalosis is unlikely to occur unless very large amounts of plant material are ingested. If a quantity large enough is ingested, the oxalates can cause hypocalcemia in addition to renal oxalate precipitation. Signs typically are limited to vomiting although hypocalcemic tetany and signs related to renal failure are possible.

CENTRAL NERVOUS SYSTEM

Brunfelsia spp.

There are a number of species in the *Brunfelsia* genus (Figure 20.23) and a variety of common names. *B. pauciflora* is known by the common names of yesterday-today-tomorrow, morning-noon-and-night or yesterday-and-today. *Brunfelsia americana* is called lady-of-the-night or Franciscan rain tree. These are primarily outdoor ornamental plants but are sometimes used indoors. Dogs seem to find the fruits appealing and as a result have a higher risk of exposure. The toxin in the plant has not been identified but neuroexitatory and neurodepressant agents are present. Typical signs include anxiety and excitement followed by coughing, gagging, sneezing, and nystagmus. Initial signs are followed within a few hours by tremors and tetanic or paddling seizures, which can be precipitated by external stimuli. Tremors and seizures can last hours to days with full recovery taking up to a week or longer. Treatment involves appropriate and timely decontamination and symptomatic and supportive care. Control of

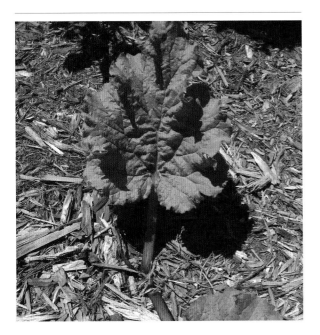

Figure 20.22. Rhubarb (*Rheum rhabarbarum*).

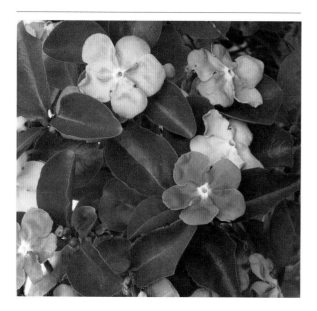

Figure 20.23. Yesterday-Today-Tomorrow (*Brunfelsia* sp.).

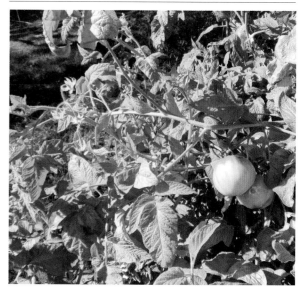

Figure 20.24. Tomato (*Lycopersicon lycopersicum*) (photo courtesy SM Gwaltney-Brant).

central nervous system excitation is achieved with diazepam or pentobarbital.

Laburnum anagyroids

This plant is also known as golden rain tree, golden chain tree, scotch laburnum, and alpine golden chain. It contains quinolizidine alkaloids, some of which are teratogenic (Burrows and Tyrl 2001). The greatest concentration of the alkaloids is found in the seeds, but the toxins are present throughout all parts of the plant. The leaves, seed pods, and seeds are toxic. Ingestion of plant material equaling 0.1%–1% body weight is toxic. Horses appear to be the most sensitive species to intoxication, but poisonings have been reported in dogs as well.

The main toxins are rapidly absorbed and excreted and clinical signs would be expected to develop rapidly after a toxic dose of the plant has been consumed. The most common signs seen in dogs are a centrally mediated vomiting and abdominal pain, and occasionally weakness, depression, ataxia, and tachycardia. Sweating, delirium, excitation, tonic-clonic convulsions, and death are reported. The signs are usually short-lived due to rapid excretion of the alkaloid, cystisine. If a large quantity of seeds has been consumed, myocardial degeneration and death can occur.

With small ingestions, treatment might not be needed. If signs do occur symptomatic and supportive care is needed to control vomiting and abdominal pain. Cleft palate and arthrogryposis are possible teratogenic effects in pregnant animals exposed to the plant more chronically.

Lycopersicon lycopersicum and *Solanum* spp.

The toxins found in tomatoes (*L. lycopersicum*, Figure 20.24) and *Solanum* spp. (many species and common names, but many are referred to as nightshades) are steroidal glycoalkaloids. These include α-solanine and α-chaconine. Although for most species all plant parts are considered potentially toxic with the exception of ripe fruits, the immature fruits typically contain the highest toxin concentrations. However, even the ripe fruits are poisonous for some *Solanum* spp. Uncooked sprouted or green potatoes are also toxic.

The glycoalkaloids are irritating to the gastrointestinal tract and large ingestions can cause dilated pupils, tachycardia, and central nervous system depression, and respiratory difficulty. In severe cases, dilated pupils, muscle tremors, and incoordination may develop. Treatment involves appropriate and timely decontamination and symptomatic and supportive care. Solanine can cause mild cholinergic effects due to cholinesterase inhibition, and atropine can be used to reverse such effects in severe cases.

Nicotiana **spp.**

Nicotiana spp., include tobacco and tree tobacco. These plants contain the pyridine alkaloids nicotine and nornicotine. The alkaloids are rapidly absorbed across skin, mucous membranes, and gastrointestinal tract. All parts of the plant are toxic. Nicotine directly affects the brain and muscles initially causing stimulation followed by paralysis due to a depolarizing blockade. The minimum lethal dose in dogs and cats is 20–100 mg. The cardiovascular, urinary, and reproductive systems can also be affected.

Initial signs include excitement, bradycardia, and a slow respiration rate. Subsequent signs can include depression, hypersalivation, vomiting, diarrhea, rapid and labored breathing, ataxia, tremors, severe weakness, muscle twitching or trembling (beginning at the shoulders and then extending to the whole body), stiff-legged gait, and protrusion of the third eyelid. Death is most typically from respiratory failure. Signs are typically short-lived and last 5–6 hours; the prognosis is good if an animal survives the first 12 hours after onset of signs. Treatment involves appropriate and timely decontamination and symptomatic and supportive care. Antacids should not be given; they increase the absorption of nicotine. Patients should be closely monitored. Oxygen, positive pressure respiration, and sedatives might be needed.

Prunus **spp.**

There are a number of *Prunus* species that contain cyanogenic glycosides. High concentrations are found in the kernels of the seeds. As a result of damage to the plant or following ingestion, cyanogenic glycosides are broken down to hydrocyanic acid (cyanide). Although many *Prunus* spp. contain cyanogenic glycosides, most do not present a significant intoxication hazard. The ingestion of intact seeds does not release cyanide, and many seed kernels would need to be crushed and ingested for a toxicosis to occur. In intoxicated animals, signs include sudden onset of apprehension and distress, weakness, ataxia, labored breathing, collapse, and lateral recumbency. Paddling and tetanic seizures may occur. Due to rapid metabolism of cyanide following absorption, signs usually last only 5–15 minutes; animals either die or recover quickly. The rapidity of onset of clinical signs and possibly death make timely initiation of treatment problematic.

Antidote kits for cyanide poisoning are available and include a nitrite salt such as sodium nitrite and sodium thiosulfate (Burrows and Tyrl 2001). Amyl nitrite, which is used in intoxicated humans, is not recommended for use in animals. Nitrite forms methemoglobin, which combines with cyanide to form cyanmethemoglobin. Thiosulfate acts as a sulfur donor for the conversion of cyanide to thiocyanate by the action of the enzyme rhodanese, which is then rapidly excreted in the urine. Hydroxycobalamin (vitamin B12a) has also been used as an effective antidote.

MULTISYSTEMIC EFFECTS

Colchicum autumnale

Colchicum autumnale is known as autumn crocus, meadow saffron, and naked lady, and should not be confused with spring-blooming crocuses (*Crocus* spp., see earlier discussion). *Colchicum autumnale* contains the toxin colchicine, which is present in all parts of the plant with the greatest concentrations in the flowers and seeds. Glory lily (*Gloriosa superba*) is also known to contain colchicine and other alkaloids similar to those in *Colchicum autumnale*. Colchicine is quite toxic. Ingestion of as little as 08 mg/kg body weight of colchicine, 1.5 to 2.0 grams of plant material, 2 to 3 seeds, or 1/2 flower can be fatal (Burrows and Tyrl 2001). Colchicine is an antimitotic and is used in human medicine to treat a number of diseases including gout. Thus, animals can be intoxicated following the ingestion of both the plant and prescription medication. Intoxication results in multiple organ failure impairing cardiovascular, pulmonary, renal, metabolic, and neuromuscular function.

Initial signs of toxicosis are related to effects on the digestive tract and include vomiting, abdominal pain, and severe hemorrhagic diarrhea. Soon after, the patient becomes weak and disoriented, and develops seizures and cardiac abnormalities. Additional signs developing within 2–12 hours and include dysphagia, paralysis, and hypovolemic shock. If the animal survives for 4 to 5 days, bone marrow depression may occur. Death is attributed to respiratory failure. Treatment involves appropriate and timely decontamination and symptomatic and supportive care. In people, colchicine poisoning has been treated successfully using colchicine-specific Fab fragments.

Humulus lupulus

Also known as hops, beer hops, European hops, and lupulin. The plant is native to Europe and Asia and contains a number of biologically active constituents including essential oils, phenolic compounds, resins, and proteins. Spent hops from beer brewing are a significant concern in dogs, because they will readily eat them. A cup of spent hops has been reported to cause malignant hyperthermia in greyhounds (the responsible compound is not known). Hops also can affect the estrus cycle, since they contain phytoestrogens, although chronic exposure would probably be necessary to interfere with reproduction. Acute signs reported within 1 hour of consumption by greyhounds include hyperthermia, restlessness, panting, vomiting, abdominal pain, and seizures. Creatinine phosphokinase (CPK) levels become markedly elevated and urine becomes dark brown, suggesting muscle necrosis. Treatment includes standard decontamination procedures. Fluids should be administered to maintain renal function. Sedatives such as benzodiazepines can be used to control excitement or seizures.

A list of other potentially toxic plants and the general signs typically attributed to them is provided in Appendix 2.

NONTOXIC PLANTS

Although it is important to know whether a particular plant is potentially toxic or not, it is equally important to know which plants, when ingested, are considered to be nontoxic. Appendix 3 provides a list of nontoxic plants. Keep in mind that mild GI upset and perhaps vomiting is not unusual even when nontoxic plants are ingested.

REFERENCES

Albretson, J.C., Gwaltney-Brant, S.M., and Khan, S.A. 2000. Evaluation of castor bean toxicosis in dogs: 98 cases. *J Am Anim Hosp Assoc* 36:229–233.

ASPCA National Animal Poison Control Center. 1998. *Household Plant Reference*. New York: ASPCA.

Barr, A.C. 2006. Household and garden plants. In Peterson, M.E., Talcott, P.A., eds. *Small Animal Toxicology*, 2nd ed., pp. 345–410. St. Louis: Saunders Elsevier.

Burrows, George E. and Tyrl, Ronald J. 2001. *Toxic Plants of North America*. Ames, Iowa State University Press.

Hare, W.R., Schutzman, H., Lee, B.R., and Knight, M.W. 1997. Chinaberry poisoning in two dogs, *Journal of the American Veterinary Medical Association* 210:1638–1640.

Langston, C.E. 2002. Acute renal failure caused by lily ingestion in six cats. *J Am Vet Med Assoc* 220(1):49–52.

Means, Charlotte. 2004. Insoluble calcium oxalates. In *Veterinary Clinical Toxicology*, edited by Konnie H. Plumlee, pp. 340–341. St. Louis: Mosby.

Mouser, P., Filigenzi, M.S., Puschner, B., Johnson, V., Miller, M.A., and Hooser, S.B. 2007. Fatal ricin toxicosis in a puppy confirmed by liquid chromatography/mass spectrometry when using ricinine as a marker. *J Vet Diagn Invest* 19:216–220.

Peterson, M.E., Talcott, P.A., eds. 2006. *Small Animal Toxicology*, 2nd ed., pp. 345–410. St. Louis: Saunders Elsevier.

Spoerke, D.G. and Smolinske, S.C. 1990. *Toxicity of Houseplants*, Boca Raton: CRC Press, Inc.

Internet Resources

ASPCA Poison Control Center: http://www.aspca.org/petcare/poison-control/

Canadian Poisonous Plants Information System: http://www.cbif.gc.ca/pls/pp/poison?p_x=px

Cornell Department of Animal Science, Poisonous plants affecting dogs: http://www.ansci.cornell.edu/plants/dogs/index.html

Humane Society of the United States: http://www.humanesociety.org/animals/resources/tips/plants_poisonous_to_pets.html

Pet Poison Helpline, Plants that are toxic to cats: http://petpoisonhelpline.com/IsThatPoisonous/plants-toxic-to-cats/

Poisonous plants of North Carolina: http://www.ces.ncsu.edu/depts/hort/consumer/poison/poison.htm

Dietary Supplements and Herbs

21

Charlotte Means

INTRODUCTION

The sales of herbal dietary supplements in 2007 totaled approximately 4.8 billion dollars. Because of the popularity of herbal supplements, dogs and cats (as well as other household pets) are exposed by accidental overdoses or by owner administration. Adverse effects can occur because of dosage, species differences in metabolism, or drug-herb interactions.

SYMPATHOMIMETICS

Sources and Formulations

Herbs that contain sympathomimetics include ma huang (*Ephedra sinica*), Indian common mallow (*Sida cordifolia*), and bitter orange (Citrus aurantium). Historically, these herbs were used to treat asthma, cough, and colds. Today, these herbs are most commonly sold as weight loss aids, decongestants, and also for illicit recreational use (such as herbal ecstasy) or to improve athletic performance (such as weightlifters). Supplements containing ma huang were among the first widely marketed and advertised herbal products. When used as a weight-loss aid, frequently caffeine-containing plants are included in the formulation, which can increase toxicity (Means 1999). The active components of *Ephedra sinica* and *Sida cordifolia* are alkaloids, including ephedrine and pseudoephedrine. Bitter orange contains synephrine (Der Marderosian 1996; Means 1999).

In 2004, the FDA issued a final rule summary declaring dietary supplements containing ephedrine alkaloids adulterated under the Federal Food, Drug and Cosmetic Act. The FDA stated that these supplements presented an unreasonable risk of illness or injury under the conditions of use recommended or stated in labeling. The rule applies to all dietary supplements containing ephedrine alkaloids, such as ephedra, ma huang, *Sida cordifolia*, and pinellia. At this time, the FDA is monitoring supplements marketed as substitutes for ephedra, such as *Citrus aurantium*. (FDA. 222.fda.gov/oc/initiatives/ephedra/February2004/qu_020604.html). Because the rule does not include traditional Chinese herbal medicines, the potential for exposure to ephedra still exists.

Citrus aurantium, also known as the Seville orange, or bitter orange, is used to make orange marmalade. The unripe peel contains synephrine, neohesperidien, and five other adrenergic amines. Proponents for bitter orange use claim that bitter orange stimulates only beta-3 receptors in the adipose tissue and liver. They claim that bitter orange will not increase blood pressure or heart rate and thus is safer and a substitute for ephedra. However, a study using healthy volunteers showed that bitter orange elevated systolic and diastolic blood pressure and heart rate following a single dose (Bui et al. 2006).

The potential for adulterated products must be kept in mind when evaluating a patient. On January 9, 2009, the FDA released a press release naming 69 different weight loss products adulterated with various drugs, including sibutramine (a controlled IV drug found in the weight loss pharmaceutical Meridia®), phenytoin, phenolphthalein, rimonabant, and bumetadine. Most of the products claimed to be natural or only herbal ingredients. (FDA Expands Warning to Consumers About Tainted Weight Loss Pills. http://www.fda.gov/bbs/topics/NEWS/2008/NEW01933.html. Accessed Feb 28, 2009).

Small Animal Toxicology Essentials, First Edition. Edited by Robert H. Poppenga, Sharon Gwaltney-Brant.
© 2011 John Wiley and Sons, Inc. Published 2011 by John Wiley and Sons, Inc.

Mechanism of Action

Pharmacologically, ephedrine and pseudoephedrine are sympathomimetic alkaloids. The alkaloids stimulate alpha- and beta-adrenergic receptors, causing the release of endogenous catecholamines at synapses in the brain and heart. This stimulation results in peripheral vasoconstriction and cardiac stimulation. This results in increased blood pressure, tachycardia, ataxia, restlessness, tremors, and seizures (Gurley et al. 1998).

Kinetics

Pseudoephedrine is excreted in urine as an unchanged drug (Means 1999). In humans, the elimination half-life varies between 2–21 hours, depending on the urine pH.

Toxicity

Clinical signs have been seen in dogs at 5–6 mg/kg and deaths have occurred at 10–12 mg/kg. Dogs have a narrow margin of safety compared to other species (Means 1999). Toxicity can be increased if other sympathomimetic substances (such as phenylpropanolomine) are taken at the same time. Underlying disease can also increase an animal's susceptibility to toxicosis. Some of these conditions include heart disease, diabetes, and seizure disorders (Brinker 1998).

Clinical Signs

Effects are generally limited to the cardiovascular and central nervous systems. Initial signs usually begin with restlessness, pacing, and agitation. Vocalization may occur. Dogs may exhibit hallucinogenic behavior. On clinical examination, mydriasis, tachycardia, hypertension, muscle tremors, and seizures may be present. Death is usually due to cardiovascular collapse. Hypertension can cause pulmonary edema, although it is rare. Once an animal becomes symptomatic, clinical signs may last for 36–48 hours (Means 1999).

Management of Exposures

For a recent ingestion (15 minutes or less) in an asymptomatic animal, emesis may be induced followed by administration of activated charcoal with a cathartic. Agitation, nervousness, and tremors are best controlled by acepromazine maleate, chlorpromazine, or if seizures develop, a barbiturate such as phenobarbital is recommended (Plumb 1999). For acepromazine and chlorpromazine, start at the low end of the dosage range and increase as needed. Dissociative effects of benzodiazepines are frequently exaggerated in dogs with pseudoephedrine toxicosis; dogs may actually become more agitated after the administration of diazepam. Serotonin syndrome may be present, and cyproheptadine is a serotonin antagonist that may aid in management of serotonergic signs (disorientation, vocalization, hyperthermia). Propranolol or another beta-blocker can be used to control tachycardia. Supportive care includes administration of intravenous fluids and monitoring the patient. Baseline blood tests, including serum potassium and glucose concentrations, should be obtained and any abnormalities corrected.

METHYLXANTHINES

Sources

Caffeine is obtained from guarana (*Paullinia cupana*) a plant containing high levels of caffeine. Guarana may contain 3%–5% caffeine by dry weight compared to coffee beans (1%–2% caffeine) and tea (1%–4% caffeine). Common names include Brazilian cocoa and Zoom. Theobromine and theophylline have also been found in the plant. Historically, guarana was used to provide energy during fasting, as an aphrodisiac, and to prevent malaria and dysentery. Guarana is frequently found in herbal weight loss aids (with or without ma huang) and in products promising increased energy (Der Marderosian 1996; PDR 1998). Because guarana contains methylxanthines, it produces a clinical syndrome similar to chocolate, coffee, or over-the-counter stimulant products, which contain caffeine.

Mechanism of Action

Caffeine is a methylated xanthine. It increases cyclic AMP, releases catecholamines, and increases muscular contractility. The net effect is a positive inotropic and chronotropic effect on the heart, cerebral vasoconstriction, renal vasorelaxation, and smooth muscle relaxation in the gastrointestinal tract (Beasley 1997).

Kinetics

Caffeine is well absorbed orally. The plasma half-life in the dog is 4.5 hours. Caffeine is metabolized in the liver and undergoes enterohepatic recirculation. Caffeine is excreted through the urine (Beasley 1997; Kisseberth and Trammel 1990). Caffeine has caused birth defects in animals (Brinker 1998).

Toxicity

The LD_{50} of caffeine in dogs is reported to be 140 mg/kg. However, serious toxicity and death have been reported at doses much lower than the LD_{50}. Signs of acute caffeine toxicity in humans appear at 15 to 30 mg/kg and the lethal dose is estimated to be 100 to 200 mg/kg (Kisseberth and Trammel 1990; Shannon 1998). For combinations of ma huang and guarana, the minimum dose at which clinical signs were reported in dogs is 1.3 mg/kg ma huang and 4.4 mg/kg guarana. The minimum dose at which death was reported was 5.8 mg/kg ma huang and 19.1 mg/kg guarana. These doses were obtained from cases reported to the ASPCA Animal Poison Control Center (Ooms et al. 2001). There are multiple drugs that can interact with caffeine. Besides pseudoephedrine and ma huang, monoamine oxidase inhibitors, aspirin, and cimetidine are commonly used medications that should not be combined with caffeine. The sedative effects of benzodiazepines may be decreased by caffeine (Brinker 1998). As with ma huang, there are several medical conditions, which may enhance toxicity. These conditions include heart and kidney disease and ulcers.

Clinical Effects

Clinical signs include vomiting, restlessness and hyperactivity, polydipsia, and polyuria. Tachycardia and other cardiac arrhythmias such as premature ventricular contractions (PVCs) are possible. Clinical signs progress to muscle tremors and seizures, and finally death (Beasley 1997; Ooms et al. 2001).

Management of Exposure

Treatment consists of early decontamination. Induce emesis in an asymptomatic animal or perform gastric lavage. Because enterohepatic recirculation occurs in caffeine toxicosis, repeated doses of activated charcoal are beneficial. Cardiac function should be monitored. Tachycardia can be treated with a beta-blocker such as metoprolol or propranolol. The dose is the same as in ma huang toxicosis. Premature ventricular contractions can be treated with lidocaine. Lidocaine is dosed as an initial bolus slowly intravenously, followed by an IV drip. Muscle tremors and seizures are treated with diazepam or a barbiturate can be used (dose as per ma huang). Intravenous fluids may enhance excretion. A urinary catheter should be placed because methylxanthines can be absorbed through the bladder wall (Beasley 1997; Ooms et al. 2001).

HYPOGLYCEMICS

Alpha Lipoic Acid

Sources

Alpha lipoic acid (ALA), also known as thioctic acid, is considered a "vitaminlike" antioxidant. ALA is found in yeast, liver, kidney, heart, skeletal muscle, spinach, broc-

coli, and potatoes. It is used in alternative veterinary practices to treat diabetic polyneuropathy, cataracts, and glaucoma. In toxicology, it has been used to treat amanita mushroom poisoning. However, the doses used in human medicine for mushroom toxicity can cause toxicity in dogs.

Toxicity

ALA is taken orally, usually in 100 or 300 mg capsules. The reported LD_{50} in dogs is 400–500 mg/kg. However, suspicious deaths have been reported at doses below 100 mg/kg, and confirmed deaths at 330 mg/kg (ASPCA 2010). Cats are about 10 times more sensitive than dogs (Hill et al. 2004). The minimum toxic dose in cats is 13 mg/kg and at 30 mg/kg neurologic signs and hepatotoxicity develop.

The therapeutic dose for cats is 1–5 mg/kg, with a maximum dose of 25 mg/day. For dogs, the therapeutic dose is up to 200 mg/day. Decontamination is recommended for all cats if the calculated dose is >5 mg/kg and dogs if the dose is >30 mg/kg.

Clinical Effects

Clinical signs include hypersalivation, vomiting, ataxia, tremors and seizures, and death. Serum chemistry abnormalities include profound hypoglycemia and increased liver enzymes. Acute renal failure has occurred in some patients. The onset of clinical signs is within 30 minutes up to several hours postingestion.

Management of Exposure

Treatment is symptomatic and supportive. Treat hypoglycemia, if present, with dextrose; support liver function; correct dehydration and control vomiting; and control tremors and seizures. Monitor blood glucose as well as renal and liver enzymes. See the section "Xylitol" in Chapter 24 for specific treatment.

Cinnamon

Sources and Formulations

Cinnamon (*Cinnamomum cassia* and *Cinnamomum zeylanicum*) is currently touted as an adjunct therapy in the treatment of type II diabetes (Chase and McQueen 2007; Baker et al. 2008). Cinnamon can be purchased in capsular form at natural food stores or wherever vitamins and supplements are sold. Most of the clinical trials reported at this time have had a small number of patients, or used rats, and some studies had conflicting results.

Cinnamon is NOT the same as cinnamon oil. Cinnamon oil is sometimes abused by teenagers, generally boys.

They report a rush or sensation of warmth, facial flushing, and oral an burning sensation (Klepser and Klepser 1999; Lee et al. 2000; Libster 1999; McGuffin and Hobbs 1997; Means 1999).

Mechanism of Action

The mechanism of action is generally described as an insulinlike effect. Cinnamon contains an active constituent classed as a methylhydroxychalcone polymer (MHCP) that may be linked to the effect. This substance, when combined with insulin, has synergistic effects. People are advised to monitor blood glucose carefully when taking cinnamon, especially when concurrent diabetic medications are used.

If a dog ingests large quantities of cinnamon, the potential for hypoglycemia exists. Cinnamon is also reported to cause hypotension in dogs. Cinnamon does have an emetic effect in large quantities, so many dogs will self-decontaminate after ingestion.

Some concerns with long-term usage do exist. Some sources of cinnamon may have significant pesticide contamination, and there have been reports of hepatic injury with long-term use. Cinnamon also contains coumarin and can have drug interactions.

Management of Exposures

In asymptomatic animals, emesis should be induced following large ingestions. Home care will be appropriate in many cases. Owners can monitor and feed small frequent meals and transport to a veterinary clinic if clinical signs develop.

MISCELLANEOUS HERBS

Griffonia simplicifolia

Sources and Formulations

Seeds from this plant are used as a source of 5-hydroxytryptophan (5-HTP). This extract is generally used to treat depression, headaches, obesity, and insomnia in humans. 5-HTP is reported to increase serotonin in the CNS. Label information may list 5-HTP, 5-hydroxytryptophan, or griffonia seed extract as an ingredient. Drug interactions with MAO inhibitors, antidepressants, and herbs such as St. John's Wort can occur (Gwaltney-Brant et al. 2000).

Kinetics and Toxicity

5-HTP is rapidly and well absorbed from the gastrointestinal tract. 5-HTP readily crossed the blood-brain barrier. Once target cells are reached, 5-HTP is converted to sero-

tonin (5-hydroxytryptamine). Serotonin is important in the regulation of sleep, cognition, behavior, temperature regulation, and other functions.

In dogs, the minimum toxic dose reported is 23.6 mg/kg and the minimum lethal dose reported in dogs is 128 mg/kg (Gwaltney-Brant et al. 2000). There is not necessarily a good correlation between severity of signs and dose ingested. Signs have been reported from 10 minutes up to 4 hours postingestion. Signs can last up to 36 hours (Gwaltney-Brant et al. 2000).

Clinical Effects

Clinical signs resemble serotonin syndrome in humans. Signs include seizures and tremors, depression, ataxia, disorientation, vocalization, and hyperesthesia. Gastrointestinal effects including vomiting, diarrhea, and drooling are common. Severe hyperthermia and blindness have been reported (Gwaltney-Brant et al. 2000).

Management of Exposures

Treatment includes early decontamination. Seizures, tremors, and other neurologic signs usually respond well to diazepam or barbiturates. Fluid therapy should be initiated. Hyperthermia can be managed with cool water baths and fans. Baseline blood and chemistry panels should be obtained. Cyproheptadine is a serotonin antagonist and can be used PO or rectally until signs resolve (Gwaltney-Brant et al. 2000)

Echinacea purpurea

Sources and Formulations

This herb is one of the most popular supplements in use today. The common names of *Echinacea* include purple coneflower, comb flower, scurvy root, and others. Echinacea is indigenous to the United States and cultivated elsewhere. The plant is a perennial herb with narrow leaves and can grow up 3 feet. It is not unusual to have echinacea confused with *Parthenium integrifolium*, a member of the same family, but one that contains no pharmacological activity. Historically, echinacea was used by Native Americans and adopted by settlers. Uses ranged from "blood purifiers" to dizziness to rattlesnake bites. Extracts were widely used as anti-infectives until antibiotics were discovered (Der Marderosian 1996; PDR 1998).

Echinacea contains essential oils, as well as glycoproteins, alkamides, and flavonoids. All parts of the plant are used in various herbal preparations. Echinacea is taken as a tincture and in capsule form, and is applied locally to wounds. Echinacea is typically used as an immune stimulant and as supportive therapy for the common cold or coughs, urinary tract infections, and stomatitis. Echinacea is recommended for chronic skin ulcers or poorly healing wounds. Because echinacea is suspected of being an immunostimulant, it should not be taken for more than 8 consecutive weeks. Echinacea is contraindicated in progressive diseases such as AIDS or multiple sclerosis, and tuberculosis (Der Marderosian 1996; Brinker 1998).

Toxicity

Echinacea has a wide margin of safety. Arabinogalactan, a purified compound found in *E. purpurea*, has been dosed at 4 gm/kg IP and IV with no toxic effects. People have reported a variety of adverse effects including hypotension, dizziness, fever, chills, nausea and vomiting, dyspnea, and dermatological effects. At least some of the effects are probably due to hypersensitivity and allergic reactions (Der Marderosian 1996; Brinker 1998; PDR 1998).

Signs

The ASPCA National Animal Poison Control Center has received 45 calls involving echinacea since 1992. In many cases, multiple herbal trades were ingested, or the capsules contained multiple ingredients. The most common clinical signs when echinacea was the only trade ingested were vomiting and drooling. In 2 cases, the animal developed a mild cough, possibly associated with retching. Both hyperactivity and lethargy were reported. Erythema was reported in 1 case. In 25 cases, no clinical signs developed (ASPCA 2010).

Management of Exposures

A small ingestion of echinacea generally does not require medical intervention. Any gastrointestinal upset is generally self-limiting and the pet owner will be able to treat with supportive care (NPO, kaolin/pectin). It is imperative to determine whether the animal ingested other herbal products or medications. Large recent ingestions can be treated with gastric decontamination. If an animal develops severe vomiting, symptomatic treatment with IV fluids and other supportive care should be initiated.

Chamomile

Sources

Chamomile refers to both German chamomile (*Matricaria recutita*) and Roman chamomile (*Chamaemelum nobile*). Common names for German chamomile include wild chamomile and pin heads. Common names for Roman chamomile include garden chamomile, sweet chamomile, ground apple, and whig plant. The plant is indigenous to Europe and northwest Asia and naturalized in America. German chamomile is an annual, and Roman chamomile is a slow-growing perennial. The plant is erect and grows to about 20–40 cm. Flowers are white with yellow centers (Eisenberg 1997; Klepser and Klepser 1999). Chamomile has been used medicinally since the Roman Empire. It was used as an antispasmodic and sedative. In folk medicine, chamomile is used for rheumatism and intestinal parasitism. Chamomile has also been used as a hair tint and cigarette flavoring (Der Marderosian 1996; Brinker 1998). In veterinary medicine, the most common uses are as a natural dewormer, sedative and as a treatment for aggression.

Chamomile contains essential oils, flavanoids, and hydroxycoumarins. Both fresh and dried flower heads are used. Some preparations will use the entire plant. Chamomile is most frequently taken as a tea. Ointments, gels, and bath salts are also available. Chamomile is used as a sedative and gastrointestinal antispasmodic. It may also be taken to treat colds, bronchitis, and fevers. In one study using rats, the development of gastrointestinal ulcers caused by indomethacin (a nonsteroidal anti-inflammatory) was prevented by chamomile (Der Marderosian 1996). Topically, chamomile is used to treat wounds and burns. Chamomile is contraindicated in pregnancy (especially early pregnancy) ((McGuffin and Hobbs 1997; Brinker 1998).

Toxicity

Bisaldolol, which accounts for 50% of the essential oils found in chamomile, has an acute LD_{50} of 15 ml/kg in rats and mice. In a 4-week subacute toxicity study, 1–2 ml/kg given orally to rats produced no significant effects Der Marderosian 1996).

Clinical Effects

Hypersensitivity and anaphylaxis has been reported. Contact dermatitis occurs in people sensitive to other plants in the family, such as ragwort. Ingestion of large quantities of the flower heads produces vomiting. The ASPCA Animal Poison Control Center has had 6 cases of ingestion in cats (ASPCA 2010). Three cases involved gastrointestinal upset (vomiting and/or diarrhea), 4 cases reported depression and lethargy, and 2 cases reported epistaxis. Of the two cats with epistaxis, one also developed hematomas. Epistaxis and hematoma development is probably due to the hydroxycoumarin content. One cat developed no clinical signs. The majority of dogs developed no clinical signs. Vomiting and hypersalivation were the most commonly reported clinical signs in dogs (ASPCA 2010).

Management of Exposures

Management of recent ingestions includes gastric decontamination. In cases of large ingestions, activated charcoal can be given. Treatment for gastric irritation is symptomatic and supportive (NPO, gastrointestinal protectants, fluid therapy if severe vomiting or dehydration occurs). If anaphylaxis occurs, standard therapy with epinephrine, steroids, and antihistamines should be initiated. For cats, or dogs with bleeding disorders such as von Willebrand's disease, a packed cell volume and activated clotting time or coagulation profile may be required. If necessary, a blood transfusion could be administered.

St. John's Wort (*Hypericum perforatum*)

Sources and Formulations

St. John's wort is also known as goatweed, rosin rose, and Klamath weed. It is a perennial native in Europe, Canada, and the United States. This plant can be found throughout much of the United States, but northwestern states have had the greatest livestock economic losses due to *Hypericum*. There are several *Hypericum* species, some with overlapping ranges, but the most important is *Hypericum perforatum*. The plant grows aggressively in roadside areas and ditches, meadows, and woods. The height is usually 2 feet. Yellow flowers bloom from June through September. The plant must be harvested between July and August and dried immediately to retain pharmacological properties.

St. John's Wort has been used since the Middle Ages. Traditionally, this herb is used as an antidepressant and to treat diarrhea and gastritis. It was also used to treat insomnia and cancer. Topically, the herb is mixed with olive oil to create "red oil" and used for inflammation (Der Marderosian 1996; PDR 1998). In veterinary medicine, this plant is well known for causing photosensitization in livestock and horses. St. John's wort has been responsible for devastating economic losses to livestock producers.

Mechanism of Action

The major active constituents are anthraquinone derivatives, hypericin, and pseudohypericin, as well as flavanoids. The concentration varies considerably depending on harvest time, drying process, and storage. St. John's wort is used primarily as an antidepressant and sedative. Studies have shown that St. John's wort inhibits serotonin uptake, accounting for the antidepressant effects. It is taken as an infusion or as dried herb. The most common preparation is a standardized 300 mg capsule. St. John's wort can interact with several medications. It decreases the activity of protease inhibitors, antagonizes reserpine, and increases stupor when consumed with alcohol. Monoamine oxidase inhibitors (MAO) such as seligiline (Anipryl®) are potentiated when taken concomitantly. Serotonin syndrome is possible if St. John's wort is taken with selective serotonin reuptake inhibitors (SSRIs) due to synergistic activity. Common SSRIs include fluoxetine (Prozac®) and sertraline (Zoloft®). Serotonin syndrome has also been noted when St. John's wort is taken with dextrometorphan and meperidine. Sympathomimetics combined with St. John's wort may lead to a hypertensive crisis (Shannon 1999).

Clinical Effects

Adverse effects occur commonly. In humans, the most frequently reported signs include gastrointestinal upset, allergic reactions, and agitation. Photosensitization has occurred, generally after large doses or long-term usage. Prior to 1994, the only cases in the ASPCA National Animal Poison Control Center databanks involved livestock and photosensitization. Almost all cases involving herbal products involve dogs (35 out of 38 cases). In almost half the cases, no signs were reported. The most commonly reported clinical signs were depression, vomiting, and diarrhea. Tremors and/or seizure were reported in three cases. Two cases developed increased liver enzymes (ASPCA 2010).

Management of Exposures

Recent ingestions are best treated by decontamination. Gastrointestinal disorders are generally easily managed with symptomatic and supportive care. In large ingestions, or unknown quantities, especially if early decontamination is not possible, baseline liver enzymes should be obtained. If evidence of serotonin syndrome develops (tremors, seizures, hyperthermia, vomiting, and diarrhea), standard therapy as discussed in the section *Griffonia simplicifolia* is initiated. If evidence of photosensitization occurs, keep the animal out of sunlight, and provide supportive care for hepatic damage.

Valerian Root (*Valeriana officianalis*)

Sources and Formulations

Valerian root is one of the most popular herbs on the market. Common names include all-heal, heliotrope, Vandal root, and Capon's tale. It is an herbaceous perennial found widely over the United States. The dried rhizome contains a volatile oil with an odor many find offensive. The fresh drug does not have an odor. The plant grows to about 50 to 100 cm high and is erect without a branching stem. Flowers are bright pink to white. The fruit is yellow with a tuft of white hair. Valerian is sometimes confused with *Veratrum album*, which is a toxic plant. There are over 200 species of valerian, with various degrees of pharmacologic activity. *Valeriana officianalis* is considered the standard genus and species used in herbal medicine (Der Marderosian 1996; PDR 1998).

The primary active ingredients are volatile oils, alkaloids, and most importantly, valepotriates. The root is the only part of the plant that is used. Valerian is classed as generally recognized as safe (GRAS) for food use. The volatile oils are used as flavoring in some food products. Valerian is used primarily as a sedative and as a sleeping aid. It has also been used in epilepsy, headaches, colic, and numerous other minor ailments. Valerian is frequently taken as a tea or as an extract. Valerian increases the length of sedation induced by pentobarbital and length of anesthesia produced by thiopental. Valerian has helped ease the effects of withdrawal from benzodiazepines due to similar receptor sites, but it increases the effects of sedatives if taken concomitantly (Der Marderosian 1996; PDR 1998).

Toxicity

Most reports of adverse effects of valerian in human literature occur after chronic use. These effects include headache, cardiac arrhthymias, and agitation. In one case report, 200 mg in a human caused fatigue, tremors, abdominal pain, and mydriasis (Shannon 1999). Animal studies included injections of 50 mg/kg intravenous in cats, which caused a drop in heart rate and blood pressure. Another study found no pharmacological effect in cats at 250 mg/kg. Mice given up to 4600 mg/kg orally produced mild clinical effects. Signs of toxicity included ataxia, hypothermia, and muscle relaxation (Der Marderosian 1996).

Clinical Effects

The ASPCA Animal Poison Control Center has had only a few calls on valerian ingestion. Most produced no clinical effects, although lethargy and sedation were seen in a cat (ASPCA 2010).

Management of Exposures

Generally, significant treatment would be unnecessary. The sedative effects are generally short-lived and can be managed by an owner at home. Large ingestions in an asymptomatic animal could be treated by decontamination.

ESSENTIAL OILS

Sources and Formulations

Essential oils are produced by a large number of plants (Wolfe 1999). The oils are a mixture of terpenes and other chemicals. Essential oils are used from food flavorings to perfumes to medications. The most commonly used essential oils in veterinary medicine include Melaleuca or tea tree oil (*Melaleuca alternifolia*), pennyroyal oil (*Mentha pulegium*), D-limonene and linalool (*Citrus spp.*), Citronella (*Cymbopgum nardus*), Thuja (*Thuja occidentalis*), and wormwood or absinthe (*Artemisia absinthium*).

In veterinary medicine, essential oils are most commonly used to treat flea infestations, hot spots or other dermatological conditions, or as wormers. Oils may be found in shampoos, dips, liniments, teas, tinctures, syrups, or other formulations (Villar et al. 1994; Bischoff and Gaule 1998; Wolfe 1999).

Kinetics

Essential oils are rapidly absorbed both orally and dermally. They are metabolized by the liver to glucuronide and glycine conjugates. Repeated exposure can cause inductions of the hepatic enzyme systems cytochrome P-450 and UPD-glycuronyl transferase systems. Thus, preexisting liver disease can increase the risk of toxicity.

Toxicity

Cats appear to be more sensitive to essential oils than dogs (Villar et al. 1994; Bischoff and Gaule 1998; Wolfe 1999). The acute LD_{50} varies significantly between various essential oils. Formulations mixed with an organic solvent, such as alcohol, can allow increased absorption and toxicity. Generally, a greater volume of fresh product is required to produce the same effects as a concentrated essence. The basic mechanism of action is unknown (Villar et al. 1994).

Clinical Effects

The most common clinical signs after dermal exposures include ataxia, muscle weakness, depression, and behavioral abnormalities. Severe hypothermia and collapse have occurred in cats. A transient paresis can occur in small breed dogs when melaleuca oil is applied down the spine as a topical flea treatment (Villar et al. 1994; Kaluzienski 2000). Cats have developed scrotal dermatitis after exposure to *d*-limonene or linalool (Power et al. 1988; Hooser 1990). Liver failure has been associated with essential oils, especially pennyroyal and melaleuca (Villar et al. 1994; Bischoff and Gaule 1998; Kaluzienski 2000; Sudekum et al. 1992).

Oral ingestions cause vomiting and diarrhea. Central nervous system depression may occur, and seizures are possible with large doses. Aspiration pneumonia can occur when essential oils are inhaled. Death can occur with sufficient doses. Signs usually develop from almost immediately up to 8 hours postexposure (Villar et al. 1994; Bischoff and Gaule 1998; Der Marderosian 1996).

Management of Exposures

Recent dermal exposures should be treated by bathing using a hand dishwashing liquid. Activated charcoal is effective in oral exposures. Emesis should not be induced due to the potential for aspiration pneumonia. Intravenous fluids help correct hypotension and aid in renal elimination. Body temperature should be monitored and regulated as needed, and electrolytes, cardiac, and respiratory function should be monitored. Seizures and tremors usually respond to diazepam. Aspiration pneumonia may require oxygen and broad-spectrum antibiotics. Hepatic damage usually responds to good supportive care, although N-acetylcysteine has been used experimentally in humans diagnosed with pennyroyal toxicosis (Poisindex® 2001). Signs usually resolve over a few hours up to a few days. Most animals do have a good prognosis with appropriate treatment. Many mild cases require only mild home treatment and observation (Villar et al. 1994; Bischoff and Gaule 1998; Poisindex® 2001; Plumb 1999).

HERBS AND PETS

One of the most important considerations in treating herbal ingestions is product quality assurance. Although most herbal companies are reputable, there are numerous reports of adulterated products (addition of substances not noted on the label). This has been particularly true of Chinese herbal products, which frequently contain pharmaceuticals. Plant identification errors occur, and entire batches of product have been mixed using the wrong herb. In some cases, labels are written in a foreign language or contain directions only for mixing, making interpretation difficult. In cases where a known ingestion produces unexpected clinical signs, the potential for adulteration or other errors should be considered. When a product is not standardized, a consumer can not be sure what dosage of active constituents or how bioavailable the product may be. Standardization also provides assurance that the actual herb is in the product (Winslow and Kroll 1998).

Clients who use herbal products should be advised to treat them as a medication, and keep them away from pets. Specifically ask clients if they take or use any natural or herbal products. Many people do not consider these substances to be drugs or assume "if natural, it is harmless." Clients should be encouraged to learn about the herbal and nutriceutical products they are taking or giving their pets. Clients need to be encouraged to discuss proper use of herbal products in pets with their veterinarian. Clients can be encouraged to discuss alternative therapies by discussing a pet's diagnosis and suggested treatments thoroughly. Discuss the client's expectations and opinions of both alternative and conventional medicine. Issues of safety and efficacy must be explained to clients. They should be encouraged to report potential adverse reactions or to discuss different routes of therapy if a pet's medical condition is not improving. Clients who want to use alternative medical treatments should be encouraged to obtain a good medical workup in order to obtain a correct diagnosis and be referred to a veterinarian trained in alternative medicine. In choosing an alternative medicine practitioner, the same criteria would be used as for any other specialist: education, training, and professionalism (Libster 1999).

REFERENCES

ASPCA Animal Poison Control Center Databanks, unpublished data, 2010.

Baker, W.L., Guiterrez-Williams, G., White, C.M., Kluger, J., and Coleman, C.I. 2008. Effect of cinnamon on glucose control and lipid parameters. *Diabetes Care* 31(1): 41–43.

Beasley, V.R. 1997. *A Systems Affected Approach to Veterinary Toxicology*, pp. 116–120. Urbana: University of Illinois.

Bischoff, K. and Gaule, F. 1998. Australian Tea Tree (Melaleuca alternifolia) oil poisoning in three purebred cats. *J Vet Diagn Invest* 10:208–210.

Brinker, F. 1998. *Herb Contraindications and Drug Interactions, 2nd ed.* Sandy, Oregon: Eclectic Medical Publications.

Bui, L.T., Nguyen, D.T., and Ambrose, P.J. 2006. Blood pressure and heart rate effects following a single dose of bitter orange. *Ann Pharmacother* 40:53–57.

Chase, C.K. and McQueen, C.E. 2007. Cinnamon in diabetes mellitus. *Am J Health Syst Pharm* 64(10):1033–1035.

Der Marderosian, A., ed. 1996. *The Review of Natural Products.* St. Louis: Facts and Comparisons Publishing Group.

Eisenberg, E.M. 1997. Advising patients who seek alternative medical therapies. *Ann Intern Med* 27(1):61–69.

Gulla, J. and Singer, A.J. 2000. Use of alternative therapies among emergency department patients. *Ann Emer Med* 35(3):226–228.

Gurley, B.J., Gardner, S.F., White, L.M., and Wang, P.L. 1998. Ephedrine pharmacokinetics after the ingestion of nutritional supplements containing Ephedra sinica (ma huang). *Ther Drug Monit* 20:439–445.

Gwaltney-Brant, S.M., Albretson, J.C., and Khan, S.A. 2000. 5-hydroxytryptophan toxicosis in dogs: 21 cases (1989–1999). *J Am Vet Med Assoc* 216(12):1937–1940.

Hill, A.S., Werner, J.A., Rogers, Q.R. et al. 2004. Lipoic acid is 10 times more toxic in cats than reported in humans, dogs, or rats. *J Anim Physiol Anim Nutr (Berl)* 88: 150–156.

Hooser, S.B. 1990. D-limonene, linalool, and crude citrus oil extracts. *Vet Clin North Am Small Anim Pract* 20(2): 383–385.

Kaluzienski, M. 2000. Partial paralysis and altered behavior in dogs treated with melaleuca oil. *Clin Tox* 38(5): 518–519.

Kisseberth, W.C. and Trammel, H.T. 1990. Illicit and abused drugs. *Vet Clin North Am Small Anim Pract* 20(2):405–417.

Klepser, T.B. and Klepser, M.E. 1999. Unsafe and potentially safe herbal therapies. *Am J Health Syst Pharm* 56:125–138.

Lee, K.W., Yamato, O., Tajima, M. et al. 2000. Hematologic changes associated with the appearance of eccentrocytes after intragastric administration of garlic extract to dogs. *Am J Vet Res* 61(11):1446–1450.

Libster, M. 1999. Guidelines for selecting a medical herbalist for consultation and referral: Consulting a medical herbalist. *J Altern Complement Med* 5(5):457–462.

McGuffin, M. and Hobbs, C. 1997. In *Botanical Safety Handbook*, edited by R. Upton and A. Goldberg. New York: CRC Press.

Means, C. 1999. Ma huang: All natural but not always innocuous. *Vet Med* 94(6):511–512.

Ooms, T.G., Khan, S.A., and Means, C. 2001. Suspected caffeine and ephedrine toxicosis resulting from ingestion of an herbal supplement containing guarana and ma huang in dogs: 47 cases (1997–1999). *J Am Vet Med Assoc* 218(2): 225–229.

PDR for Herbal Medicines. 1998. Montvale, New Jersey: Medical Economics Company.

Plumb, D.C. 1999. *Veterinary Drug Handbook, 3rd ed*. Ames: Iowa State University Press.

Poisindex® Editorial Staff. 2001. Essential oils. In *POISINDEX® System*, edited by L.L. Toll and K.M. Hurlbut. Englewood, Colorado: Micromedex, Inc. (Edition expired 2001.)

Power, K.A., Hooser, S.B. et al. 1988. An evaluation of the acute toxicity of an insecticidal spray containing linalool, D-limonene, and piperonyl butoxide applied topically to domestic cats. *Vet Human Tox* 30(3):206–210.

Shannon, M. 1999. Alternative medicines toxicology: A review of selected agents. *Clin Tox* 37(6):709–713.

Shannon, M.W. 1998. Theophylline and caffeine. In *Clinical Management of Poisoning and Drug Overdose, 3rd ed.*, edited by L.M. Haddad, M.W. Shannonm, and J.F. Winchester, pp. 1102–1104. Philadelphia: W.B. Saunders.

Sudekum, M., Poppenga, R.H., Raju, N. et al. 1992. Pennyroyal oil toxicosis in a dog. *J Am Vet Med Assoc* 200(6):817–818.

Villar, D., Knight, M.J., Hansen, S.R. et al. 1994. Toxicity of melaleuca oil and related essential oils applied topically on dogs and cats. *Vet Human Tox* 36(2):139–142.

Winslow, L.C. and Kroll, D.J. 1998. Herbs as medicines. *Arch Intern Med* 158:2192–2199.

Wolfe, A. 1999. Essential oil poisoning. *Clin Tox* 37(6): 721–727.

Zootoxins

22

Tamara Foss

HYMENOPTERA: BEES, WASPS, AND HORNETS

Sources

The Order Hymenoptera includes three medically important families of insects: bees of the family Apidae, wasps and hornets of the family Vespidae, and fire ants of the family Formicidae. Bees, wasps, and hornets are credited with being responsible for more human deaths than any other venomous animal (Cowell et al. 1991).

The family Apidae includes European honeybees, Africanized honeybees, bumblebees, and carpenter bees. All Apids feed on nectar and pollen and can sting only once because they are eviscerated and die after their barbed stinger is left behind. European honeybees, although protective of their hives, are considered to be less aggressive than their Africanized honeybee relatives and Vespids. When honeybees, especially Africanized honeybees, sting, they release an alarm pheromone that alerts and attracts other bees (Diaz 2007). Africanized honeybees are more easily agitated, experience more prolonged agitation and defend a greater distance of area around their hives than their European counterparts (Rodriguez-Lainz et al. 1999). Although bigger than honeybees, bumblebees and carpenter bees do not receive as much discussion in the literature and are considered less aggressive than honeybees (Diaz 2007).

The family Vespidae includes yellow jackets, hornets, and wasps. Vespids are predatory carnivores; they feed on other insects and are attracted to sweet foods and meats. Vespid stingers are not barbed and are therefore not left behind in the victim, so a lone vespid has the ability to sting multiple times.

Solenopsis invicta, the red imported fire ant, a member of the Formicidae family, is the primary species of concern in regard to envenomation of animals (Gwaltney-Brant et al. 2007). There are unique clinical signs that develop with fire ant envenomation, as discussed later.

Toxicity

The amount of venom delivered to a victim does not determine whether an anaphylactic reaction will result. A single sting can result in anaphylaxis. Cases involving multiple stings result in higher venom doses delivered to the victim and a greater toxic reaction (Fitzgerald and Vera 2006). The estimated lethal dose is approximately 20 stings/kg for most mammals (Fitzgerald and Flood 2006).

Toxicokinetics and Mechanism of Action

Only female bees and wasps are able to sting. The stinger is associated with venom glands within the modified ovipositor (Gwaltney-Brant et al. 2007). Hymenoptera venoms contain proteins (which are largely responsible for allergic responses), peptides, and enzymes (which are made up of proteins). The two major enzymes implicated in allergic responses in Apid envenomations are phospholipase and hyaluronidase (Gwaltney-Brant et al. 2007). Phospholipase A2 is a major allergen and is regarded as the most lethal peptide in honeybee venom (Gwaltney-Brant et al. 2007). Mellitin, which is unique to honeybee venom, is responsible for the local pain associated with a

Small Animal Toxicology Essentials, First Edition. Edited by Robert H. Poppenga, Sharon Gwaltney-Brant.

sting. Apamin peptide is also unique to honeybee venom and may have neurotoxic effects on the peripheral nerves (Gwaltney-Brant et al. 2007).

Vespid venoms contain serotonin, kinins, and acetylcholine, all of which are believed to play a role in production of the intense pain that follows envenomation (Fitzgerald and Flood 2006). Antigen 5 is the major allergenic component of vespid venom (Fitzgerald and Flood 2006; Merck 2008). Mastoparans are peptide toxins found in wasp venom, which are similar to but less potent than mast cell degranulation peptide 401 found in Apid venom (Fitzgerald and Flood 2006).

Clinical Effects

Signs

A localized reaction including pain and swelling will generally occur in all victims of envenomation. Erythema can be seen and embedded stingers can result in abscess formation. Local reactions can go unnoticed since the reaction often does not progress in severity and resolves without treatment within 24 hours (Fitzgerald and Flood 2006).

Allergic or hypersensitivity reactions can also occur and vary in their severity. They can be relatively moderate on the continuum of allergic reactions and present as more regional swelling of an area in which a sting was received (Rodriguez-Lainz et al. 1999), or they can be as severe as an anaphylactic response and result in death. Anaphylaxis occurs fairly infrequently in animals, but if it is going to occur, signs typically develop within 10–15 minutes (Rodriguez-Lainz et al. 1999; Fitzgerald and Flood 2006). Anaphylactic signs include urticaria, pruritis, angioedema, vomiting, diarrhea, lethargy, hematuria, laryngeal edema, dyspnea, hyperpnea, tachycardia, possibly hypotension in dogs and cats, ataxia, syncope, seizures, and death (Fitzgerald and Flood 2006; Akre and Reed 2002; Gwaltney-Brant et al. 2007; Rodriguez-Lainz et al. 1999). Anaphylactic reactions in cats can involve salivation and collapse (Cowell and Cowell 1995).

Nonanaphylactoid systemic or toxic reactions typically are delayed for 6 to 24 hours, or even up to several weeks or months (Akre and Reed 2002). Reactions seen include serum sickness, vasculitis, glomerulonephritis, neuropathy, disseminated intravascular coagulation, and arthritis (Fitzgerald and Flood 2006). Other possible conditions include acute lung injury/acute respiratory distress syndrome (Walker et al. 2005) and immune-mediated hemolytic anemia (Noble and Armstrong 1999). Specific signs include ataxia, prostration, convulsions, CNS depression, shock, hyperthermia, bloody diarrhea, bloody vomiting,

hematuria, leukocystosis, intravascular hemolysis, increased blood urea nitrogen (BUN) and elevated alanine transaminase (ALT) (Gwaltney-Brant et al. 2007). Cats can develop hepatic injury following hornet envenomation (Gwaltney-Brant et al. 2007).

Laboratory

When systemic reactions or anaphylaxis occur, it is important to monitor laboratory values including urinalysis and various blood chemistries such as alanine amino transaminase (ALT), total bilirubin, electrolyte levels, blood urea nitrogen (BUN), creatinine, arterial blood gases, and serum creatine kinase. Urine can be red or brown and might contain granular casts (Cowell and Cowell 1995). Blood hemograms reflect an inflammatory leukogram: leukocytosis with a left shift. Anemia may occur with marked spherocytosis (Cowell and Cowell 1995). Rhabdomyolysis and acute renal failure can occur. Electrocardiograph monitoring may be necessary.

Differential Diagnoses

In cases that develop anaphylaxis, it is prudent to rule out other potential toxicological causes such as spiders or other insects. Rule-outs to keep in mind include infection, abscess, trauma, neoplasia, allergy, abscessed tooth, or foreign object (Fitzgerald and Vera 2006). Another possible differential diagnosis is heatstroke (Cowell et al. 1991). Differential diagnoses for animals presenting with respiratory distress should also include acute lung injury/acute respiratory distress syndrome, aspiration pneumonia, interstitial pneumonia, congestive heart failure, and pulmonary thromboembolism (Walker et al. 2005). A potential diagnosis for sudden unexplained death is insect sting, especially when death occurs outdoors (Diaz 2007).

Diagnostics

Antemortem

Evidence of stingers is diagnostic of Apid envenomation. Stingers will not be present with Vespid envenomation. Areas most commonly stung in animals include the head and neck, oral cavity, and limbs and paws (Oliveira et al. 2007).

Postmortem

Postmortem findings include facial edema, gastric hemorrhage, petechiation of the epicardium, and red-black urine (Noble and Armstrong 1999). Facial cellulitis, lung and liver congestion, and pulmonary hemorrhage might also be noted (Noble and Armstrong 1999). Bees and wasps can be found in the gastrointestinal tract (Rodriguez-Lainz et al. 1999).

Management of Exposures

Single sting envenomations can cause pain and swelling. In most cases, treatment will not be necessary (Fitzgerald and Flood 2006). If the incident is witnessed and a stinger is located, it can be removed by scraping away from the injection site. The pet should be monitored for anaphylaxis for the first 10–15 minutes following an envenomation.

Anaphylaxis must be treated intensively. Epinephrine should be administered subcutaneously (Cowell and Cowell 1995). Cardiac monitoring and respiratory support are vital. Intubation and administration of oxygen may be needed. Fluid administration with a crystalloid solution is important to avoid vascular collapse (Fitzgerald and Flood 2006). Antihistamine and corticosteroid administration is recommended (Gwaltney-Brant et al. 2007). Diazepam can be used for convulsions (Gwaltney-Brant et al. 2007).

Cases involving more severe regional reactions and multiple stings should be hospitalized and closely monitored. Corticosteroid administration of prednisolone sodium succinate followed by prednisolone orally and then tapered over 3–5 days may be beneficial in alleviating progression of an envenomation syndrome (Fitzgerald and Flood 2006). If hypotension develops, an intravenous bolus of normal saline should be given (Fitzgerald and Flood 2006). Since hymenopterid venom can be nephrotoxic, it is important to provide continuous fluid administration to ensure normal urine output (Fitzgerald and Flood 2006). Additional treatment including continued fluid and electrolyte therapy and prevention of vascular stasis will be required if signs progress. Toxic reactions, most often associated with massive envenomations, also require closer monitoring of major systems including hematologic profiles, cardiac and respiratory function and renal sufficiency for several days (Fitzgerald and Flood 2006). The more rapidly a patient can be stabilized and provided with supportive care, the better chance for a positive outcome. Even after resolution of signs, monitoring should continue for 24 hours in patients suffering anaphylactic or massive envenomation responses (Fitzgerald and Flood 2006).

Prognosis

Most animals that are victims of single-sting Hymenoptera envenomation will not develop serious signs, so overall, prognosis is very good. Patients that develop anaphylaxis have a better chance of full recovery if they survive the first 60 minutes of the initial envenomation (Fitzgerald and Flood 2006). The chance of recovery increases for animals that experience anaphylaxis or develop severe reactions from multiple sting envenomation if treatment is sought immediately.

HYMENOPTERA: IMPORTED FIRE ANTS

Sources

Fire ants belong to the order Hymenoptera in the family Formicidae. Two species of imported fire ants, *Solenopsis richteri* (black imported fire ants) and *Solenopsis invicta* (the red imported fire ant), are the most problematic and dangerous formicids to humans, agriculture, companion animals, livestock, and wildlife. Due to its greater distribution as compared to *Solenopsis richteri*, *Solenopsis invicta* is the primary species of concern.

Toxicity

Anaphylaxis can occur after fire ant envenomation and is not predictable based on dose or the number of stings received (Fitzgerald and Vera 2006). Although uncommon overall, human fatalities associated with fire ant envenomation are largely due to anaphylaxis (Fitzgerald and Vera 2006). However, there are no known reports of animal deaths from fire ant stings as a result of anaphylaxis (Gwaltney-Brant et al. 2007; Conceicao et al. 2006). Since fire ant envenomations generally occur en masse due to their aggressive and swarming nature, multiple stings leading to systemic toxicity is possible. There is no established lethal number of stings for mammals.

Toxicokinetics and Mechanism of Action

Formicid venom is unique compared to bee, wasp, and hornet venom. It is comprised of 95% water insoluble alkaloids (Akre and Reed 2002). The alkaloid portion includes solenopsin A (trans-2-methyl-6-n-undecylpiperidine), which is a piperidine alkaloid derivative (Conceicao et al. 2006). The dermal necrosis that occurs with envenomation is attributed to the alkaloid portion of the venom (Akre and Reed 2002; Rakich et al. 1993). The alkaloid component is also the cause of most of the local sting reactions that occur (Akre and Reed 2002). The alkaloids have cytotoxic, hemolytic, fungicidal, insecticidal and bactericidal properties (Gwaltney-Brant et al. 2007; Rakich et al. 1993). Unlike the high protein content in bee, wasp, and hornet venom, only approximately 1%–5% of fire ant venom is proteinaceous (Gwaltney-Brant et al. 2007; Akre and Reed 2002; Cowell and Cowell 1995; Elgart 1990). The proteinaceous component of fire ant venom includes hyaluronidase and phospholipase, and is the cause of allergic and anaphylactic responses that occur (Rakich et al. 1993; Akre and Reed 2002).

Fire ants bite and sting their victims. The stingers are not barbed, so they are capable of delivering multiple stings. Fire ants initially bite and then rotate about their fixed heads in a circular fashion as they repeatedly sting (Fitzgerald and Vera 2006).

Clinical Effects

Signs

Clinical signs range from mild dermatologic reactions to anaphylaxis and possibly death. It is unclear as to the annual incidence of bites involving pets or livestock. Generally, signs in dogs are associated with local sting reactions and may include erythema, pruritis, pain, swelling, and dermal necrosis. It is debatable as to whether pustules develop in dogs, but pustule formation is characteristic and diagnostic in humans (Akre and Reed 2002; Gwaltney-Brant et al. 2007; Rakich et al. 1993; Conceicao et al. 2006; Fowler 1993).

There are no reported deaths in animals attributed to anaphylaxis secondary to fire ant stings (Gwaltney-Brant et al. 2007). An anaphylactic reaction is associated with urticaria, cutaneous and laryngeal edema, bronchospasm, and vascular collapse and is mediated by IgE (Fitzgerald and Vera 2006). Typically, anaphylaxis will develop a short time after an envenomation, whereas systemic toxicity from massive envenomations can result in death more than 24 hours postencounter (Fitzgerald and Vera 2006).

Laboratory

There are no laboratory tests that will confirm or determine fire ant exposure (Fitzgerald and Vera 2006).

Differential Diagnoses

Primary diagnoses to keep in mind are similar to those noted in the earlier discussion of bees, wasps, and hornets. Other differential diagnoses to consider include subcorneal pustular dermatosis, pustular psoriasis, and other skin diseases manifested by pustules (Conceicao et al. 2006).

Diagnostics

Antemortem

In humans, the unique circular pattern of stings and the resulting wheal and flare that develop are diagnostic (Elgart 1990). Typically, the wheals progress into papules that fill with fluid, which then develop into pustules within 24 hours (Elgart 1990; Gwaltney-Brant et al. 2007). It is

suggested that rather than developing pustules, dogs develop erythematous pruritic papules that commonly resolve within 24 hours (Gwaltney-Brant et al. 2007).

Postmortem

No postmortem diagnostics are specifically described for fire ant evenomation.

Management of Exposures

Generally, fire ant exposures involving a small number of stings will not require treatment. Multiple sting envenomations involving neonatal or geriatric patients may require veterinary treatment. Severe systemic reactions or anaphylaxis, should they develop, are treated as noted in the previous bees, wasps, and hornets discussion. If live fire ants are observed when an animal is presented for treatment, they should be removed as soon as possible to limit further venom delivery. A soapy water bath or application of a low-toxicity insecticide (e.g., pyrethrin) might be required (Drees et al. 2002).

Fire ants target areas on animals with minimal hair growth and/or moist areas including the muzzle, eyes, ears, ventral abdomen, and perineum (Drees et al. 2002). Animals lick or bite at areas where fire ants congregate and sting; in so doing they may ingest a number of fire ants and potentially suffer stings in the oral cavity or gastrointestinal tract (Drees et al. 2002). Gastrointestinal protectants and nutritional supplementation might be indicated (Drees et al. 2002).

If the eyes are bitten, excessive lacrimation, blepharospasm, and mucopurulent exudates can be observed (Drees et al. 2002). Focal necrotic ulcers can be present on the cornea and conjunctiva (Drees et al. 2002). Topical ophthalmic antibiotic solutions should be administered. Corticosteroids should be avoided in cases involving corneal ulcers (Drees et al. 2002).

Prognosis

Overall, the prognosis is very good. In most cases, a local reaction involving mild swelling and pain may be the extent of clinical signs. In many cases, owners will not be aware that their pet was stung.

BUFO TOADS

Sources

Bufo marinus (cane toad, giant toad, or marine toad) gained access to the United States from Puerto Rico via Hawaii. It now additionally resides in the southern tip of Florida and Texas (Eubig 2001). *Bufo alvarius*

(Colorado River toad) inhabits southern Arizona, southeastern California and southwestern New Mexico (Eubig 2001).

Toads have mucous and granular glands that aid in defense against predators. *Bufo* toads have a pair of parotid glands, which begin caudal to the tympanum and continue over the shoulders (Fowler 1993; Palumbo 1983; Eubig 2001). The parotid glands serve as the primary release site of a thick, creamy, poisonous secretion through pinhole orifices on the surface of the skin (Fowler 1993; Palumbo 1983; Eubig 2001). *Bufo alvarius*, although considered less toxic than *Bufo marinus*, is equipped with an additional pair of poison glands on the forelimbs and several pairs on the hindlimbs (Eubig 2001).

Toxicity

Bufo marinus that reside in Florida are equipped with a more potent toxin than those residing in Hawaii; the mortality of dogs exposed to *Bufo marinus* in Florida that subsequently receive no treatment is almost 100% compared to about only 5% for those exposed to *Bufo marinus* in Hawaii (Palumbo 1983; Beasley 1999). The entire content of both parotid glands, which is approximately equivalent to 0.1 g of venom, is considered a potentially lethal oral dose for a dog (Reeves 2004). However, toxicity varies (Peterson and Roberts 2006). The size of the animal exposed and size of the toad delivering the venom, coupled with the length of time subjected to the venom, will largely impact the outcome of exposure (Peterson and Roberts 2006). Typically, a bite and release exposure is not as severe as one involving holding and chewing, or ingestion of a toad (Peterson and Roberts 2006). Clinical signs are expected in exposures involving a dose of 1 mg/kg (Peterson and Roberts 2006).

Toxicokinetics and Mechanism of Action

Bufo toad secretions contain two primary components: bufogenins and bufotoxins (Peterson and Roberts 2006; Fowler 1993; Eubig 2001). The secretions also contain bufotenines (serotonin and 5-hydroxytryptophan), catecholamines (dopamine, epinephrine, and norepinephrine), and indolealkylamines (Peterson and Roberts 2006; Eubig 2001). Bufogenins are similar in activity to cardiac glycosides and, along with bufotoxins, are responsible for arrhythmias such as ventricular fibrillation that develop (Eubig 2001; Beasley 1999; Fowler 1993). Bufotenines are associated with vomiting, diarrhea, depression, tremors, seizures, hyperthermia and hypersensitivity to sensory stimuli (Eubig 2001). Tachycardia, hypertension, anxiety, and respiratory distress can develop as a result of the cat-

echolamine activity in the secretions (Eubig 2001). Indolealkylamines, along with serotonin and 5-hydroxytryptophan, have hallucinogenic effects (Beasley 1999; Peterson and Roberts 2006; Reeves 2004).

Clinical Effects

Signs

Initial signs after oral exposure include profuse salivation, deep red mucous membranes, pawing at the mouth, and vocalizing (Peterson and Roberts 2006). Vomiting and anxiety can also be noted (Roder 2004a). Commonly, signs include ataxia, seizures, stupor, coma, nystagmus, recumbency or collapse, and tachypnea (Eubig 2001; Roberts et al. 2000; Roder 2004a). Signs can worsen quickly and death can occur within 15 minutes (Eubig 2001; Roder 2004a). Various arrhythmias and hyperthermia or hypothermia can develop (Eubig 2001). Although exposures to *Bufo marinus* or *Bufo alvarius* are more likely to result in development of serious signs, exposure to any *Bufo* species is potentially toxic, especially for smaller, older pets or those with underlying health conditions (Eubig 2001).

Laboratory

Serum potassium may be elevated (Peterson 2000; Morgan 1997). Elevated packed cell volume, hemoglobin, blood glucose, serum urea nitrogen, and serum calcium might be observed (Palumbo 1983; Reeves 2004). Serum sodium and chloride concentrations drop minimally while serum inorganic phosphorus dramatically decreases (Palumbo 1983).

Differential Diagnoses

Signs associated with *Bufo* toad exposures are similar to those assicuated with seizure disorders, ataxic conditions, heat stroke, and trauma (such as hit by car) (Eubig 2001). Exposure to insecticides in organophosphorous, carbamates, pyrethroids, metaldehyde or chlorinated hydrocarbons can cause similar signs (Eubig 2001). Sympathomimetic, methylxanthine, β-blocker, β-agonist and various antidepressant medication exposures should be ruled out (Eubig 2001). Ingestion of outdoor plants such as rhododendron (*Rhododendron* sp.), oleander (*Nerium oleander*), and foxglove (*Digitalis purpurea*) can result in development of signs seen in *Bufo* exposures. Additionally, exposure to caustic agents such as liquid potpourri and various cleaning agents, orally irritating agents such as topical flea and tick products, and plants containing insoluble calcium oxalates such as *Diffenbachia* and *Philodendron*, can cause copious salivation (Eubig 2001;

Peterson 2000). Seizure disorders to rule out include idiopathic epilepsy, inflammatory meningoencephalitis (secondary to an infection, immune-mediated reaction, or neoplasm), and internal masses (Peterson and Roberts 2006). Ataxia is often reported in peripheral and central vestibular diseases (Peterson and Roberts 2006).

Diagnostics

Antemortem

Since *Bufo* toad toxicosis is similar in presentation to a variety of other potential exposures ranging from insecticides to various medications, the only truly beneficial antemortem diagnostic information is a witnessed exposure to a *Bufo* toad (Fowler 1993).

Postmortem

No specific postmortem diagnostics are suggested. However, necropsy might reveal pulmonary edema and, if ingested, toad parts can be identified in stomach contents (Fowler 1993).

Management of Exposures

If a toad exposure is suspected or was witnessed, and the pet is showing no or only minor signs (such as excessive salivation and gagging), the mouth should be irrigated with large volumes of water (such as with a garden hose) to minimize any further secretion absorption via the mucous membranes. If more severe signs are present, initial decontamination should take place under the care of a veterinarian, following stabilization and preferably intubation of the pet (Gwaltney-Brant et al. 2007; Eubig 2001). It is best to flush the mouth rostrally, to avoid ingestion of the water (Eubig 2001). In areas in which *Bufo marinus* resides, especially Florida, it is important to seek veterinary care immediately.

Ingestion of an entire toad warrants inducing emesis under the direct supervision of a veterinarian (Eubig 2001). For those pets with more serious signs, it might be necessary to remove the toad endoscopically or surgically after stabilizing the patient (Eubig 2001). Another option is to administer multiple doses of charcoal with a cathartic (Eubig 2001). Activated charcoal has not specifically been assessed for its effectiveness in adsorbing *Bufo* toxins but it is nonetheless indicated in situations involving serious signs or observed ingestion of a toad (Eubig 2001).

Pets presented in areas in which *Bufo marinus* or *Bufo alvarius* reside should be thoroughly examined, including auscultation of the heart. Continuous monitoring of an electrocardiogram is indicated if any cardiac

abnormalities are detected or if severe neurologic signs or shock develop (Eubig 2001; Roder 2004a). Electrolytes should be monitored and corrected as needed (Eubig 2001).

Patients experiencing severe toxicosis should receive intensive symptomatic support. Diazepam or a barbiturate may be administered to control seizures, tremors, and agitation (Eubig 2001). Electrolytes, especially potassium, should be monitored, and corrected as needed (Gwaltney-Brant et al. 2007; Eubig 2001). Intravenous fluids should be given to provide additional cardiovascular support (Gwaltney-Brant et al. 2007). Atropine is contraindicated for treatment of hypersalivation due its potential to contribute to arrhythmias; however, it is indicated to treat severe bradycardia (Eubig 2001; Roder 2004a). Arrhythmias (such as tachycardia, ventricular and supraventricular arrhythmias) that do not respond to fluids may be treated using propranolol or esmolol (Gwaltney-Brant et al. 2007; Eubig 2001). Body temperature should be continuously monitored in those patients with severe signs since it is common for secondary hypothermia to develop (Eubig 2001).

Digoxin-specific antigen-binding fragments (digoxin immune Fab) have proven to be valuable in the treatment of humans exposed to *Bufo* species glandular toxins (Eubig 2001). This treatment is especially beneficial for those patients experiencing severe arrhythmias, significant hyperkalemia, and marked neurologic signs (Eubig 2001; Gwaltney-Brant et al. 2007). Fab is expensive and might not be readily available, so its use might not be a feasible option in many veterinary cases (Eubig 2001; Gwaltney-Brant et al. 2007).

Prognosis

The prognosis is good when early decontamination and symptomatic treatment is effectively administered in cases involving *Bufo marinus* or *Bufo alvarius* exposure (Roder 2004a; Eubig 2001). However, death is more likely in cases involving advanced signs where treatment is delayed (Eubig 2001). Generally, exposure to *Bufo* species other than *Bufo marinus* or *Bufo alvarius* involve only mild signs that respond to oral decontamination and resolve without veterinary assistance (Eubig 2001).

ARACHNIDS—*LATRODECTUS* AND *LOXOSCELES*

Sources

There are more than 20,000 species of spider that live in the United States (Graudins 2007). Although most spiders are venomous, they are not all physically able to deliver the venom to humans or pets or the venom may not be potent enough to be of medical concern (Graudins 2007; Mullen 2002; Fowler 1993). Spiders belonging to the *Latrodectus* (widow spiders) and *Loxosceles* (recluse spiders) genera are of primary veterinary importance in the United States (Graudins 2007).

Latrodectus—Widow Spiders

Only female black widow spiders have the characteristic, well-rounded abdomen. Males have an oval-shaped abdomen that is flatter than the females. The species generally prefers outdoor living. *Latrodectus mactans* (black widow) seems to be the most common species found indoors (Mullen 2002). With its proclivity for unheated indoor areas such as barns, sheds, and garages, there is a greater potential for human and animal interaction (Mullen 2002).

Toxicity

A single bite can deliver enough venom to cause death in domestic animals (Peterson and McNalley 2006a). *Latrodectus geometricus*, with a median lethal dose (LD_{50}) of 0.43 mg/kg body weight, has the most potent venom of the five native *Latrodectus* species in the U.S. (Peterson and McNalley 2006a). Comparatively, *Latrodectus mactans* has an LD_{50} of 1.39 mg/kg of body weight (Peterson and McNalley 2006a). Cats are very sensitive to black widow spider venom (Peterson and McNalley 2006a; Gwaltney-Brant et al. 2007). Dogs are considered more resistant but often develop severe clinical signs (Peterson and McNalley 2006a). The prevalence of *Latrodectus* envenomation of domestic animals is not known (Peterson and McNalley 2006a).

Toxicokinetics and Mechanism of Action

Both males and females are venomous but only the females are physically able to envenomate an animal or human (Poppenga 2002; Peterson and McNalley 2006a). The venom is supplied from two venom glands located behind the eyes. Venom is delivered via the paired fangs at the terminal ends of the chelicera (Fowler 1993). Not all bites are associated with venom transfer to the victim; black widows are capable of controlling the amount of venom they deliver (Peterson and McNalley 2006a). Approximately 15% of the bites inflicted in humans are nonenvenomating (Peterson and McNalley 2006a). The venom of black widow spiders is made up of 5 or 6 proteinaceous toxins, most notably alpha-latrotoxin, a powerful mammalian neurotoxin (Peterson and McNalley 2006a).

Clinical Effects

Signs

Latrodectism is the syndrome associated with black widow spider envenomation (Gwaltney-Brant et al. 2007). The signs are generally central nervous system or muscular in origin due to the neurotoxic nature of the venom (Roder 2004b). The bite itself may not be felt and local reactions such as swelling and tissue changes are uncommon (Forrester and Stanley 2003; Peterson and McNalley 2006a). Clinical signs develop within 8 hours of envenomation and are generally serious (Peterson and McNalley 2006a). Dogs may display progressive muscle pain and fasciculation (Peterson 1997). A rigid abdomen without noted tenderness is a unique clinical sign associated with black widow spider bites (Peterson and McNalley 2006a). The pain associated with the condition worsens with the severity of the envenomation (Peterson and McNalley 2006a). Restlessness and other signs associated with severe pain such as contortions and writhing may develop (Peterson 1997). Excessive production of runny nasal secretions, hypersalivation, hyperesthesia, regional numbness and facial swelling may be noted (Peterson 1997). Hypertension and tachycardia commonly develop and seizures can occur (Peterson and McNalley 2006a). Muscle cramping might be evident and can result in major respiratory difficulty (Peterson and McNalley 2006a). When death occurs, it is due to respiratory or cardiovascular failure (Peterson and McNalley 2006a).

Cats might develop early and severe signs of paralysis (Peterson 1997). Howling and other loud vocalizations are common and hypersalivation, restlessness, diarrhea, and vomiting may occur (Peterson 1997). Muscle tremors, cramping, ataxia, and difficulty standing due to muscle weakness may be noted and often occur prior to paralysis. Respiratory collapse often precedes death (Peterson 1997).

Laboratory

Complete blood cell count and a serum chemistry panel is recommended. A leukocytosis is often noted A (Peterson and McNalley 2006a). Creatine kinase can be elevated, especially when severe muscle spasms are noted (Peterson 1997). Hyperglycemia, oliguria, albuminuria, and elevated specific gravity might be noted.

Differential Diagnoses

Acute abdomen, intervertebral disk disease, and bromethalin toxicosis are the primary differential diagnoses to consider (Peterson and McNalley 2006a). Additionally, in cats, rabies should be considered.

Diagnostics

There are no specific tests to confirm black widow spider bite.

Antemortem

A rigid abdomen without tenderness and accompanied by markedly severe pain in cases of severe envenomation is a unique clinical sign associated with black widow spider bites (Peterson and McNalley 2006a). Cats might vomit the spider (Peterson 1997).

Postmortem

No postmortem diagnostics are characteristic for latrodectism.

Management of Exposures

Treatment is focused on alleviation of clinical signs (Gwaltney-Brant et al. 2007; Graudins 2007; Roder 2004b). Diazepam and methocarbamol are recommended to alleviate muscular effects as well as seizures. Opioids are best utilized for pain management (Gwaltney-Brant et al. 2007).

There is a specific antivenin of equine origin (Lyovac®, available from Merck and Co.) that can be administered. It is generally reserved for use in high-risk patients (neonatal or geriatric or those with underlying health conditions) or in those that are not responding to symptomatic treatment (Gwaltney-Brant et al. 2007). If needed, it might be available from a hospital pharmacy or a regional poison control center (Roder 2004b). Although the risk is generally low, anaphylaxis can develop upon administration of antivenin (Peterson and McNalley 2006a). It is best to give it slowly, and administration of diphenhydramine might provide a calming effect and potentially prevent an allergic reaction (Peterson and McNalley 2006a).

Prognosis

The prognosis is difficult to determine because patients may not fully recover until weeks after envenomation (Peterson and McNalley 2006a). Due to their increased sensitivity to black widow spider bites, cats generally will have a guarded prognosis even with administration of antivenin (Peterson and Roberts 2006). The average survival time reported for 20 of 22 felines that died subsequent to envenomation was 115 hours (Gwaltney-Brant et al. 2007; Peterson and McNalley 2006a).

Loxosceles—Brown Recluse Spiders

The *Loxosceles* genus includes an estimated 70 species, 14 of which reside in the United States (Mullen 2002). *Loxosceles* spiders are also known as violin or fiddle-back spiders. The most distinguishing feature of this genus is the violin shape located on the dorsal cephalothorax. They are more likely to be found indoors than black widow spiders. They are reclusive and prefer dark, warm, dry, undisturbed areas (Mullen 2002). The most notorious and medically important is *Loxosceles reclusa* (Gwaltney-Brant et al. 2007; Mullen 2002).

Brown recluse spiders do not inhabit the Pacific Northwest. However, *Tegenaria agrestis*, the hobo spider or aggressive house spider, resides in that area and its bite can result in similar skin lesions as those seen following brown recluse envenomation (Peterson and McNalley 2006b).

Toxicity

Male *Loxosceles* spiders have a smaller venom capacity than do females (Peterson and McNalley 2006b). Lethal envenomation can occur as the result of a single bite (Peterson and McNalley 2006b). An estimated 40 mcg of venom-proteins are delivered per bite (Roder 2004b). Less than 5 mcg of venom may potentially result in clinical lesions (Poppenga 2002). The bigger and more mature a spider is, the larger the venom volume (Peterson and McNalley 2006b).

Toxicokinetics and Mechanism of Action

Brown recluse venom contains a number of necrotizing enzymes, most notably, sphingomyelinase D (Gwaltney-Brant et al. 2007; Graudins 2007). Other enzymes include hyaluronidase, which acts as a spreading factor for the venom, lipase, proteases, esterases, and alkaline phosphatases (Gwaltney-Brant et al. 2007; Roder 2004b). Sphingomyelinase D binds to cell membranes and causes damage to small blood vessels and aggregation of platelets (Roder 2004b). Serum hemolytic complement is inactivated, which results in intravascular coagulation, small capillary occlusion, and tissue necrosis (Gwaltney-Brant et al. 2007; Peterson and McNalley 2006b; Beasley 1999). Activated partial thromboplastin time (PTT) is prolonged, and clotting factors VIII, IX, XI, and XII are exhausted (Gwaltney-Brant et al. 2007; Peterson and McNalley 2006b). In the presence of serum C-reactive protein and calcium, sphingomyelinase causes hemolysis (Gwaltney-Brant et al. 2007; Peterson and McNalley 2006b). Free lipids in the blood, caused by the lipases, serve as inflammatory intermediaries and cause embolization (Peterson and McNalley 2006b; Gwaltney-Brant et al. 2007).

Clinical Effects

Signs

Loxoscelism is the syndrome associated with brown recluse spider envenomation (Mullen 2002). There are two general manifestations of loxoscelism: tissue necrosis (most common) or systemic effects (which are rare but can be life-threatening) (Peterson and McNalley 2006b). Dogs are especially sensitive to brown recluse bites. The severity of a bite is dependent on the amount of venom injected, the size of the bite, and the immune status of the victim (Peterson and McNalley 2006b).

The bite might not be felt or a mild stinging sensation might be evident for up to 8 hours (Peterson and McNalley 2006b). Blood vessels constrict, resulting in diminished supply of blood to the bite area, and pruritus and soreness may develop. Swelling of the bite area and a characteristic bull's-eye lesion, with a dark necrotic center, develops (Peterson and McNalley 2006b). Gravity can displace venom further and result in irregular expansion of the lesion (Peterson and McNalley 2006b). A scab forms that sloughs in 2 to 5 weeks and results in a slow-healing ulcer (Peterson and McNalley 2006b). Generally, ulcers will not extend into muscle but if they extend into fatty tissue, they can become extensive and take months to heal while potentially leaving a deep scar (Peterson and McNalley 2006b).

Loxoscelism with systemic signs is generally uncommon. Systemic signs, when they occur, typically develop 24–72 hours postenvenomation and can be serious (Gwaltney-Brant et al. 2007; Peterson and McNalley 2006b). The most predominant systemic sign is hemolytic anemia with prominent hemoglobinuria (Peterson and McNalley 2006b). Other potential but infrequent systemic signs include tachycardia, fever, muscle pain, vomiting, difficulty breathing, disseminated intravascular coagulation, and coma (Gwaltney-Brant et al. 2007).

Laboratory

Assessment of a complete blood cell count (CBC) and a serum chemistry panel with electrolytes is recommended (Peterson and McNalley 2006b). The CBC may indicate leukocytosis, anemia, and thrombocytopenia (Peterson 1997). Urinalysis may reveal hemoglobinuria (Peterson 1997). A Coombs-negative hemolytic anemia may be noted (Roder 2004b). A coagulation profile to monitor prothrombin time, partial thromboplastin time, platelet count, and fibrinogen is recommended (Peterson and McNalley 2006b).

Differential Diagnoses

Differential diagnoses include pyoderma (such as *Staphylococcus* spp.) or mycobacterial infection, decubital ulcer, and third-degree burn; all are potentially present with a necrotizing wound (Peterson and McNalley 2006b; Peterson 1997). Causes of hemolytic anemia, such as immune-mediated conditions, zinc poisoning, and onion poisoning, should be considered (Peterson and McNalley 2006b). Other rule-outs for the systemic manifestations are snakebite, insect sting, erlichiosis, jaundice, unexplained fever, and red blood cell parasitism (Peterson 1997; Peterson and McNalley 2006b).

Diagnostics

There are no specific tests available in the United States to confirm brown recluse spider bite (Peterson and McNalley 2006b).

Antemortem

There is a characteristic bull's-eye lesion, with a dark necrotic center, that develops in association with brown recluse spider envenomation (Peterson and McNalley 2006b).

Postmortem

No postmortem findings are characteristic for loxoscelism.

Management of Exposures

Treatment is primarily symptomatic and supportive because there is no specific antidote for loxoscelism (Poppenga 2002). Necrotic wound care involves measuring and monitoring the size of the wound, debridement with aluminum acetate or hydrogen peroxide, and bandaging (Gwaltney-Brant et al. 2007). Dapsone, a leukocyte inhibitor, might reduce the severity of dermal lesions and also has antibacterial properties, although its efficacy is questionable (Gwaltney-Brant et al. 2007; Peterson and McNalley 2006b; Hahn and Lewin 2006). If pain is evident, nonsteroidal anti-inflammatory medications or opioids may be given (Gwaltney-Brant et al. 2007). If dapsone is not being administered and infection is suspected, broad-spectrum antibiotics should be given (Gwaltney-Brant et al. 2007; Peterson and McNalley 2006b). Pruritis may be treated with diphenhydramine (Gwaltney-Brant et al. 2007).

Prognosis

The prognosis for patients with advanced systemic signs is guarded (Peterson and McNalley 2006b). Patients with dermonecrotic lesions generally recover but typically endure an extended healing process of weeks to months.

ARACHNIDS—SCORPIONS

Sources

Of the approximately 45 species of scorpions worldwide that are considered health risks, only *Centruroides sculpturatus*, or the Arizona bark scorpion, is of great concern to people and pets in the United States (Thomas et al. 2007; Mullen 2002). Although *Centruroides sculpturatus* is considered the most dangerous scorpion in the United States, it is mostly a threat to young children (Mullen 2002).

Toxicity

Scorpion envenomation typically presents as one of two conditions (Bryson 1996). With the less toxic scorpions, signs beyond those associated with a local reaction are uncommon. The risk of anaphylaxis does exist, but does not often occur (Goddard 2003). With the more dangerous scorpions such as *Centruroides sculpturatus*, local effects are not typically noted. More severe, systemic signs associated with the neurotoxins in the venom are more prevalent. The venom composition varies among species as well as by the age and health of the scorpion and the time of year (Thomas et al. 2007). The size of a scorpion does not correlate with its toxicity; therefore, larger scorpion species are not automatically more toxic than smaller ones (Thomas et al. 2007; Mullen 2002).

Toxicokinetics and Mechanism of Action

Scorpions generally sting once but are capable of stinging multiple times (Mullen 2002). Proteins are common constituents of all scorpion venoms and include phospholipase A2 (Fowler 1993). Other enzymes like hyaluronidase and acetylcholinesterase are present in some species but not in others. Serotonin may also be present and is typically associated with the pain felt after envenomation (Mullen 2002). The *Hemiscorpius* genus is equipped with a cytotoxic venom that can cause serious tissue injury upon evenomation (Mullen 2002).

All scorpions are equipped with chelicerae and pedipalps with pincers that are utilized to capture their prey (Thomas et al. 2007; Fowler 1993). Scorpions with more slender pedipalps are generally more toxic than those with thicker pedipalps. The stinger is supplied with venom from the telson, both of which are located in the terminal end of the tail.

Clinical Effects

Signs

The occurrence of localized reactions is dependent on the scorpion species. If they occur, localized reactions include immediate pain at the injection site and edema that may or may not be associated with discoloration (Goddard 2003). Envenomation by *C. sculpturatus* is typically not associated with localized reactions. However, a tap test, which involves lightly tapping on the envenomation site, can cause increased pain in human victims of *Centruroides sculpturatus* stings (Mullen 2002).

Additional signs include enlargement of regional lymph nodes, pruritis, atypical skin sensation such as numbness and tingling, fever, nausea, and vomiting. A systemic anaphylactic reaction can occur but is rare (Goddard 1993). Systemic signs associated with neurotoxic venoms include difficulty swallowing, salivation, nystagmus, sweating, difficulty breathing, hypertension, cranial nerve dysfunction, tremors, myocardial failure, and pulmonary edema (Fowler 1993). Ferrets and cats can develop seizures.

Laboratory

Hyperkalemia and hyponatremia might be noted (Fowler 1993).

Differential Diagnoses

Rule-outs for painful local reactions include other insect stings (Fowler 1993; Mullen 2002; Heard 2000). When neurologic signs are present, rule-outs should include acute dystonic reaction, central nervous system (CNS) stimulants, cholinergic agents, strychnine toxicosis, head trauma, CNS infections, botulism, and tetanus (Mullen 2002).

Diagnostics

There are no specific antemortem or postmortem tests available in the United States to confirm scorpion envenomation. The only test that is useful for the diagnosis of *Centruroides sculpturatus* envenomation in humans is the tap test (Trestrail 1981).

Management of Exposures

Treatment of the majority of scorpion stings in the United States involves local wound management and administration of analgesics for pain (Gwaltney-Brant et al. 2007). Narcotic analgesics are contraindicated due to their apparent enhancement of scorpion venom effects (Trestrail 1981). Treatment of systemic signs is symptomatic and supportive. Special attention should be given to cardiovascular monitoring and management of hypertension and neurologic signs (Gwaltney-Brant et al. 2007).

Prognosis

The prognosis is generally good for most pets envenomated by scorpions. Pet fatalities are not common and signs typically improve within 24 hours of the envenomation (Fowler 1993).

SNAKES—*ELAPIDS*

Sources

Coral snakes belong to the family Elapidae. There are two genera of coral snake indigenous to the United States: *Micruroides* and *Micrurus* (Peterson 2006a). Coral snakes of the *Micrurus* genus are more clinically significant (Peterson 2006a).

All species of coral snakes in the United States have a similar color pattern that starts with a black snout and consists of small yellow (may be vibrant yellow or pale, almost white) bands, and larger red and black bands (Peterson 2006a). Sayings such as "red on yellow, kill a fellow" or "if caution (yellow) touches danger (red)" can prove to be helpful in the identification of poisonous coral snakes in the United States versus nonpoisonous snakes that have the same colors but in a different pattern (Peterson 2006a). The saying "red touches black, friend of Jack" can be helpful in identification of the similarly colored, nonpoisonous snakes in the United States.

Coral snakes have round (generally black) eyes, small, nontriangular heads, and small mouths (Peterson 2006a). They have short, fixed fangs that are not as efficient and streamlined for venom delivery as pit viper fangs. Coral snakes often employ a chewing action to deliver their venom (Peterson 2006a). Victims of coral snake bites may have to shake or pull the snake off, or it may still be attached upon presentation.

Toxicity

The toxicity of a coral snake bite is dependent on the size of the coral snake involved, the volume of venom injected, and the size of the victim (Peterson 2006a). Larger snakes are capable of delivering larger volumes of venom. Up to 20 mg of venom may be delivered from a large coral snake; 4 to 5 mg of venom may be lethal to a human (Peterson 2006a). Coral snakes deliver non-envenomating bites about 60% of the time. Human fatality percentages from coral snake bites are believed to be about 10% (Peterson 2006a).

Toxicokinetics and Mechanism of Action

Coral snake venom is primarily neurotoxic. The venom consists of polypeptides and enzymes including hyaluronidase, proteinase, ribonuclease, desoxyribonuclease, phosphodiesterase, phospholipase A, and cholinesterase (Peterson 2006a; Gwaltney-Brant et al. 2007; Poppenga 2002). The peptides in coral snake venom have similar effects in humans and dogs as does curare in that they create a nondepolarizing, postsynaptic neuromuscular block (Peterson 2006a; Gwaltney-Brant et al. 2007; Chrisman et al. 1996). Phospholipase A is believed to play a role in the hemolysis and hemoglobinurea that are often noted in dogs following coral snake envenomation (Peterson 2006a). Paralysis, central nervous system depression, and vasomotor effects are also common.

Clinical Effects

Signs

Clinical signs are not the same for all species. Signs associated with coral snake bites in dogs include acute depression, vomiting, hypersalivation, quadriplegia involving diminished spinal reflexes in all the limbs, and respiratory paralysis (Peterson 2006a; Chrisman 1996). Anemia, intravascular hemolysis, hemoglobinuria, morphologic red blood cell effects, hypotension, and ventricular tachycardia with or without pulse deficits may also be noted (Peterson 2006a; Chrisman 1996). Other signs noted in dogs include difficulty breathing, difficulty swallowing, and muscle fasciculations (Gwaltney-Brant et al. 2007).

Signs associated with coral snake envenomation in cats include acute, ascending, flaccid quadriplegia, depression, reduced spinal reflexes, and inhibited recognition of painful stimuli (Gwaltney-Brant et al. 2007; Peterson 2006a). Other signs include unequal pupil size, hypothermia, hypotension, respiratory depression, and lack of cutaneous trunci reflex (Peterson 2006a; Chrisman 1996). Unlike with dogs, no clinical evidence of hematuria or hemoglobinuria has been observed in cats (Peterson 2006a; Chrisman 1996).

Laboratory

It is recommended that baseline data be obtained from a CBC, serum electrolytes, and serum chemistries (Peterson and Roberts 2006). Abnormalities that might be noted include hyperfibrinogenemia, moderate leukocytosis, and early and high increases in creatine kinase (Peterson 2006a). The only laboratory findings considered highly suggestive of coral snake envenomation are an early increase in creatine kinase and burring and spherocytosis of canine red blood cells (Peterson and Roberts 2006).

Differential Diagnoses

Rule-outs for coral snake bite include tick-associated paralysis, macadamia nut exposure in dogs, botulism, bromethalin toxicosis, ionophore toxicosis, acute polyneuritis, myasthenia gravis, polyradiculoneuritis, organophosphate toxicosis, and various drugs that might be associated with neurologic signs (Peterson 2006a; Chrisman 1996).

Diagnostics

There are no specific antemortem or postmortem tests to confirm coral snake envenomation (Peterson 2006a).

Management of Exposures

Although development of signs can be delayed 10–18 hours after envenomation, it is important to seek medical treatment as soon as possible once signs develop. Antivenin is suggested in animals showing evidence of puncturing fang marks or in which an exposure to coral snakes other than the Sonoran coral snake (for which the antivenin is ineffective) have been witnessed (Peterson 2006a). Unfortunately, production of antivenin has been discontinued so it may not be available (Peterson 2006a).

Hospitalization for at least 48 hours, with special attention given to preventing aspiration pneumonia and respiratory collapse is of utmost importance (Peterson 2006a). It is prudent to take radiographs to monitor development of aspiration pneumonia (Peterson 2006a). Endotracheal intubation is recommended at the onset of respiratory difficulty to prevent aspiration. Maintenance intravenous fluid administration is recommended.

In the absence of antivenin (or in cases involving Sonoran coral snakes, since no antivenin is available), treatment is generally symptomatic and supportive and may require respiratory support (Peterson 2006a). Assisted mechanical ventilation may be necessary for up to 48 to 72 hours. Broad-spectrum antibiotics are recommended because pathogenic bacteria are prevalent in the mouths of snakes.

Antivenin administration is the only definitive treatment for coral snake envenomation (Peterson 2006a). Antivenin is most effective when administered as soon as possible following envenomation. The amount required to treat a patient is generally higher in smaller pets since the dose of venom per kilogram of body weight is higher. It is recommended that 1 to 2 vials be administered initially

and additional doses be given as required based on progression of signs. Since coral snake antivenin contains equine proteins, an allergic reaction is possible, albeit rare (Peterson 2006a). Anaphylaxis, an anaphylactoid reaction or delayed serum sickness may occur in response to an allergic reaction. Anaphylaxis is generally treated by cessation of antivenin administration and administration of epinephrine, corticosteroids, and crystalloid fluid infusion. More commonly experienced anaphylactoid reactions are best treated by ceasing antivenin administration and giving intravenous or subcutaneous diphenhydramine, waiting five minutes, and restarting antivenin infusion at a slower rate (Peterson 2006a). Delayed serum sickness usually develops 7 to 14 days postantivenin treatment and is best treated with antihistamines and/or corticosteroids. There is no known predilection of development of an allergic reaction in patients with a history of having received antivenin therapy in the past (Peterson 2006a).

Prognosis

Overall, the prognosis is guarded. It is dependent on variables such as where the bite occurred, the severity of envenomation, and the time at which treatment is initiated (Peterson 2006a). Some pets have recovered without administration of antivenin. Smaller pets are at greater risk due to their smaller body weight and therefore higher dosage of venom.

SNAKES—PIT VIPERS

Sources

The family Viperidae includes three genera of snakes that are collectively referred to as pit vipers. These include rattlesnakes, water moccasins, cottonmouths, and copperheads. All three genera are indigenous to the United States and include *Crotalus*, *Sistrurus*, and *Agkistrodon* (Peterson 2006b). The only states in the United States that are not home to a venomous snake of some kind are Maine, Alaska, and Hawaii (Peterson and Roberts 2006).

All pit vipers are similar in appearance. They have heat-sensing pits located between their vertical pupil and nostril, triangular-shaped heads, retractable fangs, and a single row of subcaudal scales distal to the anal plate (Peterson 2004). Rattlesnakes in the United States all have hollow, dried skin segments at the end of their tails that rattle when the snakes vibrate their tails (Peterson 2004). Rattlesnakes are most responsible for deaths in humans and animals (Peterson 2006b). Pit vipers are believed to be involved in 99% of snakebites delivered to animals in North America (Peterson 2004).

Toxicity

There is significant variation of venom toxicity both between and within various species of pit vipers (Peterson 2006b). Some rattlesnake venoms can be toxic at less than 2 mg/kg body weight, whereas copperhead venom toxicity requires a dose of greater than 10 mg/kg (Poppenga 2002). The three main types of pit vipers arranged in order of greatest toxicity to least are rattlesnakes, water moccasins, and copperheads (Peterson 2006b). The Eastern diamondback rattlesnake is the most dangerous snake in the United States based on its size, strength, and long fang length, which all contribute to its high venom volume delivery (Meerdink 1983).

Venom composition varies considerably among rattlesnakes. The venom from 9 species and 12 subspecies contains proteins that are similar to those found in mojave toxin, which is a powerful neurotoxin (Peterson 2006b). During the hottest summer months, when the daylight hours are at their maximum, snakes are more active and aggressive and contain the highest venom yields compared to other times during the year (Peterson 2006b). A nonenvenomating bite occurs about 25% of the time (Peterson 2004).

The amount of venom delivered can be controlled by pit vipers (Peterson 2006b). Bites initiated in response to pain are the most deadly because the maximum amount of venom available is delivered (Peterson 2006b). Toxicity is also dependent on the number of strikes and the depth of fang penetration per bite (Meerdink 1983). It is possible for multiple fangs to be present per side; so a bite might have two fang marks or up to six. Older snakes might have more potent venom and larger snakes typically have a larger amount of venom to deliver (Gwaltney-Brant et al. 2007).

Species vary in their sensitivity to pit viper venoms; cats are considered more resistant (Gwaltney-Brant et al. 2007). The size and health status of the victim, the site of the bite and the immediacy with which treatment is sought also impact the severity of the envenomation (Gwaltney-Brant et al. 2007). Bites to the thoracic area result in more rapid venom uptake, bites to the tongue are equivalent to intravenous envenomation, and bites to the muzzle area are capable of inducing life-threatening facial swelling and airway obstruction (Gwaltney-Brant et al. 2007).

Toxicokinetics and Mechanism of Action

Pit viper venom is delivered from venom glands via muscular contractions that force the venom through the hollow fangs and into the victim (Gwaltney-Brant et al. 2007). The venom is 90% water while the remaining portion consists of enzymatic and nonenzymatic proteins, peptides, cytotoxins, myotoxins, cardiotoxins, neurotoxins, coagulants and anticoagulants, lipids, nucleosides and nucleotides, organic acids, and cations (Peterson 2004, 2006b; Gwaltney-Brant et al. 2007). Venom makeup varies among species but generally consists of at least 10 of the previously named components (Gwaltney-Brant et al. 2007). Rattlesnake envenomation typically results in one of three presentations. Diamondback rattlesnake venom is representative of the classic syndrome of significant tissue destruction, coagulopathy, and hypotension (Gwaltney-Brant et al. 2007). Mojave A rattlesnake venom contains neurotoxins and does not impact tissues or result in coagulopathy (Gwaltney-Brant et al. 2007). Other venoms contain a combination of both classic and neurotoxic venom components (Gwaltney-Brant et al. 2007).

Clinical Effects

Signs

Dogs most commonly receive bites to their front legs or head (Peterson 2004). In contrast, cats most commonly are presented with bites to their torso (Gwaltney-Brant et al. 2007). Cats often present later for treatment due to their tendency to run and hide following injury (Gwaltney-Brant et al. 2007). Signs will vary because they are dependent on dose of venom, bite location, age, health status and species of victim, and the physical activity of the victim following envenomation (Poppenga 2002). Commonly, signs will include severe pain in the area of the bite, fang marks, swelling, possibly profuse bleeding in the bite area, salivation, abnormally deep or rapid breathing, tachycardia, and mydriasis (Poppenga 2002). Secondary infection can develop. Additional signs that might be noted include petechiae, ecchymoses, cyanosis, discolored skin and possibly sloughing tissue, hypotension, shock, vomiting, diarrhea, lethargy, nausea, muscle fasciculations, reduced alertness, and enlarged lymph nodes (Paul 2007; Peterson 2004). Serious signs can be delayed over a few hours postenvenomation (Peterson 2004). Local tissue response cannot be the sole predictor of severity of envenomation; severe systemic signs can develop with only mild tissue effects, and neurotoxic venom typically has little tissue effect (Peterson 2004). More severe, systemic developments include hemolysis, rhabdomyolysis, thrombocytopenia, and coagulopathy (Gwaltney-Brant et al. 2007).

Laboratory

Baseline data including a CBC with differential and platelet count, serum chemistries, urinalysis, and coagulation

Table 22.1. Snakebite severity score

Pulmonary System

0	Signs within normal limits
1	Minimal: slight dyspnea
2	Moderate: respiratory compromise, tachypnea, use of accessory muscles
3	Severe: cyanosis, air hunger, extreme tachypnea, respiratory insufficiency or respiratory arrest from any cause

Cardiovascular System

0	Signs within normal limits
1	Minimal: tachycardia, general weakness, benign dysrhythmia, hypertension
2	Moderate: tachycardia, hypotension (but tarsal pulse still palpable)
3	Severe: extreme tachycardia, hypotension (nonpalpable tarsal pulse or systolic blood pressure <80 mmHg), malignant dysrhythmia or cardiac arrest

Local Wound

0	Signs within normal limits
1	Minimal: pain, swelling, ecchymosis, erythema limited to bite site
2	Moderate: pain, swelling, erythema involves less than half of extremity and may be spreading slowly
3	Severe: pain, swelling, ecchymosis, erythema involves most or all of one extremity and is spreading rapidly
4	Very severe: pain, swelling, ecchymosis, erythema extends beyond affected extremity, or significant tissue slough

Gastrointestinal System

0	Signs within normal limits
1	Minimal: abdominal pain, tenesmus
2	Moderate: vomiting, diarrhea
3	Severe: repetitive vomiting, diarrhea, or hematemesis

Hematologic System

0	Signs within normal limits
1	Minimal: coagulation parameters slightly abnormal, PT < 20 sec, PTT < 50 sec, platelets 100,000–150,000/mm^3
2	Moderate: coagulation parameters abnormal, PT 20–50 sec, PTT 50–75 sec, platelets 50,000–100,000/mm^3
3	Severe: coagulation parameters abnormal, PT 50–100 sec, PTT 75–100 sec, platelets 20,000–50,000/mm^3
4	Very severe: coagulation parameters markedly abnormal with bleeding present or the threat of spontaneous bleeding, including PT unmeasurable, PTT unmeasurable, platelets <20,000/mm^3

Central Nervous System

0	Signs within normal limits
1	Minimal: apprehension
2	Moderate: chills, weakness, faintness, ataxia
3	Severe: lethargy, seizures, coma

Total Possible Score	0–20

profiles should be obtained (Peterson 2006b). Red blood cell morphology should be examined; transient echinocytosis may be evident within 48 hours in dogs and is indicative of pit viper envenomation (Peterson 2006b). Urinalysis should include free protein, hemoglobin, and myoglobin evaluation (Peterson 2006b). Coagulation profile tests should include activated clotting times (ACT), prothrombin time (PT), activated partial thromboplastin time (PTT), fibrinogen, and fibrin degradation products. Animals with severe envenomations might require electrocardiogram monitoring (Peterson 2006b). These tests should be repeated on a periodic basis to follow progression of envenomation and provide feedback regarding treatment success (Peterson and Roberts 2006).

Complete blood counts often show hemoconcentration, leukocytosis, or thrombocytopenia (Paul 2007). Increased creatine phosphokinase and myoglobinuria might be noted as a result of rhabdomyolysis from rattlesnakes equipped with neurotoxins (Peterson 2006b). Hematuria can be noted as well (Paul 2007). Transient hypokalemia that responds to intravenous fluid and antivenin treatment may be evident following pit viper snake envenomation (Peterson 2006b). Coagulation profiles often reveal increased ACT, PT, and PTT as well as increased fibrinogen degradation products (Paul 2007).

Differential Diagnoses

Rule-outs for pit viper snake bite include trauma, insect bites or stings, animal bites, draining abscess, and penetrating wound (Peterson 2006b; Paul 2007).

Diagnostics

There are no specific antemortem or postmortem tests to confirm pit viper snake envenomation (Peterson 2006b).

Management of Exposures

Development of significant signs, other than the immediate pain felt at the time of bite, can be delayed. It is imperative that treatment be sought as soon as possible because major irreversible complications can develop if too much time has elapsed (Peterson 2006b). It is important to keep the animal calm after being bitten because physical activity and anxiousness could promote more rapid uptake of the venom. Additionally, if possible, the bite site should be kept below heart level and the animal should be transported to a veterinary medical facility as soon as possible so that treatment, including antivenin therapy, can be initiated (Peterson 2006b). Pit viper bite victims should be hospitalized for a minimum of 8 hours

so that they can be closely monitored. A severity score sheet should be initiated upon presentation and periodically updated (Peterson 2006b) (Table 22.1). The severity score is a more objective method for assessing the patient's condition at any given point in time or assessing trends over time. In addition, it is important to take circumferential measurements at, above, and below the bite area so development of swelling can be methodically tracked (Peterson 2006b).

Administration of a crystalloid fluid drip via intravenous catheter should be initiated. Corticosteroids are contraindicated. Broad-spectrum antibiotic therapy is recommended in veterinary patients due to the plethora of pathogenic bacteria that may be introduced during the bite (Peterson 2006b).

Antivenin therapy is the only proven therapy for pit viper envenomation. Crotalidae polyvalent immune Fab Ovine is the antivenin of choice because it is FDA approved (Peterson 2006b). This antivenin is less likely to produce an allergic response, it efficiently and effectively penetrates tissues, and it has a high affinity for venom antigens (Peterson 2006b). Repeated administration may be required.

Prognosis

Although pit viper envenomation varies in severity, most dogs and cats treated promptly and aggressively, generally recover (Peterson 2006b; Paul 2007). Administration of antivenin increases the likelihood of recovery but does not ensure recovery; some pets have died despite antivenin treatment (Paul 2007). Smaller pets are at greater risk. The prognosis is poor in animals receiving high-volume envenomation or in those that experience shock, severe cardiac arrhythmias, hematologic effects, and infection (Paul 2007).

REFERENCES

Akre, R.D. and Reed, H.C. 2002. Ants, wasps, and bees (Hymenoptera). In *Medical and Veterinary Entomology*. edited by G. Mullen and L. Durden, pp. 383–409. New York: Academic Press.

Beasley, V.R. 1999. *A Systems Affected Approach to Veterinary Toxicology*. Urbana: University of Illinois College of Veterinary Medicine.

Bryson, P.D. 1996. Scorpions. In *Comprehensive Review in Toxicology for Emergency Clinicians*, *3rd ed.*, pp. 736–738. Washington, D.C.: Taylor and Francis.

Chrisman, C.L., Hopkins, A.L., Ford, S.L. et al. 1996. Acute flaccid quadriplegia in three cats with suspected coral snake envenomation. *J Am Anim Hosp Assoc* 32: 343–349.

Conceicao, L.G., Haddad Jr., V., and Loures, F.H. 2006. Pustular dermatosis caused by fire ant (*Solenopsis invicta*) stings in a dog. *Eur Soc Vet Dermatol* 17:453–455.

Cowell, A.K. and Cowell, R.L. 1995. Management of bee and other hymenoptera stings. In *Kirk's Current Veterinary Therapy XII: Small Animal Practice*, edited by J.D. Bonagura, pp. 226–228. Philadelphia: W.B. Saunders.

Cowell, A.K., Cowell, R.L., Tyler, R.D. et al. 1991. Severe systemic reactions to hymenoptera stings in three dogs. *J Am Vet Med Assoc* 198(6):1014–1016.

Diaz, J.H. 2007. Hymenopterid bites, stings, allergic reactions and the impact of hurricanes on Hymenopterid-inflicted injuries. *J La State Med Soc* 159:149–157.

Drees, B.M., Jensen, J.M., Joyce, J.R. et al. 2002. *Diagnosing and treating animals for red imported fire ant injury*. Available at: http://fireant.tamu.edu/materials/factsheets_pubs/pdf/FAPFS022.2002rev.pdf

Elgart, G.W. 1990. Ant, bee and wasp stings. *Dermatol Clin* 229–236.

Eubig, P.A. 2001. *Bufo* species toxicosis: Big toad, big problem. *Vet Med* 96(1):595–599.

Fitzgerald, K.T. and Flood, A.A. 2006. Hymenoptera stings. *Clin Tech Small Anim Pract* 21:194–204.

Fitzgerald, K.T. and Vera, R. 2006. Insects—Hymenoptera. In *Small Animal Toxicology*, 2nd ed., edited by M.E. Peterson and P.A. Talcott, pp. 744–767. St. Louis: Elsevier Saunders.

Forrester, M.B. and Stanley, S.K. 2003. Black widow spider and brown recluse spider bites in Texas from 1998 through 2002. *Vet Hum Toxicol* 45(5):270–273.

Fowler, M.E. 1993. *Veterinary Zootoxicology*, pp. 41–46; 69–80; 81–86. Boca Raton: CRC Press, Inc.

Goddard, J. 2003. Scorpions. In *Physician's Guide to Arthropods of Medical Importance*, 4th ed., pp. 301–308. Washington, D.C.: CRC Press, Inc.

Graudins, A. 2007. Venomous arthropods. In *Haddad and Winchester's Clinical Management of Poisoning and Drug Overdose*, 4th ed., edited by M.W. Shannon et al., pp. 433–439. St. Louis: Elsevier Saunders.

Gwaltney-Brant, S., Dunayer, E.K., and Youssef, H.J. 2007. Terrestrial zootoxins. In *Veterinary Toxicology Basic and Clinical Principles*, edited by R.C. Gupta. pp. 794–807. New York: Academic Press.

Hahn, I., Lewin, N.A. 2006. Arthropods. In *Goldfrank's Toxicologic Emergencies*, edited by N.E. Flomenbaum et al., pp. 1603–1622. New York: McGraw-Hill.

Heard, K. 2000. Scorpion envenomation. In *5-Minute Toxicology Consult*, edited by R.C. Dart, pp. 624–625. Philadelphia: Lippincott Williams and Wilkins.

Meerdink, G.L. 1983. Bites and stings of venomous animals. In *Kirk's Current Veterinary Therapy VIII Small Animal Practice*, edited by J.D. Bonagura, pp. 160–162. Philadelphia: W.B. Saunders.

Merck Online Medical Library for Healthcare Professionals accessed September 23, 2008, at http://www.merck.com/mmpe/print/sec21/ch325/ch325c.html.

Morgan, R.V. 1997. Toad poisoning. In *Handbook of Small Animal Practice*, 3rd ed., p. 1288. Philadelphia: W.B. Saunders.

Mullen, G.R. 2002. Spiders. In *Medical and Veterinary Entomology*, edited by G.R. Mullen and L. Durden, pp. 427–444. Philadelphia: Academic Press.

Noble, S.J. and Armstrong, P.J. 1999. Bee sting envenomation resulting in secondary immune-mediated hemolytic anemia in two dogs. *J Am Vet Med Assoc* 214(7):1026–1027.

Oliveira, E.C., Pedroso, P.M.O., Meirelles, A.E.W.B. et al. 2007. Pathological findings in dogs after multiple Africanized bee stings. *Toxicon* 49:1214–1218.

Palumbo, N.E. 1983. Toad poisoning. In *Kirk's Current Veterinary Therapy VIII Small Animal Practice*, edited by J.D. Bonagura, pp. 160–162. Tokyo: W.B. Saunders.

Paul, A. 2007. Snakebite. In *Clinical Veterinary Advisor Dogs and Cats*, edited by E. Cote and E. Rozanski, pp. 1012–1014. St Louis: Mosby Elsevier.

Peterson, M.E. 1997. Spider venom toxicosis—Brown recluse family. In *5-Minute Veterinary Consult*, edited by L.P. Tilley and F.W.K Smith Jr., p. 1207. Philadelphia: Williams and Wilkins.

———. 2000. Toad venom toxicosis. In *5-Minute Veterinary Consult Canine and Feline*, 2nd ed., edited by L.P. Tilley and F.W.K. Smith Jr., pp. 1252–1253. Philadelphia: Lippincott Williams and Wilkins.

———. 2004. Reptiles: Pit vipers. In *Clinical Veterinary Toxicology*, edited by K.H. Plumlee, pp. 106–111. St Louis: Mosby.

———. 2006a. Snake bite: Coral snakes. In *Small Animal Toxicology*, 2nd ed., edited by M.E. Peterson and P.A. Talcott, pp. 1039–1047, St Louis: Elsevier Saunders.

———. 2006b. Snake bite: North American pit vipers. In *Small Animal Toxicology*, 2nd ed., edited by M.E. Peterson and P.A. Talcott, pp. 1017–1038. St. Louis: Elsevier Saunders.

Peterson, M.E. and McNalley, J. 2006a. Spider evenomation: Black recluse. In *Small Animal Toxicology*, 2nd ed., edited by M.E. Peterson and P.A. Talcott, pp. 1063–1069. St. Louis: Elsevier Saunders.

———. 2006b. Spider evenomation: Brown recluse. In *Small Animal Toxicology*, 2nd ed., edited by M.E. Peterson and P.A. Talcott, pp. 1070–1075. St. Louis: Elsevier Saunders.

Peterson, M.E. and Roberts, B.K. 2006. Toads. In *Small Animal Toxicology*, 2nd ed., edited by M.E. Peterson and P.A. Talcott, pp. 1083–1093. St. Louis: Elsevier Saunders.

Poppenga, R.H. 2002. Zootoxins, Western Veterinary Conference, February, Las Vegas, Nevada.

Rakich, P.M., Latimer, K.S., Mispagel, M.E. et al. 1993. Clinical and histologic characterization of cutaneous reactions to stings of the imported fire ant (*Solenopsis invicta*) in dogs. *Vet Path* 30:555–559.

Reeves, M.P. 2004. A retrospective report of 90 dogs with suspected cane toad (*Bufo marinus*) toxicity. *Aust Vet J* 82(10):608–611.

Roberts, B.K. et al. 2000. *Bufo marinus* intoxication in dogs: 94 cases (1997–1998). *J Am Vet Med Assoc* 216(12): 1941–1944.

Roder, J.D. 2004a. Biotoxins: Toads. In *Clinical Veterinary Toxicology*, edited by K.J. Plumlee, pp. 113. St. Louis: Mosby.

———. 2004b. Biotoxins: Spiders. In *Clinical Veterinary Toxicology*, edited by K.J. Plumlee, pp. 111–113. St. Louis: Mosby.

Rodriguez-Lainz, A., Fritz, C.L., and McKenna, W.R. 1999. Animal and human health risks associated with Africanized honeybees. *J Am Vet Med Assoc* 215(12): 1799–1804.

Thomas, J.D., Thomas, K.E., Kazzi, Z.N. 2007. Scorpions and stinging insects. In *Haddad and Winchester's Clinical Management of Poisoning and Drug Overdose*, 4th ed., edited by M.W. Shannon et al., pp. 440–447. St. Louis: Elsevier Saunders.

Trestrail III, J.H. 1981. Scorpion envenomation in Michigan: Three cases of toxic encounters with poisonous stowaways. *Vet Hum Toxicol* 23(1):8–11.

Walker, T., Tidwell, A.S., Rozanski, E.A., DeLaforcade, A., and Hoffman, A.M. 2005. Imaging diagnosis: Acute lung injury following massive bee envenomation in a dog. *Vet Radiol Ultrasound* 46(4):300–303.

Mycotoxins and Mushrooms

23

Joyce Eisold and Michelle Mostrom

INTRODUCTION

Mushroom poisonings are common in dogs and infrequent in cats. Poisonings probably occur more frequently because ingestions may not be observed by owners and few analytical laboratories can confirm mushroom toxicosis. Therefore, many mushroom-induced toxicoses are likely attributed to other causes. According to the ASPCA Animal Poison Control Center, most of the documented cases of mushroom poisonings occur in California. Of 700 cases reported to the ASPCA between 2002 and 2007, 11% were from California (Puschner 2007).

When dealing with a possible mushroom toxicosis, it is important to verify whether the mushroom was purchased from a store for medicinal or ingestion purposes or if it was obtained from mushroom hunting. If the owner suspects mushrooms, request a description of the mushroom (size, color) and whether the dog or cat ate the cap or stem. Whenever possible, the mushroom should be positively identified as to genus and species. If the owner has access to the mushroom it should be placed in a paper bag and refrigerated. The best way to bag it is to place the mushroom with the cap down on a white sheet of paper that has the site and the conditions written on it. It is sometimes important to include known trees in the environment because certain mushrooms are associated with specific trees (Spoerke 2006).

There are many different types of mushrooms containing a variety of toxins that cause differing clinical signs. The mushrooms that will be covered in this chapter include the mushrooms affecting the gastrointestinal system; muscarine-containing mushrooms, which cause classic cholinergic signs (SLUDD); isoxazole- and psilocybin-containing mushrooms, which cause hallucinogenic signs; and amanitin- and gyromitin-containing mushrooms, which are hepatotoxic (Table 23.1). Each category of mushroom, their mechanisms of action, their associated clinical signs, and medical management of intoxications will be covered separately because they have widely varying symptoms and degrees of toxicity.

MUSHROOMS CAUSING GASTROINTESTINAL SIGNS

Sources

A large number of mushrooms cause gastrointestinal upset in animals. The species involved are members of the genera *Agaricus, Albatrellus, Armillaria, Boletus, Chlorophyllum, Entoloma, Gomphus, Hebeloma, Laccaria, Lactarius, Laetiporus, Lampteromyces, Meripilus,* and *Omphalotus.* The specific toxins for many of them have not been identified. Some possible toxins include illuden S (*Omphalotus illudents, Omphalotus olearuis,* and *Lampteromyces japonica*), monoterpenes (*Albatrellus* spp.), norcaperatic acid (*Gomphus* spp.), hebeleomic acid A (cytotoxic triterpene, *Hefeloma crustuliniforme*), cucurbitane triterpene glycosides (*Hebeloma vinosphyllum*), lectins (*Laccaria amethystine*), marasmane/lactarane sesquitrpenes (*Russula* spp. and *Lactarius* spp.), and phenolethylamines (*Lactiprus sulphureus,* and Meripilus spp.) (Spoerke 2001; Tegzes and Puschner 2002a). These mushrooms are widely distributed throughout the United States and grow in a variety of substrates and environments.

Small Animal Toxicology Essentials, First Edition. Edited by Robert H. Poppenga, Sharon Gwaltney-Brant.
© 2011 John Wiley and Sons, Inc. Published 2011 by John Wiley and Sons, Inc.

Table 23.1. Mushrooms of veterinary importance in North America

Mushroom	Toxin	Clinical Signs
Agaricus, Albatrellus, Armillaria, Boletus, Chlorophyllum, Entoloma, Gomphus, Hebeloma, Laccaria, Lactarius, Lampteromyces, Omphalotus, Rhodophyllus, Ramaria, Suillus	No specific toxin identified	**Gastrointestinal irritation** Vomiting Abdominal pain Diarrhea Lethargy Weakness Dizziness
Inocybe spp. *Clitocybe* spp. *Entoloma*	Muscarine	**S**alivation **L**acrimation **U**rination **D**iarrhea Miosis Tachycardia Hypotension Bronchoconstriction Vomiting
Amanita muscaria (fly agaric) *Aminata pantherina* (panther or warted agaric)	Isoxazole: ibotenic acid, muscimol	**Behavioral changes** (disoriented, agitated, depression) Somnolence/ coma Lethargy Vomiting Ataxia/paresis Dyspnea Hyperactivity Salivation Diarrhea Miosis Tremors/seizures 2nd-degree atrioventricular block
Psilocybe *Conocybe* *Gymnopilus, Panaeolus* *Stropharia* (hallucinogenic or magic mushrooms)	Psilocybin Psilocin	**CNS derangement** **Altered behavior** Agitation Aggression Vocalization Weakness/ataxia Tachycardia Hyperreflexia Mydriasis Seizures Hyperthermia Hypertension Drowsiness

Table 23.1. *Continued*

Mushroom	Toxin	Clinical Signs
Gyromitra spp. (false morels) *Helvella* spp. *Verpa bohemica*	Monomethylhydrazine	Vomiting Watery diarrhea Dehydration Abdominal pain Lethargy Fever Liver and renal damage Hemolysis Methemoglobinemia Hypoglycemia Seizures
Amanita spp. (*A.phalloides* or death cap) *Galerina* *Lepiota*	Cyclopeptides: amatoxins (α- , β- , γ- , ε-amanitins), phallotoxins, virotoxins	Irreversible cytotoxicity of liver and kidney Severe hypoglycemia Gastroeneteritis **Death**

Kinetics

Kinetic information on these species has not been established because the toxic principle of most GI irritant mushrooms is not known.

Mechanism of Action

A variety of mechanisms are thought to be responsible for causing clinical signs, including hypersensitivity, local irritation, and enzyme defiencies (Spoerke 2001).

Toxicity

The toxicity of these mushrooms varies. One-half of a cap from an *Agaricus* spp. caused foaming, vomiting, diarrhea, and disorientation in a 1-year-old cat (Spoerke 2001). Ingestion of one *Scleroderma citrinum* in a 7-month-old potbellied pig resulted in persistent vomiting, depression, weakness, recumbency, hypothermia, abdominal splinting, and death within 5 hours despite treatment with dexamethasone and fluids. An unknown species of *Russula* was eaten by a cat that subsequently developed hematemesis (Spoerke 2001). Precise toxicity information specific to pet animals or livestock is not available.

Clinical Signs

The most common clinical effect seen is gastrointestinal upset, including vomiting and diarrhea (possibly bloody), salivation, abdominal discomfort, and lethargy. The gastrointestinal effects can result in dehydration and rarely cause electrolyte imbalances, hypovolemia, collapse, and death. Onset of signs is within 15 minutes to several hours and the duration is a few hours to a couple of days. If the onset of gastrointestinal signs is 6–24 hours after ingestion there is a possibility that the animal ingested an amanitin-containing mushroom, which is a much more serious intoxication.

Differential Diagnoses

The differential diagnoses for the GI class of mushrooms includes bacterial or viral gastroenteritis, dietary indiscretion, pancreatitis, hepatotoxic mushroom ingestion, irritant plant ingestion, or tremorgenic mycotoxin ingestion.

Diagnostics

In a live animal the vomitus should be examined for evidence of mushrooms, and at a necropsy mushrooms may be found in the gastric contents. Fragments of mushrooms found in vomitus or gastric contents might be suitable for identification purposes. If the client can provide fresh, fairly intact samples of the suspected mushrooms, they can be sent to qualified mycologists for identification.

Management of Exposures

The medical management of a GI toxin mushroom consists of inducing emesis if vomiting has not already occurred. Emesis can be achieved by having the owners use 3% hydrogen peroxide at home with the dose based on the weight of the animal, or a veterinarian can induce emesis using conjunctival or injectable apomorphine. After calming the GI tract, activated charcoal should be administered. A complete blood count, liver/renal panels, electrolytes, and acid/base evaluation should be obtained if hepatotoxic mushroom ingestion has not been ruled out. Parenteral fluid administration to combat dehydration due to excessive vomiting may be needed along with stomach protectants and antiemetics. Symptomatic and supportive care should be provided as needed.

Prognosis

Ingestion of these mushrooms is rarely fatal, but it is essential to differentiate GI-toxic mushrooms from hepatotoxic ones.

MUSCARINIC MUSHROOMS

Sources

The agent in muscarinic mushrooms is muscarine, which is heat stable; only the L(+) isomer is active. *Inocybe* spp. and *Clitocybe* spp. species of mushrooms contain this agent and are nondescript small brown mushrooms. Very low concentrations of muscarine can be found in many other genera including *Entoloma* and *Mycena*. These mushrooms are found throughout the United States and Canada and prefer to grow in hardwood and coniferous forests, parks, lawns, and gardens. They fruit in late fall and early winter.

Kinetics

The oral absorption of muscarine is poor, but some species (e.g., rabbits) have negligible absorption of muscarine (Benjamin 1995). Muscarine is not affected by digestive enzymes. It does not cross the blood-brain barrier, so any CNS signs are attributed to secondary effects from hypoxia due to hypotension.

Mechanism of Action

Muscarine binds to muscarinic (acetylcholine) receptors in the parasympathetic nervous system, stimulating postsynaptic neurons. It is not degraded by acetylcholinesterase so the action is prolonged. The specific target organs are gland cells, cardiac nodal muscle fibers and smooth muscle. Effects are peripheral, not central (Spoerke 2006).

Toxicity

Species differ in their sensitivity to intoxication. Rabbits are relatively resistant due to poor oral absorption of mus-

carine. Cat and mouse cardiovascular systems are particularly sensitive to muscarine. In cats, as little as 0.01 mg/kg IV can cause hypotension (Benjamin 1995).

Clinical Signs

The clinical signs are typically cholinergic signs (e.g., salivation, lacrimation, urination, defecation, and dyspnea or SLUDD) without nicotinic or significant CNS effects. The most common signs seen are hypersalivation (with thick ropy saliva), vomiting, diarrhea, lacrimation, and wet bronchial sounds. There is frequently abdominal pain, urinary incontinence, and anxiety; occasionally, tachycardia, miosis, hypotension, and dyspnea; and rarely, animals exhibit respiratory and cardiac arrest. Onset of signs is usually within 5–30 minutes of ingestion and almost never beyond 2 hours (Benjamin 1995). Signs can persist for several hours if not treated, but they quickly subside when atropine is administered. There are no laboratory abnormalities expected.

Differential Diagnoses

The differential diagnoses include organophosphorus or carbamate insecticide, anatoxin-a, or slaframine intoxications.

Diagnostics

Muscarine can be detected in urine and this has been used to confirm exposure, but the best diagnostic parameter is response to treatment (i.e., administration of atropine).

Management of Exposures

Induction of emesis is advised if the animal has not already vomited and the time from ingestion to presentation is not prolonged. Emesis can be achieved by having the owners use 3% hydrogen peroxide at home with a dose based on body weight of the animal, or a veterinarian can induce emesis using conjunctival or injectable apomorphine. Gastric emptying is followed by activated charcoal without a cathartic since muscarine causes increased peristalsis and diarrhea in many patients (Spoerke 2006). Symptomatic and supportive care is always needed. Oxygen can be administered if dyspnea is noted. Intravenous fluid therapy can be administered for possible hypotension. The specific antagonist for muscarine is atropine. Atropine competitively dislodges muscarine from receptor sites without stimulating postsynaptic neurons. A preanesthetic atropine dose should be administered and, if no signs of atropinization occur, additional atropine may be given to effect. The starting dose is 0.04 mg/kg (1/4 IV with the remainder IM).

The end point is not mydriasis, but cessation of secretions (Spoerke 2006).

Prognosis

The prognosis is usually good since ingestions are rarely fatal.

HALLUCINOGENIC MUSHROOMS

Sources

Hallucinogenic mushrooms or "magic mushrooms" contain psilocybin and psilocin. Psilocin is the dephosphorylated form of psilocybin and can be the primary form present in the bloodstream. It is a methyltryptamine derivative and is heat stable and resists drying. Psilocybe spp., Panaeolus spp., Conocybe spp., Gymnophilus spp. and some Stropharia spp. also contain this type of toxin. Stems of some psilocybin-containing mushrooms will turn blue when handled.

These mushrooms are found in North America, especially in the Pacific Northwest and Gulf Coast. They thrive in manure although some prefer mulch and rotting wood. (Benjamin 1995). They will grow in lawns, gardens, parks, roadsides, and open woods. These mushrooms are used recreationally for hallucinogenic effects. Their sale and use is illegal in the United States, but the sale of the mycelia of the "magic mushrooms" is not illegal. The mushrooms have been put in capsules in a powdered form and added to soups, stews, milkshakes, and other edible products in order to mask the bitter taste (Benjamin 1995).

Kinetics

The bioavailability of pysilocybin is ~50% in rats (Benjamin 1995). It is widely distributed throughout the body and it crosses the blood-brain barrier and concentrates in the liver and adrenals. Within 4 hours of ingestion it cannot be detected in blood, but it remains in the liver and adrenals for up to 48 hours (Benjamin 1995). It does not appear to be metabolized via monoamine oxidase. Approximately 66% is excreted in urine within the first 24 hours while the remainder in the liver and adrenals is gradually eliminated over 7 days (Benjamin 1995).

Mechanism of Action

The chemical acts as a serotonin agonist. It is thought to stimulate serotonin receptors (e.g., 5-HT2A) within the CNS and PNS. The mechanism may also involve norepinepherine-mediated pathways (Beasley 1999).

Toxicity

Doses of about 4–8 mg psilocybin/2 g of dried mushrooms or 20 fresh mushrooms can produce signs. In humans the initial signs consist of relaxation and detachment and can occur at a psilocybin dose of 4 mg. In humans, 6–12 mg psilocybin results in perceptual alteration and visual distortions. Greater than 12 mg psilocybin or 1 to 4 large fresh mushrooms can cause hallucinations in humans (Benjamin 1995).

Clinical Signs

The most common clinical effects from ingestion of these mushrooms are alteration of behavior and mentation, ataxia, and vocalization. Frequently, there will also be mydriasis and hyperthermia and possibly tachycardia, seizures, and muscle weakness. Rarely, death has occurred. There are no specific laboratory abnormalities expected.

Differential Diagnoses

Differentials include serotonergic/psychotropic drug, alcohol, marijuana, or LSD intoxications.

Diagnosis

Tests are available to detect psilocybin, but the signs will probably have subsided by the time test results are obtained. No specific laboratory or necropsy/histopathologic alterations are expected.

Management of Exposures

Decontamination via emesis and lavage can be performed and activated charcoal given for recent ingestions. Emesis can be induced by having the owners use 3% hydrogen peroxide at home with a dose based on the weight of the animal, or a veterinarian can induce emesis using conjunctival or injectable apomorphine. Aspiration is a risk that needs to be taken into consideration in animals showing neurologic signs. Gastric emptying is followed by administration of one dose of activated charcoal. Seizures can be controlled with diazepam or, if no response, barbiturates, propofol, or isoflurane can be used as needed. The body temperature needs to be regulated and all sensory stimuli needs to be kept to a minimum. Cyproheptadine, while not an antagonist, can block the effects of serotonergic drugs and may also be helpful for hyperthermia.

Prognosis

The prognosis is generally good and most animals survive with supportive and symptomatic care.

IBOTENIC ACID AND MUSCIMOL-CONTAINING MUSHROOMS

Sources

Ibotenic acid and muscimol are isoxazoles. Muscimol is the decarboxylation product of ibotenic acid (Benjamin 1995).

Amanita gemmata, Amanita muscaria (fly agaric mukhomor, woodpecker-of-Mars), *Amanita pantherina* (panther mushroom), *Amanita smithiana, Amanita strobilformis,* and *Tricholoma muscarium. A. muscaria* and *A. pantherina* are responsible for most animal and human poisonings (Benjamin 1995).

A. muscaria has a cap that ranges from bright orange to bright crimson ("looks like a candy apple with a bad case of dandruff") (Benjamin 1995). It grows from summer to fall and fruiting most commonly occurs in fall and early winter. In the eastern United States it can fruit in the summer and again in late fall. It is found primarily in coniferous and deciduous forests, but can also be found on roadsides, in parks and open forests, and on edges of pastures (Benjamin 1995; Spoerke 2001). It is abundant in the Pacific Northwest in association with Douglas fir trees and is widespread throughout the United States and Canada. It is often found in association with beech and aspen. *A. muscaria* has been used as a fly attractant/poison (Benjamin 1995) and as an inebriant for recreational and religious purposes.

A. pantheris is found more commonly in the western United States, especially the western coastal plain (Benjamin 1995). It fruits in the spring and early summer and again in the fall and is associated with conifers and sometimes hardwoods.

Kinetics

Muscimol and ibotenic acid cross the blood-brain barrier

Mechanism of Action

Isoxazoles cause fluctuating CNS excitation and depression due to opposing effects of muscimol and ibotenic acid. The mechanism of action for the cholinergic-like effects is not known. Muscimol is formed by the decarboxylation of ibotenic acid, which binds GABA receptors in the central nervous system. This binding is irreversible and leads to prolonged activity, which results in central nervous system depression. Ibotenic acid acts on glutamate receptors in the brain, which results in CNS stimulation. It may also have direct neurotoxic effects, which can cause neuronal necrosis. Tricholomic acid from *Tricholoma muscarium* has a similar structure and mechanism of action as ibotenic acid.

Toxicity

The toxicity of these mushrooms can be difficult to quantify because it depends on many factors. Six mg of muscimol causes CNS effects in adult humans (Benjamin 1995). This amount is found in a single cap of *A. pantherina* and some *A. muscaria*. A lethal dose (human) is approximately 15 caps. Spring and summer fruiting caps may have higher levels of toxins. Ibotenic acid is 5 to 10 times less potent than muscimol in humans (Benjamin 1995). Drying mushrooms containing ibotenic acid results in spontaneous decarboxylation to muscimol. Dried mushrooms are more toxic than fresh, but prolonged storage results in degradation of the toxins so they become less toxic over time (>1 year).

Clinical Signs

The most common clinical signs are vomiting, ataxia, and disorientation. Frequently one can see hallucinations, vocalizations, alternating lethargy and agitation, hyperesthesia, recumbency, somnolence, and fasciculations. There is also the possibility of tremors, seizures, bradycardia, hypotension, and hypothermia. Rarely, one can see respiratory depression and death. The onset of signs is almost always within 30 minutes to 2 hours, but can sometimes be delayed for up to 6 hours. The duration of signs can be for 8–24 hours. There are no long-term sequela expected and no laboratory abnormalities expected, but if the vomiting and diarrhea are prolonged there can be electrolyte abnormalities.

Diagnosis

There are no diagnostic tests available and there are no diagnostic lesions that develop.

Differential Diagnoses

Differential diagnoses include ethylene glycol, alcohol, marijuana, serotonergic or dopaminergic drug, opiate, barbiturate or other CNS depressants intoxications, and viral or bacterial encephalitis.

Management of Exposures

Decontamination is useful in asymptomatic animals and consists of induction of emesis if ingestion has been within 4 hours. Emesis can be achieved as previously discussed followed by activated charcoal. Symptomatic and supportive care is required. Intravenous fluids are needed for cardiovascular support. If seizures develop, diazepam and barbiturates can be used. Injectable methocarbamol is best for tremors. Providing an environment that minimizes external stimuli can reduce the tendency to seizure or tremor. Thermoregulation is needed and antiemetics and GI protectants are part of the supportive care needed. Atropine is contraindicated because it may worsen the clinical effects of isoxazoles (Benjamin 1995).

Prognosis

The prognosis is generally excellent provided good supportive care is provided.

GYROMITRIN-CONTAINING MUSHROOMS

Sources

Gyromitrin is heat-labile, volatile, and water soluble (Tegzes and Puschner 2002s). Cooking the mushroom causes a decrease in toxicity, although the cooking liquid is toxic. Species containing gyromitrin include *Gyromitra* spp. (false morels), *Helvella crispa* and *H. lacuose*. These mushrooms grow throughout North America, usually near conifers, aspens, and melting snow banks. They are commonly found in the spring.

Kinetics

Gyromitrin is metabolized to methyl-formylhydrazine and then to monomethylhydrazine (Poisindex® 2003). The mushrooms contain a monomethylhydrazine precursor that is toxic (Spoerke 2006). Monomethylhydrazine inhibits γ-aminobutyric acid (GABA) synthesis with decreased GABA inhibition. The monomethylhydrazine also reacts with pyridoxal 5-phosphate to form a hydrazone. Depletion of tissue pyridoxal 5-phosphate results in decreased glutamic acid decarboxylase inhibition and GABA synthesis. Decreased GABA synthesis predisposes to seizures. The inhibition of a diamine oxidase in the intestinal mucosa may be responsible for the GI signs. The mechanism of hepatic damage is hypothesized to involve inhibition of certain mixed function oxidases in the liver, resulting in the formation of free radicals and causing lipid peroxidation. The mechanism of hemolysis is not clearly defined but might be secondary to other metabolic disruptions (Benjamin 1995).

Toxicity

There is a wide variation of gyromitrin in individual mushrooms and species of mushrooms and thus mushroom toxicity varies. Monomethylhydrazine precursor varies from 50–300 mg/kg and gyromitrin varies from 0.06–1.6 g/kg in fresh mushrooms. Cooking removes over 99% of the gyromitrin and drying also removes it. Five mg of monomethylhydrazine caused vomiting in monkeys and 7 mg caused death (Benjamin 1995).

Clinical Signs

The mushrooms cause a gastrointestinal effect followed by neurologic, hepatoarenal, and/or hemolytic syndromes. Onset of signs can be delayed from 6–24 hours after ingestion, but in some cases the signs occur as late as 53 hours postingestion. In one dog vomiting began 3 hours following ingestion (Beasley 1999). There is a 2–8-hour latent period following spore inhalation. Onset of GI signs is often sudden and may last for 2 days (Spoerke 2006). The GI phase involves nausea, vomiting, watery and possibly bloody diarrhea, along with abdominal discomfort, lethargy, and possibly fever. No additional signs might occur and there may be spontaneous recovery in a few days to a week.

For the hepatorenal syndrome, signs may develop by 36–48 hours and consist of icterus, hepatomegaly, and possibly splenomegaly. Rarely renal failure develops secondary to hypotension, dehydration, and hemolysis.

The hemolytic syndrome occurs rarely and appears to be more prevalent in dogs, who appear to be more susceptible to hemolysis and methemoglobinemia (Benjamin 1995). Sometimes there is methemoglobinemia without hemolysis.

There can be a neurologic syndrome that is a terminal phase. This phase consists of delirium, fasciculations, mydriasis, stupor that progresses to coma, circulatory collapse, and respiratory arrest. Rabbits intoxicated with gyromitrin developed loss of activity, seizures, anorexia, hemoglobinuria, and weight loss (Spoerke 2001). In one case a dog developed vomiting 2–3 hours after chewing on *Gyromitra esculenta* and in the course of 6 hours developed lethargy, followed by coma and death.

The most common signs are vomiting, diarrhea, and abdominal pain with fever. More severe signs can occur, but are very rare and occur mainly in dogs. The duration of signs varies. The GI effects can last for up to a week; hepatic and renal signs can last for weeks before recovery or, conversely, deterioration and death. Hemolytic and liver and kidney effects can be chronic.

Differential Diagnoses

Differential diagnoses include amanitin, zinc, iron, and acetaminophen toxicosis.

Diagnosis

Diagnostically one has to rely on the history of ingestion of mushrooms and any clinical signs consistent with exposure (i.e., latent period followed by GI, and/or hepatic and renal signs and hemolysis). Clinical pathology tests can show elevations in PT, AST, ALT, BUN, serum bilirubin, and creatinine (Spoerke 2006). On postmortem, histopathology can show renal tubular necrosis, periacinar hepatic degeneration and necrosis, and cerebral edema (Benjamin 1995; Tegzes and Puschner 2002a).

Management of Exposures

Management starts with early decontamination using emesis and activated charcoal. Emesis can be achieved as specified previously. It is necessary to correct fluid and electrolyte imbalances, so it is important to monitor electrolytes, acid/base balance, hydration, PCV, and renal and liver function. Hemolysis and methemoglobinemia can also be factors and need to be monitored (Spoerke 2006). Antiemetics can be used to control vomiting and antiseizure medications, such as diazepam, for control of seizures (Tegzes and Puschner 2002a). Intravenous fluid therapy at twice a maintenance rate might be required; a blood transfusion might be required for patients experiencing hemolysis. For liver and renal damage, antibiotics, lactulose, and SAMe (S-adenosylmethionine) can be employed. Pyridoxine (vitamin B_6) is a specific antagonist (Tegzes and Puschner 2002a). It is used to counter the neurologic signs caused by gyromitrin (Spoerke 2001).

Prognosis

The prognosis is guarded in patients progressing beyond GI effects.

HEPATOTOXIC MUSHROOMS

Sources

Hepatotoxic mushrooms, *Amanita*, *Galerina* and *Lepiota* genera, contain amanitins. There are nine amatoxins of which α-, β- and γ-amanitins are of major importance (Puschner 2007). The highest concentration of toxin is in the gills (46%) followed by the stems (23%) and cap (23%).

The most frequently reported poisoning results from ingestion of *A. phalloides* (Tegzes and Puschner 2002a). *A. phalloides* (death cap, deadly amanita) is found in Maryland, Pennsylvania, Delaware, New Jersey, Virginia, Rhode Island, Massachusetts, California, Oregon, and Washington. The Midwest, Southeast, and mountain states appear to be free of *A. phalloides*. It fruits from August to

January in California and from August to November in the eastern states. *A. phalloides* requires tree roots to grow, so it is not often found in grassy areas unless they contain mature trees with an extensive root system (Tegzes and Puschner 2002a). *A. phalloides* mushrooms are most often associated with birch and oak trees and can be in woodlands, parks, and golf courses. This mushroom species is the most toxic of the amatoxin-containing mushrooms and responsible for about 90%–95% of human deaths from mushroom poisonings worldwide (Donnelly and Wax 2005).

Amanita bisporigera (destroying angel) can be found across the northern tier states and in eastern Canada (Benjamin 1995). It is found in hardwood forests and mixed woodlands and is associated with oaks, birches, and aspens.

Amanita verna (spring destroying angel, spring amanita, white death cap, fool's mushroom) is associated with oak trees and fruits in spring, summer, and early fall.

Amanita virosa is found throughout southeast Canada and eastern coastal United States and is especially abundant along Lake Ontario shores. It is found in hardwood and mixed forests.

Amanita ocreata is found primarily along the coast of California, fruits in the spring, and is associated with oak trees. The remaining *Amanita* spp. are found primarily in southern and southeastern United States.

Kinetics

The bioavailability of amanitins in dogs and cats ranges from 10 to 20% (Benjamin 1995). Amanitins are taken up by epithelial cells of the GI tract and by hepatocytes, where they cause injury to GI mucosa and liver, respectively. Uptake into the hepatocytes can be blocked by bile salts, prednisolones, antanamide, and silibinin. There is no evidence of the amanitins crossing the placental barrier. They undergo extensive enterohepatic recirculation, and excretion occurs in dogs via the urine. Within 6 hours 90% of the amanitins are eliminated via the kidneys. The concentration of amanitins may be 100–150 times higher in the urine than in the blood (Benjamin 1995). Urinary excretion can continue for up to 72 hours due to the persistence of the mushrooms in the GI tract and extensive enterohepatic recirculation.

Mechanism of Action

Amanitins inhibit nuclear RNA polymerase II and interfere with DNA and RNA transcription (Benjamin 1995), which results in inhibition of ribosomal protein synthesis. Cells that have a high rate of metabolism are affected the

Table 23.2. Typical clinical phases of cyclopeptides or *Amanita phalloides* toxicosis[a]

	Description	Time Period	Clinical Effects
Initial	Latent period	6 to 12 (to 24) hours after exposure	
Phase I	Gastroenteritis (can detect amanitins in serum and urine)	±12 to 24 hours duration	Nausea Vomiting Bloody diarrhea Abdominal pain Lethargy Twitching Dehydration
Phase II	Severe gastroenteritis	±18 to 24 hours duration	Bloody diarrhea Hemolysis Electrolyte imbalance Hyperthermia Tachycardia Bradycardia
Latency	Latent period (continue monitoring liver and kidney function)	2 to 48 hours duration	Apparent recovery
Phase III	Final/terminal	Begins 36 to 84 hours after exposure	Liver, kidney, and multiorgan failure Severe hypoglycemia Icterus Coagulopathy Encephalopathy Seizures Azotemia Anuria Metabolic acidosis Cerebral edema Coma Sepsis Death

[a]Note that with large amanintin ingestions or ingestions by puppies, death may occur within 2 hours postexposure.

most, such as hepatocytes and intestinal crypt cells, but all cells in the body are susceptible. Blocking uptake by the hepatocytes might predispose other cells to damage through increased circulating amanitin concentration. The kidneys can be damaged in a similar way.

Toxicity

Toxicity varies with species. Rodents and rabbits seem to be unaffected by ingestion of the amanitins. The oral LD_{50} for a dog is approximately 1 mg amanitin (Benjamin 1995). This is about equivalent to one "decent-sized" mushroom cap. The IV LD_{50} for α-amanitin is 0.1 mg/kg.

Clinical Effects

Signs

Signs typically occur in phases (Puschner 2007). Following a latent period of 6–12 hours, there is a triphasic syndrome (Table 23.2). Phase 1 consists of GI signs: vomiting, diarrhea, abdominal pain, dehydration, and lethargy. Anorexia may also be seen. Phase 2 is characterized by severe GI upset manifested as nausea, vomiting, bloody diarrhea, and severe abdominal pain. In this phase there is hepatotoxic damage with signs and lab values that point to liver failure leading to coagulopathy. These signs can include icterus, tachycardia,

Table 23.3. Treatment of mushroom ingestion

Treatment	Recommendation	Dose
Emesis	Apomorphine	0.02 to 0.04 mg/kg IV, IM, or subconjunctival sac in the dog
	3% hydrogen peroxide	1 to 5 ml/kg PO (generally do not exceed 50 ml for dogs or 10 ml total for cat)
		Can repeat once after 15 min
Gastric lavage	Water at body temperature	10 mg/kg body weight
Adsorbent	Activated charcoal	2 to 5 g/kg body weight PO (1 g activated charcoal in 5 ml water); repeat dose every 4 to 6 hours; may be used to up 48 hours
Cathartic	Sorbital	3 ml/kg (70%) PO
Gastroeneteritis	GI protectants: kaolin/pectin	1 to 2 ml/kg every 6 to 12 hours
	Sucralfate	Dogs: 0.5 to 1 g PO every 8 to 12 h cats: 0.25 g PO every 8 to 12 h
Dehydration	Crystalloid fluids	As needed
	Glucose	
Hepatic damage	Acetylcysteine	140 mg/kg PO followed by 70 mg/kg PO every 6 hr
Seizures	Diazepam	0.5 to 2 mg/kg IV
	Phenobarbital	6 mg/kg IV to effect
	Propofol	0.1 mg/kg/min IV constant rate infusion
Dyspnea	Oxygen	
	Mechanical ventilation	
Sepsis	Broad-spectrum antibiotics	Parenteral as needed
Severe hemorrhage	Vitamin K_1	2.5 to 5 mg/kg daily
	Packed red blood cells	As needed
	Whole blood	
Amatoxin hepatic damage	Penicillin G	300,000 to 40 million U/day (human dose)
	Silymarin (herbal milk thistle—check label for concentration)	1.4 to 4.2 g/day PO for 4 to 5 days
Cholinergic stimulation	Atropine	0.2 to 2 mg/kg; give 50% of dose IV and 50% IM or SC to effect of drying secretions
Tremors	Methocarbamol	50 mg/kg IV q 8 hr
Hydrazine	Pyridoxine (vitamin B_6)	25 mg/kg by slow IV infusion over 15–30 min

acidosis, hypotension, and hypoglycemia. This can be followed by another latent phase in which the animal appears to have recovered. This latent period requires diligent monitoring of liver and renal values to determine whether damage is being done and to assess liver and kidney function. Phase 3 involves hemorrhages, seizures, fulminant hepatic failure, and renal failure leading to death in 4 to 7 days (Enjalbert et al. 2002). Fifty percent of dogs given amanitins in lethal doses died from hypoglycemia within 1 to 2 days of exposure. The onset of signs is generally 6 to 12 hours for GI signs and 24 to 72 hours for hepatic failure. The duration of signs can be a few days for mild cases and in severe cases death in 4–10 days. In beagles experimentally given sublethal doses of amanitins, vomiting, and diarrhea began in 16 hours and subsided 60 hours later. In beagles given lethal doses, an initial hyperglycemia was followed by hypoglycemia. Glucose was administered, which culminated in hepatic dystrophy and was fatal in 1–2 days (Spoerke 2006).

Laboratory

Significant elevations in serum AST, ALT, alkaline phosphatase, and bilirubin are commonly observed. Severe hypoglycemia is also characteristic (Tegzes and Puschner 2002b). Coagulopathy as evidenced by prolonged clotting times occurs in a high percent of affected dogs.

Differentials

Differentials include blue-green algae, acetaminophen, cycad, iron, aflatoxin, and phenolic compounds intoxications, leptospirosis, infectious hepatitis, and hepatic neoplasia.

Diagnosis

Antemortem

Liver biopsies can be done to detect evidence of hepatic injury; hepatic necrosis would be the expected finding. Urine samples can be tested for the presence of amanitin.

Postmortem

On necropsy one would expect to find evidence of hepatic necrosis, gastrointestinal mucosal injury, and renal tubular necrosis. Acute tubular necrosis is believed to the result of reabsorption of the toxins by renal tubules after glomerular filtration (Puschner 2007). Liver and kidney samples can be tested for amanitin to confirm exposure (Puschner 2007).

Management of Exposures

Early detection appears to be critical because survival rates were greatly improved with prompt therapeutic intervention (Tegzes and Puschner, 2002b; Puschner 2007). Standard decontamination is recommended if initiated soon after exposure. Emesis can be achieved as previously specified. After gastric emptying, activated charcoal should be administered. Giving repeated doses every 2 to 6 hours for 2 to 3 days is recommended to decrease enterohepatic recirculation (Puschner 2007). With this frequency of activated charcoal administration, serum sodium levels should be monitored because there is a high probability for hypernatremia.

Baseline serum chemistries, CBC, acid/base, and electrolytes, especially Na, should be obtained, and glucose, liver enzymes, renal values, and coagulation parameters should be monitored. Coagulation abnormalities have occurred in animals that develop GI signs within 24–48 hours of ingesting mushrooms. Levels are expected to be normal for the first 24 hours. ALT and AST begin to elevate and peak within 72–96 hours, with severe elevation evident within 72 hours. Supportive and symptomatic care is needed consisting of fluid therapy (diuresis without use of diuretics), temperature management, GI protectants, vitamin K_1, blood replacement therapy, special dietary food, and diazepam for seizures.

Liver protectants are recommended. N-acetylcysteine and silibinin (or silymarin, an herbal milk thistle protectant) appear to be equally efficacious. N-acetylcysteine and silibinin are free radical scavengers (Benjamin 1995). SAMe has also been recommended because it acts as a membrane stabilizer, hinders amatoxins penetration of cell, scavenges free radicals, and favors regeneration of damaged livers (Enjalbert et al. 2002).

Both silibinin and penicillin G interfere with enterohepatic recirculation of amatoxins. Cephalosporins may also be as, or even more, effective. (Enjalbert et al. 2002). Table 23.3 lists some of the therapeutic agents and dosages used for mushroom toxicosis in pets.

Prognosis

The prognosis is poor, especially if there is a short latent period with an early rise in liver enzyme concentrations, presence of a coagulopathy, and persistent hypoglycemia.

MYCOTOXINS

Mycotoxins are secondary chemical metabolites produced by various species of fungi in numerous commodities, foods, and feed. These compounds have diverse chemical structures and may cause biological and pathological changes in animals. Numerous fungi do not produce mycotoxins, and the presence of mold in feed or food does not guarantee that mycotoxins were or will be produced. Once produced, mycotoxins are fairly stable compounds, are not readily destroyed by processing, and can be found in cereal by-products (e.g., corn and wheat gluten, distiller's grains, etc.) and pet foods. Three genera of fungi—*Fusarium*, *Penicillium*, and *Aspergillus*—are primarily responsible for invasion of crops, particularly cereal grains, in the field and during harvest, transportation, processing, and storage of foods and feeds. Each fungus has specific requirements for matrix, oxygenation, temperature, and moisture for mold growth and subsequent mycotoxin development.

Mycotoxins frequently associated with pet food contamination include aflatoxins, *Fusarium* mycotoxins—particularly vomitoxin or deoxynivalenol (DON)—and ochratoxin A (Table 23.4). The tremorgenic mycotoxins associated with moldy food (bread, walnuts, cream

Table 23.4. Mycotoxins in pet food (adapted from CAST, 2003)

Mycotoxin	Fungi	Environment for Mold Growth	Commodity	Effects in Animals
Aflatoxins (B₁, B₂, G₁, G₂, M₁, M₂)	*Aspergillus* flavus and *A. parasiticus*	Warm days and nights (78 to 90°F), high grain moisture (16 to 28%), drought stress, insect damage	Corn Rice Peanuts/nuts Cottonseed	Liver damage Liver tumors Hemorrhage Death
Vomitoxin (trichothecene mycotoxin)	*Fusarium* spp.	Alternating warm days and cool nights (40 to 80°F), and humid	Cereals (wheat, corn, barley, oats)	Digestive disorders (vomiting, feed refusal, diarrhea)
Zearalenone	*Fusarium graminearum* (primarily)	Moderating temps (45 to 70°F) and high grain moisture (22 to 25%)	Cereals (wheat, corn, barley)	Estrogenic effects (edema of vulva, vagina, uterus)
Fumonisin	*Fusarium veriticilliodes* (syn. *Moniliforme*)	Drought during growing season followed by cool, wet weather during pollination	Corn Corn screenings	Liver insult *Note:* Horses are very sensitive to fumonisins and can develop brain necrosis (leukoencephalomalacia) and die
Ochratoxin A	*Aspergillus* ochraceus *Penicillilum verrucosum*	Cooler weather (54 to 77°F) and grain moisture >16%	Corn Wheat Dried beans Dried fruits	Kidney tubular necrosis
Roquefortine Penitrem A (tremorgens)	*Penicilium roqueforti* and others *Penicillium crustosum*		Walnuts Cream cheese Bread Rice Cheese Garbage	Tremors Incoordination Death

cheese, and garbage), such as penitrem A and roquefortine, are discussed in Chapter 24, "Food-Associated Intoxications."

Cereal grains, cereal by-products, and nuts are often incorporated into commercial food for dogs, cats, birds, rabbits, and other companion animals. These commodities can be contaminated with mycotoxins and may be diverted from use in human food to use in animal feeds. A majority of larger pet food companies test commodities for mycotoxins prior to incorporation into pet food; however, deviations in testing protocols may not detect mycotoxins and smaller, local mills may not test pet food ingredients prior to use. The end result can be pet food contamination with mycotoxins.

In a worldwide review of the prevalence of mycotoxins in pet foods, a majority of reported mycotoxin outbreaks in pets were related to aflatoxins, a few cases were related to tremorgenic mycotoxins, and several in Europe and the United Kingdom were associated with ochratoxin A (Leung et al. 2006). No natural outbreaks of aflatoxicosis have been reported in cats (Böhm and Razzazi-Fazeli 2005). This chapter focuses on two mycotoxins—aflatoxins and vomitoxin.

AFLATOXINS

Aflatoxins are polycyclic furan compounds produced by *Aspergillus* molds both in the field prior to harvest and in storage. Aflatoxins are hepatotoxic and potent liver carcinogens. Cases of fatal hepatitis in dogs during the 1950s and turkeys in 1960, termed "hepatitis X" and "X disease," respectively, were likely caused by aflatoxins.

Sources

Aspergillus flavus, *A. parasiticus*, and *A. nomius* can produce a number of aflatoxins. Aflatoxins identified include B_1 and B_2 (fluoresce blue in ultraviolet light), G_1 and G_2 (fluoresce green in ultraviolet light, and M_1 and M_2 (animal metabolites from hydroxylation of aflatoxins B_1 and B_2, respectively). Aflatoxin B1 is the most toxic mycotoxin in this group, generally found at the highest concentration, and the most important member of the aflatoxins for analytical purposes in feeds. Aflatoxins M_1 and M_2 can be found in tissues, meat, milk, and eggs. Fungal growth and aflatoxin production are favored when grain moisture is >15%, relative humidity is >75%, and temperatures are warm (78 to 90+°F). Aflatoxins may occur in corn, nuts, cottonseed, rice, and other crops during years of drought, warm-to-hot temperatures, and insect damage to crops. Large portions of crops in a region can be affected with widespread aflatoxin contamination in animal feeds.

Kinetics

Aflatoxin absorption is by passive diffusion from the small intestine (Meerdink 2004). Absorption is rapid and complete in numerous animal species, with a higher rate of absorption in young animals. Aflatoxins are eliminated from the body through the bile, urine, and feces, and into milk and eggs. Aflatoxins can undergo enterohepatic circulation. Generally, most of the toxin is excreted within 24 hours after exposure. Dogs given a single oral 100μg aflatoxin B_1/kg body weight dose in corn oil showed some vomiting postdosing, but no additional adverse effects, and over 90% of total aflatoxin M1 was found in the urine 12 hours postdosing; by 48 hours postdosing aflatoxin M1 was almost undetectable in urine (Bingham et al. 2004). Aflatoxins do not accumulate in body tissues, but repeated exposure may result in lasting adverse effects in tissues.

A majority of aflatoxin is biotransformed in the liver, with smaller amounts biotransformed in the kidney and small intestine. A critical metabolic step is the transformation of aflatoxin B_1 to a reactive epoxide intermediate by the cytochrome P450 system. Rapid formation of the reactive 8,9-epoxide of aflatoxin B1 can overwhelm detoxification mechanisms by depleting intracellular glutathione (Dereszynski et al. 2008). Dogs as a species have low liver glutathione concentrations, compared with other species. The unstable aflatoxin expoxides can bind covalently to intracellular molecules such as DNA, RNA, and proteins forming adducts, which can result in cellular damage and hepatic necrosis. As mentioned earlier, aflatoxin M_1 is formed from hydroxylation of aflatoxin B1 and is the major excretion product in several species via urine and milk (Meerdink 2004).

Mechanism of Action

The epoxide of aflatoxin B_1 binds cellular macromolecules, nucleic acids, subcellular organelles, and regulatory proteins that disrupt normal cellular processes and organ function. The outcome may result in cellular necrosis, cancer, immunosuppression (both humoral and cell-mediated immunity), mutagenesis, and teratogenesis.

Toxicity

In naturally occurring cases, the concentration of aflatoxin in the feed (dose) and the duration of exposure may not be known. It is very important to retain a sample of the suspect pet food that the animals have been consuming and test for aflatoxins in an analytical laboratory. Dogs are considered sensitive to aflatoxins, with a LD_{50} from 0.5 to 1.0 mg/kg body weight, and death may occur within 3 days after exposure. The LD_{50} of aflatoxins in cats ranges from 0.3 to 0.6 mg/kg body weight and in rabbits is approximately 0.4 mg/kg body weight. Mice, rats, and hamsters are more resistant to aflatoxins, with a single-dose oral LD_{50} greater than 5 mg/kg body weight. Following consumption of aflatoxin contaminated food, dogs can show peracute to acute, subacute, and chronic clinical signs. In a subacute study, young beagle dogs were orally dosed with an aflatoxin mixture (37.5% B_1, 5.4% B_2, 17.1% G_1, and 1.0% G_2) at dosages of 1, 5, and 20 μg/kg body weight, with the duration of dosing lasting for 10 weeks at 5 days a week (Armbrecht et al. 1971). Clinical signs of icterus, inappetence, yellow-orange colored urine, and increased prothrobin time were noted in dogs at the high dosage of 20 μg/kg body weight. Histological changes were observed in only the high-dosed group and consisted of moderate bile duct proliferation, bile pigment accumulation in the liver portal areas, and multiple vascular channels around central and portal liver veins. Therefore, the toxic dose for aflatoxins in dogs is estimated to be less than 20 μg/kg body weight.

Clinical Signs

Clinical features of aflatoxicosis in dogs are not unique to this condition and may not be recognized antemortem. Pathological changes in the liver are more indicative of aflatoxicosis, and analytical detection of elevated aflatoxins B_1 in the feed and M_1 in hepatic tissue can confirm aflatoxicosis. Sudden deaths in kennel dogs fed a similar pet food may serve as sentinels of aflatoxicosis (Dereszynski et al. 2008). Dogs may be reluctant to eat the contaminated food (aflatoxins are considered odorless and tasteless), but may consume noncontaminated feeds. The clinical signs of aflatoxicosis are related to liver damage and failure, which may be acute or chronic in nature. In a retrospective case study of dogs exposed to aflatoxin-contaminated pet food in 2005 to 2006, the order of onset of clinical signs was anorexia, lethargy, vomiting, jaundice, diarrhea frequently associated with melena progressing to hematochezia, abdominal effusion (usually a transudate), peripheral edema, and terminal encephalopathy associated with hemorrhagic diathesis (Table 23.5) (Dereszynski et al. 2008). Dogs may develop polyuria and polydipsia and show depression. The severity of clinical signs can vary among dogs, probably related to differences in dose and duration of aflatoxin exposure, biotransformation of aflatoxins, nutritional status, and preexisting health conditions. Poor survival of dogs affected by aflatoxins in pet food was linked with severe enteric hemorrhage. Afla-

toxicosis in dogs may induce disseminated intravascular coagulation that can deplete coagulation factors.

Good early markers of aflatoxicosis in dogs are hypocholesterolemia and lower plasma protein C and antithrombin activities (Dereszynski et al. 2008). Commonly, dogs have coagulopathies, such as prolonged activated partial thromboplastin time (aPTT)and prothrombin time (PT), and lower fibrinogen concentrations and plasma coagulation factor VII (FVII:C). Because of vomiting, diarrhea, or abnormal body fluid distribution (i.e., abdominal effusion), electrolyte disturbances occur, such as lower serum concentrations of sodium and calcium and elevated serum phosphate. Dogs also had lowered serum albumin and total protein, and increased liver enzyme activities and hyperbilirubinemia. The magnitude of liver enzyme activities did not correlate with the severity of hepatocellular damage noted at necropsy (Dereszynski et al. 2008). No significant differences were observed in urine specific gravity, (between survivor and nonsurvivor dogs), but dogs with granular casts, specifically with cylindruria (renal casts or tiny, tube-shaped particles) died from aflatoxicosis, while few of these dogs were azotemic (Dereszynski et al. 2008). The presence of granular casts in the urine of dogs dying from aflatoxicosis could be related to aflatoxin adduct injury to tissue, altered redox status, or impaired renal perfusion from systemic effects of aflatoxins; the cause-effect relationship is only speculated.

Needle aspirates of liver from dogs that died from aflatoxicosis were processed for cytology examination and revealed diffuse hepatocyte lipid vacuolation, hepatocyte degeneration, and minor inflammatory cell infiltrates. These findings are not pathognomonic for aflatoxins and a full necropsy is recommended.

Diagnosis

Diagnosis is based on compatible clinical signs and clinical pathology changes, particularly related to liver failure or sudden death. A complete necropsy is recommended in suspect aflatoxicoses. Histopathologic findings consistent with aflatoxicoses include hepatic lipidosis; portal fibroplasias; magelocytosis of hepatocytes; biliary hyperplasia; and, in chronic hepatopathy cases, marked lobular atrophy, bridging portal fibrosis, and regenerative hepatocellular nodules (Newman et al. 2007).

Suspect food consumed by the animal should be tested in analytical laboratories for aflatoxins, in particular aflatoxin B_1, for confirmation of exposure to aflatoxins. Aflatoxins are notorious for occurring in localized hot spots in feeds; multiple samples of the suspect food should be

Table 23.5. Clinical signs and clinicopathologic changes in dogs associated with aflatoxin exposure (adapted from Dereszynski et al., 2008)

Clinical Signs	Clinicopathologic Changes
Sudden death	Coagulopathic disturbances: low plasma anticoagulant proteins (protein C, antithrombin)
Anorexia	Hypocholesterolemia
Lethargy	Hypoproteinemia (↓total protein and albumin)
Vomiting	ä serum liver enzyme activities
Jaundice	Hyperbilirubinemia
Diarrhea (melena, hematochezia)	↓ serum electrolytes (Na^+, Ca^+)
Dehydration	Granular casts in urine (cylindruria or renal casts)
Abdominal effusion, peripheral edema	Liver needle aspirates cyto prep: diffuse hepatocyte lipid vacuolation
Polyuria, polydipsia	
Terminal encephalopathy	
Hemorrhagic diathesis	

taken and can be held and frozen for future analysis. If the animal has been consuming the suspect food recently, liver samples can be frozen for subsequent analysis for aflatoxin M_1; however, the half-life of aflatoxins in dogs has not been determined and is thought to be very short. Aflatoxin M_1 may be cleared from the liver within 7 days after a suspect food has been discontinued in the diet, so analysis of liver tissue may be of value only with recent exposure to a suspect food (Newman et al. 2007). Dog foods associated with outbreaks of aflatoxicosis had greater than 60 μg aflatoxin/kg and from to 100 to 300+ μg aflatoxin/kg of food (Leung et al. 2006). Analysis of some dog feed associated with aflatoxicosis in the eastern United States during 2005 and 2006 revealed high concentrations of aflatoxin B_1 in a range of 223 to 579 μg/kg (ppb or parts per billion) of feed, and hepatic tissue of affected dogs contained high concentrations of aflatoxin M_1, from 0.6 to 4.4 μg/kg liver (Newman et al. 2007). The US Food and Drug Administration's action level for maximum aflatoxin in feed for pets (dogs, cats, horses) is 20 μg/kg or ppb (FDA 1994).

Differential Diagnoses

Differential diagnoses would include acetaminophen, cyanobacterial toxin—microcystins, iron, phenolic compounds, *Penicillium islandicum* mycotoxin—leutoskyrin, and pyrrolizidine alkaloid intoxications, leptospirosis, infectious hepatitis, and hepatic neoplasia from other causes.

Treatment

If aflatoxin is suspected from food exposure, identify the potential aflatoxin-contaminated food source(s) and stop further exposure. Ensure that possible contaminated food sources are retained and frozen for analytical testing for aflatoxins. There is no antidote for aflatoxin.

There is no definitive treatment protocol for aflatoxicosis in animals. General supportive treatment and care are the main focus. Dogs may require intravenous fluids and blood component treatment; vitamins K and E may be administered to replenish the coagulation cofactor and to inhibit membrane lipid peroxidation, respectively (Dereszynski et al. 2008). The dose of vitamin E was limited to ≤10 U/kg/d (≤4.5 U/lb/d) because of concerns that higher dosages may inhibit gamma-carboxylation of vitamin K dependent coagulants. In the 2005/2006 outbreak of aflatoxicosis in dogs, one therapeutic approach was to provide hepatic supportive care with thiol donors for 2 months after the initial aflatoxin diagnosis; glutathione was considered important for aflatoxin detoxification mechanisms

(aflatoxin metabolites undergo enterohepatic circulation) and glutathione can be depleted in dogs with spontaneous liver disease (Dereszynski et al. 2008). Initial thiol replacement was by intravenous n-acetylcysteine but was changed to oral s-adenosylmethionine when the dogs could tolerate oral treatment. Dogs with persistent vomiting were given antiemetics, but gastric atony, detected in several affected dogs, did not respond to antiemetic or prokinetic treatment and some dogs were euthanized.

Dogs suspected of developing gastric ulcers and esophagitis secondary to protracted vomiting were treated with a histamine-2 receptor blocking agent famotidine and a gastric cytoprotective drug sucralfate. Silybin, considered a hepatic protective flavanoid from herbal milk thistle, was given to enhance glutathione-S-transferase activity and promote glutathione synthesis (Dereszynski et al. 2008). Broad-spectrum antibiotics are recommended to protect against systemic infections from possible immunosuppression. L–carnitine was provided to dogs to combat hepatic lipidosis, which has been shown to be beneficial in experimental aflatoxicosis in several species. Treated dogs frequently deteriorated despite treatment (Dereszynski et al. 2008).

Prognosis

The prognosis depends on the severity of liver damage. Severe liver damage suggests a guarded to poor prognosis. Monitoring coagulation (particularly aPTT and PT, plasma protein C, and antithrombin activity), serum liver enzyme activities, serum biochemistry panel, and electrolytes can be indicative of the hepatic damage. The presence of granular casts, specifically for cylindruria, has been associated with fatality. The finding of enteric blood has been associated with the onset of hepatic encephalopathy and terminal stages of aflatoxicosis and death.

VOMITOXIN OR DEOXYNIVALENOL (DON)

Fusarium molds invade a variety of cereal plants resulting in widespread plant diseases, such as "*Fusarium* head blight" or "scab" in wheat and barley and "*Giberella* ear rot" of corn. Moderate temperatures during flowering and higher humidity favor *Fusarium* growth in cereals and mycotoxin production in the field (see Table 23.4). A group of mycotoxins produced by *Fusarium* spp. are the trichothecenes, sesquiterpenoid compounds with an epoxy ring at C12-13 that is considered essential for toxicity. The trichothecenes include a number of mycotoxins, vomitoxin, 15- and 3-acetyldeoxynivalnol, nivalenol, scirpenol, T-2 toxin, HT-2 toxin, diacetoxyscirpenol, etc., with a broad range of toxicity. Reports of adverse effects in dogs and cats are not common from trichothecene-contaminated pet food. This chapter is focused on vomitoxin, the most common trichothecene contaminant identified in grain.

Sources

Trichothecenes are produced by several genera of fungi, including *Fusarium*, *Stachybotrys*, *Myrothecium*, *Trichothecium*, and others. Trichothecene production by *Fusarium* fungi is heavily dependent on oxygen, environmental pH, osmotic tension, and temperature. For example, vomitoxin is produced under conditions of low oxygen tension, whereas zearalenone production by the same fungi requires oxygen saturation, usually occurring after field crops senesce. *F. graminearum*, the primary producer of vomitoxin in North America, has an optimum temperature range for growth of 78 to 82°F (26 to 28°C) at a water activity (a_W) greater than 0.88. Vomitoxin is a stable chemical and is not destroyed by high temperatures and pressure treatments.

Kinetics and Toxicity

The kinetics of vomitoxin have not been described in dogs and cats. In other monogastric animals, vomitoxin is rapidly and nearly completely absorbed in the stomach and proximal small intestine after oral exposure. Distribution to all body tissues is fairly rapid, and most of the vomitoxin is eliminated in the urine and feces in less than 24 to 48 hours. Vomitoxin is not accumulated in tissues. In a feeding trial with mature Brittany and beagle dogs and American shorthair cats, naturally contaminated wheat was incorporated into pet foods at increasing concentrations of vomitoxin from 0 to 10 mg/kg or ppm (parts per million) (Hughes et al. 1999). Dogs previously exposed to vomitoxin-contaminated pet food preferentially selected uncontaminated food. When the vomitoxin concentration in feed was >4.5 ±1.7 mg/kg in dog food and >7.7 ±1.1 mg/kg in cat food, feed intake was reduced in dogs and cats, respectively. Vomitoxin concentrations greater than 8 to 10 mg/kg in the diet caused vomiting in dogs and cats.

Mechanism of Action

Trichothecene mycotoxins have multiple effects on eukaryotic cells, including inhibition of protein, RNA, and DNA synthesis, alteration of membrane structure and mitochondrial function, stimulation of lipid peroxidation, induction of programmed cell death or apoptosis, and activation of cytokines and chemokines. Typical effects from trichothecene exposure are anorexia, vomiting, gastrointestinal irritation, and immunosuppression.

Table 23.6. Clinical signs in dogs associated with vomitoxin exposure

Feed refusal
Vomiting
Weight loss
Diarrhea
Poor feed conversion
Gastrointestinal irritation

Clinical Signs

The predominant clinical signs from vomitoxin exposure in pet food are feed refusal, vomiting, and weight loss in dogs (Table 23.6). In a study of mature beagle dogs fed *Fusarium* mycotoxin-contaminated diets (2.7 and 3.9 ppm vomitoxin with low concentrations [<0.5 ppm] of 15-acetyldeoxynivalenol and zearalenone, and 8 to 10 ppm fusaric acid), rapid onset of reduced feed intake was reported (Leung et al. 2007). Only one dog vomited on these diets; however, weight loss was reported in dogs fed the vomitoxin-contaminated diets. Vomitoxin has been reported to delay gastric emptying through peripheral action at serotonin receptors in rodents (Fioramonti et al. 1993). Additional clinical signs from vomitoxin exposure could include gastrointestinal irritation and diarrhea, and poor feed conversion. Dogs can show individual susceptibility to mycotoxins, and younger animals may be more susceptible to adverse effects at lower concentrations of vomitoxin in food.

Diagnosis

The clinical signs associated with vomitoxin exposure are common to many conditions and generally no significant changes are observed in clinicopathologic parameters. Vomitoxin, and other trichothecene mycotoxins, can be analyzed for in pet foods by numerous veterinary diagnostic labs. The FDA advisory levels for vomitoxin on grains and grain by-products for pets are not greater than 5 mg/kg (ppm) and not to exceed 40% of the diet or not to exceed 2 mg/kg (ppm) of their final diet (FDA 2010).

Differential Diagnoses

Clinical signs of feed refusal, vomiting, weight loss, and diarrhea could be attributed to bacterial or viral intestinal infections and garbage or irritant plant ingestion.

Treatment

As with any mycotoxin exposure in feed, the first recommendation is to stop the exposure and switch to a diet with low or nondetectable concentrations of vomitoxin. Feed samples can be taken of the suspect pet food, frozen, and submitted to veterinary diagnostic laboratories for analysis. Generally, treatment is not required; if the animals are dehydrated from fluid loss through vomiting or diarrhea, fluid therapy should be instituted.

Prognosis

After exposure to the vomitoxin-suspect diet is discontinued, rapid recovery to normal status should occur. The prognosis is good for recovery.

OTHERS

Numerous mycotoxins can be produced in natural infections of mold in grains, feed, and food. Zearalenone, a resorcyclic acid lactone, is a mycotoxin produced by *Fusarium* species in corn and other crops, and it is often found with vomitoxin. Zearalenone, and related metabolites zearalenols and zearalanols, are estrogenic compounds that can affect the reproductive system causing edema of the vulva and uterus, enlargement of mammary glands, and possibly ovarian dysfunction. The concern for adverse reproductive effects in dogs would be the breeding bitches; however, no case reports of zearalenone toxicosis have been adequately documented in dogs. Additional mycotoxins produced by *Fusarium* species are the fumonisins, particularly fumonisin B_1. Dogs and cats are not considered sensitive to fumonisins and toxicoses have not been reported for dogs and cats; on the other hand, horses are very sensitive to fumonisins and can develop brain malacia and necrosis. All species have the potential to have some liver damage from fumonisins. The FDA guidance levels for total fumonisins in corn and corn by-products intended for pets are not greater than 10 mg/kg (ppm) and not to exceed 50% of the diet or not to exceed 5 mg/kg (ppm) of their final diet (FDA 2001). The FDA guidance level for equids and rabbits is not to exceed 1 ppm of the final diet.

Particularly in Europe and the United Kingdom, ochratoxin A is an important nephrotoxin mycotoxin. The molds *Aspergillus ochraceus* and *Penicillium verrucosum* produce ochratoxins in cereal grains under cooler weather, 54 to 77°F, and moist conditions. Dogs are sensitive to ochratoxin A and can develop anorexia, vomiting, polyuria, polydipsia, bloody feces, paralysis, and die (Böhn and Razzazi-Fazeli 2005). Daily oral doses of 0.2 to 0.3 mg ochratoxin A/kg body weight can be lethal to dogs within 10 to 14 days. Necropsy lesions related to ochratoxin A exposure include necrosis of proximal renal tubules, mucohemorrhagic enteritis, and necrosis of lymphoid tissue. No cases of ochratoxin A toxicosis in pets have been reported in North America.

REFERENCES

Armbrecht, B.H., Geleta, J.N., and Shalkop, W.T. 1971. A subacute exposure of beagle dogs to aflatoxin. *Toxicol Appl Pharmacol* 18:579–585.

Beasley, V.R. 1999. *A Systems Affected Approach to Veterinary Toxicology*. Urbana: University of Illinois College of Veterinary Medicine.

Benjamin, D.R. 1995. *Mushrooms: Poisons and panaceas*. New York: W.H. Freeman and Company.

Bingham, A.K., Huebner, H.J., Phillips, T.D. et al. 2004. Identification and reduction of urinary aflatoxin metabolites in dogs. *Food Chem Toxicol* 42:1851–1858.

Böhm, J. and Razzazi-Fazeli, E. 2005. Effects of mycotoxins on domestic pet species. In *The Mycotoxin Blue Book*, edited by Diaz, D., pp. 77–91. Nottingham, UK: Nottingham University Press.

CAST (Council for Agricultural Science and Technology). 2003. *Mycotoxins: Risks in Plant, Animal and Human Systems*. Task Force Report No. 139. Ames, Iowa.

Dereszynski, D.M., Center, S.A., Randolph, J.E. et al. 2008. Clinical and clinicopathologic features of dogs that consumed foodborne hepatotoxic aflatoxins: 72 cases (2005–2006). *J Am Vet Med Assoc* 232:1329–1337.

Donnelly, M. and Wax, P. 2005. Cyclopeptide-containing mushrooms: the deadly amanita mushrooms. In *Critical Care Toxicology: Diagnosis and Management of the Critically Poisoned Patient*, edited by Brent, J., Wallace, K.L., Burkhart, K.K., Phillips, S.D., Donovan, J.W., pp. 1277–1285. New York: Elsevier Mosby.

Enjalbert, F., Rapior, S., Nouguier-Soulè, J. et al. 2002. Treatment of amatoxin poisoning 20 year retrospective analysis. *J Toxicol Clin Toxicol* 40(6):715–757.

FDA (Food and Drug Administration). 1994. CPG Sec. 683.100 Action Levels for Aflatoxins in Animal Feeds. Revised 8/28/94. http://www.fda.gov/ICECI/Compliance Manuals/CompliancePolicyGuidanceManual/ucm074703. htm.

———. 2001. Guidance for Industry: Fumonisin Levels in Human Foods and Animal Feeds; Final Guidance. Revised 11/9/2001. http://www.fda.gov/Food/GuidanceCompliance RegulatoryInformation/GuidanceDocuments/ChemicalCo ntaminantsandPesticides/ucm109231.htm.

———. 2010. Guidance for Industry and FDA: Advisory Levels for Deoxynivalenol (DON) in Finished Wheat Products for Human Consumption and Grains and Grain By-products Used for Animal Feed. Revised 7/7/2010. http:// www.fda.gov/Food/GuidanceComplianceRegulatoryInfor mation/GuidanceDocuments/NaturalToxins/ucm12018 4.htm.

Fioramonti, J., Dupuy, C., Dupuy, J. et al. 1993. The mycotoxin, deoxynivalenol, delays gastric emptying through serotonin-3 receptors in rodents. *J Pharmacol Exp Ther* 266:1255–1260.

Hughes, D.M., Gahl, M.J., Graham, C.H. et al. 1999. Overt signs of toxicity to dogs and cats of dietary deoxynivalenol. *J Anim Sci* 77:693–700.

Leung, M.C., Diaz-Llano, G., and Smith, T.K. 2006. Mycotoxins in pet food: A review on worldwide prevalence and preventative strategies. *J Agric Food Chem* 54:9623–9635.

Leung, M.C., Smith, T.K., Karrow, N.A. et al. 2007. Effects of foodborne *Fusarium* mycotoxins with and without a polymeric glucomannan mycotoxin adsorbent on food intake and nutrient digestibility, body weight, and physical and clinicopathologic variables of mature dogs. *Am J Vet Res* 68:1122–1129.

Meerdink, G.L. 2004. Aflatoxins. In *Clinical Veterinary Toxicology*, edited by Plumlee, K.H., pp. 231–235. St. Louis: Mosby.

Newman, S.N., Smith, J.R., Stenske, K.A. et al. 2007. Aflatoxicosis in nine dogs after exposure to contaminated commercial dog food. *J Vet Diagn Invest* 19:168–175.

Poisindex CD-ROM Editorial Staff. 2003. Mushrooms (Toxicologic Managements) Poisindex System Vol 114 Micromedex, Englewood, Colorado. Expires 12-20-2003.

Puschner, B. 2007. Mushrooms toxins. In *Veterinary Toxicology, Basic and Clinical Principles*, edited by Gupta, R.C., pp. 915–923. New York: Elsevier Academic Press.

Spoerke, D. 2001. Mushroom exposure. In *Small Animal Toxicology*, edited by Peterson, M.E., Talcott, P.A., pp. 571–592. St. Louis: Saunders.

———. 2006. Mushrooms. In *Small Animal Toxicology*, edited by Peterson, M.E., Talcott, P.A., pp. 860–888. St. Louis:Saunders.

Tegzes, J.H. and Puschner, B. 2002a. Toxic mushrooms. *Vet Clin North Am Small Anim Pract* 32:397–407.

———. 2002b. Amanita Poisoning: efficacy of aggressive treatment of two dogs. *Vet Hum Toxicol* 11:96–99.

Food-Associated Intoxications

24

Mindy Bough

ALLIUM SPECIES

Sources

There are a number of plants in the *Allium* genera. Some common examples include *Allium cepa*, cultivated onion; *Allium validum* and *Allium canadense*, wild onion; *Allium sativum*, garlic; *Allium schoenoprassum*, chives; and *Allium porrum*, leek. These plants are frequently used by humans as food, flavoring agents, and as medicinal herbs. Cull onions have been used as livestock feed.

Companion animals may have access to *Allium spp.* in the yard or garden, from the feeding of table food, from foods left unattended, or when pet owners give the food or supplements to their pets directly. Regardless of the source of exposure, dogs, and especially cats, may demonstrate signs of toxicosis.

Kinetics

The crushing or chewing of *Allium spp.* produces changes leading to the production of allicin; this compound has pharmacologic and toxicologic properties and produces the characteristic garlic odor. The oil, which contains the pharmacological and toxic components, is readily absorbed through the gastrointestinal tract. Garlic oil is eliminated both through the urine and through the lungs (Okuyama et al. 1989). The half-life of allin in rats who were given 30 mg/kg was approximately 0.7 hours (Guo et al. 1990).

Mechanism of Action

When crushed or chewed, the sulfur compounds in *Allium spp.* are hydrolyzed to thiosulfinates that then decompose to disulfides. These disulfide compounds are oxidating agents, which can cause hemolysis of erythrocytes. The most toxic disulfide is reported to be dipropenyl disulfide also known as n-propyl disulfide (Cheeke 1998). These disulfides oxidize erythrocyte membranes. The result is the formation of Heinz bodies, methemoglobinemia, and anemia (Ogawa et al. 1986). Cats are more sensitive to the effects of *Allium spp.* because their hemoglobin is more sensitive to oxidative damage than other species. They have 8 free sulfhydryl groups on their hemoglobin, which is twice the amount that dogs have and four times the amount that humans have. In addition, feline hemoglobin dissociates into dimers 10 times more readily than other species (Robertson et al. 1998).

A different mechanism of action may be involved with sheep and other ruminants. Selim et al. (1999) reported that rumen bacteria may be involved in the production of toxic metabolites.

Toxicity

Pantoja et al. (1991) reported natriuresis, diuresis, and hypotension in anesthetized dogs that were given 2.5 to 15 mg/kg of encapsulated garlic powder. Transient bradycardia was present in dogs at doses of 15 and 20 mg/kg of encapsulated garlic. Erythrocyte effects and decreased

Small Animal Toxicology Essentials, First Edition. Edited by Robert H. Poppenga, Sharon Gwaltney-Brant.
© 2011 John Wiley and Sons, Inc. Published 2011 by John Wiley and Sons, Inc.

hemoglobin concentrations were seen in dogs that were given an extract equal to 5 g of whole garlic per kg of body weight once a day for 7 days. Cats and some dog breeds, particularly Japanese breeds such as Akitas, Shibas, and Tosas, are at an increased risk for toxicosis to Allium spp. because their erythrocytes are more susceptible to oxidative damage (Christopher et al. 1990).

Large animals can be affected by *Allium spp.* Beasley (1999) reports sensitivity ratings among these animals, with cattle being the most sensitive followed by horses, and then sheep, and then goats. Feeding more than 25% of the diet in the form of onions will be hazardous to cattle. Onion toxicosis has been reported in calves and yearling cattle. An average of 11.8 kg/head per day was fed, and signs developed in 26% of the animals within 5 days (Verhoeff et al. 1985). Sheep have been fed cull onions without toxicity (Cheeke 1998). However, Selim et al. (1999) reported Heinz body hemolytic anemia when sheep were fed 50 g/kg/day for 15 days.

Clinical Effects

Signs

Hematological changes may occur from 12 hours to 5 days postexposure. The primary concern, in *Allium spp.* exposure cases, is for Heinz body hemolytic anemia and methemoglobinemia. Secondarily, in serious cases renal damage occurs from hemoglobinuria. In dogs, the most common signs reported to the American Society for the Prevention of Cruelty to Animals (ASPCA) Animal Poison Control Center (APCC) are depression, decreased hematocrit, vomiting, elevated WBC count, anorexia, hemolysis, and weakness. Less commonly reported signs include salivation, diarrhea, ataxia, hemoglobinuria, Heinz bodies, methemoglobinemia, abnormal breath, and abnormal feces. Cats most frequently exhibited vomiting, salivation, and anorexia. Ogawa et al. (1986) reported that hematocrits returned to normal in 10–14 days after oral exposure.

Differential Diagnoses

If *Allium spp.* ingestion is suspected but specific evidence is unavailable, other potential causes of hemolysis or Heinz body anemia should be ruled out. Other toxicoses that may produce similar signs include zinc, copper, propylene glycol in cats, red maple in horse, Brassica spp. in ruminants, phenothiazines, and mothballs. Additional differentials may include auto immune hemolytic anemia, blood parasites (e.g., *Haemobartonella felis*, *Babesia canis*, and *Eperythrozoon suis*), and hereditary diseases that affect red blood cells.

Diagnostics

Antemortem

Hematological testing should be performed with evaluations for Heinz body hemolytic anemia, methemoglobinemia, reticulocytes, icterus, and bilirubin, and chemistry evaluation of renal values. Urine output and presence of hemoglobinuria should be evaluated.

Postmortem

If death occurs, postmortem findings can include onion odor in the gastrointestinal contents, hemoglobin in the urine, pale or icteric tissues, and renal tubular degeneration and necrosis.

Management of Exposures

Small animals presenting with significant exposure to *Allium spp.* should be decontaminated. Induction of vomiting may be induced if the exposure was recent and the animal is asymptomatic. However, caution should be exercised in determining whether contraindications to vomiting exist and whether it is safe to have the pet owner induce vomiting at home. Activated charcoal should be given once vomiting is controlled. A cathartic such as sorbitol can be given with the first dose of activated charcoal, but not with subsequent doses. When repeat doses of activated charcoal are used as part of decontamination, electrolyte values should be monitored, since electrolyte shifts can occur.

Symptomatic treatment should be provided and may include administration of oxygen, blood transfusion(s) or Oxyglobin®, intravenous fluids, and control of gastrointestinal signs. Selim et al. (1999) reported that Heinz body hemolytic anemia in sheep was less severe when animals were fed ampicillin along with onions. Therefore, it may be beneficial to treat sheep with oral antibiotics to reduce oxidative damage. Treatment should continue until clinical signs are resolved.

Prognosis

The prognosis is generally good for animals that are decontaminated and treated early. However, the prognosis may be compromised in animals that develop renal damage secondary to hemolytic anemia.

AVOCADO

Sources

Avocados are in the family Lauraceae. They originate from southern Mexico to Central America but are now also grown in the warm climate of the southern United States.

The genus *Persea* includes approximately 150 species and is the only edible genus. *Persea americana* is the only species known to have toxicological significance (Burrows and Tyrl 2001). *Persea americana* includes 3 ecological races or varieties, Guatemalan, Mexican, and West Indian or Columbian. Of the avocado races, there are a number of hybrids.

Kinetics

The toxic compound in avocados, persin, is absorbed quickly from the gastrointestinal system. The peak plasma level of persin with oral ingestion is 1–2 hours. Elimination of persin can occur through the milk in lactating animals. Other forms of elimination are unknown, but mice that were dosed orally with persin eliminated the persin within 24 hours (Burrows and Tyrl 2001).

Mechanism of Action

The mechanism of action for avocado toxicosis is unknown (Pickrell et al. 2004).

Toxicity

The Guatemalan avocado and its hybrids have been shown to be toxic. Other races/varieties have not been implicated in toxicoses to date (Burrows and Tyrl 2001). Mammalian species that are known to be affected include cattle, goats, horses, mice, rabbits, rats, and sheep. Lower doses are associated with mammary gland effects, and higher doses are associated with cardiac effects, including acute cardiac failure and chronic cardiac insufficiency (Pickrell et al. 2004). There are no reliable literature reports of mammary gland or cardiac effects in dogs and cats. *Persea americana* has also caused signs of toxicosis in caged birds, ostriches, and fish (Burger et al. 1994; Hargis et al. 1989). Persin doses of 60 to 100 mg/kg may cause mastitis and agalactia. Doses of persin over 100 mg/kg may lead to cardiac effects (Oelrichs et al. 1995).

Clinical Effects

Signs

Lactating sheep, horses, cattle, rabbits, goats, rats, and mice may show signs of mastitis and agalactia. Reported signs include hard, swollen udders; a decrease in milk production; and watery, cheesy, curdled milk. Cardiac effects may include edema of the head, neck, brisket, and chest; cough; weakness; depression; hesitancy to move; respiratory distress; cardiac arrhythmias; acute cardiac failure; and chronic cardiac insufficiency. Sudden death has also been reported in rabbits, caged birds, and goats (Burrows and Tyrl 2001; Pickrell et al. 2004).

Mammary and cardiac signs have been reported to occur within 15 hours to 3 days of exposure (Hargis et al. 1989; Craigmill et al. 1984; McKenzie and Brown 1991). Gastrointestinal signs in dogs and cats are expected to occur within 1–3 hours of exposure.

Laboratory

Blood chemistries and electrolytes should be monitored in these cases. Elevated creatine phosphokinase and alanine aminotransferase are consistent with damage to the cardiac muscle (Pickrell et al. 2004). Hepatic enzymes may also be elevated (Burrows and Tyrl 2001). Electrolyte imbalances could occur due to the administration of activated charcoal.

Differential Diagnoses

Other toxicoses and disease processes may produce similar signs and should therefore be considered, especially if there is no known history of *Persea americana* exposure. Differentials include exposure to ionophones, gossypol, cardiac glycosides, and *Taxus spp.* as well as primary congestive heart failure and acute hepatic disease.

Diagnostics

Antemortem

A history of exposure along with expected clinical signs provide adequate diagnostic evidence (Pickrell et al. 2004).

Postmortem

Clots may be present in the mammary ducts. Edema may be present in tissues such as the subcutis and the lungs. Congestion is apparent in the lungs, liver, and spleen. Free fluid may be visible in the heart sac, thorax, and abdomen. The gallbladder and perirenal tissues may be edematous. The heart tissue appears pale (Burrows and Tyrl 2001).

Management of Exposures

Emesis may be induced in dogs and potentially cats with significant exposure if the exposure is recent, no signs are present, and no other contraindications to emesis exist. Caution should be exercised in determining whether contraindications to vomiting exist and whether it is safe to have the pet owner induce vomiting at home. Activated charcoal may be given to dogs and cats once vomiting is controlled. Other animal species at risk for toxicoses may also be administered activated charcoal. A cathartic, such as sorbitol or mineral oil may be given with or after the first dose of activated charcoal but not with subsequent doses. When repeat doses of activated charcoal are used as part of decontamination, electrolyte values should be monitored, since electrolyte shifts may occur. In cattle, sheep, and goats, rumenotomy may be considered to remove plant material prior to the administration of activated charcoal.

Treatment is primarily symptomatic, because no specific antagonist exists. Crystalloid or colloid fluid support may be required. Administration of oxygen may be necessary. Anti-inflammatories and diuretics may be useful, and antibiotics may help to control secondary infections of the mammary glands (Burrows and Tyrl 2001).

Prognosis

The risks will vary depending on the level of intoxication and the signs that develop. Animals with mastitis may fully recover; however, milk production may be reduced. Animals with cardiac effects have a more guarded prognosis (Pickrell et al. 2004).

GRAPES AND RAISINS

Sources

The grape family contains 11–13 genera and 700–735 species. Most species grow on woody vines, but a few species grow on shrubs or small trees. Grapes are an important crop because they are eaten for food in whole fresh form and are used for raisins, currants, juice, and wine. In addition, some taxa are used as ornamentals (Burrows and Tyrl 2001).

Kinetics

Grapes and raisins are ingested orally. It is not known how the toxic component is absorbed, distributed, metabolized, or eliminated from the body.

Mechanism of Action

The mechanism of action for grapes and raisins is not known.

Toxicity

A retrospective evaluation of cases, involving dogs that ingested grapes or raisins, reported to the ASPCA Animal Poison Control Center indicated that a range of doses may produce toxicosis. Raisin dosages that produced renal effects ranged from 2.8 to 36.4 g/kg. Grape dosages ranged from 19.6 to 148.4 g/kg. In this study, there was not a statistically significant difference in survival rates in dogs with varying dosages (Eubig et al. 2005).

Per unpublished information from the ASPCA Animal Poison Control Center, the lowest documented grape dosage leading to renal failure in dogs is 0.7 oz/kg, and the lowest documented raisin dosage leading to renal failure is 0.11 oz/kg.

Grapes and raisins from multiple sources have been involved in the cases reported to the ASPCA Animal Poison Control Center. Grapes from grocery stores as well as homegrown and still-on-the-vine grapes have been implicated alike. Commercial brands of raisins as well as homegrown and organic varieties have been involved. Fruits have been evaluated for pesticides, heavy metals and mycotoxins to determine whether these substances could be a factor in the toxicities, and the results to date have been negative. It is possible that individual animals may be more susceptible to toxicosis than other animals, because reports from pet owners indicate that some dogs never became ill with ingestions of grapes or raisins. More research is needed to determine whether grape and raisin characteristics or animal characteristics or both are involved in this syndrome.

It is possible that other species of animals may also experience toxicoses with ingestion of grapes and raisins. The ASPCA Animal Poison Control Center has had minimal reports on other species, so more evidence is needed.

Clinical Effects
Signs

The typical presentation involves vomiting within 12 to 15 hours of ingestion. The grapes and raisins are often seen in the vomitus and may be seen in fecal material as well. The dogs may exhibit lethargy, abdominal pain, anorexia, and diarrhea. These signs may be present for a few days or, in some cases, weeks. The kidney damage may progress leading to oliguria and finally to anuria.

Laboratory

Blood chemistry panels may begin to show changes as early as 12 hours after exposure, but changes may not be noted for several days. Elevations of calcium, blood urea nitrogen, creatinine, and phosphorus have been documented. Elevations of pancreatic and liver enzymes have been documented in some cases as well.

Differential Diagnoses

Other toxicoses and disease processes produce similar signs and should therefore be considered, especially if there is no known history of *Vitis sp.* exposure. Differentials include exposure to ethylene glycol, lilies in cats, and aminoglycosides as well as leptospirosis, bacterial pyelonephritis, and chronic renal failure. Diseases that increase the risk for acute renal failure may include pancreatitis, heat stroke, hepatic failure, Rickettsia, bacterial endocarditis, and disseminated intravascular coagulation (Lane 2001).

Diagnostics

Antemortem

A history of exposure along with consistent clinical signs provide adequate diagnostic evidence for a diagnosis. Biopsy of the kidney might provide additional information relevant for determining the prognosis.

Postmortem

Histopathological evaluation of tissues in the retrospective study demonstrated that the most consistent renal changes involved diffuse renal tubular degeneration, particularly affecting the proximal renal tubules. Other renal lesions were present in some cases. In addition, histopathology in some cases revealed congestion or edema of the liver, lungs, spleen, pancreas, and abdominal lymph nodes and occasional fibrinoid vasculitis or vascular necrosis (Eubig et al. 2005).

Management of Exposures

Emesis may be induced in dogs that have ingested grapes or raisins if the exposure is recent, no signs are present, and no other contraindications to emesis exist. Caution should be exercised in determining whether contraindications to vomiting exist and whether it is safe to have the pet owner induce vomiting at home. Activated charcoal may be given to dogs once vomiting is controlled in an effort to bind any toxic principle remaining in the gastrointestinal tract. A cathartic, such as sorbitol may be given with or after the first dose of activated charcoal but not with subsequent doses. When repeat doses of activated charcoal are used as part of decontamination, electrolyte values should be monitored, since electrolyte shifts may occur.

Baseline chemistries, complete blood count, electrolytes, and urinalysis should be performed and monitored throughout the course of treatment. Treatment is primarily symptomatic, because no specific antagonist exists. Vomiting may be treated with metoclopramide, H2 antagonists, and/or sucralfate.

Fluid support is required. Dehydration should be corrected and then fluid diuresis should be initiated. Hydration status, lung sounds, body weight, and urine output should be monitored. Diuretics such as mannitol and furosemide may be useful to treat oliguria. Dopamine has also been used in the treatment of oliguria. If hyperphosphate-mia occurs, aluminum hydroxide may be beneficial. If uremia occurs, hemodialysis or peritoneal dialysis may be beneficial. Treatment should continue until signs are resolved.

Prognosis

In the retrospective study mentioned above, ataxia, decreased urine output, and weakness were associated with a negative prognosis. In the same study, 53% of the dogs fully recovered or had mild residual azotema, 12% died, and 35% were euthanized (Eubig et al. 2005).

MACADAMIA NUTS

Sources

Macadamia integrifolia and *Macadamia tetraphylla* trees produce macadamia nuts. These trees have been cultivated in Hawaii since the late 1800s. These nuts are commonly eaten by humans. They may be eaten whole as snack foods, but they are also used in baking and in a variety of recipes.

Kinetics

Macadamia nuts are ingested orally. It is not known how the toxic component is absorbed, distributed, metabolized, or eliminated from the body.

Mechanism of Action

The mechanism of action for macadamia nut toxicosis is unknown.

Toxicity

Dogs are the only reported species to develop toxicosis from ingestions of macadamia nuts. Signs have been reported with macadamia nut ingestions of 2.4 g/kg of body weight to 62.4 g/kg of body weight. Signs may develop within 2 to 12 hours of ingestion and generally resolve within 48 hours (Hansen et al. 2000).

Clinical Effects

Signs

The most common signs from cases reported to the ASPCA Animal Poison Control Center include weakness, depression, vomiting, ataxia, tremors, and hyperthermia. A laboratory study involving 4 dogs confirmed the syndrome, which had been reported to the ASPCA Animal Poison Control Center. Weakness, stiffness, and ataxia appear to be most apparent in the rear limbs. Dogs may be reluctant to stand and have difficulty walking (Hansen et al. 2000).

Laboratory

White blood cell counts were high for all 4 dogs listed in the study above. One dog maintained an elevated white blood cell count 48 hours after ingestion. Numbers of segmented neutrophils including immature forms were increased. A few toxic neutrophils containing vacuoles were noted. The only other laboratory abnormality was alkaline phosphatase. Three of the dogs had high values 24 hours after ingestion, and the values were still elevated 48 hours after exposure (Hansen et al. 2000).

Differential Diagnoses

Other toxicoses may produce similar signs and should therefore be considered, especially if there is no known history of *Macadamia sp.* exposure. Differentials include exposure to ivermectin, milbemycin, moxidectin, or other avermectins; ethylene glycol; 5-hydroxytryptophan; benzodiazepines; barbiturate overdose; ethanol or other alcohols; and bromethalin.

Diagnostics

Antemortem

History of exposure along with expected clinical presentation provide adequate diagnostic evidence. Consistent laboratory findings may help to confirm diagnosis.

Postmortem

No deaths have been reported from *Macadamia spp.* exposures.

Management of Exposures

Emesis may be induced in dogs that have ingested macadamia nuts if the exposure is recent, no signs are present, and no other contraindications to emesis exist. Caution should be exercised in determining whether contraindications to vomiting exist and whether it is safe to have the pet owner induce vomiting at home. Activated charcoal may be given to dogs once vomiting is controlled in an effort to bind any toxic principle remaining in the gastrointestinal tract. A cathartic, such as sorbitol, may be given with or after the first dose of activated charcoal but not with subsequent doses. When repeat doses of activated charcoal are used as part of decontamination, electrolyte values should be monitored, since electrolyte shifts may occur.

Most cases of macadamia nut toxicosis do not require treatment. When treatment is needed, it is primarily symptomatic and supportive, because no specific antagonist exists. If continued vomiting occurs, it may be treated with anti-emetics. Subcutaneous or intravenous fluid support may be required if dehydration is present from vomiting and oral fluids are not tolerated.

Close monitoring is required. Confinement may be necessary to prevent injury in ataxic animals and to reduce sensory stimuli. Body temperature should be monitored, and thermoregulation provided if needed. Monitoring should continue until signs have resolved.

Prognosis

Dogs with macadamia nut toxicosis have a good prognosis. No deaths have been reported, and no sequelae have been noted.

METHYLXANTHINES

Sources

Methylxanthines are naturally occurring alkaloids. They occur naturally in some foods. They are also used as medications. Theobromine and caffeine are the methylxanthines of toxicological significance in chocolate (Table 24.1). Caffeine is also naturally present in coffee and some teas and is added to a number of commercial beverages. Pets are frequently attracted to these foods and beverages and may ingest amounts significant to produce toxicosis. Most methylxanthine toxicoses in dogs occur as a result of chocolate ingestion, so this chapter will focus on chocolate (Beasley 1999).

Kinetics

Methylxanthines are well absorbed from the gastrointestinal tract (Serafin 1995). Signs can develop within 2 hours

Table 24.1. Approximate methylxanthine levels in different forms of chocolate [a]

Chocolate	Total Methylxanthine[b] (mg/oz)
White chocolate	1.1
Milk chocolate	64
Semisweet chocolate chips	160
Baker's chocolate (unsweetened)	440
Dry cocoa powder	800

[a]Levels of methylxanthines in chocolates vary due to natural variations in methylxanthine content of the chocolate base, as well as differences in manufacturing processes.

[b]Includes levels of theobromine and caffeine.

Source: Gwaltney-Brant 2001.

of exposure but onset may be longer especially if the animal ingests the wrappers.

Methylxanthines are distributed throughout the body, cross the placenta, and are passed into the milk of lactating females. The liver metabolizes methylxanthines (Beasley 1999). Enterohepatic recirculation and reabsorption from the urinary tract has been reported (Serafin 1995). The half-life of caffeine and theobromine in dogs is 4.5 and 17.5 hours respectively (Beasley 1999). ASPCA Animal Poison Control Center data indicate that recovery generally occurs within 24–48 hours after exposure provided that the signs are controlled. Drugs that can affect methylxanthine elimination include propranolol, erythromycin, corticosteroids, and cimetidine (Serafin 1995).

Mechanism of Action

A definitive mechanism of action has not been identified, but clinical signs in animals are believed to be related to competitive inhibition of cellular adenosine receptors. Other mechanism of actions may include cellular calcium reuptake inhibition and competition for benzodiazepine receptors (Serafin 1995; Beasley 1999).

Toxicity

Both caffeine and theobromine are present in chocolate. The darker chocolates contain higher levels of methylxanthines than lighter chocolates such as milk chocolate. Toxicosis is possible with either type of product and is dependent upon the dose of methylxanthines ingested.

It is important to determine the combined dose of methylxanthines ingested. The worst case scenario should be utilized for dose calculations. At combined caffeine and theobromine doses of 10–15 mg/kg or less, signs of toxicosis generally do not occur. However, chocolate often contains a significant amount of fat, so gastrointestinal upset and/or pancreatitis may occur with any chocolate exposure. Combined doses of caffeine and theobromine that are greater than 15 mg/kg should be considered significant and may require decontamination and/or treatment. Doses of 50 mg/kg or more may induce signs of cardiotoxicity.

Clinical Effects

Signs

The most commonly observed signs associated with significant chocolate ingestion in dogs and cats include vomiting, restlessness, hyperactivity, tachycardia and other cardiac arrhythmias, tachypnea, polyuria, hyperthermia, tremors, and seizures. Weakness, coma, cyanosis, hypertension, bradycardia, and ataxia may also occur. Death

occurs from heart rhythm disturbances or respiratory failure (Beasley 1999).

Laboratory

Hypokalemia may coincide with diuresis and vomiting (Beasley 1999). Chemistries associated with the pancreas may be elevated 1–3 days after the exposure indicating pancreatitis.

Differential Diagnoses

Other toxicoses produce similar signs and should therefore be considered, especially if there is no known history of chocolate exposure. Differentials include exposure to caffeine tablets, other medications that contain methylxanthines, pseudoephedrine, amphetamines, antihistamines, cocaine, and other products that may cause seizures.

Diagnostics

Antemortem

History of exposure along with expected clinical presentation provide adequate diagnostic evidence. Some laboratories can test for methylxanthines in the serum, plasma, and urine.

Postmortem

Stomach contents can be evaluated grossly for wrappers and may be collected and submitted for methylxanthine testing. Special request for methylxanthine or other toxicology testing is usually required (Hooser and Beasley 1986).

Management of Exposures

Emesis may be induced in dogs and cats that have ingested chocolate if the exposure is recent, no signs are present, and no other contraindications to emesis exist. Caution should be exercised in determining whether contraindications to vomiting exist and whether it is safe to have the pet owner induce vomiting at home. Gastric lavage may be indicated in some cases because chocolate may form a firm mass in the stomach, and lavage may break the mass down and allow for more complete removal than emesis. Activated charcoal may be given to dogs once vomiting is controlled or may be given by stomach tube after gastric lavage is performed. Activated charcoal may bind any methylxanthines remaining in the gastrointestinal tract. Multiple doses of activated charcoal over 3 days may be required (Hooser and Beasley 1986; Shannon 1998). A cathartic such as sorbitol may be given daily if diarrhea is not present. When repeat doses of activated charcoal are used as part of decontamination, electrolyte values should be monitored, since electrolyte shifts may occur.

Close monitoring and nursing care should be provided. Intravenous fluid therapy should be initiated when significant exposure has occurred. Other treatments should be provided as needed based on signs that occur. Tremors may be controlled with diazepam or methocarbamol. Seizures may require diazepam, phenobarbital, or gas anesthesia. Beta blockers or lidocaine may be beneficial for treating tachyarrhythmias, and bradycardias can be treated with atropine (Beasley 1999).

Prognosis

The prognosis is good for animals that receive timely decontamination and treatment.

TREMORGENIC MYCOTOXINS

Sources

Mycotoxins are secondary fungal metabolites, which are toxic to species such as animals, plants, or other microbes. The effects of mycotoxins differ based upon the toxin and its chemical structure (Boysen et al. 2002). Approximately 20 mycotoxins have been identified as tremorgens. The most frequently reported tremorgenic mycotoxins affecting pets are petitrem-A and roquefortine C, both of which are produced by *Penicillium* species (Schell 2000).

Reports of tremorgenic mycotoxin exposures have involved moldy foods including dairy foods, moldy walnuts or peanuts, stored grains, and moldy pasta, as well as compost material (Schell 2000; Boysen et al. 2002). Dogs may ingest moldy food from the garbage or from composting areas. Young et al. (2003) reported on two cases, one involving the ingestion of moldy cream cheese and the other involving the ingestion of moldy macaroni and cheese. Another report described an exposure that involved four dogs from one household that ingested material from a compost pile (Boysen et al. 2002).

Kinetics

Tremorgenic mycotoxins are rapidly absorbed from the gastrointestinal tract, with onset of action occurring from 15 minutes to several hours after the exposure (Young et al. 2003). Reports on distribution and elimination are not available.

Mechanism of Action

A definitive mechanism of action has not been identified, but several have been proposed. One potential mechanism of action is the interference of inhibitory neurotransmitters such as glycine and GABA (Cole 1977; Pitt 1994; Beasley 1999). Additional studies will be required to determine a confirmed mechanism of action.

Toxicity

Severe tremors have been reported in dogs with penitrem A exposure to dosages of 0.175 mg/kg of body weight (Abramson 1997). In a clinical environment, dosage calculation may not be possible, so determining the risk based on dose may not occur.

Clinical Effects

Signs

Common signs reported to the ASPCA Animal Poison Control Center include hyperthermia, salivation, vomiting, ataxia, tachycardia, fasciculation, tremors, seizures, and death. Signs from exposure often begin within 15 minutes to 2 hours after the exposure, but signs may occur after this time frame. Young et al. (2003) reported on an 11-year-old Labrador retriever exposed to moldy cream cheese from the garbage. Signs were noted to occur the morning after the dog ingested the food. In this case penitrem A and roquefortine C were identified by the laboratory when cream cheese from the wrapper was analyzed. Signs in this case included: generalized muscle fasciculation and hyperextension of the extremities, blepharospasms, vocalization, weakness, tachypnea, hyperexcitation, and tachycardia.

A second case documented in this report involved a dog that developed status epilepticus associated with tremorgenic mycotoxin ingestion. Further complications occurred for this dog with the development of aspiration pneumonia potentially associated with emesis or the gastric lavage procedure performed on the dog (Young, et al. 2003). Signs from tremorgenic mycotoxins frequently resolve within 48 hours, but residual fasciculations or intention tremors may persist for longer periods (Young et al. 2003).

Laboratory

Diagnostic laboratories utilize chromatography or mass spectrometry to identify tremorgenic mycotoxins. Electrolytes and other blood values should be monitored based on presenting signs.

Differential Diagnoses

Other toxicoses can produce similar signs and should therefore be considered especially if there is no known history of mold exposure. Differentials include exposure to strychnine, metaldehyde, ethylene glycol, cholinesterase inhibitors, methylxanthines, pseudoephedrine, amphetamines, and cocaine.

Diagnostics

Antemortem

A tentative diagnosis can be made based upon the exposure history and the resulting signs. Confirmation of the diagnosis is dependent on the results of laboratory tests. Suspect food or vomitus may be collected and submitted for tremorgenic mycotoxin evaluation. Food samples should be sent chilled; vomitus should be frozen.

Postmortem

No characteristic postmortem lesions are expected. Suspect food, vomitus, or stomach contents may be submitted for tremorgenic mycotoxin evaluation. Food samples should be sent chilled; vomitus and stomach contents should be frozen.

Management of Exposures

Emesis may be induced in dogs that have ingested moldy food or compost if the exposure is recent, no signs are present, and no other contraindications to emesis exist. Caution should be exercised in determining whether contraindications to vomiting exist and whether it is safe to have the pet owner induce vomiting at home. Gastric lavage may be indicated in some cases. Activated charcoal may be given to dogs once vomiting is controlled or may be given by stomach tube after gastric lavage is performed. Activated charcoal binds organic compounds and is expected to help prevent the absorption of toxins. Multiple doses of activated charcoal may be required. A cathartic, such as sorbitol may be given with the first dose of activated charcoal if diarrhea is not present. When repeat doses of activated charcoal are used as part of decontamination, electrolyte values should be monitored, since electrolyte shifts may occur.

Close monitoring and nursing care should be provided. The patient should be stabilized and signs should be managed. Intravenous fluid therapy should be initiated to prevent or treat dehydration associated with vomiting and to help regulate electrolytes. Other treatments should be provided as needed based on signs that occur. Tremors may be controlled with diazepam or methocarbamol. Seizures may require diazepam, phenobarbital, phenobarbital, or gas anesthesia (Boysen etet al. 2002; Young et al. 2003). Body temperature should be monitored and thermoregulation provided.

Prognosis

The prognosis is good for animals that receive timely decontamination and treatment. Death may occur in untreated animals.

ALCOHOL

Sources

Alcohol toxicosis most frequently occurs when animals are exposed to alcoholic beverages or raw yeast dough but may also occur with ingestion of certain drug formulation or rubbing alcohol.

Kinetics

Ethanol is fully and quickly absorbed from all parts of the gastrointestinal tract generally within 30 to 60 minutes (Ellenhorn and Barceloux 1988; Osborn 1994; Rall 1990). Absorption may be enhanced if the stomach is empty, the concentration of the substance ingested is dilute, or the substance ingested is carbonated (Rangno et al. 1981; Osborn 1994). Absorption may be delayed if there is food in the stomach, gastrointestinal disease is present, certain drugs are in the system, the concentration of alcohol is high, or if there is decreased gastrointestinal motility (Lin et al. 1976; Osborn 1994). Peak plasma levels in humans are 30 minutes to 2 hours after ingestion (Osborn 1994). Ethanol is primarily metabolized in the liver. The remainder is excreted unchanged in the breath, urine, feces, and sweat (Ellenhorn and Barceloux 1988; Osborn 1994).

Mechanism of Action

A definitive mechanism of action has not been identified, but the mechanism of action is believed to be related to dissolution of lipid membranes affecting ion channels and their proteins, which causes depressant effects on the CNS. Another potential mechanism of action suggests that ethanol can also augment GABA-mediated synaptic inhibition as well as changes in chloride ions.

Toxicity

Any dose of alcohol has the potential to cause serious effects in pet animals. Effects will vary based upon the amount ingested and the absorption rate. The minimum lethal dosage in children is 3 g/kg of body weight.

Clinical Effects

Signs

Alcohol intoxication leads to central nervous system (CNS) depression (Rall 1990). The signs most commonly reported to the ASPCA Animal Poison Control Center include ataxia, lethargy, vomiting, recumbency, hypothermia, disorientation, and vocalization. Signs that have been reported but are less common include tremors, tachycardia, acidosis, diarrhea, dyspnea, coma, and seizures. Signs usually resolve within 12 hours of exposure.

Laboratory

Abnormal laboratory values may occur. Complete blood count, chemistry panel, and blood gases should be performed.

Differential Diagnoses

Other toxicoses produce similar signs and should therefore be considered, especially if there is no known history of alcohol exposure. Differentials include exposure to iron, isoniazid, lactic acidosis, diabetes, ethylene glycol, salicylic acid, toluene, and marijuana. Additional differentials may include uremia, diabetic ketoacidosis, or cardiovascular accident.

Diagnostics

Antemortem

Diagnosis may be determined based upon the exposure history and the resulting signs. Blood alcohol levels can be obtained to confirm exposure.

Postmortem

Toxicology tests may be performed on blood or tissues to confirm exposure and cause of death.

Management of Exposures

Emesis may be induced in dogs and cats that have ingested ethanol if the exposure occurred within the previous 25 minutes, no signs are present, and no other contraindications to emesis exist. Caution should be exercised in determining whether contraindications to vomiting exist and whether it is safe to have the pet owner induce vomiting at home. Activated charcoal may be given to dogs once vomiting is controlled. Care should be taken to avoid aspiration of activated charcoal in inebriated animals. When repeat doses of activated charcoal are used as part of decontamination, electrolyte values should be monitored, since electrolyte shifts may occur.

Close monitoring and nursing care including thermoregulation should be provided. Confinement may be required to prevent injury. Heart rate, blood pressure, and electrocardiogram should be obtained. Intravenous fluid and electrolyte therapy should be initiated. Sodium bicarbonate should be included if metabolic acidosis occurs,

and dextrose should be added if hypoglycemia occurs. Other treatments should be provided as needed based on signs that occur. Cardiac drugs that may be of benefit include epinephrine, atropine, lidocaine, and yohimbine. Ventilation and seizure control may be required.

Prognosis

The prognosis is good for animals that receive timely decontamination, supportive care, and treatment.

YEAST DOUGH

Sources

Dogs may ingest raw yeast dough if it is available (Thrall et al. 1984; Suter 1992). A commonly reported scenario involves a dog ingesting yeast bread or roll dough left out to rise on a countertop. Two potential syndromes may occur independently or concurrently, the first being ethanol intoxication and the second being foreign body obstruction of the gastrointestinal tract (Means 2003).

Kinetics

See Kinetics section for ethanol toxicosis.

Mechanism of Action

Foreign body obstruction may occur in the gastrointestinal tract due to dough that expands while in the stomach. See Mechanism of Action section for ethanol toxicosis.

Toxicity

See Toxicity section for ethanol toxicosis.

Clinical Effects

Signs

See Clinical Effects section for ethanol toxicosis. In addition to signs of alcohol intoxication, the ingestion of bread dough has been theorized to cause foreign body obstruction, gastric dilatation and volvulus (GDV), or even gastric rupture. The dough expands in the warm, moist environment of the stomach. Vomiting, abdominal pain, retching, and recumbency may occur.

Laboratory

See Laboratory section for ethanol toxicosis.

Differential Diagnoses

See Differential Diagnoses section for ethanol toxicosis. Other potential causes of gastrointestinal signs and foreign body obstruction should be evaluated.

Diagnostics

Antemortem

History of exposure along with expected clinical presentation provide adequate diagnostic evidence. See Antemortem section for ethanol toxicosis.

Postmortem

See Postmortem section for ethanol toxicosis. Necropsy may reveal dough mass in the stomach, GDV, or gastric rupture.

Management of Exposures

See Management of Exposures section for ethanol toxicosis. Emesis may be recommended with caution, because the stomach may rupture if the dough mass blocks the esophageal sphincter. A stomach tube may be passed to help expel gas within the stomach. A lavage with cold water may help to decrease fermentation and remove some of the dough. Surgical removal of the dough may be required in severe cases. If bloat or GDV occurs, stabilization and standard treatment should be provided (Means 2003).

Prognosis

The prognosis is good for animals that receive timely decontamination, supportive care, and treatment.

XYLITOL

Sources

Xylitol, a sugar alcohol, is a natural sweetener found in plants. It is commonly obtained from birch bark. Xylitol has comparable sweetness to table sugar (Dunayer 2004). It is a nutritive sweetener that provides calories and is found in many human and pet products, e.g., sugar-free gum, dental spray, dental lozenges, and toothpaste. It is also used as a sweetener in products for diabetics, is found in some dietary supplements and chewable vitamins, and in other products designed to be low in carbohydrates.

Kinetics

When ingested, xylitol is absorbed readily from the gastrointestinal tract with peak plasma levels occurring 30 minutes after ingestion (Kuzuya et al. 1969). It may be converted to glucose and then glycogen in the liver (WHO 1978). The liver is where 80% of xylitol metabolism occurs (Froesch and Jakob 1974).

Mechanism of Action

Xylitol is metabolized intracellularly to D-xylulose, which is then metabolized via the Pentose-Phosphate Pathway (PPP). The PPP is believed to control insulin release (Kuzuya et al. 1969). The mechanism of action for liver effects is not known, but has been theorized by Dunayer and Gwaltney-Brant (2006) to be related to either depletion of ATP during the metabolism of xylitol or to the production of reactive oxygen species.

Toxicity

One report involved a dog that ingested 2.96 g of xylotol/kg of body weight. This dog showed signs of lateral recumbency, nonresponsiveness, and gas in the gastrointestinal tract (Dunayer 2004). Unpublished data from the ASPCA Animal Poison Control Center indicates that signs of hypoglycemia may occur at doses of 0.1 g/kg and greater. Dunayer and Gwaltney-Brant (2006) report that 1.4 to 2.0 g of xylitol/kg of body weight has been associated with hepatic failure.

Clinical Effects

Signs

Reported signs include hypoglycemia, vomiting, lethargy, and ataxia. The animal's condition may advance to include recumbency, seizures, and coagulopathy (Dunayer 2004; Dunayer and Gwaltney-Brant 2006).

Laboratory

Abnormal lab values may include low potassium, low phosphate, elevated bilirubin, and elevated liver enzymes (Dunayer 2004; Dunayer and Gwaltney-Brant 2006).

Differential Diagnoses

Additional differentials may include insulinoma, insulin overdose, oral hypoglycemic agents (e.g., sulfonylureas), hunting dog hypoglycemia, juvenile hypoglycemia, and prolonged starvation.

Diagnostics

Antemortem

History of exposure along with expected clinical presentation provide adequate diagnostic evidence.

Postmortem

Xylitol is not expected to remain in the tissues, since it is metabolized quickly.

Management of Exposures

Emesis may be induced in dogs that have ingested xylitol-containing products if the exposure was within 15–30 minutes, no signs are present, and no other contraindications to emesis exist. Caution should be exercised in determining whether contraindications to vomiting exist and whether it is safe to have the pet owner induce vomiting at home.

Close monitoring is required. Glucose should be monitored every 2–4 hours for the first 12–24 hours, and blood chemistries and electrolytes should be monitored. If liver enzymes begin to elevate, coagulation parameters should be monitored. Confinement may be necessary to prevent injury in ataxic animals. Symptomatic and supportive care should be provided and may include administration of intravenous fluids with dextrose, nutritional support, and potassium supplementation. Hepatoprotective agents such as SAM-e, silymarin (milk thistle), or n-acetylcysteine may be given. Monitoring and treatment should continue until signs have resolved.

Prognosis

When treatment is provided and doses that affect the liver are not achieved, the prognosis is good. When hepatic necrosis and coagulopathy occur, the prognosis is guarded.

REFERENCES

Abramson, D. 1997. Toxicants of the genus Penicillium. In *Handbook of Plant and Fungal Toxicants*, edited by Felix, J.P., pp. 303–317. Boca Raton, Florida: CRC Press, Inc.

Beasley, V.R. 1999. *A Systems Affected Approach to Veterinary Toxicology*, pp. 116–120. Urbana: University of Illinois College of Veterinary Medicine.

Boysen, S., Rozanski, E., Chan, D., Grobe, T., Fallon, M., Rush, J. 2002. Tremorgenic mycotoxicosis in four dogs from a single household. *Journal of the American Veterinary Medical Association* 221(10):1441–1444.

Burger, W.P., Naude, T.W., Van Rensburg, I.B., Botha, C.J., Pienaar A.C. 1994. Cardiomyopathy in ostriches (*Struthio camelus*) due to avocado (*Persea americana var Guatemalensis*) intoxication. *Journal of the South African Veterinary Association* 65(3):113–118.

Burrows, G.E. and Tyrl, R.J. 2001. *Toxic Plants of North America*, pp. 744–747. Ames: Iowa State Press.

Cheeke, P. 1998. *Natural Toxicants in Feeds, Forages, and Poisonous Plants*, 2nd ed. Danville, Illinois: Interstate Publishers.

Christopher, M.M., White, J.G., Eaton, J.W. 1990. Erythrocyte pathology and mechanisms of Heinz body–mediated hemolysis in cats. *Veterinary Pathology* 27:299–310.

Cole, R.J. 1977. Tremorgenic mycotoxins. *Mycotoxins in Human and Animal Health, Conference Proceedings*, edited by Rodricks, Hesseltine, and Mehlman, pp. 583–595. Park Forest South, Illinois: Pathotox Publishers.

Craigmill A.L., Eide, R.N., Shultz, T.A., Hedrick, K. 1984. Toxicity of avocado (*Persea americana* [Guatemalan var]) leaves: Review and preliminary report. *Veterinary and Human Toxicology* 26(5):381–384.

Dunayer, E.K. 2004. Hypoglycemia following canine ingestion of xylitol-containing gum. *Veterinary and Human Toxicology* 46:87–88.

Dunayer, E.K. and Gwaltney-Brant, S.M. 2006. Acute hepatic failure and coagulopathy associated with xylitol ingestion in eight dogs. *Journal of the American Veterinary Medical Association* 229:1113–1117.

Ellenhorn, M.J. and Barceloux, D.G. 1988. Ethanol. In *Medical Toxicology: Diagnosis and Treatment of Human Poisoning*, edited by Ellenhorn, M.J. and Barceloux, D.G. New York: Elsevier.

Eubig, P.A., Brady, M.S., Gwaltney-Brant, S.M., Khan, S.A., Mazzaferro, E.M., Morrow, C.K. 2005. Acute renal failure in dogs subsequent to the ingestion of grapes or raisins: A retrospective evaluation of 43 dogs (1992–2002). *Journal of Veterinary Intern Medicine* 19:663–674.

Froesch, E.R. and Jakob, A. 1974. The metabolism of xylitol. In *Sugars in nutrition*, edited by Sipple, H.L., McNutt, K.W., pp. 241–258. New York: Academic Press.

Guo, Z., Muller, D., and Pentz, R. 1990. Bioavailability of sulphur—containing ingredients of garlic in the rat. *Planta Medica* 56:692.

Gwaltney-Brant, Sharon. 2001. Chocolate intoxication. *Veterinary Medicine* 96(2):108–111.

Hansen, S.R., Buck, W.B., Meerdink, G., Khan, S.A. 2000. Weakness, tremors, and depression associated with macadamia nuts in dogs. *Veterinary and Human Toxicology* 42(1):18–21.

Hargis, A.M., Stauber, E., Casteel, S. 1989. Avocado (*Persea americana*) intoxication in caged birds. *Journal of the American Veterinary Medical Association* 194(1):64–66.

Hooser, S.B. and Beasley, V.R. 1986. Methylxanthines. In *Current Veterinary Therapy IX*, edited by Kirk, R.W., pp. 191–192. Philadelphia: Saunders Co.

Kuzuya, T., Kanazawa, Y., Kosaka, K. 1969. Stimulation of insulin secretion by xylitol in dogs. *Endocrinology* 84:200–207.

Lane, I.F. 2001. Treatment of urinary disorders. In *Small Animal Clinical Pharmacology and Therapeutics*, edited by Boothe, D.M., pp. 528–540. Philadelphia: Saunders Co.

Lin, Y.J., Weidler, D.J., and Garg, D.C. 1976. Effects of solid food on blood levels of alcohol in man. *Research Communications in Chemistry, Pathology, and Pharmacology* 13:713–722.

McKenzie, R.A. and Brown, O.P. 1991. Avocado (Persea americana) poisoning of horses. *Australian Veterinary Journal* 68(2):77–78.

Means, C. 2003. Bread dough toxicosis in dogs. *Journal of Veterinary Emergency and Critical Care* 13(1):39–41.

Oelrichs, P.B., Pearce, C.M., Zhu, J., Filippich, L.J. 1995. Isolation and identification of a compound from avocado (Persea Americana) leaves which causes necrosis of the acinar epithelium of the lactating mammary glad and the myocardium. *Natural Toxins* 3(5):344–349.

Ogawa, E., Shinoki, T., Akahori, F., Masaoka, T. 1986. Effect of onion ingestion on anti-oxidizing agents in dog erythrocytes. *Japanese Journal of Veterinary Science* 48: 685–691.

Okuyama, T., Fujita, K., and Shibata, S. 1989. Effects of Chinese drugs "Xiebai" and "Dasuan" on human platelet aggregation (Allium bakeri, A. sativum). *Planta Medica* 55:242–244.

Osborn, H. 1994. Ethanol. In *Goldfrank's Toxicologic Emergencies*, *5th ed.*, edited by Goldfrank, L.R., Flomenbaum N.E., Lewin, N.A., pp. 813–824. Norwalk, Connecticut: Appleton and Lange.

Pantoja, C.V., Chiang, L.C., Norris, B.C., Concha, J.B. 1991. Diuretic, natriuretic and hypotensive effects produced by Allium sativum (garlic) in anaesthetized dogs. *J Ethnopharmacol* 32(3):325–331.

Pickrell, J.A., Oehme, F., Mannala, S.A. 2004. Avocado. In *Clinical Veterinary Toxicology*, edited by Plumlee, K.H., pp. 424–425, St. Louis: Mosby.

Pitt, J.I. 1994. Penicillium. In *Foodborne Disease Handbook*, Vol. 2, edited by Hui, Y.H., Gorham, J.R., Murrell, K.D., Cliver, D.O., pp. 517–630. New York: Marcel Dekker, Inc.

Rall, T.W. 1990. Hypnotics and sedatives; Ethanol. In *The Pharmacological Basis of Therapeutics*, edited by Goodman and Gilman. New York: Pergamon Press.

Rangno, R.E., Kreeft, J.H., Sitar, D.S. 1981. Ethanol dose dependent elimination: Michaelis-Menten v classical kinetic analysis. *British Journal of Clinical Pharmacology* 12:667–673.

Robertson, J.E., Christopher, M.M., Rogers, Q.R. 1998. Heinz body formation in cats fed baby food containing onion powder. *Journal of the American Veterinary Medical Association* 212:1260–1266.

Schell, M.M. 2000. Tremorgenic mycotoxin intoxication. *Veterinary Medicine* 95(4):283–286.

Selim, H.M., Yamato, O., Tajima, M., Maede, Y. 1999. Rumen bacteria are involved in the onset of onion-induced hemolytic anemia in sheep. *Journal of Veterinary Medical Science* 61:269–374.

Serafin, W.E. 1995. Methylxanthines. In *Goodman and Gilman's The Pharmacological Basis of Therapeutics*, *9th ed.*, edited by Hardman, J.G., Limbird, L.E., pp. 672–679. New York: McGraw-Hill.

Shannon, M.W. 1998. Methylxanthines. In *Clinical Management of Poisoning and Drug Overdose*, *3rd ed.*, edited by Haddad, L.M., pp. 1093–1106. Philadelphia: W.B. Saunders Company.

Suter, R.J. 1992. Presumed ethanol intoxication in sheep dogs fed uncooked pizza dough. *Aust Vet J* 69(1):20.

Thrall, M.A., Freemyer, F.G., Hamar, D.W., Jones, R.L. 1984. Ethanol toxicosis secondary to sourdough ingestion in a dog. *Journal of the American Veterinary Medical Association* 184(12):1513–1514.

Verhoeff, J., Hajer, R., van den Ingh, T.S. 1985. Onion poisoning in young cattle. *Veterinary Record* 117:497–498.

WHO (World Health Organization). 1978. WHO Food Additives Series 12. *Xylitol*. Retrieved December 30, 2008, from http://www.inchem.org/documents/jecfa/jecmono/v18je16.htm

Young, K., Villar, D., Carson, T., Ierman, P., Moore, R., Bottoff, M. 2003. Tremorgenic mycotoxin intoxication with penitrem a and roquefortine in two dogs. *Journal of the American Veterinary Medical Association* 221(1):52–53.

Drugs of Abuse

25

Sharon Gwaltney-Brant

ALCOHOL

Ethanol is the most commonly abused drug, and accidental ingestion of ethanol by pets is not an uncommon event. A complete discussion of ethanol toxicosis can be found in Chapter 28.

AMPHETAMINES

Sources/Formulations

Amphetamines encompass a wide variety of drugs, both legal and illicit. The high level of dependency and abuse that these drugs can elicit has resulted in them being designated controlled substances by the U.S. Drug Enforcement Agency. Amphetamines are prescribed legally for the treatment of obesity, narcolepsy, and attention deficit disorder in humans (Volmer 2006). Methamphetamine does have therapeutic uses, but is most infamous as the street drug also known as "crystal," "crank," "meth," and "glass." Pseudoephedrine, an over-the-counter decongestant, is a precursor to illicitly manufactured methamphetamine, and the features of pseudoephedrine overdose will be similar to those seen with amphetamines. Companion animals are generally exposed to amphetamines through the accidental ingestion of prescription or illicit medication.

Kinetics

Most amphetamines are quickly absorbed into the blood stream, and clinical signs can occur very quickly after ingestion (Volmer 2006). Amphetamines are lipophilic and cross the blood-brain barrier to enter the central nervous system. They are metabolized in the liver and both parent compound and its metabolites are excreted in the urine. Elimination by the urine is enhanced in acidic urine.

Mechanism of Action

Amphetamines produce their stimulatory activity through several neurotransmitters, including norepinephrine, dopamine, and serotonin in the central nervous system and through direct stimulation of α- and β-adrenergic receptors in the peripheral nervous system (Bischoff 2007). Amphetamines also inhibit monoamine oxidase and inhibit neuronal reuptake of catecholamines, both of which can result in accumulation of excess neurotransmitters such as serotonin and norepinephrine at the postsynaptic neuron.

Toxicity

Although the oral LD_{50} for amphetamine sulfate in dogs is listed as 20–27 mg/kg, serious and life-threatening clinical signs can occur at much lower levels.

Clinical Effects

Signs

Signs associated with amphetamine intoxication include agitation, restlessness, hyperactivity, aggression, vocalization, hyperthermia, tachycardia, tachypnea, ataxia, tremors, and seizures.

Laboratory

No specific clinical pathology abnormalities are expected, although acidosis, electrolyte imbalances, and hypoglycemia may be seen in severe cases.

Small Animal Toxicology Essentials, First Edition. Edited by Robert H. Poppenga, Sharon Gwaltney-Brant.
© 2011 John Wiley and Sons, Inc. Published 2011 by John Wiley and Sons, Inc.

Differential Diagnoses

Other CNS stimulants such as cocaine, methylxanthines, other sympathomimetics (e.g., pseudoephedrine, phenyl-propanolamine), metaldehyde, antidepressants, tremorgenic mycotoxins, organochlorine insecticides, organophosphorous and carbamate insecticides, 5-fluorouracil, hypernatremia, ephedra (e.g., ma huang/guarana preparations), 5-hydroxytryptophan, or lead should all be considered when presented with a patient with severe CNS and cardiovascular stimulation.

Diagnostics

Blood, saliva, and urine can be analyzed by most veterinary diagnostic laboratories for the presence of amphetamine, although the turnaround time may make the diagnostic laboratory of limited usefulness in diagnosing an acute toxicosis. Over-the-counter drug test kits have the advantages of being inexpensive and readily available at most pharmacies, and providing rapid results (Teitler 2009). These tests utilize urine and appear to be reasonably reliable for amphetamine exposures in dogs. These kits are not validated in nonhumans, so further testing by a veterinary diagnostic laboratory may be needed in legal cases.

Management of Exposures

The goals of managing amphetamine exposures are to stabilize the patient, manage clinical signs, decontaminate (if feasible), and provide supportive care. Agitation, hyperactivity, and other stimulatory signs tend to respond well to phenothiazine tranquilizers such as acepromazine or chlorpromazine. Benzodiazepines should be avoided, because paradoxical worsening of the neurologic effects has been reported (Volmer 2006). Seizures are best controlled with injectable anesthetics (pentobarbital or propofol). Hyperthermia should be managed by external cooling measures (ice packs, fans, etc.). For tachycardia that persists after sedation, a beta blocker such as propranolol should be used. Intravenous fluid therapy will aid in stabilizing the cardiovascular system as well as enhancing elimination of amphetamine via the urine. Although acidification of the urine can increase urinary excretion of amphetamine, severely symptomatic animals may already be acidotic, so urinary acidification is not recommended until it has been established that acidosis doesn't already exist.

In animals that have presented following recent exposure and are asymptomatic, induction of emesis and administration of activated charcoal is recommended. The patient should then be monitored in-hospital for a minimum of 3–4 hours (prompt release products) or up to 12 hours following the ingestion of delayed-release products (i.e., extended release, sustained release, controlled release products). It is important to realize that amphetamines can cause a very rapid onset of signs, so close monitoring during and after decontamination is recommended.

Prognosis

The prognosis for animals ingesting amphetamine depends on the dose ingested, the severity and duration of clinical signs at presentation and the response to appropriate therapy. Complications from severe cases can include injury due to hyperthermia, hypoxia, trauma, uncontrolled seizure activity, or cerebral edema.

BARBITURATES

Sources/Formulations

Barbiturates are derivatives of barbituric acid that are used therapeutically as anticonvulsants and sedatives. Barbiturates are also the primary component of most euthanasia solutions. Most barbiturate poisonings in companion animals are the result of accidental ingestion of human or veterinary prescription products, although ingestion of illicit medications, iatrogetic overdoses, accidental injection of euthanasia solutions, and ingestion of meat from carcasses euthanized with barbiturate-based solutions are other means of exposure (Bischoff 2007; Volmer 2006).

Kinetics

Barbiturates are well absorbed orally. Barbiturates are classified according to their duration of action as ultra–short-acting (less than 3 hours), short-acting (3–6 hours) and long-acting (6–12 hours), which is related to their lipid solubility (Volmer 2006). Highly lipid-soluble barbiturates rapidly distribute throughout the body, including the CNS, and then are very rapidly redistributed into fat and total body water, which terminates their anesthetic effect. Barbiturates undergo hepatic metabolism, and metabolites as well as parent compound are eliminated in the urine. Chronic barbiturate use results in induction of their metabolic enzymes, which can result in accelerated metabolism of barbiturates and other compounds that are normally biotransformed by those enzymes.

Mechanism of Action

In the CNS, barbiturates stimulate γ-aminobutyric acid (GABA), an inhibitory neurotransmitter, receptors and inhibit glutamate, a stimulatory neurotransmitter, receptors, causing CNS depression. Some of the CNS depressive effects of barbiturates relate to their inhibition of the release of other neurotransmitters such as norepinephrine and acetylcholine. Very high doses of barbiturates depress respiration and cardiac contractility, leading to respiratory depression and hypotension.

Toxicity

Barbiturates have a narrow margin of safety and even small overdoses can result in significant CNS depression. The lowest reported oral lethal dosage of phenobarbital in cats is 125 mg/kg (Volmer 2006). The oral LD_{50} (dosage at which 50% will die) for phenobarbital in dogs is 150 mg/kg.

Clinical Effects

Signs

The clinical effects of barbiturates relate to CNS depression, so the signs that can be seen include lethargy, ataxia, weakness, disorientation, recumbency, coma, respiratory depression, tachycardia or bradycardia, hypothermia, and death.

Laboratory

Although a minimum database should be established for patients in order to determine any preexisting conditions (e.g., renal or hepatic insufficiency) that may interfere with elimination of the drug, no specific clinical pathologic abnormalities are expected in patients with barbiturate overdose. Severely comatose animals with compromised respiration may develop respiratory acidosis.

Differential Diagnoses

Other agents that can cause CNS and respiratory depression resembling barbiturate toxicosis include benzodiazepines, macrolide antiparasiticides (e.g., ivermectin, moxidectin), amitraz, ethanol and other alcohols, ethylene glycol, propylene glycol, other sedatives (opioids, phenothiazines, sleep aids such as zolpidem, etc.), and marijuana. Nontoxicologic rule-outs include hypoglycemia, encephalopathy (infectious vs. metabolic), encephalitis, CNS trauma, and cerebral vascular accident.

Diagnostics

Blood, urine, stomach content, and feces can be analyzed by most veterinary diagnostic laboratories for the presence of barbiturates, although the turnaround time may make the diagnostic laboratory of limited usefulness in diagnosing an acute toxicosis. Over-the-counter drug test kits have the advantages of being inexpensive and readily available at most pharmacies, and providing rapid results (Teitler 2009). These tests utilize urine and appear to be reasonably reliable for rapid identification of barbiturates exposures in dogs in a clinical setting. These kits are not validated in nonhumans, so further testing by a veterinary diagnostic laboratory may be needed in legal cases.

Management of Exposures

The goals of managing a patient exposure to barbiturates are to minimize absorption of the drug and provide symptomatic and supportive care to animals experiencing CNS depression. For exposures with no-to-minimal signs, emesis may be induced followed by administration of activated charcoal and monitoring in-hospital for 4–6 hours. Animals that present with severe CNS depression should not have vomiting induced due to the risk of aspiration; in these patients, gastric lavage should be considered. Activated charcoal administration should be repeated every 12 hours until the animals are ambulatory, because redistribution of barbiturate after activated charcoal has been eliminated from the GI tract may result in recurrence of severe depression. Activated charcoal has been shown to act as a "sink" in enhancing movement of barbiturates from the circulation into the gastrointestinal tract, and therefore it is of benefit even in cases where the barbiturate was administered parenterally (Volmer 2006).

Animals experiencing severe coma will need intensive supportive care. Endotracheal tube placement may be indicated in those animals with severe coma and subsequent respiratory depression; in some cases mechanical ventilation may be necessary. Oxygen and intravenous fluids should be administered, and standard nursing care for comatose animals (prevention of hypothermia and decubital ulcers) is important in those animals experiencing severe toxicosis. Depending on the lipid solubility of the barbiturate involved, intravenous lipid solutions may assist in removal of barbiturates from the circulation (see Chapter 8).

Prognosis

The prognosis of barbiturate intoxication depends on the amount ingested and the severity and duration of signs at presentation. Comatose animals provided with prompt and appropriate supportive care have a reasonable expectation of recovery, although it may take up to several days.

BENZODIAZEPINES

Sources/Formulations

Benzodiazepines are used in human and veterinary medicine as sedatives, anxiolytics, and anticonvulsants. There are a large number of different benzodiazepines that are distinguished by their onset and duration of action. Benzodiazepines can trigger dependency in human patients and are widely abused in certain populations, especially psychiatric and substance-abuse patients (Longo and Johnson 2000). Additionally, flunitrazepam (Rohypnol®) has been used illicitly as a "date rape" drug.

Kinetics

Benzodiazepines are well absorbed from the GI tract and are widely distributed throughout the body. They are highly protein bound and highly lipophilic. Most are metabolized in the liver via glucuronide conjugation. Some benzodiazepines have pharmacologically active metabolites with half-lives exceeding those of the parent compound (Volmer 2006).

Mechanism of Action

Benzodiazepines act on GABA receptors, triggering inhibitory impulses in the CNS and resulting in CNS depression.

Toxicity

Although benzodiazepines can produce intoxications that require veterinary care, they tend to have a wide margin of safety, and death is not common unless very large amounts have been ingested or there is coingestion of other CNS depressants. However, even low doses can cause sedation and ataxia. Dosages greater than or equal to a dosage equivalent to 20 mg/kg of diazepam can cause more severe clinical effects and will need veterinary intervention (ASPCA Animal Poison Control Center, unpublished data).

Clinical Effects

Signs

Clinical effects of benzodiazepines can occur as rapidly as 10 to 15 minutes following exposure. The clinical signs associated with benzodiazepine toxicosis include sedation, ataxia, and disorientation. Severely affected animals may become comatose, hypothermic, and hypotensive. Seizures are possible, although uncommon, in comatose patients. Some animals exposed to benzodiazepines present with paradoxical agitation and hyperactivity; in the author's experience, this is most commonly seen with large ingested doses or with juvenile animals (dogs and cats <6 months of age). Rarely, liver necrosis has been reported following therapeutic use of diazepam in cats (Volmer 2006); whether this is an issue with acute intoxications is not known.

Laboratory

No significant clinical pathological abnormalities are expected with benzodiazepine overdose. With large exposures, a baseline minimum database is recommended.

Differential Diagnoses

Other CNS depressants that can cause signs similar to those of benzodiazepines include barbiturates, opioids, alcohols, ethylene glycol, marijuana, amitraz, xylitol, antidepressants, centrally acting skeletal muscle relaxants (e.g., baclofen), macrolide antiparasiticides (e.g., ivermectin), sleep aids such as zolpidem, and marijuana. Nontoxicologic rule outs would include encephalopathy, encephalitis, head trauma, hypoglycemia, and cerebral vascular accident.

Diagnostics

Blood and urine can be analyzed by most veterinary diagnostic laboratories for the presence of benzodiazepines, although the turnaround time may make the diagnostic laboratory of limited usefulness in diagnosing an acute toxicosis. Over-the-counter drug test kits have the advantages of being inexpensive and readily available at most pharmacies, and providing rapid results (Teitler 2009). These tests utilize urine and appear to be reasonably reliable for rapid identification of benzodiazepines exposures in dogs. These kits are not validated in nonhumans, so further testing by a veterinary diagnostic laboratory may be needed in legal cases.

Management of Exposures

Because benzodiazepines have wide margins of safety, animals ingesting small doses (e.g., one tablet) generally can be managed at home provided they can be kept in a secure area away from obstacles (e.g., furniture or stairs) to avoid accidental trauma. Owners should be instructed to keep the animal in a quiet area to reduce the likelihood of paradoxical excitation. Mild ataxia can be dealt with at home, but if the animal becomes recumbent or develops paradoxical excitation, it should be taken to the veterinary hospital for monitoring and further care.

The goals of therapy in benzodiazepine exposures are to minimize absorption and provide symptomatic and supportive care. Because of the potential for rapid onset of signs, decontamination should be performed in the veterinary hospital under veterinary supervision. Ataxic and disoriented animals may be at risk of aspiration if vomiting is induced. For animals showing no or very mild signs, induction of emesis may be considered; otherwise, careful administration of activated charcoal is recommended.

Most animals do very well with decontamination and careful monitoring. In the rare event that severe CNS depression develops, respiratory function should be closely monitored, and flumazenil, a benzodiazepine antagonist, may be used for those patients experiencing respiratory depression. Because flumazenil has a short duration of action, animals must be closely monitored for return of respiratory depression when the effects of flumazenil subside. Recumbent animals require careful nursing and supportive care including IV fluid therapy, thermoregulation (hypothermia is common in comatose animals), and prevention of decubital ulcers. Animals experiencing paradoxical excitation should be given a very low dose of acepromazine (0.01 to 0.02 mg/kg) with the caveat that once the excitation has resolved, the CNS depression may be quite pronounced. Anecdotally, cyproheptadine has also been effective in managing the paradoxical excitation of benzodiazepines. The duration of signs will vary with the type of benzodiazepine, the dose ingested, and the effectiveness of decontamination measure instituted.

Prognosis

Most benzodiazepine overdoses have excellent outcomes, provided patients receive prompt and appropriate care.

COCAINE

Sources/Formulations

Cocaine is an alkaloid extracted from the leaves of the shrub *Erythroxylon coca*, which grows in Central and South America as well as Indonesia and the West Indies. Therapeutically, cocaine is used as a topical local anesthetic for oral and nasal mucous membranes. However, the most common exposures to cocaine in companion animals occur when they are exposed to illicitly obtained cocaine.

Kinetics

Cocaine is very rapidly absorbed across all mucosal surfaces, and clinical effects can be seen within minutes of exposure. Cocaine is metabolized in the serum and liver and is excreted as parent compound and metabolites in the urine.

Mechanism of Action

Cocaine is a potent sympathomimetic that blocks the reuptake of norepinephrine and serotonin in the CNS, causing accumulation of these neurotransmitters in the synapse and resulting in prolonged stimulation of postsynaptic neurons. It also sensitizes the myocardial cells to endogenous catecholamines, resulting in tachycardia.

Toxicity

The LD_{50} for cocaine in dogs is 3 mg/kg IV, and it is reported that dogs can tolerate oral doses 2–4 times that level (Bischoff 2007).

Clinical Effects
Signs

Signs of cocaine intoxication occur quickly following ingestion and include hyperactivity, hyperthermia, agitation, ataxia, mydriasis, vomiting, vocalization, tachycardia, tremors, and seizures. Severe seizures may result in myoglobinemia or disseminated intravascular coagulopathy secondary to hyperthermia.

Laboratory

Metabolic acidosis and electrolyte abnormalities may be seen with cocaine toxicosis. As with most intoxications, a minimum database should be established, including complete blood count, serum chemistries, and electrolyte status.

Differential Diagnoses

Other intoxications from CNS stimulants such as amphetamines, methylxanthines, other sympathomimetics (e.g., pseudoephedrine, phenylpropanolamine), metaldehyde, antidepressants, tremorgenic mycotoxins, organochlorine insecticides, organophosphorous and carbamate insecticides, 5-fluorouracil, hypernatremia, ephedra (e.g., ma huang/guarana preparations), 5-hydroxytryptophan, or lead should all be considered when presented with a patient with severe CNS and cardiovascular stimulation.

Diagnostics

Blood, stomach contents, and urine can be analyzed by most veterinary diagnostic laboratories for the presence of cocaine, although the turnaround time makes the diagnostic laboratory of limited usefulness in diagnosing an acute toxicosis. Over-the-counter drug test kits have the advantages of being inexpensive and readily available at most pharmacies, and providing rapid results (Teitler 2009). These tests utilize urine and appear to be reasonably reliable for rapid identification of cocaine exposures in dogs. These kits are not validated in nonhumans, so further testing by a veterinary diagnostic laboratory may be needed in legal cases.

Management of Exposures

The goals of managing cocaine intoxications include stabilization of the symptomatic patient, decontamination (when feasible) and providing symptomatic and supportive care to minimize complications.

Because of the potential for very rapid onset of severe signs with cocaine ingestion, emesis should only be induced in a veterinary setting and only in asymptomatic animals. Attempting emesis in even mildly symptomatic animals may trigger a seizure. Sedation and gastric lavage should be considered, especially if animals have begun to show clinical signs of intoxication. Activated charcoal should follow emesis or lavage. Police dogs that have ingested bags of cocaine or dogs with surgically implanted bags (cocaine "mules") should be anesthetized and the bags carefully extracted surgically or via endoscopy to avoid rupture and spillage of cocaine onto tissues (Bischoff 2007).

Diazepam should be used to manage existing seizures. Barbiturates should be used for seizures refractory to diazepam. Acepromazine or chlorpromazine may work better than diazepam at managing agitation in nonseizing animals. Cyproheptadine has been recommended by some to block the effects of excess serotonin caused by cocaine; this often helps with disorientation, hyperthermia, and vocalization (ASPCA Animal Poison Control Center, unpublished data). Severe tachycardia may be treated with propranolol once the agitation and hyperactivity is under control. Intravenous fluids will help with hyperthermia as well as provide cardiovascular support.

Prognosis

The prognosis will depend on the amount of cocaine ingested and the duration and severity of signs at presentation. Animals experiencing seizures have a more guarded prognosis.

MARIJUANA

Sources/Formulations

Marijuana is the dried leaves, seeds, and stems of the *Cannibis sativa* plant. The major active ingredient of marijuana is the cannabinoid delta-9-tetrahydrocannabinol (THC). Marijuana is most commonly used as an illicit recreational drug, but it is also used medicinally in humans to limit nausea in chemotherapy patients and to lower intraocular pressure in glaucoma patients (Janczyk et al. 2004). Marinol®, a tablet form of synthetic THC has recently been approved for the relief of nausea and vomiting in chemotherapy cancer patients and assist with loss of appetite in AIDS patients. Most companion animals are exposed when they ingest a "stash" of illicit marijuana, although exposures to medicinal agents or, rarely, through

inhalation of smoke from marijuana cigarettes intentionally blown into their faces are possible (Janczyk et al. 2004).

Kinetics

THC is rapidly absorbed after ingestion or inhalation, with onset of effects occurring within 6 to 12 minutes of inhalation and 30 to 60 minutes of ingestion (Donaldson 2002). THC is highly lipid-soluble and highly protein-bound and undergoes a significant first pass effect when ingested. Because of high levels of storage of THC in body fat, the half-life is relatively long (25–30 hours), with 80% to 90% being eliminated by 5 days after exposure.

Mechanism of Action

The cannabinoids in marijuana act on cannabinoid-specific receptors within the CNS, which trigger most of the psychoactive effects of marijuana. Cannabinoids also interact with a variety of CNS neurotransmitters, stimulating the release of dopamine, enhancing GABA turnover, and enhancing the synthesis of norepinephrine, dopamine and serotonin (Donaldson 2002).

Toxicity

The minimum toxic dosage of marijuana in dogs is reported to be 84.7 mg/kg of dry leaves, which is the equivalent of approximately 1/2 teaspoon of dry leaves in a 30 kg dog (Gwaltney-Brant 2004). Although marijuana can produce significant clinical effects at low exposure levels, it does have a wide margin of safety with the lethal dose being over 1000 times the behaviorally effective dose (Volmer 2006). Doses of 3 to 28 g/kg of marijuana did not result in deaths in dogs. Deaths from marijuana ingestion may be more likely the result of accidental misadventure (e.g., trauma) or leading to complications of preexisting serious health issues (e.g., prior cardiac dysfunction) than from a direct effect of the cannabinoids in marijuana.

Clinical Effects
Signs

The most common clinical effects seen in marijuana toxicosis in dogs and cats are depression, ataxia, and bradycardia. Other common signs include agitation, disorientation, vocalization, vomiting, hyperesthesia, hypothermia, mydriasis, hypersalivation, diarrhea, recumbency, coma, and seizures, although the latter three signs are relatively uncommon (Bischoff 2007; Donaldson 2002; Gwaltney-Brant 2004). A single case of atopic dermatitis in a dog thought to be associated with marijuana has been reported (Evans 1989).

Laboratory

As with most intoxications, a baseline minimum database consisting of serum chemistry and complete blood count is recommended to identify any concurrent disease issues. Marijuana is not expected to cause any specific laboratory abnormalities.

Differential Diagnoses

Intoxication from other CNS depressants such as macrolide anitparasiticides (e.g., ivermectin), amitraz, benzodiazepines, barbiturates, opioids, alcohols, ethylene glycol, centrally acting skeletal muscle relaxants, sedatives, and isoxazole and hallucinogenic mushrooms should all be considered in the differential list if marijuana exposure is suspected but cannot be confirmed historically. Nontoxic differentials include head trauma, encephalopathy, encephalitis, and hypoglycemia.

Diagnostics

Stomach contents and urine can be analyzed by most veterinary diagnostic laboratories for the presence of cannabinoids, although the turnaround time makes the diagnostic laboratory of limited usefulness in diagnosing an acute toxicosis. Over-the-counter drug test kits, which work so well on other drugs of abuse, appear to be less reliable in the detection of marijuana exposures (Teitler 2009). It is possible that the metabolite that many of these tests detect is not one that is excreted by dogs in sufficient quantities for the test to identify. However, some veterinary emergency clinics have reported to the author that they have found some brands of test kits that do appear to work. So, when using the kits it is important to remember that a negative test does not completely rule out marijuana exposure and confirmation from an analytical laboratory should be considered. The OTC kits are not validated in nonhumans, so further testing by a veterinary diagnostic laboratory may be needed in legal cases.

Management of Exposures

Fortunately, marijuana exposures are rarely life-threatening, and providing good supportive care and decontamination is generally all that is needed for successful recovery. Emesis should be induced in animals with mild or no clinical signs. Repeated doses of activated charcoal are recommended (monitor electrolytes for hypernatremia) to attempt to reduce the duration of signs. Central nervous stimulation can be managed with diazepam. Body temperature should be monitored and hypothermia corrected as needed. Intravenous fluids will assist in cardiovascular support but will not enhance elimination of marijuana.

Prognosis

The prognosis in most uncomplicated cases of marijuana intoxication is excellent and most patients will make full recoveries within 2 to 5 days. Once the patient's disorientation has largely resolved and the patient is able to maintain normal body temperature and heart rate, it may be discharged from the hospital. Close supervision is recommended for 5 days after ingestion to avoid accidental injury from any residual ataxia.

OPIATES AND OPIOIDS

Sources/Formulations

There are many opiates and opioids used in human and veterinary medicine. *Opiates* are natural extracts derived from the opium poppy, *Papaver somniferum*. *Opioids* are semisynthetic or fully synthetic compounds that act on opiate receptors. Opiates include morphine and codeine, while semisynthetic opioids include oxymorphone, hydromorphone, hydrocodone, oxycodone, heroin, etorphine, and buprenorphine. Fully synthetic opioids include fentanyl, methadone, propoxyphene, and tramadol. For ease of this discussion, the term *opioid* will be used to include both opiates and opioids.

Opioids are used in veterinary and human medicine for their analgesic effects. Apomorphine is used in veterinary medicine as an emetic. Fentanyl suckers, lozenges, and transdermal patches are becoming more frequently used in both human and veterinary medicine. The lozenges or suckers contain fentanyl citrate in a sucrose and liquid glucose base and are attractive to animals. Companion animals are most commonly exposed when they ingest their own or their owner's medication, lozenges, or discarded fentanyl patches.

Kinetics

Most opioids are well absorbed from the GI tract. Although fentanyl in transdermal patches has poor absorption from the GI tract due to first pass effect, significant amounts of fentanyl can be absorbed transmucosally when animals chew the patches. Metabolism varies, but opioids generally undergo hepatic metabolism with some form of conjugation, hydrolysis, oxidation, glucuronidation, or dealkylation. The requirement for metabolism via glucuronidation may account for the relative sensitivity of cats to opioids.

Mechanism of Action

Opioids are generally classified by their ability to exert effects at the different opioid receptors (mu, kappa, delta, sigma), and by their agonist or antagonist effects on those receptors. Partial agonists act as agonists at one or more opioid receptors and as antagonists at others. Opioids act centrally to elevate the pain threshold and to alter the psychological response to pain. Most of the clinically used opioids exert effect at the mu receptor (mu$_1$ subtype mediates analgesic effects, mu$_2$ mediates respiratory depression). Opioids also can induce emesis through stimulation of the dopamine receptors in the chemoreceptor trigger zone (Volmer 2006). Opioids can, paradoxically, sometimes cause CNS excitation in overdose situations. The exact mechanism is not known but is postulated to involve stimulation of dopaminergic, adrenergic, cholinergic, and/or serotonergic receptors, possibly associated with inhibition of GABA receptors (Kukanich and Papich 2009; Tashakori and Afshari 2010).

Toxicity

The toxicity of individual opioid compounds varies considerably. The minimum lethal dosage of morphine in laboratory dogs is between 110 and 210 mg/kg (Bischoff 2007). Heroin given at 0.20 mg/kg to dogs (route not specified) caused sedation and respiratory depression. The minimum lethal dosage of heroin is 25 mg/kg subcutaneously in dogs and 20 mg/kg orally in cats. Oxymorphone, fentanyl, and etorphine have approximately 10, 80, and 10,000 times the potency of morphine, respectively.

Clinical Effects

Signs

In dogs, CNS signs include depression, ataxia, and seizures. Respiratory depression, vomiting, bradycardia, and hypotension may also be seen. Cats may show excitatory behavior and urinary retention. Some opioids, such as tramadol can result in serotonin syndrome in overdose situations (see Chapter 27 for further information on serotonin syndrome).

Laboratory

As with most intoxications, a baseline minimum database consisting of serum chemistry and complete blood count is recommended to identify any concurrent disease issues.

Differential Diagnoses

Intoxication from other CNS depressants such as macrolide anitparasiticides (e.g., ivermectin), amitraz, benzodi-azepines, barbiturates, alcohols, ethylene glycol, centrally acting skeletal muscle relaxants, sedatives, and isoxazole and hallucinogenic mushrooms should all be considered in the differential list if opioid exposure is suspected but cannot be confirmed historically. Nontoxic differentials would include head trauma, encephalopathy, encephalitis, and hypoglycemia.

Management

The goals in management of opioid overdoses include stabilizing and decontaminating the patient, providing ventilatory support, and providing supportive care until recovery. Treatment in an asymptomatic animal may include emesis if the ingestion is recent. Activated charcoal with cathartic should be administered and the patient monitored for up to 12 hours. If the animal becomes symptomatic, respiratory support may need to be given. If severe respiratory depression is seen, naloxone (a pure competitive antagonist with activity at the mu receptors) can be administered to reverse respiratory effects. As the duration of action of naloxone is much shorter than that of the opioids, repeat dosages may be necessary. Naloxone may not result in the animal regaining full consciousness. Partial agonists/antagonists (i.e., butorphanol) may be used to partially reverse the effects of pure agonists if no naloxone is available. Animals exhibiting signs of serotonin syndrome (agitation, vocalization, disorientation) may benefit from the use of cyproheptadine. Monitoring of temperature, cardiac function, and blood gases is important. Treatment times will vary with the half-life of the opioid.

Prognosis

If respiratory and cardiovascular function can be maintained, the prognosis is good. For those cases that experience seizures, prognosis is more guarded.

REFERENCES

Bischoff, Karen. 2007. Toxicity of drugs of abuse. In *Veterinary Toxicology: Basic and Clinical Principles*, edited by Ramesh C. Gupta, pp. 391–410. New York: Elsevier.

Donaldson, Caroline. 2002. Marijuana exposures in animals. *Veterinary Medicine* 97(6):437–439.

Evans, A.G. 1989. Allergic inhalant dermatitis attributed to marijuana exposure in a dog. *Journal of the American Veterinary Medical Association* 195:1588–1590.

Gwaltney-Brant, Sharon. 2004. Ataxia and depression in a Newfoundland dog, *NAVC Clinician's Brief* 2(10):29–30.

Janczyk, Pawel, Donaldson, Caroline W., and Gwaltney, Sharon M. 2004. Two hundred and thirteen cases of marijuana toxicoses in dogs. *Veterinary and Human Toxicology* 46(1):19–21.

Kukanich, Butch, and Papich, Mark G. 2009. Opioid analgesic drugs. In *Veterinary Pharmacology and Therapeutics*, *9th ed.*, edited by Jim E. Riviere and Mark G. Papich, pp. 302–335. Ames, Iowa: Blackwell.

Longo, Lance P., and Johnson, Brian. 2000. Addiction: Part 1. Benzodiazepines—Side effects, abuse risk and alternatives. *American Academy of Family Physicians* 61:2121–2128.

Tashakori, A., and Afshari, R. 2010. Tramadol overdose as a cause of serotonin syndrome: A case series. *Clinical Toxicology* 45(4):337–341.

Teitler, Joan B. 2009. Evaluation of a human on-site urine multidrug test for emergency use with dogs. *Journal of the American Animal Hospital Association* 45(2): 59–66.

Volmer, Petra A. 2006. Recreational drugs. In *Small Animal Toxicology*, *2nd edition*, edited by Michael E. Peterson and Patricia A. Talcott, pp. 273–311. St. Louis: Saunders.

OTC Drugs

26

Mary M. Schell and Sharon Gwaltney-Brant

ACETAMINOPHEN

Sources/Formulations

Acetaminophen (Tylenol®, nonaspirin pain reliever, APAP) is a synthetic nonopiate derivative of p-aminophenol. Acetaminophen is available as an over-the-counter drug found in a variety of medications. When dealing with a potential exposure to acetaminophen, it is important to verify the exact ingredients in a product, because many medications have nonsteroidal anti-inflammatory drugs (e.g., ibuprofen) rather than acetaminophen as their "nonaspirin" component. Additionally, many of the other ingredients found in combination products (e.g., antihistamines, decongestants) may also contribute to the toxicosis and their potential adverse effects need to be addressed. Acetaminophen is used as an analgesic and antipyretic drug but has little anti-inflammatory action. Most companion animals are exposed through accidental ingestion of medication, although many cats are poisoned when owners are unaware of the hazards of administering acetaminophen to cats.

Kinetics

Acetaminophen is rapidly and almost completely absorbed from the GI tract (Roder 2004). Peak plasma levels are seen at 10–60 minutes for regular release products and at 60–120 minutes for extended release forms. At therapeutic dosages, acetaminophen is metabolized in the liver by sulfation and glucuronidation to nontoxic metabolites that are eliminated in the urine. Because cats cannot effectively glucuronidate acetaminophen, they are particularly sensi-

tive to its toxic effects. The serum half-life in dogs and cats is dose-dependent, increasing as the ingested dosage increases.

Mechanism of Action

Pharmacologic Action

The exact mechanism of pharmacologic action of acetaminophen is unknown but it is believed to act primarily in the CNS to increase the pain threshold through cannabinoid receptors, and it may also inhibit chemical mediators that sensitize the pain receptors to mechanical or chemical stimulation (Ottani et al. 2006). The antipyretic activity of acetaminophen is achieved by blocking the effects of endogenous pyrogens by inhibiting prostaglandin synthesis through inhibition of cyclooxygenase 2 or 3 (Burke et al. 2005).

Mechanism of Toxicity

Acetaminophen itself is of low toxicity. When normal hepatic sulfation and glucuronidation pathways are saturated (e.g., in overdose situations), cytochrome P450 enzymes convert acetaminophen to the oxidative metabolite, N-acetyl-para-benzoquinoneimine (NAPQI). Intracellular glutathione acts as a scavenger to conjugate and neutralize NAPQI, but when glutathione stores are depleted, NAPQI binds to sulfhydryl groups on tissue macromolecules leading to hepatocellular necrosis. At very high doses, the same mechanism occurs in renal tubules, resulting in nephrotoxicity.

Acetaminophen is also deacetylated to p-aminophenol (PAP), which causes oxidative damage to red blood cells

Small Animal Toxicology Essentials, First Edition. Edited by Robert H. Poppenga, Sharon Gwaltney-Brant.
© 2011 John Wiley and Sons, Inc. Published 2011 by John Wiley and Sons, Inc.

resulting in methemoglobinemia (McConkey et al. 2009). Cats are more susceptible to acetaminophen-induced methemoglobinemia because they are deficient in the enzyme that converts PAP back to acetaminophen, allowing buildup of high levels of PAP. Additionally, PAP causes methemoglobinemia by binding to sulfhydryl groups on hemoglobin. As cats have more sulfhydryl groups on their hemoglobin (8 –SH compared to 4 in dogs and 2 in humans) and are deficient in methemoglobin reductase, they are inherently more susceptible to oxidative injury to hemoglobin (Bischoff 2007).

Toxicity

Hepatotoxicity has been reported in dogs at 100 mg/kg and 200 mg/kg can cause clinically evident methemoglobinemia (Talcott 2006). In dogs, dosages of >40 mg/kg have resulted in keratoconjunctivitis sicca 72 hours after ingestion (ASPCA Animal Poison Control Center, unpublished data). In cats, methemoglobinemia has been reported at dosages as low as 10 mg/kg and hepatotoxicity is possible if dosages exceed 40 mg/kg.

Clinical Effects

In cats, methemoglobin values increase within 1–4 hours of ingestion, followed by Heinz body formation within 72 hours. Methemoglobinemia in dogs may occur within 4–12 hours or may be delayed up to 48 hours following exposure (Bischoff 2007). Liver injury may not become clinically apparent for 24–72 hours following exposure. In general, dogs typically develop liver injury while cats develop methemoglobinemia, although at acetaminophen doses over 200 mg/kg, dogs can develop both. Rare cases of cats developing liver injury without initial methemoglobinemia have been reported, but cats most often succumb to methemoglobinemia before liver injury develops.

Signs

Clinical signs seen in patients with methemoglobinemia can include depression, vomiting, weakness, hypersalivation, chocolate brown mucous membranes, hyperventilation, cyanosis, dyspnea, facial or paw edema, tachycardia, hypothermia, hemolysis, shock, and death. Clinical signs of methemoglobinemia may last 3–4 days.

Clinical signs associated with liver injury include vomiting, anorexia, depression, abdominal pain, icterus, tachycardia, tachypnea, and death. Other less common clinical effects include renal insufficiency/damage, myocardial damage, hemolytic anemia and coma. Hepatic injury may not resolve for several weeks.

Laboratory

Methemoglobinemia, Heinz bodies, hemolytic anemia, metabolic acidosis, hemoglobinemia, hemoglobinuria, and hyperbilirubinemia have been reported with acetaminophen toxicosis in both dogs and cats. Changes consistent with liver damage include elevated alanine transaminase (ALT; the most reliable indicator of liver injury), elevated aspartate transaminase (AST), hyperbilirubinemia, bilirubinuria, decreased serum cholesterol and albumin, elevated prothrombin (PT), and elevated partial thromboplastin times (PTT).

Differential Diagnoses

Other causes of methemoglobinemia and Heinz body anemia include onions/garlic, naphthalene, hydroxyurea, chlorates, benzocaine, zinc, skunk spray, and propylene glycol (cats) toxicoses (Plumlee 2004; Stockham and Scott 2008).

Other causes of liver injury include hepatotoxic mushrooms, blue-green algae, iron salts, xylitol, alpha lipoic acid, aflatoxin, cycad palms, castor beans, and idiopathic NSAID hepatopathy (Moeller 2004).

Diagnostics

There are no in-house tests for acetaminophen for animals, and diagnosis is often made based on history and clinical signs. Most human hospitals have the ability to measure acetaminophen levels in serum or plasma, and may be helpful in determining whether an exposure has occurred if the turnaround time for obtaining the results is reasonably short. Veterinary diagnostic laboratories can also measure acetaminophen levels, but turnaround times can be long, making them less useful for diagnosis of acute exposure.

Management of Exposures

The goals of managing acetaminophen exposures include stabilization, prevention of liver damage and methemoglobinemia, decontamination (when feasible) and providing supportive care. Symptomatic patients need initial stabilization, including oxygen if dyspneic. To aid in replenishing glutathione stores, n-acetylcysteine (Mucomyst®, NAC) is used. Adverse effects of the oral route of NAC administration include nausea and vomiting; NAC at concentrations over 5% can be corrosive to oral and esophageal tissue. Recently, an IV formulation of NAC (Acetadote®) has become available. For hepatic injury, a new therapy that shows potential is s-adenosylmethionine (SAMe, Denosyl-SD4®). Early studies and anecdotal reports show a positive effect for treatment of acetaminophen toxicosis. Over-the-counter formulations of SAMe have variable potency and prescription quality, enteric coated products are recommended (round the dose to nearest whole tablet and do not break tablet).

Intravenous fluid therapy is used to correct dehydration and for maintenance needs, but not for diuresis. Whole blood transfusions or Oxyglobin® may be necessary to increase oxygen-carrying capacity in patients with methemoglobinemia. Ascorbic acid provides a reserve system for the reduction of methemoglobin back to hemoglobin; however, ascorbic acid has questionable efficacy and when given orally may irritate the stomach. Cimetidine is an inhibitor of the cytochrome P-450 oxidation system in the liver and may help reduce the metabolism of acetaminophen, although its use is coming into question (Bischoff 2007). Cimetidine is not recommended for cats, because it may increase the accumulation of p-aminophenol responsible for methemoglobinemia.

Decontamination of asymptomatic patients includes induction of emesis and administration of activated charcoal (repeat doses with large exposures) and cathartic. In most cases where overdose is expected to cause severe signs and only oral NAS is available, the administration of a loading dose of NAC is recommended 30 to 40 minutes prior to the first dose of activated charcoal in order to achieve efficacious NAC concentrations as quickly as possible. A 2- to 2-hour interval between subsequent activated charcoal and per os NAC is recommended, because activated charcoal could adsorb NAC as well as acetaminophen.

Liver function and methemoglobin concentrations should be monitored. Liver enzymes and bilirubin may rise within 24 hours after ingestion and peak within 48 to 72 hours. Serum albumin concentrations may decrease significantly after 36 hours and continue to decrease if liver failure occurs (providing a true index of liver function).

Prognosis

The prognosis is good if the animal is treated promptly. Animals with severe signs of methemoglobinemia or with hepatic damage have a more guarded prognosis.

ANTIHISTAMINES

Sources/Formulations

Antihistamines are found in many over-the-counter allergy relief products, both as single drugs and in combination with decongestants and/or analgesics. They are also marketed to prevent motion sickness and as sleep aids. A wide variety of antihistamines are available. These include first-generation agents (FGAs) diphenhydramine, brompheniramine, dimenhydrinate, and chlorpheniramine, and second-generation agents (SGAs) loratadine and cetirizine. Other ingredients in antihistamine medications (e.g., pseudoephedrine) may pose higher risk for severe toxicosis, so it is important to verify all of the active ingredients in a product when an exposure occurs.

Kinetics

Antihistamines are absorbed rapidly when ingested, reaching peak blood levels within 1–3 hours (Gwaltney-Brant 2004). FGAs are small and lipophilic molecules are able to cross the blood brain barrier and cause central nervous system signs such as extensive drowsiness. Other central effects are the result of increased cholinergic activity and include dry mouth and decreased tear release. SGAs are less lipophilic, less able to cross the blood-brain barrier, and thus less likely to cause CNS and cholinergic side-effects (Gonzalez and Estes 1998).

Mechanism of Action

Antihistamines are reversible, competitive inhibitors of the pharmacologic actions of histamine. Cetirizine and loratadine also decrease histamine release from basophils (Boothe 2006). The mechanism of the adverse effects of antihistamine is an exacerbation of normal pharmacologic action.

Toxicity

Antihistamines vary considerably in their toxicity, and many can cause mild adverse effects (e.g., lethargy) at therapeutic doses. Specific toxic doses have not been established for companion animals, although most will tolerate twice therapeutic doses with little more than sedation.

Clinical Effects

First-generation agents are more likely to cause sedation within 30 minutes of ingestion (Gwaltney-Brant 2004). If no clinical signs are apparent at 2 hours following ingestion, development of significant signs is unlikely. At higher doses, especially in animals under 6 months, initial sedation may progress to agitation, tremors, tachycardia, hypotension, and seizures.

Differential Diagnoses

Many conditions can cause signs similar to antihistamine toxicosis. Differentials include systemic infectious/

inflammatory disorders, ingestion of CNS depressants or stimulants, ethylene glycol, alcohol, and marijuana.

Diagnostics

No specific biochemical alterations are expected with antihistamine intoxication. Diagnosis is based on a history of exposure and development of consistent clinical signs. Antihistamine serum concentrations are not routinely measured, although most veterinary diagnostic laboratories would be able to perform the analysis.

Management of Exposures

If the ingested dose is above suggested therapeutic ranges and exposure was within half an hour, induction of emesis should be considered for decontamination. Activated charcoal is indicated in large ingestions. The patient should be monitored for at least 2 to 3 hours following decontamination. Additional care, if needed, is supportive and includes parenteral fluids for marked hypotension and diazepam for seizures or hyperactivity.

Prognosis

The prognosis for most exposures is good provided veterinary care is provided. Clinical signs can persist for up to 72 hours in severe cases. Animals exhibiting seizures or coma have more guarded prognoses.

ASPIRIN AND OTHER SALICYLATES

Sources/Formulations

Salicylates are found in many products. Aspirin (acetylsalicylic acid, ASA) is available alone or in combination with other drugs as tablets, capsules, powders, effervescent tablets, and oral liquid preparations. Bismuth subsalicylate (Pepto-Bismol®, Kaopectate®) is used to treat and prevent diarrhea. Pepto Bismol® (bismuth subsalicylate) contains 9 mg/ml of salicylate. Thus 2 tablespoons of bismuth subsalicylate is equivalent to 1 regular-strength aspirin. Salicylate ointments are used for the anti-inflammatory effects in arthritis and for their keratolytic properties in dermal conditions such as psoriasis. Topically applied salicylic acid can be absorbed through the skin and cause systemic problems. Oil of wintergreen is used as a flavoring for candy and contains approximately 98% methyl salicylate. Salicylates are used in some teething ointments, sunscreens, and topical wart removal products.

Kinetics

Aspirin is rapidly absorbed from the stomach and proximal small intestines in monogastric animals (Gwaltney-Brant 2001). Aspirin is metabolized in the liver and excreted through the urine. The elimination half-life increases with the dosage. In dogs, the half-life at therapeutic doses is 8.6 hours. Cats are deficient in glucuronyl transferase and have prolonged half-lives due to decreased aspirin metabolism. Feline dosages of 5–12 mg/kg have a half-life of 22–27 hours; dosages of 25 mg/kg have a half-life of approximately 44 hours. Elimination is also slower in neonates and geriatric animals.

Mechanism of Action

Aspirin reduces pain and inflammation by reducing prostaglandin and thromboxane synthesis through inhibition of cyclooxygenase. Decreased prostaglandin production results in a decrease secretion of the protective mucous layer in the stomach and small intestine and causes vasoconstriction in gastric mucosa. At very high dosages, aspirin and other salicylates uncouple oxidative phosphorylation, leading to fever and seizures. Salicylates also impair platelet aggregation. Unlike other NSAIDs, salicylate toxicosis does not commonly produce renal injury; instead the liver is the target organ (Gwaltney-Brant 2001).

Toxicity

In dogs, toxicosis has occurred at dosages of 100–300 mg/kg/day PO for 1–4 weeks. Doses of 325 mg twice a day were lethal to cats.

Clinical Effects

Clinical effects of salicylate overdoses include metabolic acidosis with respiratory alkalosis, gastrointestinal ulceration, liver necrosis, and coagulopathy.

Signs

Signs may include vomiting (±blood), hyperpnea, abdominal pain, lethargy, weakness, pallor, diarrhea, pyrexia, increased bleeding times, dehydration, icterus, coma, and seizures. Renal insufficiency is uncommon with salicylate toxicoses but could develop secondary to rhabdomyolysis (from seizuring) or hypotension.

Laboratory

Laboratory abnormalities expected with salicylate toxicosis include high anion gap metabolic acidosis, respiratory alkalosis, anemia, hypoproteinemia, elevated liver enzymes, and elevated white blood cell count.

Differential Diagnoses

Differential diagnoses include ethylene glycol, alcohol, or metaldehyde toxicoses, inflammatory and infectious disorders, hemorrhagic gastroenteritis, viral enteritis, hypoadrenocorticism, gastrointestinal foreign body, anticoagulant rodenticide toxicosis, and other causes of liver failure (acetaminophen, iron, or blue-green algae toxicosis, among others).

Diagnostics

Serum salicylate levels can be measured by veterinary diagnostic laboratories or human hospitals but turnaround times need to be considered when trying to confirm acute toxicosis.

Management of Exposures

The primary goals of treatment are to prevent or treat gastric ulceration, acidosis, hepatopathy, and coagulopathy. Decontamination of asymptomatic patients includes induction of emesis and administration of activated charcoal (repeat dosages with large exposures) and cathartic. Peritoneal dialysis can be effective in removing salicylates. Liver values, glucose, acid base status and electrolytes should be monitored. Gastrointestinal protectant therapy should be initiated to help manage and/or prevent gastric ulcers and should include sucralfate and an acid reducer (H2 blocker or proton pump inhibitor). Misoprostol could be considered in patients at higher risk for GI bleeding (e.g., higher exposure levels, prior NSAID or corticosteroid use). In the asymptomatic patient, gastric protectants should be continued for a minimum of 5–7 days. Bismuth subsalicylate antacid formulations and corticosteroids are contraindicated. Assisted ventilation and supplemental oxygen may be required if the animal is comatose. Seizures should be treated with diazepam. Intravenous fluids, whole blood, and electrolytes should be given as needed to control hypotension and hemorrhage, manage acute bleeding ulcers, maintain hydration, and correct electrolyte abnormalities. Acid base imbalances should be corrected. Hyperpyrexia should be treated conservatively because ice baths or cold water enemas could result in hypothermia.

Prognosis

In most cases of salicylate toxicosis, the prognosis is good if the animal is treated promptly and appropriately.

DECONGESTANTS

Sources/Formulations

Decongestants are found in cold and flu medications, allergy products, and eyedrops intended to decrease redness. The most common decongestants in over-the-counter oral medications are the sympathomimetics pseudoephedrine and phenylephrine. These compounds are often found in combination with antihistamines or analgesics for cold and allergy relief. Because of the similarities with amphetamine, the reader is directed to the amphetamine discussion in Chapter 25, "Drugs of Abuse," for further information on these compounds.

The most common active ingredients in ocular and nasal decongestants are imidazoline compounds such as oxymetazoline or tetrahydrozoline. These compounds work as topical vasoconstrictives and are used to decrease ocular redness associated with conjunctivitis and to decrease nasal congestion due to colds, allergies, and sinusitis. Companion animals are most commonly exposed by chewing on bottles of medication and ingesting the contents.

Kinetics

Imidazoline decongestants are well absorbed from the GI tract as well as across mucosal surfaces. It is thought that the imidazolines are metabolized in the liver, although some fraction is excreted unchanged in the urine. In humans, the half-life is 2–4 hours.

Mechanism of Action

In the central nervous system, imidazolines bind to alpha-2-adrenergic receptors, which inhibits norepinephrine release and decreases sympathetic effects. This results in hypotension, bradycardia, and sedation (Means 2004). Peripherally, stimulation of alpha-2 receptors results in vasoconstriction and hypertension. With oral intoxications the central effects usually predominate.

Toxicity

Imidazoline decongestants have very low margins of safety, with even small exposures resulting in significant clinical signs.

Clinical Effects

Clinical effects can be seen as quickly as 10 minutes after exposure and include vomiting, lethargy or sedation, weakness, collapse, bradycardia, and coma. Hypotension is commonly seen, although occasionally hypertension occurs, often accompanied by hyperactivity and muscle tremors.

Differential Diagnoses

Other causes of hypotension and sedation include alpha-2 agonist (e.g., amitraz, xylzine, medetomidine), calcium channel blocker, cardiac glycoside, and beta adrenergic blocker toxicosis, and primary cardiac dysfunction.

Diagnostics

No laboratory tests to detect these drugs are readily available and no specific clinical pathology changes are expected with imidazoline toxicosis.

Management of Exposures

Decontamination following exposure is generally impractical due to the rapidity of onset of signs and the small volume of liquid medication that is involved. Exposed asymptomatic animals should be monitored for the development of signs for a minimum of 4 hours following exposure. Symptomatic animals should be administered intravenous fluids. If needed, atropine, yohimbine, or atipamezole may be used to increase heart rate and blood pressure. The latter two drugs are preferred because they are alpha antagonists and can reverse many of the clinical effects.

Prognosis

Animals receiving appropriate treatment have a good prognosis for recovery.

NONSTEROIDAL ANTI-INFLAMMATORY MEDICATIONS

This section covers the nonsalicylate NSAIDs. Aspirin and other salicylates are discussed elsewhere in this chapter.

Sources/Formulations

Nonsteroidal anti-inflammatory medications (NSAIDs) are commonly used to treat pain and inflammation and to reduce fevers. Many are also available in combination with antihistamines and/or decongestants in cold, flu, and allergy products. It is important to verify the active ingredients in over-the-counter products because clients are sometimes confused as to which NSAID (e.g., ibuprofen vs. naproxen) the product contains, and there may be additional ingredients such as caffeine, antihistamines, or decongestants that might contribute to adverse effects. There are several NSAIDs approved for use in veterinary medicine. Most exposures to NSAIDs in companion animals are due to accidental ingestion of human or veterinary formulations, although iatrogenic exposures through overzealous administration by pet owners are common.

Kinetics

In general, over-the-counter NSAIDs are well absorbed from the stomach and upper small intestine, and are highly (>90%) protein-bound (Burke et al. 2005). They exhibit a higher degree of toxicity when other highly protein-bound drugs are coingested. Most NSAIDs undergo liver metabolism, with metabolites excreted primarily via the urine. One exception is naproxen, which is excreted via the bile in dogs, undergoes extensive enterohepatic recirculation, and has a long half-life (74 hours).

Mechanism of Action

NSAIDs inhibit prostaglandin synthesis by blocking the conversion of arachidonic acid to various prostaglandins through the inhibition of the enzyme cyclooxygenase (COX). Although many modern NSAIDs are marketed as being specific for certain forms of COX (e.g., COX-2), the fact that COX specificity is lost in overdose situations minimizes the importance of this distinction (Talcott 2006). The NSAIDs decrease secretion of the protective mucous layer in the stomach and small intestine and cause vasoconstriction in gastric mucosa. Renal effects include inhibition of renal blood flow, glomerular filtration rate, tubular ion transport, renin release, and water homeostasis. Some NSAIDs also affect platelet aggregation and possibly hepatic function, although unlike salicylates, serious hepatotoxicosis does not appear to be a common problem with acute NSAID overdoses.

Toxicity

There is tremendous variation in the degree of toxicity among the many NSAIDs, as well as significant species and individual variation in sensitivity to the different NSAIDs (Table 26.1). Many over-the-counter NSAIDs (e.g., naproxen and ibuprofen) pose risk for gastrointestinal injury at commonly suggested doses, especially when given repeatedly. Larger overdoses can result in renal tubular injury. Ibuprofen can cause severe neurologic dysfunction when dosages exceed 400 mg/kg (Dunayer 2004).

A rough rule of thumb for dogs is that GI toxicity may be seen at 4–5 times the therapeutic dose of a given NSAID and renal injury may occur at doses 8–10 times the therapeutic doses. Cats are considered to be 2–4 times more sensitive than dogs (Dunayer 2004).

Clinical Effects

The onset of GI upset is generally within the first 2–6 hours after ingestion, with GI hemorrhage and ulceration occurring 12 hours to 4 days postingestion. In severe cases, gastrointestinal perforation may occur, causing septic peritonitis and shock. The onset of renal failure

Table 26.1. Therapeutic and toxic dosages for selected NSAIDs in dogs and cats

NSAID	Therapeutic Dosage	Toxic Dosage (GI)[a]	Toxic Dosage (Renal)[a]
Ibuprofen	Dogs: 5 mg/kg q 24 h	Dogs: >25 mg/kg	Dogs: >175 mg/kg(>400 mg/kg associated with CNS signs)
	Cats: None	Cats: >10 mg/kg	Cats: Not known but thought to be twice as sensitive as dogs
Naproxen	Dogs: 2 mg/kg q 48 h	>5 mg/kg	>20 mg/kg
	Cats: None		
Carprofen	Dogs: 4.4 mg/kg PO q 24 h or 2.2 mg/kg PO q 12 h	Dogs: >20 mg/kg	Dogs: >40 mg/kg
	Cats: 1–2 mg/kg SQ once or 2 mg/kg PO q 12 h for 48 h	Cats: >4 mg/kg	Cats: >8 mg/kg
Deracoxib	Dogs: 1–2 mg/kg q 12 h	Dogs: 15 mg/kg	Dogs: 30 mg/kg
	Cats: None	Cats: 4 mg/kg	Cats: 8 mg/kg

[a]These dosages are for young adult, healthy animals; pediatric animals, geriatric animals, or animals with prior health issues may be more susceptible to the effects of NSAID overdose.

Sources: Plumb 2005; Dunayer 2004; Gwaltney-Brant 2010.

usually occurs within the first 12 hours after massive exposure to an NSAID but may be delayed for 3–5 days.

Signs

Clinical signs include vomiting, hematemesis, depression, anorexia, hyperthermia, melena, abdominal pain, and hematochezia. Polydipsia, polyuria, dehydration, lethargy, hematuria, and oliguria have been reported in animals experiencing renal injury from NSAIDs. Central nervous signs include depression, ataxia, tremors, seizures, coma, and hypothermia.

Laboratory

Complete blood counts may reflect GI hemorrhage and inflammation, with elevations in white blood cell and segmented neutrophil counts and decreases in hematocrit noted. Patients with renal failure will have increases in BUN and creatinine as well as isosthenuria. With larger overdoses of NSAIDs, transient elevations in liver enzymes (especially ALT) may be noted.

Differential Diagnoses

Other potential causes of gastrointestinal upset and hemorrhage include hemorrhagic gastroenteritis, hypoadrenocorticism, gastrointestinal foreign bodies, viral enteritis, and gastrointestinal neoplasia. Other causes of renal failure include leptospirosis and ingestion of grapes/raisins, lilies(cats), ethylene glycol, and heavy metals.

Diagnostics

Antemortem

Serum measurements for many NSAIDs can be performed at veterinary diagnostic laboratories and many human hospitals, but turnaround time may be too long to assist in diagnosis of an acute case. Diagnosis is generally based on history of exposure and development of consistent clinical signs.

Postmortem

Lesions associated with ibuprofen overdose include perforations, erosions, ulcers, and hemorrhages in the upper (stomach and duodenum) and, on occasion, lower (colon) gastrointestinal tract. Renal damage includes renal tubular necrosis and/or papillary necrosis.

Management of Exposures

Decontamination includes emesis if it can be performed within an hour of ingestion and activated charcoal if within 4 hours postingestion. Activated charcoal should not be administered if there is evidence of gastrointestinal bleeding, because the charcoal may impede healing of ulcerated areas. Gastrointestinal protectants (H2 blocker or proton pump inhibitor, sucralfate, and misoprostol) should be maintained for 5–10 days or longer if evidence of GI bleeding occurs. For animals ingesting potentially nephrotoxic doses, intravenous (IV) fluid therapy at 2× maintenance rate for a minimum of 48 hours (72 hours for naproxen) is recommended to protect renal tubules. Animals with evidence of renal insufficiency should be managed as for any type of acute renal failure. Central nervous system signs should be treated symptomatically (i.e., diazepam for seizures, oxygen and thermoregulation for coma).

Prognosis

The prognosis is dependent upon the dose ingested, species of animal involved, and promptness of treatment. Those with mild GI and renal effects can be expected to make full recoveries; patients with gastrointestinal perforation or severe renal insufficiency have more guarded prognoses.

PHENYLPROPANOLAMINE

Sources/Formulations

Phenylpropanolamine (PPA) is a sympathomimetic agent that has been withdrawn from the human market due to an association with increased stroke risk, but it is still used in veterinary medicine for controlling urinary incontinence in dogs. Chewable veterinary formulations are extremely palatable, especially to dogs, which may increase the risk of accidental overdose.

Kinetics

Phenylpropanolamine is quickly absorbed orally, although extended release products may have a delayed onset of action (Means 2004).

Mechanism of Action

Sympathomimetics like PPA stimulate α- and β-adrenergic receptors, resulting in the release of endogenous catecholamines in the brain and heart. This results in peripheral vasoconstriction, cardiac stimulation and bronchodilation (Means 2004).

Toxicity

Signs can be seen at therapeutic doses in some dogs, and serious signs appear at dosages above 20 mg/kg (Means 2004).

Clinical Effects

Signs normally start within 30–90 minutes and may continue up to 72 hours, depending on the dose ingested.

Signs of PPA toxicosis include tachycardia, hypertension, panting, agitation, hyperesthesia, piloerection, hyperthermia, tremors, seizures, and secondary depression. Bradycardia may result in response to hypertension; therefore, dogs may present either depressed, bradycardic, and hypertensive OR agitated, tachycardic, and hypertensive.

Differential Diagnoses

Differential diagnoses include intoxication from other CNS stimulants such as other sympathomimetics (e.g., pseudoephedrine, amphetamine), metaldehyde, cocaine, ethylene glycol, albuterol, strychnine, and 5-hydroxytryptophan.

Diagnostics

Diagnosis is based on clinical signs and history. Serum levels can be measured at a veterinary diagnostic laboratory, but turnaround times may be too long to assist in prompt diagnosis of an acute case.

Management of Exposures

Because of the potential for rapid onset of signs, emesis should be induced at the veterinary hospital and within 30 minutes of exposure. Activated charcoal should be given if no contraindications exist. Heart rate and blood pressure should be closely monitored. Phenothiazines (acepromazine or chlorpromazine) may be used to control agitation, and may also help to lower the blood pressure. Cyproheptadine has been found to be useful for alleviating some of the central nervous system signs. Nitroprusside or other pressor agents may be used to manage severe hypertension. Managing the blood pressure often results in correction of the reflex bradycardia. Atropine is contraindicated in the management of bradycardia because it will worsen the hypertension. Beta-blockers should not be used on bradycardic animals because they will worsen the bradycardia. In tachycardic animals very low doses of metoprolol (preferred due to beta-1 selectivity and short half-life) or propranolol may be considered but should be used with caution and only after CNS signs (agitation, hyperactivity) have been controlled. Intravenous fluids are recommended to promote excretion, protect renal function, and aid in thermoregulation. Fluid rates should be adjusted accordingly in hypertensive animals.

Prognosis

The prognosis will depend on the dose ingested, severity of clinical signs, elapsed time between onset of signs and institution of therapy, and response to therapy. Animals experiencing seizures have a more guarded prognosis.

VITAMINS

Sources/Formulations

Vitamin supplements are widely available and include multivitamins as well as products containing single vitamins as ingredients. Many vitamin supplements also contain a variety of minerals (e.g., iron, selenium, etc.). Most products are designed to provide the minimum daily requirement (MRA) of vitamins, but some products have higher potencies and contain several times the MRA in each tablet or capsule. For instance, most vitamin supplements contain vitamin D_3 at 400 IU per serving, but high-potency products containing 1000 to 50,000 IU have become available and these pose a higher risk of acute toxicosis.

Toxicity

Ingredients of concern in vitamin supplements include iron and vitamin D. Water-soluble vitamins (B vitamins, vitamin C) are not likely to cause significant clinical effects because excess vitamins are eliminated through the urine. However, formulations with B vitamins can result in benign orange discoloration of the urine. High doses of niacin (vitamin B3) can cause a self-limiting flushing of the skin of the face and ear pinnas in some dogs (though transiently uncomfortable, no serious harm will occur). Vitamin C can be irritating to the gastrointestinal tract and result in mild, transient vomiting, or diarrhea.

Vitamin D is of concern if the ingested dosage exceeds 0.1 mg/kg (4000 IU/kg). (See to the cholecalciferol section of Chapter 17 for information on risks and management of vitamin D exposures.) Iron dosages above 20 mg/kg can cause vomiting and diarrhea; dosages over 60 mg/kg can cause corrosive injury to the intestinal mucosa and liver injury. (see the iron section in Chapter 29 for further information on iron toxicosis.)

REFERENCES

Bischoff, Karen. 2007. Toxicity of over-the-counter drugs. In *Veterinary Toxicology: Basic and Clinical Principles*, edited by Ramesh C. Gupta, pp. 363–390. San Diego: Elsevier.

Boothe, Dawn M. 2006. *Small Animal Pharmacology and Therapeutics*. St. Louis: Saunders.

Burke, Anne, Smyth, Emer, and FitzGerald, Garret A. 2005, Analgesic-antipyretic and antiinflammatory agents: Pharmacotherapy of gout. In *Goodman & Gilman's The Pharmacological Basis of Therapeutics, 11th edition*, edited by Laurence Brunton, John Lazo, and Keith Parker, pp. 671–716. New York: McGraw-Hill Professional.

Dunayer, Eric K. 2004. Ibuprofen toxicosis in dogs, cats, ferrets. *Veterinary Medicine* 99(7):580–586.

Gonzalez, M.A., and Estes, K.S. 1998. Pharmacokinetic overview of oral second-generation H1 antihistamines. *International Journal of Clinical Pharmacology and Therapeutics* 36(5):292–300.

Gwaltney-Brant, Sharon M. 2010. *Toxicology of Pain Medication*. Proceedings from the CVC Baltimore, Baltimore, MD, April 11, 2010.

———. 2004. Antihistamines. In *Veterinary Clinical Toxicology*, edited by Konnie H. Plumlee, pp. 309–311. St. Louis: Mosby.

———. 2001. Salicylate toxicosis in dogs and cats. *Standards of Care: Emergency and Critical Care Medicine* 4(7):1–5.

McConkey, S.E., Grant, D.M., and Cribb A.E. 2009. The role of para-aminophenol in acetaminophen-induced methemoglobinemia in dogs and cats. *Journal of Veterinary Pharmacology and Therapeutics* 32(6):585–595.

Means, Charlotte. 2004. Decongestants. In *Veterinary Clinical Toxicology*, edited by Konnie H. Plumlee, pp. 309–311. St. Louis: Mosby.

Moeller, Robert B. 2004. Hepatobiliary system: Toxic response of the hepatobiliary system. In *Veterinary Clinical Toxicology*, edited by Konnie H. Plumlee, pp. 61–68. St. Louis: Mosby.

Ottani, A., Leone, S., Sandrini, M., Ferrari, A., and Bertolini, A. 2006. The analgesic activity of paracetamol is prevented by the blockade of cannabinoid CB1 receptors, *European Journal of Pharmacology*, 531(1–3): 280–281.

Plumb, Donald C. 2005. *Veterinary Drug Handbook, 5th edition*. Ames, Iowa: Blackwell.

Plumlee, Konnie H. 2004. Hematic system. In *Clinical Veterinary Toxicology*, edited by Konnie H. Plumlee, p. 59. St. Louis: Mosby.

Roder, Joseph D. 2004. Analgesics. In *Clinical Veterinary Toxicology*, edited by Konnie H. Plumlee, pp. 282–284. St. Louis: Mosby.

Sellon, Rance K. 2006. Acetaminophen. In *Small Animal Toxicology, 2nd edition*, edited by Michael E. Peterson and Patricia A. Talcott, pp. 550–558. St. Louis: Saunders.

Stockham, Steven L. and Scott, Michael A. 2008. *Fundamentals of Veterinary Clinical Pathology, 2nd edition*, p. 186. Oxford: Blackwell.

Talcott, Patricia A. 2006. Nonsteroidal antiinflammatories. In *Small Animal Toxicology, 2nd edition*, edited by Michael E. Peterson and Patricia A. Talcott, pp. 902–933. St. Louis: Saunders.

Prescription Drugs

27

Sharon Gwaltney-Brant

ALBUTEROL

Sources/Formulations

Albuterol (salbutamol) and albuterol sulfate are bronchodilators available as tablets (immediate- and extended-release forms), oral syrups, liquids for nebulization, and aerosols for inhalation (Rosendale 2004). Bronchodilators are used for the management of airway diseases such as asthma. Companion animals are most commonly exposed when they accidentally ingest tablets or liquids or when they bite into pressurized inhalers.

Kinetics

Albuterol is rapidly absorbed via inhalation or ingestion. Albuterol crosses the blood brain barrier and placenta; it is not known whether albuterol distributes into milk. Albuterol is metabolized to inactive metabolites in the liver and is excreted as metabolites and parent compound in the urine.

Mechanism of Action

The pharmacologic action of albuterol is due to stimulation of β_2 adrenergic receptors on bronchial smooth muscle, causing bronchodilation (Mensching and Volmer 2007). In overdose situations, the β_2 selectivity is lost and β_1 receptors are also stimulated resulting in increased rate and force of contraction of the heart. Peripheral vasodilation results in hypotension, potentiating the tachycardia and increasing the likelihood of more severe cardiac arrhythmias such as premature ventricular contraction,

atrioventricular block, etc. Stimulation of β_2 receptors on skeletal muscle results in muscle tremors.

Toxicity

Toxic doses for albuterol have not been established, but adverse clinical effects can be seen in some dogs at therapeutic dosages (0.05 mg/kg for dogs) (Rosendale 2004). Animals biting into inhalers could have the entire contents expelled into the oral cavity and pharynx, resulting in exposures many times the therapeutic levels (Mensching and Volmer 2007).

Clinical Effects

Aerosolized products can have an almost immediate effect; tablets and liquids may have some delay in onset of clinical signs.

Signs

Clinical signs of albuterol toxicosis include tachycardia or other arrhythmia, weakness, lethargy, tachypnea, aggression, agitation, hyperactivity, vomiting, and tremors (Mensching and Volmer 2007). Seizures, although uncommon, can occur.

Laboratory

Hypokalemia and hypophosphatemia have been reported in dogs with albuterol toxicosis (Mensching and Volmer 2007). Although the hypophosphatemia generally resolves on its own, hypokalemia may require potassium supplementation.

Small Animal Toxicology Essentials, First Edition. Edited by Robert H. Poppenga, Sharon Gwaltney-Brant.
© 2011 John Wiley and Sons, Inc. Published 2011 by John Wiley and Sons, Inc.

Differential Diagnosis

Other central nervous system and cardiovascular stimulants such as methylxanthines, amphetamines, cocaine, antidepressants, ethylene glycol, metaldehyde, pseudoephedrine, and phenylpropanolamine can cause signs resembling albuterol toxicosis.

Diagnostics

Plasma albuterol levels can be measured but require submission to a specialty laboratory, so they would not be helpful in making a prompt diagnosis.

Management of Exposures

The goals of management of albuterol toxicosis are control of clinical signs, correction of electrolyte abnormalities, and supportive care until full recovery. Decontamination is inadvisable, and likely to be unrewarding, in cases involving aerosol or liquid formulations due to the rapidity of onset of clinical signs (Rosendale 2004). Intravenous fluid therapy is key to providing cardiovascular support in patients with albuterol toxicosis. In mild toxicosis, fluid therapy may be sufficient to manage hypotension; however, with more severe intoxications, more aggressive treatment will be necessary. Diazepam should be utilized first to manage central nervous system stimulation, because some tachycardia may be due to the agitated state of the patient. Propranolol is the beta blocker of choice in treating tachycardia that persists after central nervous system stimulation has been managed; propranolol also often assists in normalizing serum potassium. Once the heart rate is within reasonable levels, the serum should be analyzed for hypokalemia and potassium supplementation administered as needed.

Prognosis

Most animals receiving prompt and appropriate care will recover within 12 hours of exposure, but large overdoses may result in signs that last for 24–48 hours.

ANTIDEPRESSANTS

Introduction

The use of psychotropic drugs to alter behavior of humans and animals has dramatically increased in the last decade. The behaviors that these types of drugs are intended to alter include depression, anxiety, obsessive/compulsive behavior, and undesirable impulses such as smoking in humans. With the increased usage of these drugs, the potential for accidental overdosage in companion animals has increased. This is especially true for dogs, who due to

Table 27.1. Classes of antidepressants

Tricyclic Antidepressants
Amitriptyline (Elavil®)
Clomipramine (Clomicalm®)
Doxepin (Sinequin®)
Imipramine (Tofranil®)
Nortriptyline (Pamelor®)

Selective Serotonin Reuptake Inhibitors
Citalopram (Celexa®)
Escitalopram (Lexapro®)
Fluoxetine (Prozac®)
Paroxetine (Paxil®)
Sertraline (Zoloft®)

Nonselective Serotonin Reuptake Inhibitors
Desvenlafaxine (Pristiq®)
Venlafaxine (Effexor®)

Monoamine Oxidase Inhibitors
Phenylzine (Nardil®)
Selegiline (Eldepryl®, Anypril®)

Atypical Antidepressants
Bupropion (Wellbutrin®)
Mirtazapine (Remeron®)
Nefazodone (Serzone®)
Trazodone (Desyrell®)

their inquisitive nature and often indiscriminate eating habits, may ingest entire prescriptions of psychotropic drugs in one sitting. Table 27.1 gives examples of the various classes of psychotropic drugs used in human and veterinary medicine.

Serotonin and Serotonin Syndrome

Early psychotropic drugs were nonselective and frequently targeted a variety of areas of the central nervous system (CNS). Over time, it became apparent that certain neurotransmitters in the CNS were more influential in altering undesirable behaviors, and drugs that more selectively targeted those neurotransmitters were developed. Serotonin is one neurotransmitter that appears to be extremely important in managing many CNS disorders and older drugs that targeted a variety of neurotransmitters (e.g., tricyclic antidepressants) have, in human medicine, largely given way to drugs that more selectively alter CNS serotonin levels, including selective serotonin reuptake inhibitors (SSRIs) and nonselective serotonin reuptake inhibitors (NSSRIs).

Table 27.2. Mechanism of action of serotonergic drugs

Increase Serotonin Synthesis
L-tryptophan
5-hydroxytryptophan
 	
Increase Serotonin Release
Amphetamine
Cocaine
Fenfluramine (Pondimin®)
Reserpine
Dextromethorphan
 	
Decrease Serotonin Metabolism
Amphetamine (metabolites)
Monoamine Oxidase Inhibitors
   Phenylzine (Nardil®)
   Selegiline (Eldepryl®, Anypril®)
 	
Serotonin Receptor Agonist
Buspirone (Buspar®)
Lysergic acid diethylamide (LSD)
Sumatriptan (Imitrex®)
	Inhibit Serotonin Reuptake
	Tricyclic Antidepressants
	   Amitriptyline (Elavil®)
	   Clomipramine (Clomicalm®)
	   Doxepin (Sinequin®)
	   Imipramine (Tofranil®)
	   Nortriptyline (Pamelor®)
	Selective Serotonin Reuptake Inhibitors
	   Citalopram (Celexa®)
	   Escitalopram (Lexapro®)
	   Fluoxetine (Prozac®)
	   Paroxetine (Paxil®)
	   Sertraline (Zoloft®)
	Nonselective Serotonin Reuptake
	   Inhibitors
	   Venlafaxine (Effexor®)
	Other Serotonin Reuptake Inhibitors
	   Amphetamine
	   Cocaine
	   Dextromethorphan
	   Meperidine (Demerol®)
	   Nefazodone (Serzone®)
	   Tramadol (Ultram®)
	   Trazodone (Desyrell®)

Source: Mills 2005.

Enhancing serotonin levels in the CNS can result in dramatic and favorable alterations in behaviors of humans and animals. However, excessive levels of serotonin can result in a severe and potentially life-threatening condition termed *serotonin syndrome*. Many CNS stimulants that primarily affect other neurotransmitters such as norepinephrine and/or dopamine (e.g., amphetamines and cocaine), also have some degree of serotonergic action, so at least part of the clinical effects seen may be due to serotonin excess (Table 27.2). In humans, serotonin syndrome is most commonly seen when two different serotonergic drugs are administered simultaneously, or when insufficient time has elapsed between discontinuation of one class of serotonergic drug and institution of therapy with a different class of serotonergic drug. In dogs, serotonin syndrome has been associated with excessive ingestion of 5-hydroxytryptophan as well as a variety of serotonergic drugs (Gwaltney-Brant 2004; Wismer 2000).

Clinical Effects
Serotonin syndrome is characterized by a variety of effects including altered mental status (agitation or depression,

aggression, vocalization, seizures, etc.), altered neuromuscular activity (rigidity, myoclonus, tremors, hyperreflexia, ataxia, etc.), hyperthermia, autonomic derangements, and diarrhea. Death can be due to hyperthermia, respiratory compromise or disseminated intravascular coagulopathy.

General Management of Serotonin Syndrome
Management of serotonin syndrome includes managing any severe CNS effects with diazepam or a phenothiazine; refractory seizures may require general anesthesia (Merola and Dunayer 2006; Gwaltney-Brant 2004; Wismer 2000). Due to its serotonin-blocking effects, cyproheptadine may be beneficial in managing the agitation, hyperthermia, and vocalization. Once animals have been stabilized and severe signs managed (or in asymptomatic animals), decontamination should be attempted. If the animal has not already vomited, induction of emesis or gastric lavage might be performed. Administration of activated charcoal is recommended in most cases and is especially important if extended- or sustained-release products have been ingested. Severe tachycardia may be managed with beta-blockers such as propranolol. Fluid therapy is important

to provide cardiovascular support and protect the kidney from hypotension-related injury. Acid/base status should be monitored and managed as needed.

Differential Diagnosis

Other agents that may cause signs resembling serotonin syndrome (or have a serotonergic component themselves) include amphetamines, cocaine, methylxanthines, pseudoephedrine, albuterol, metaldehyde, ethylene glycol, strychnine, organophosphorous or carbamate insecticides, and zinc phosphide.

Diagnosis

Most human hospitals can run quick screens for antidepressants and may be able to provide results on a STAT basis. Antidepressants can also be detected in blood and urine by a veterinary diagnostic laboratory.

Prognosis

The prognosis of serotonin syndrome is generally good if prompt veterinary medical care is obtained. In cases involving immediate-release products, signs of serotonin syndrome usually resolve within 12 to 36 hours, while extended-release (including controlled- and sustained-release) products may have signs that persist up to 72 hours (Gwaltney-Brant 2004).

Tricyclic Antidepressants

Kinetics

Tricyclic antidepressants (TCA) are rapidly absorbed from the GI tract and widely distributed throughout the body. The half-lives of these drugs vary considerably between individuals, and half-lives can be extended during a toxicosis. Delayed gastric emptying and enterohepatic recirculation are features of TCA intoxication that can also prolong the clinical effects (Wismer 2000).

Mechanism of Action

Tricyclic antidepressants block the reuptake of norepinephrine and serotonin by the presynaptic neuron, resulting in increased levels of these drugs within the CNS. These drugs also have significant antihistiminic and cholinergic effects, as well as cardiac sodium channel blocking action, resulting in significant cardiovascular effects.

Toxicity

Many TCAs have narrow margins of safety, with signs of toxicosis possible at 2–5 times therapeutic doses. Amitrip-

tyline at 15 mg/kg may be lethal to dogs. The oral lethal dosage of clomipramine is 100 mg/kg (Wismer 2000).

Clinical Effects

Signs of TCA intoxication may occur as soon as 30 minutes following exposure and include initial lethargy and ataxia that progresses to agitation, vocalization, hyperesthesia, hyperthermia, vomiting, tachycardia, hypotension, cardiac arrhythmia, dyspnea, pulmonary edema, seizures, coma, and death. Death due to cardiac arrhythmia may occur as early as 2 hours of ingestion in untreated animals (Wismer 2000).

Management

Management of TCA overdosage includes decontamination of clinically stable animals (emesis or gastric lavage followed by activated charcoal with cathartic). Management of clinical signs would be as above for serotonin syndrome, but cardiac arrhythmias in TCA overdoses may be pronounced and require further treatment. The use of hypertonic saline has been recommended to manage severe cardiac arrhythmias, because the arrhythmias are thought to be due to blockade of sodium channels within the myocardium.

Selective Serotonin Reuptake Inhibitors

Mechanism of Action

Selective serotonin reuptake inhibitors (SSRI) are classed by function rather than structure; this class of drugs blocks the reuptake of serotonin by the presynaptic neuron, resulting in increased serotonin levels at the postsynaptic receptors.

Kinetics

Selective serotonin reuptake inhibitors are well absorbed orally and are highly protein-bound. They tend to have rapid onsets of action, although delayed onset may occur when extended- or controlled-release products are ingested. (Gwaltney-Brant 2004).

Toxicity

At therapeutic levels, SSRI have fewer histaminic, cardiovascular, and sedative side effects compared to TCAs or monoamine oxidase inhibitors (MAOIs); in overdose situations these effects, while present, tend to be less severe than the other two classes of antidepressants. At therapeutic and low overdose levels (<5 times therapeutic), these drugs tend to cause sedation; at higher doses, more severe signs, including CNS stimulation, may be seen.

Management

Because these agents tend to exert primarily a direct serotonin effect, the treatment outlined above for serotonin syndrome is the recommended management when overdosages occur. Sustained- or extended-release products tend to have signs that may persist for up to 72 hours.

Nonselective Serotonin Reuptake Inhibitors

Nonselective serotonin reuptake inhibitors (NSSRI) act similarly to SSRI to block serotonin reuptake but also block the reuptake of other amines, such as dopamine or norepinephrine. Venlafaxine capsules appear to be appealing to cats, who will readily ingest them (Merola and Dunayer 2006). Dosages of venlafaxine of 1 mg/kg can cause sedation, and tremors may be seen at 10 mg/kg of immediate-release products (Wismer 2000). The clinical effects of NSSRI overdose include serotonin syndrome as well as a potential cardiovascular stimulation, resulting in tachycardia or other cardiac arrhythmias. Management is the same as for SSRI, but symptomatic treatment of cardiac arrhythmias may be needed.

Monoamine Oxidase Inhibitors

Monoamine oxidase is an enzyme that breaks down various amines including epinephrine, dopamine, and serotonin. Monoamine oxidase inhibitors (MAOI) therefore inhibit the breakdown of these amines, resulting in an increase in their concentrations both within the presynaptic neuron and at the synapse (Wismer 2000). Signs of MAOI overdose in companion animals include hypo/hypertension, tachycardia or other arrhythmias, depression, ataxia, agitation, hyperthermia, tremors, seizures, coma, and respiratory depression. The onset of signs may vary from 2 to 24 hours depending on dosage ingested and the form of the drug (immediate- vs. sustained-release). Management is as for serotonin syndrome. It is recommended that animals ingesting large doses of MAOIs have liver enzyme values monitored as elevations in these values can sometimes occur with MAOI overdose.

Atypical (Novel) Antidepressants

The atypical, or novel, antidepressants comprise a class of drugs of varying structure and mechanism of action; essentially, they do not fit well into the previous categories and are lumped together as "atypical" (Wismer 2000). Signs expected from this class of antidepressant vary, but still tend to fall in line with signs seen with other antidepressants. Similarly, treatment of toxicoses will be the same as that of the other antidepressants outlined above.

BACLOFEN

Sources/Formulations

Baclofen is a centrally acting skeletal muscle relaxant that is used to control spasticity and pain in humans with musculoskeletal disorders and to treat urethral resistance in dogs with urinary retention.

Kinetics

Baclofen is well absorbed orally and can have a very rapid onset of action. Baclofen is lipid-soluble and crosses the blood brain barrier in overdose situations (but not at therapeutic levels) (Gwaltney-Brant 2004a). Baclofen is excreted largely unchanged in the urine. The half-life is dose-dependent and increases significantly in overdose situations.

Mechanism of Action

At therapeutic levels, baclofen mimics GABA within the spinal cord, blocking excitatory responses to sensory input (Gwaltney-Brant 2004a). In overdose situations, baclofen enters the central nervous system where it inhibits substance P, a stimulatory compound within the brain stem. The mechanism of baclofen-induced seizures is thought to be due to decreased GABA release from presynaptic neurons, causing excessive postsynaptic firing.

Toxicity

In dogs, dosages of 1.3 mg/kg have resulted in clinical signs, and deaths have occurred at dosages over 8 mg/kg (Wismer 2004).

Clinical Effects

Clinical signs of baclofen toxicosis include vomiting, ataxia, vocalization, disorientation, depression, hypersalivation, weakness, recumbency, coma, hypothermia, hypotension or hypertension, bradycardia, hyperactivity, agitation, tremors, mydriasis, dyspnea, respiratory arrest, pulmonary edema, and death (Wismer 2004). Seizures and respiratory compromise secondary to paralysis of the diaphragm and intercostal muscles are the most life-threatening signs.

Differential Diagnosis

Other compounds that can cause signs similar to baclofen include other central nervous system depressants (barbiturates, benzodiazepines, sleep aids such as zolpidem, etc.), ethylene glycol, isoxazole mushrooms, antidepressants, macrolide antiparasiticides (e.g., ivermectin, moxidectin, etc.) and marijuana.

Diagnosis

Baclofen blood levels can be measured at a human hospital or veterinary diagnostic laboratory, although unless STAT results can be obtained, they may be of little value when dealing with the emergent patient.

Management

Treatment goals for baclofen exposures are managing clinical signs, maintaining respiration, decontamination, and supportive care. Patients developing respiratory compromise may need mechanical ventilation. Comatose animals should be monitored closely for respiratory insufficiency and hypothermia. Seizures generally respond to diazepam, but the lowest dose necessary to control seizures should be used in order to prevent exacerbating the central nervous system depression that will follow seizure control. Intravenous fluid therapy is helpful in correcting hypotension and providing cardiovascular support. Vocalization and disorientation sometimes respond to cyproheptadine. Anecdotally, some clinicians have found the use of intravenous lipid solutions to be helpful in managing baclofen toxicoses. Decontamination (emesis and single dose of activated charcoal) can be considered in asymptomatic animals, but patients displaying even mild central nervous system effects may be at risk of aspiration, so decontamination should be done with care.

Prognosis

Resolution of clinical signs can take up to several days in severe cases. Patients provided with prompt supportive care have a reasonable prognosis of recovery as long as adequate ventilatory support can be maintained. Patients experiencing seizures have a more guarded prognosis (Wismer 2004).

CARDIAC DRUGS

ACE Inhibitors

Sources/Formulations

Angiotensin-converting enzyme (ACE) inhibitors include drugs such as enalapril, lisinopril, benazepril, and captopril. These drugs are used in human and veterinary medicine to manage heart failure or hypertension. These drugs are available as tablets and capsules alone or combined with other medication (e.g., diuretics).

Kinetics

ACE inhibitors are well absorbed orally. Food in the gastrointestinal tract can reduce bioavailability of captopril by 30% to 40% (Plumb 2005). Some ACE inhibitors (e.g., enalapril and benazepril) are prodrugs that are converted to an active metabolite following absorption. In dogs, the half-lives of benazepril and captopril are 3.5 hours and 2.8 hours. Enalapril has a slower onset of action (4–6 hours) but longer duration of action (12–14 hours) compared to benazepril and captopril (Plumb 2005). The half-life of benazepril in cats is 16–23 hours. Half-lives of all are increased in patients with renal failure.

Mechanism of Action

ACE inhibitors prevent the conversion of angiotensin I to angiotensin II by competing with angiotensin I for the ACE enzyme. The ACE enzyme has a higher affinity for ACE inhibitors than for angiotensin I. Decreased angiotensin II levels result in decreased aldosterone secretion and increased renin secretion, causing peripheral vasodilation.

Toxicity

Compared to other cardiac drugs, ACE inhibitors have a relatively wide margin of safety, with hypotension expected only at high doses. Generally dosages equivalent to <20 mg/kg of lisinopril are not likely to cause any serious clinical problems in healthy adult dogs (ASPCA Animal Poison Control Center, unpublished data).

Clinical Effects

The primary clinical effect of ACE inhibitor overdose is hypotension, which can result in nausea, vomiting, and weakness.

Differential Diagnosis

Other causes of hypotension include primary cardiovascular disease, cardiac glycosides (drugs, plants, *Bufo* toads), calcium channel blockers, nitroglycerine, alpha2 agonists (e.g., amitraz, xylazine), imidazoline decongestants, beta blockers, and muscarinic mushrooms.

Diagnosis

Serum or plasma levels of ACE inhibitors are not readily available. Diagnosis of toxicosis is based on history and clinical signs.

Management

Large ingestions of ACE inhibitors should be managed with decontamination (emesis followed by activated charcoal) and monitoring for hypotension. Patients developing hypotension should be treated with intravenous fluids to assist in maintaining blood pressure.

Prognosis

The prognosis for patients ingesting overdoses of ACE inhibitors is excellent because serious consequences are rare.

Calcium Channel Blockers

Sources/Formulations

Calcium channel blockers include verapamil, diltiazem, nifedipine, and nimodipine. These drugs have been used to manage a variety of cardiovascular disorders in human and veterinary medicine.

Kinetics

Calcium channel blockers are rapidly absorbed from the gastrointestinal tract and undergo significant first pass effect (Roder 2004a). These drugs are metabolized in the liver and metabolites are excreted through the urine. The half-life of diltiazem in cats is 2 hours and the half-life of verapamil in the dog is 0.8 to 2.5 hours (Plumb 2005).

Mechanism of Action

Calcium channel blockers prevent the opening of voltage-gated calcium channels within the heart, slowing the influx of calcium into the myocardiocyte and inhibiting calcium-dependent processes in the myocardium (Miller and Adams 2009; Roder 2004a). This results in coronary and peripheral vasodilation, decreased cardiac contractility, and decreased activity of cardiac pacemaker nodes. The net effect is slowing of heart rate and lowering of blood pressure. These effects are exaggerated in overdose situations.

Toxicity

Calcium channel blockers have a narrow margin of safety and doses 2–3 times therapeutic doses can cause adverse reactions (Roder 2004a).

Clinical Effects

The clinical effects of calcium channel blockers include bradycardia and hypotension resulting in weakness, recumbency, coma, vomiting, depression, and disorientation (Roder 2004a). Severe cardiac conduction disturbances (e.g., second- and third-degree AV blockade) and pulmonary edema are possible. Hyperglycemia may also occur (Plumb 2005).

Differential Diagnosis

Other causes of hypotension and/or bradycardia include primary cardiovascular disease, cardiac glycosides (drugs, plants, *Bufo* toads), calcium channel blockers, nitroglycerine, alpha2 agonists (e.g., amitraz, xylazine), imidazoline decongestants, beta blockers, and muscarinic mushrooms.

Management

Prompt decontamination of recent ingestions is recommended, including induction of emesis and administration of activated charcoal. Patients should be monitored a minimum of 6 hours following ingestion of immediate-release products and 12 hours following ingestion of sustained-, controlled- or extended-release products. Mild hypotension and bradycardia may be manageable with intravenous fluids alone, but more severe cardiovascular effects need more intensive treatment, including administration of intravenous calcium salts. Treatment for refractory cases includes pressor agents (dopamine, norepinephrine, isoproterenol, etc.), atropine, and cardiac pacing. Intravenous lipid solutions have been reported to be helpful in managing severe toxicosis from calcium channel blockers (Cave and Harvey 2009).

Prognosis

Prognosis will depend on dose ingested, time to presentation for veterinary care, severity of clinical signs, and response to therapy. Patients with poor response to appropriate therapy have a guarded to poor prognosis.

Cardiac Glycosides

Sources/Formulations

Cardiac glycoside drugs include digoxin and digitoxin. Cardiac glycoside compounds are also found in a variety of plants including foxglove (*Digitalis purpura*), oleander (*Nerium oleander*), and lily of the valley (*Convallaria* spp.), as well as the secretions of several species of *Bufo* toads.

Kinetics

Cardiac glycosides are well absorbed orally. Protein binding varies, with digitoxin being highly protein-bound and digoxin having low protein binding (Roder 2004a). These drugs are metabolized in the liver.

Mechanism of Action

Cardiac glycosides interfere with normal functioning of Na+/K+-ATPases, increasing intracellular sodium and extracellular potassium. The final result is an increase in force of contraction, increase in cardiac output, and decrease in heart rate.

Toxicity

Cardiac glycosides have a very narrow margin of safety, and adverse effects with chronic therapeutic use are not uncommon. Doses 2 to 3 times therapeutic doses can cause significant adverse cardiovascular effects (Roder 2004a).

Clinical Effects

Clinical Signs

Clinical signs of cardiac glycoside toxicosis include vomiting and diarrhea as well as cardiac effects (Roder 2004a). Cardiac effects can be seen without any initial gastrointestinal signs and can include just about any known arrhythmia. Clinical signs associated with the cardiovascular effects in acute intoxications include weakness, collapse, pale or gray mucous membrane color, hypotension, hypothermia, coma, and death. Pulmonary edema and renal failure may occur secondarily.

Laboratory

Serum potassium should be monitored because hyperkalemia is commonly seen with cardiac glycoside toxicosis.

Differential Diagnosis

Other causes of cardiac dysfunction include primary cardiovascular disease, calcium channel blockers, nitroglycerine, alpha2 agonists (e.g., amitraz, xylazine), imidazoline decongestants, beta blockers, and muscarinic mushrooms.

Diagnosis

Diagnosis is based on history of exposure and clinical signs. Most human hospitals can run serum digoxin levels on a STAT basis.

Management

Prompt decontamination of recent ingestions is recommended, including induction of emesis and administration of activated charcoal. Patients should be monitored a minimum of 6 hours following ingestion. There is a wide range of arrhythmias that can be seen with cardiac glycoside toxicosis, so the cardinal rule of treatment is to "treat the patient, not the poison," and manage the arrhythmias symptomatically (e.g., atropine for bradyarrhythmias). For patients that are not responding to appropriate antiarrhythmic therapy, the use of digoxin immune Fab may be considered (for further information, see Chapter 8, "Antidotes"). Management of hyperkalemia may include the use of potassium-free fluids and/or insulin therapy.

Prognosis

The prognosis will depend on the dose ingested, time to presentation for veterinary care, severity of clinical signs and response to therapy. Patients with poor response to appropriate therapy have a guarded to poor prognosis.

5-FLUOROURACIL

Sources/Formulations

5-Fluorouracil is a pyrimidine analog in the class of antineoplastic dugs termed antimetabolites. 5-Fluorouracil is used to treat a variety of cancers in human and veterinary medicine. Topical creams and solutions are used to treat dermal disorders such as solar keratosis in humans (Roder 2004).

Kinetics

5-Flurouracil is well-absorbed both orally and following topical application.

Mechanism of Action

5-Fluorouracil inhibits DNA synthesis, resulting in interference with cell division, so it is more toxic to rapidly dividing cells of the gastrointestinal tract and bone marrow (Albretsen 2001). Metabolites of 5-fluorouracil are thought to contribute to the seizures that are frequently seen with 5-fluorouracil toxicosis in dogs (Yamashita et al. 2004).

Toxicity

The minimum lethal dosage of 5-fluorouracil in dogs is 20 mg/kg, although serious clinical effects can be seen at dosages well below this (Albretsen 2001). Any exposure should be considered potentially serious and merit evaluation of the patient by a veterinarian.

Clinical Effects

Clinical signs in dogs exposed to 5-fluorouracil include vomiting, lethargy, tremors, seizures, cardiac arrhythmias, and respiratory depression (Albretsen 2001). Severe vomiting can begin within minutes of exposure; seizures may occur quickly or can be delayed up to several hours. Patients surviving the acute crisis may develop evidence of bone marrow suppression and/or alimentary tract mucosal necrosis within days of exposure.

Differential Diagnosis

Other toxicants that can cause acute onset of signs similar to 5-fluorouracil include CNS stimulant drugs (amphetamines, cocaine, antidepressants, etc.), organophosphorous or carbamate insecticides, strychnine, methylxanthines, ethylene glycol, nicotine, and zinc phosphide.

Diagnosis

Diagnosis is based on history of exposure and clinical signs. Serum levels of 5-fluorouracil are not readily available.

Management

Management of 5-fluorouracil toxicosis entails managing life-threatening clinical signs, seizure control, gastrointestinal protection, supportive care, and monitoring for bone marrow suppression. Decontamination is indicated only in recent, asymptomatic exposures. Once clinical signs develop, decontamination is less rewarding and may add the risk of aspiration. Seizures are often refractory to diazepam alone, but a dose of pentobarbital followed by a constant-rate-infusion of diazepam has been found to be helpful in managing seizures (ASPCA Animal Poison Control Center, unpublished data). Antiemetics should be used to manage vomiting, and gastrointestinal protectants should be provided. Cardiac arrhythmias should be managed as they occur. General supportive care includes intravenous fluid administration, pain management (patients experiencing alimentary tract necrosis are quite painful), thermoregulation, and antibiotics to prevent infection from the eroded GI mucosa. Serum chemistry, complete blood count, acid/base, and electrolytes should all be monitored. Animals that survive beyond a few days should have serial complete blood counts twice weekly for 4 weeks to detect evidence of bone marrow suppression. Patients with bone marrow suppression may need to be treated with bone marrow stimulants (e.g., filgrastim for leukopenia).

Prognosis

The prognosis for patients with 5-fluorouracil exposures is guarded, and mortality rates of >50% have been reported, despite intensive care (Albretsen 2001). Positive prognostic indicators include no seizures or seizures that respond well to therapy. Negative prognostic indicators include being a cat and poor response to anticonvulsant therapy.

ORAL DIABETIC MEDICATIONS

Sulfonylureas

Sources/Formulations

Sulfonylureas are oral hypoglycemic drugs used in the treatment of diabetes in human and veterinary medicine. Included in this class are glimepiride, glipizide, glyburide, chlorpropamide, and tolazamide (Rosendale 2004a).

Kinetics

Sulfonylureas are rapidly absorbed from the gastrointestinal tract and are highly protein-bound. They are metabolized in the liver and excreted via the urine. Half-life information in nonhumans is not available but glimepiride and glyburide appear to have duration of action of approximately 24 hours in cats, while glipizide has a hypoglycemic effect in cats lasting less than 60 minutes at therapeutic levels (Plumb 2005).

Mechanism of Action

Sulfonylureas are thought to act by triggering the endogenous release of insulin and may enhance the binding of insulin to receptors (Rosendale 2004a).

Toxicity

In normoglycemic animals, hypoglycemia can be seen at therapeutic doses (Rosendale 2004a).

Clinical Effects

Clinical signs of sulfonylurea toxicosis are primarily those of hypoglycemia. Liver dysfunction has been reported with therapeutic use of sulfonylureas in cats, but whether liver injury would occur following acute overdose is not known.

Clinical Signs

Vomiting, anorexia, lethargy, ataxia, weakness, behavioral changes, seizures and coma can occur in patients experiencing hypoglycemia. Icterus, vomiting, and diarrhea were reported in cats experiencing adverse hepatic effects from glipizide (Rosendale 2004a).

Laboratory

Hypoglycemia is the primary laboratory abnormality expected with sulfonylurea overdose.

Differential Diagnosis

Other causes of hypoglycemia that should be considered include juvenile hypoglycemia, xylitol (dogs), alpha-lipoic acid (dogs), primary liver disease, sepsis, iatrogenic insulin overdose, and insulinoma.

Diagnosis

Sulfonylurea serum levels can be determined by a veterinary diagnostic laboratory but turnaround times can be long, making determination of serum levels of little use for diagnosing the acute patient.

Management

Management of sulfonylurea overdose should focus on managing serious clinical effects (coma, seizures), normalization of serum glucose, decontamination, and monitoring for return of hypoglycemia. Because of the potential for rapid onset of signs of hypoglycemia, emesis should only be induced in a hospital setting once serum glucose levels have been determined and, if necessary, corrected. Monitoring of serum glucose should be done for a minimum of 24 hours following exposure. Small, frequent meals may help in management of mild intoxications. As needed, intravenous dextrose solutions should be administered to maintain blood glucose in patients experiencing more severe hypoglycemia. Seizing animals may also require diazepam. Baseline liver values should be obtained and repeated at 24 and 48 hours; patients showing increasing liver values should continue to have levels repeated every 24 hours until it is apparent that the enzyme values have leveled off or started to decline.

Prognosis

Most cases of sulfonylurea overdose will have a good prognosis provided prompt veterinary care has been obtained. Patients with protracted hypoglycemia prior to presentation have a more guarded prognosis.

Metformin

Sources/Formulations

Metformin is a biguanide antidiabetic agent with the trade name Glucophage®. Metformin is used to treat non–insulin-dependent diabetes mellitus in humans and cats (Rosendale 2004a; Plumb 2005).

Kinetics

Metformin is slowly absorbed in humans and variably absorbed in cats (Plumb 2005). Metformin is eliminated unchanged in the urine (Rosendale 2004a). The half-life of metformin in cats is 11.5 hours.

Mechanism of Action

Metformin is thought to lower blood glucose by improving peripheral sensitivity to insulin and increasing insulin uptake by peripheral cells (Rosendale 2004a). Unlike sulfonylureas, metformin does not increase serum insulin levels.

Toxicity

No toxic doses exist for dogs or cats ingesting metformin; doses ranging from 58 to 170 mg/kg in dogs and cats did not result in hypoglycemia (Heller 2007). Unlike sulfonylureas, ingestion of metformin is not expected to cause hypoglycemia in euglycemic animals (Rosendale 2004a). Animals with inadequate caloric intake or with recent excessive exercise could be at risk for hypoglycemia. Although gastrointestinal signs have been seen with metformin overdoses in animals, serious life-threatening signs have not been reported.

Clinical Effects
Clinical Signs

Clinical signs of metformin are primarily related to gastrointestinal upset: nausea, vomiting, abdominal bloating, diarrhea, flatulence, and anorexia (Heller 2007).

Laboratory

Hypoglycemia is not anticipated with metformin exposures in most animals. Animals in a negative energy balance or those with recent excessive exercise without adequate food intake could develop hypoglycemia following metformin exposure (Rosendale 2004a). Lactic acidosis has been reported in humans taking metformin and in severe overdose situations, but this condition has not been reported in animals.

Differential Diagnosis

Differential diagnoses for signs of metformin exposure include other causes of gastrointestinal upset such as dietary indiscretion, infectious gastroenteritis, gastrointestinal foreign body, etc.

Diagnosis

Metformin serum levels can be measured, but because metformin is not expected to cause serious issues, measuring is not generally recommended.

Management

Management of metformin overdoses primarily involves managing gastrointestinal upset. Antiemetics can be utilized in vomiting patients. Decontamination is recommended in large exposures, including induction of emesis if within 1 hour of exposure followed by administration of activated charcoal. Animals appearing to be in a negative energy balance (e.g., emaciated, cachexic) should have blood glucose monitored; small frequent meals may help keep blood glucose within normal limits. With large ingestions, monitoring for lactic acidosis may be prudent.

Prognosis

Most cases develop no more than gastrointestinal upset that is responsive to symptomatic care, so the prognosis in most cases is excellent.

REFERENCES

Albretsen, Jay C. 2001. 5-Fluorouracil toxicosis in dogs. *Veterinary Medicine* 96(4):270–274.

Cave, G. and Harvey, M. 2009. Intravenous lipid emulsion as an antidote beyond local anesthetic toxicity: A systematic-review. *Academic Emergency Medicine* 16(9):815–824.

Gwaltney-Brant, Sharon M. 2004. Antidepressants. In *Clinical Veterinary Toxicology*, edited by Konnie H. Plumlee, pp. 286–291. St. Louis: Mosby.

———. 2004a. Muscle relaxants. In *Clinical Veterinary Toxicology*, edited by Konnie H. Plumlee, pp. 326–330. St. Louis: Mosby.

Heller, Jacqueline B. 2007. Metformin overdose in dogs and cats. *Veterinary Medicine* 102(4):231–234.

Mensching, Donna and Volmer, Petra A. 2007. Breathe easier when managing beta$_2$ agonist inhaler toxicoses in dogs. *Veterinary Medicine* 102(6):369–373.

Merola, Valentina M. and Dunayer, Eric D. 2006. The 10 most common toxicoses in cats. *Veterinary Medicine* 101(6): 339–342.

Miller, Matthew W. and Adams, H. Richard. 2009. Digitalis, positive inotropes and vasodilators. In *Veterinary Pharmacology and Therapeutics, 9th edition*, edited by Jim E. Riviere and Mark G. Papich, pp. 541–574. Ames, Iowa: Wiley-Blackwell.

Mills, Kirk C. 2005. Serotonin syndrome. In *Critical Care Toxicology*, edited by Jeffrey Brent, Kevin L. Wallace, Keith K. Burkhart, Scott D. Phillips, and J. Ward Donovan, pp. 281–290. Philadelphia: Mosby.

Plumb, Donald C. 2005. *Veterinary Drug Handbook, 5th ed.* Ames, Iowa: Blackwell.

Roder, Joseph D. 2004. Antineoplastics. In *Veterinary Clinical Toxicology*, edited by Konnie H. Plumlee, pp. 299–302. St. Louis: Mosby.

———. 2004a. Cardiovascular drugs. In *Veterinary Clinical Toxicology*, edited by Konnie H. Plumlee, pp. 307–309. St. Louis: Mosby.

Rosendale, Marcy. 2004. Bronchodilators. In *Veterinary Clinical Toxicology*, edited by Konnie H. Plumlee, pp. 305–306. St. Louis: Mosby.

———. 2004a. Diabetes medications. In *Veterinary Clinical Toxicology*, edited by Konnie H. Plumlee, pp. 311–319. St. Louis: Mosby.

Wismer, Tina A. 2000. Antidepressant overdoses in dogs. *Veterinary Medicine* 95(7):520–525.

Wismer, Tina A. 2004. Baclofen overdose in dogs. *Veterinary Medicine* 99(5):406–410.

Yamashita, K., Yada, H., and Yariyoshi, T. 2004. Neurotoxic effects of alpha-fluoro-beta-alanine (FBAL) and fluoroacetic acide (FA) in dogs. *Journal of Toxicologic Science* 29:155–166.

Household and Industrial Toxicants

28

Rhian Cope

ASPIRATION

Sources

Aspiration is the accidental introduction of liquid into the lungs. It may occur either directly or as a consequence of vomiting. It is a common complication of ingestion of many low viscosity household products. Petroleum distillates with a kinematic viscosity of less than $19\,mm^2/s$ @ 40°C (e.g., kerosene, diesel/gas oil fuels, gasoline, Stoddard cleaning solvent, light lubricating oils, light hydraulic fluids), glycols, and many other low viscosity household products are significant aspiration hazards.

In general, the potential for aspiration depends on the viscosity, surface tension and volatility of the ingested material. Viscosity, however, provides the best estimate of the aspiration potential of a material and determines the rate and extent of penetration into deeper lung structures. Any substance with low viscosity has low resistance to flow and can readily spread in the respiratory tract. Consequently, even a small volume may cause widespread tissue damage. The viscosity of baby oil is an approximate high cut-off viscosity for a high risk of aspiration.

Mechanism

Aspiration may occur silently and insidiously (most commonly) or occur secondarily to vomiting. Aspirated hydrocarbons (and other potential aspirants) impair lung fluid surfactant function, leading to alveolar instability, early distal airway closure, and ventilation/perfusion mismatches with subsequent hypoxemia. If the aspirated hydrocarbon is highly volatile, it may also displace alveolar oxygen leading to temporary transient hypoxia or in some cases to asphyxia due to rapid displacement of air. In addition, many aspirated materials can damage pulmonary capillaries directly, producing pathological findings ranging from chemical pneumonitis, hemorrhages, and bronchopneumonia to gross pulmonary edema.

CLINICAL EFFECTS

Signs

It is wise to always assume that pulmonary aspiration has occurred following ingestion of low viscosity materials, even when there is no clinical history or signs of vomiting, coughing, or choking. Many patients who aspirate low viscosity materials are often initially asymptomatic and may not be presented for treatment until significant respiratory compromise is present. In the majority of cases, aspiration is a quiet and insidious process that goes unrecognized until respiratory distress develops. In relatively rare instances, patients may present with initial symptoms such as gagging, choking, coughing, and dyspnea.

Examination of the patient may show tachypnea, intercostal retractions, diminished breath sounds, tachycardia, and fever. Some patients will show few or no signs until respiratory compromise becomes evident.

Patients with a history of ingestion of a potentially aspiratable material should always be monitored for aspiration pneumonia/pneumonitis and other respiratory system complications by continuous monitoring of peripheral hemoglobin oxygen saturation by pulse oximetry/co-oximetry. It is important to use periodic diagnostic

Small Animal Toxicology Essentials, First Edition. Edited by Robert H. Poppenga, Sharon Gwaltney-Brant.

imaging of the thorax starting at 6 hours postingestion/ aspiration and continuing for at least 48–72 hours postingestion.

A high proportion of patients with aspiration (particularly of hydrocarbon distillates) will develop acute respiratory distress syndrome. Pulmonary involvement is usually progressive during the first 24–48 hours. Reversible bronchial hyperresponsiveness and restrictive ventilatory limitation may be demonstrated.

If the patient survives, the pulmonary involvement often gradually subsides over days to weeks. Other complications may include pulmonary edema, pneumomediastinum, emphysema, pneumatoriles, cysts, and secondary infectious pneumonia. Nonpulmonary organ toxicity is rare with simple petroleum distillate aspiration, but may occur with other materials.

Laboratory Findings

Typically, a progressive decline in peripheral blood hemoglobin oxygen saturation (as measured by pulse oximetry/ co-oximetry) occurs. The lowered peripheral blood hemoglobin oxygen saturation is most commonly due to the development of a ventilation-perfusion mismatch.

Bronchoalveolar lavage commonly demonstrates inflammatory responses characterized by neutrophilia and foamy macrophages (foamy cytoplasmic vacuolization of macrophages)

Differential Diagnosis

Common and important differential diagnoses include paraquat poisoning, inhalation of superheated air, and acute viral and/or bacterial pneumonia.

Diagnostics

Antemortem

A history of exposure/ingestion is usually the most important antemortem diagnostic clue. Occasionally, it may be possible to smell petroleum distillates on the animal's breath or the facial coat or paws. Aspiration of stomach contents via small-bore nasogastric tube may yield valuable diagnostic samples if performed within about an hour following ingestion. Diagnostic imaging evidence of pneumonitis is usually present within 6–12 hours. The most common radiographic pattern is pulmonary edema, although various radiographic opacities may occur.

Postmortem

Gross findings of a necropsy range from frank chemical pneumonitis, hemorrhages, and bronchopneumonia to gross pulmonary edema. In some cases, it may be possible to smell petroleum distillates in the fluid present in the airways and lungs.

Histopathological changes in the lung in these cases include interstitial inflammation, bronchial and bronchiolar necrosis, intra-alveolar hemorrhage, and inflammatory cell exudate.

Management of Exposures

In cases where the patient has ingested material and is at risk of aspiration, induction of vomiting and gastric lavage, even with a secure airway, are ineffective, increase the morbidity and mortality, and are directly contraindicated.

Insufficient data either to support or exclude the effectiveness of simple small-bore nasogastric aspiration is available. In cases where significant volumes of material have been ingested and the animal presents for treatment within 30 to 60 minutes of ingestion, simple small-bore nasogastric aspiration may be of some benefit.

Medical treatment of aspiration is symptomatic. Conservative fluid management, avoidance of overaggressive fluid therapy, and overhydration are critical in minimizing the affects of the acute respiratory distress syndrome that may develop following aspiration. In humans, conservative fluid management has been definitively shown to contribute to improved outcomes in patients with acute respiratory distress.

Pharmaceutical interventions for acute respiratory distress syndrome have so far been proven ineffective and thus cannot be recommended. The use of high-dose corticosteroids is controversial and large-scale trials in humans have demonstrated a lack of effectiveness. Prophylactic corticosteroids may increase the death rate among human patients at risk for acute respiratory distress syndrome. Because of the controversy and lack of data demonstrating clear benefit in animals, the use of corticosteroids in the treatment of aspiration in domestic animals remains one of individual judgment.

Prognosis

The prognosis for confirmed cases of aspiration is always guarded, particularly if acute respiratory distress is present.

ALCOHOLS

Ethanol

Synonyms include alcohol, ethyl; denatured alcohol; distilled spirits; ethyl alcohol, undenatured; ethanol; ethyl alcohol; ethylcarbinol.

Sources

Ethanol is a ubiquitous household and industrial chemical. A partial list of common sources of ethanol in households includes alcoholic beverages, fermenting organic waste materials (particularly fruit, food waste in garbage), bread dough and related fermenting yeast doughs, automotive deicers, window cleaners, antifogging solutions, dental mouthwashes, toothpastes, perfumes, fragrances, after-shaves, cosmetics, paints, varnishes, polishes, shellacs, sealers, degreasers, design and sketch art markers, paints, tinctures (e.g., tincture of iodine), cough syrups, cosmetics, adhesive removers, liquid detergents, stain removers, disinfectants, deodorizers, shampoos, hair conditioners, antiperspirants, thermometers, and insect repellents. An extensive list of U.S. household products that contain ethanol can be found on the U.S. Department of Health and Human Services' Household Products Database (Health and Safety Information on Household Products). Alcohol content in household products can be surprisingly high. It should be noted that the percentage of ethanol in distilled alcoholic beverages is half of its "proof value." Pungent fermenting fruits, grains, and vegetable matter are often attractive to several domestic and wildlife species and are commonly voluntarily consumed to excess.

In industrial situations, ethanol is an extensively used solvent and transported intermediate. Industrial-grade ethanol is typically high purity (>98% by mass). In the context of veterinary medicine, acute poisoning is the most common of the various ethanol toxidromes.

Kinetics

The most common route of exposure in domestic animals is via ingestion, although inhalation exposures can occur under some rare circumstances (prolonged inhalation of ethanol vapors). Ethanol is rapidly absorbed from the gastrointestinal tract and the onset of clinical signs is generally correlated with blood ethanol concentration. The presence of food in the stomach or small intestine delays systemic absorption, as can the type of formulation containing the ethanol. However, the onset of clinical signs will typically occur within an hour following ingestion.

Ethanol is metabolized by three basic mechanisms: (1) first-pass metabolism of ethanol to acetaldehyde by gastric alcohol dehydrogenase; (2) first-pass metabolism of ethanol to acetaldehyde by liver alcohol dehydrogenase IB followed by conversion of the acetaldehyde to acetic acid by liver aldehyde dehydrogenase, and acetic acid is then converted to acetyl CoA that is consumed as an energy source via the citric acid cycle or for the synthesis of lipids; and (3) conversion of ethanol to acetaldehyde by hepatic CYP 2E1. In domestic animals that are not normally regularly exposed to ethanol, mechanisms (1) and (2) are usually the most important.

Clearance of ethanol from the bloodstream is mostly via hepatic metabolism, but small amounts of ethanol (<10% of the ingested amount) are exhaled or excreted in urine. Whole body elimination follows zero order kinetics.

Mechanism of Action

Ethanol, particularly concentrated ethanol, is a skin, respiratory, eye, and gastrointestinal irritant. Its irritancy on the gastric mucosa is associated with its well-known capacity to induce vomiting. Consumption of concentrated industrial ethanol produces significant damage to the gastric mucosa and bleeding into the stomach.

Within the CNS, ethanol and many of the anesthetics and narcotic hydrocarbon solvents appear to have a common site of action on CNS neurotransmitter receptors. Ethanol has agonistlike effects on CNS GABA-A and glycine receptors and inhibitory effects on glutamate NMDA receptors (particularly in the hippocampus). These mechanisms help to explain the CNS depressive, aestheticlike effects and its amnesic actions. Importantly, the CNS depressive effects also include the loss of central cardiovascular/respiratory drive and the loss of normal airway-protective reflexes. The loss of normal airway-protective effects, plus the ethanol-induced decreased pulmonary secretion clearance, plus ethanol's propensity for inducing vomiting creates a substantial risk of aspiration pneumonia.

Ethanol suppresses the release of antidiuretic hormone (arginine vasopressin) by the posterior pituitary. This reduces water reabsorption in the distal convoluted tubules and collecting tubules in the nephrons of kidneys and increased urine production.

Doses of ethanol that produce inebriation typically sensitize the myocardium to the effects of catecholamines and fatal cardiac arrhythmias may develop. The hypothermia that is common in ethanol intoxication exacerbates these effects and increases the difficulty of treating any cardiac arrhythmias that develop. Hypothermia develops in ethanol poisoning due to a combination of peripheral vasodilation (increased heat loss), and a central loss of the ability to thermoregulate. Acute ethanol poisoning may also trigger acute pancreatitis. Ethanol is a proven teratogen in animals.

With chronic exposure, ethanol has a myriad of other effects. However, most of these are rarely of relevance to veterinary medicine.

Toxicity

The lowest dosage expected to produce death in dogs following ingestion is around 5.5 g/kg. However, clinical signs of toxicity may occur at much lower dosages.

Clinical Effects
Signs

Clinical signs of acute ethanol poisoning in companion animals resemble the classical signs in humans: vomiting, an initial period of paradoxical behavioral excitation followed by CNS depression, ataxia, lethargy, and sedation. Significant ingestions are associated with coma and hypothermia. Signs of abdominal pain may be present due to ethanol's irritant effects on the gastric mucosa and its ability to trigger acute pancreatitis. Dehydration may occur because of an inability to concentrate urine due to decreased antidiuretic hormone. Pupillary reflexes may be variable in their response. Tachycardia or myocardial depression and hypotension may be present. Death is typically from cardiovascular respiratory arrest combined with hypothermia. Cardiac arrhythmias are common. Hypoglycemic seizures may occur, particularly in young animals.

Importantly, many patients lose their airway protective reflexes. Thus aspiration of vomitus is an important delayed effect of ethanol poisoning. Sequential diagnostic imaging should be performed if aspiration is suspected.

Laboratory Findings

Determination of whole blood or serum alcohol concentration is the most effective method of confirming the diagnosis. However, ethanol levels can be determined in most body fluids and vomitus. Osmolar gap metabolic acidosis is a common finding in acute ethanol poisoning. An elevated anion gap may also be occasionally present in acute ethanol poisoning. Hypoglycemia, serum electrolyte disturbances, and evidence of hemoconcentration are common. Blood pCO_2 measurement may be useful if respiratory depression is present. Evidence of acute pancreatitis such as elevated serum amylase and lipase may be present.

Because the early stages of ethanol poisoning and ethylene glycol poisoning are clinically similar, blood ethylene glycol levels should also be measured.

Differential Diagnoses

The most critical differential diagnosis is ethylene glycol poisoning. Other alcohols (methanol, isopropyl alcohol), hydrocarbon solvents, chemsols, marijuana, macrolide antiparasitics, and amitraz produce similar effects to ethanol in domestic animals, as do most benzodiazepine, barbiturate, antipsychotic, antiseizure, and antidepressant human prescription drugs.

Diagnostics
Antemortem

The patient's history plus the presence of the typical clinical signs/laboratory findings of the ethanol toxidrome are usually the best diagnostic clues. Definitive diagnosis typically requires the determination of whole blood or serum ethanol. Alternatively, ethanol levels can be determined in most body fluids and in vomitus. Aspirating stomach contents using a small-bore nasogastric tube can often yield useful samples for ethanol testing if performed within about 1 hour following ingestion. Samples of the material suspected of being ingested, preferably in the original container, are always particularly valuable.

Postmortem

Ethanol levels can be measured in most body fluids and in the gastric contents. Detection of significant amounts of ethanol provides the most definitive diagnosis. Hyperemia and inflammation of the gastric mucosa may be present. Inflammation of the esophagus and bleeding from the gastric mucosa may be present if concentrated ethanol solutions have been ingested. The presence of pneumonia is strongly suggestive of aspiration.

Management of Exposures

Given that absorption of ethanol from the gastrointestinal tract is rapid, attempts at decontamination of the upper intestinal tract are usually ineffective. Because of the potential loss of airway reflexes, induction of vomiting should only be used with extreme caution in asymptomatic patients with a history of very recent ingestion (within 15 minutes). Gastric lavage is no longer used in cases of human ethanol poisoning since it has been shown to be ineffective and to increase the risk of severe complications. Activated charcoal does not bind ethanol and is ineffective. Evacuation of stomach contents using a small-bore nasogastric tube may be of some value if the patient presents within 1 hour of ingestion.

Intravenous fluid therapy should be used to correct/prevent dehydration, support kidney function, maintain circulation and blood pressure, correct/prevent hypoglycemia (dextrose intravenous fluids), and correct any electrolyte/acid base disturbances present. Treatment of acidosis may include sodium bicarbonate administration. Regular monitoring of the patient's blood pressure, serum electrolytes, and acid base status is recommended. Vasopressors, such as dopamine, and plasma expanders may be useful if significant hypotension is present.

Regular monitoring of cardiac electrical activity, particularly if the patient is hypothermic, is recommended. Hypothermia is a common and serious problem in ethanol toxicoses and supplementary heat may be required. Given that animals with ethanol toxicoses have poor thermoregulation, it is also important to avoid iatrogenic hyperthermia.

Yohimbine has been recommended to treat CNS depression in dogs with ethanol poisoning. Careful dose selection is required to avoid producing overdose effects under these circumstances.

Prognosis

Most cases in domestic animals are relatively mild and involve consumption of relatively dilute alcoholic materials. In this situation, most uncomplicated cases will recover within 24–48 hours provided close monitoring and supportive care is available. The prognosis for patients with severe CNS signs, significant hypothermia, significant cardiovascular respiratory depression, or metabolic acidosis is much more guarded. The presence of aspiration pneumonia always warrants a guarded prognosis.

Methanol

Synonyms include alcohol, methyl carbinol, methyl alcohol, and wood alcohol

Sources/Formulations

Methanol is typically used in the same range of household products as ethanol. It is no longer used in cosmetics or personal care products in most jurisdictions. Any product containing methanol is usually required to have a child-proof cap or closure. However, the lack of a childproof cap or closure on a product is not an absolute guarantee that methanol is not present in it. An extensive list of US household products that contain methanol can be found on the U.S. Department of Health and Human Services' Household Products Database (Health and Safety Information on Household Products). Most automotive windshield deicers contain from 20–86% methanol; dogs are commonly exposed when they chew on the plastic bottles. A potential cause of methanol poisoning is home brewing and home distillation of alcohol.

Kinetics

The kinetics of methanol resemble that of ethanol. Importantly, significant toxicoses have been reported following exposure of the skin, as well as following ingestion and inhalation. Methanol is rapidly metabolized by alcohol dehydrogenase to formaldehyde that is then oxidized to formic acid by formaldehyde dehydrogenase. In all domestic nonprimate animals, formic acid rapidly converts to CO_2 and water. Formic acid is metabolized much more slowly in humans, leading to blindness and other effects. These effects do not occur in domestic companion or production animals.

Mechanism of Action

The mechanisms of action of methanol in the CNS in nonprimates are presumed to be similar to those of ethanol. However, the methanol is generally a less potent inebriant than ethanol. Methanol is generally more irritating to the gastrointestinal tract than ethanol. Acute pancreatitis is common in acute methanol poisoning. Methanol is a proven teratogen.

Toxicity

The minimum lethal dosage in dogs is between 5.0 and 11.25 mg/kg. Methanol is far more toxic to primates, where blindness and neuronal necrosis can occur after exposure to relatively small amounts.

Clinical Effects

The effects of methanol in nonprimate companion animals essentially resemble those of ethanol. Importantly, methanol does not produce blindness in nonprimates. Unlike ethanol, an increased anion gap is typically present in methanol toxicoses.

Differential Diagnoses

Important differential diagnoses are similar to those of ethanol, but also include other potential causes of anion gap metabolic acidosis. Common causes of anion metabolic acidosis can be memorized using the following mnemonic AT MUD PILES: **A**lcohols, **T**oluene; **M**ethanol, **U**remia, **D**iabetic ketoacidosis (alcoholic ketoacidosis, starvation ketoacidosis; **P**araldehyde (phenformin), **I**ron (isoniazid), **L**actic acidosis, **E**thylene glycol and **S**alicylates (nonsteroidal anti-inflammatory drugs).

Diagnostics

Ante- and postmortem diagnostic techniques are essentially the same as for ethanol.

Management of Exposures

In nonprimate companion animals, the management of methanol poisoning resembles that of ethanol poisoning.

Prognosis

In nonprimate domestic animals, the prognosis is similar to ethanol toxicoses.

Isopropanol

Synonyms include 1-methylethanol; 2-hydroxypropane; 2-propanol; 2-propyl alcohol; dimethylcarbinol; isopropyl alcohol; isopropyl alcohol, rubbing alcohol.

Sources/Formulations

Isopropanol is typically used in the same range of household and industrial products as ethanol. Seventy percent aqueous isopropanol is extensively used in medicine as an antiseptic and cleansing agent, and isopropanol is used as the base in alcohol-based flea and tick sprays.

Kinetics

Isopropanol is rapidly absorbed from the gastrointestinal tract: approximately 80% of an oral dose is absorbed within 30 minutes. Except in the case of massive overdose, absorption is usually complete within 2 hours. Isopropanol is rapidly metabolized to acetone via alcohol dehydrogenase. Acetone is metabolized relatively slowly compared with the metabolites of ethanol and methanol.

Mechanism of Action

Isopropanol is a potent CNS depressant and its metabolite, acetone, potentiates this effect. Acetone, by itself, is also a CNS depressant. The mechanisms of action of isopropanol in the CNS are assumed to be similar to that of ethanol.

Toxicity

Isopropanol is approximately two times more toxic than ethanol. This is due to a combination of the innate properties of isopropanol, plus the potentiating effect and long half-life of its main metabolite, acetone.

Clinical Effects

Acute isopropanol toxicosis following voluntary consumption is relatively uncommon in domestic animals because of its bitter taste. The clinical effects resemble those of ethanol. Given an identical dose, CNS signs will generally be more severe in isopropanol poisoning compared with ethanol poisoning.

Differential Diagnoses

Differential diagnoses are as per ethanol.

Diagnostics

Ante- and postmortem diagnostic techniques are essentially the same as for ethanol.

Management of Exposures

The management of isopropanol poisoning resembles that of ethanol poisoning.

Prognosis

In nonprimate domestic animals, the prognosis is similar to ethanol toxicoses.

Benzyl Alcohol (Benzoid Acid, Sodium Benzoate, Potassium Benzoate)

Synonyms include benzyl alcohol, benzenemethanol, alphahydroxytoluene, phenol carbinol, phenyl carbinol, phenylmethanol, and phenylmethyl alcohol.

Sources/Formulations

Benzyl alcohol is most commonly encountered in veterinary medicine as an excipient and antibacterial preservative in pharmaceutical preparations, particularly those designed for intravenous delivery. Significant exposures may occur during repeated drug infusions or when bacteriostatic water or sodium chloride solutions are used to flush IV lines.

Benzoic acid and its benzoate salts are common food additives/preservatives. Benzyl alcohol is a natural constituent of a number of plants. It occurs, for example, in some edible fruits (up to 5 mg/kg) and in green and black tea (1–30 and 1–15 mg/kg, respectively). Benzyl alcohol is added as a flavoring substance to some foods and beverages at a level up to about 400 mg/kg (chewing gum 1254 mg/kg). Benzyl alcohol is extensively uses as a preservative in cosmetics and personal care products.

Among domestic animals, toxicity has most commonly been reported in cats administered lactated Ringer's solution containing benzyl alcohol as a preservative.

Kinetics

Benzyl alcohol is rapidly metabolized to benzyl aldehyde by alcohol dehydrogenase. Alcohol dehydrogenase then converts benzyl aldehyde to benzoic acid. In all domestic species except cats, benzoic acid is either glucuronidated to form benzyl glucuronide or conjugated to glycine to form hippuric acid. These metabolites are then largely excreted in urine.

Mechanism of Action

Domestic cats lack the ability to rapidly glucuronidate benzoic acid and primarily slowly metabolize benzoic acid to hippuric acid. Under these circumstances, benzoic acid accumulates, resulting in anion-gap metabolic acidosis. Benzoic acid has been shown to be extremely toxic to cats.

Toxicity

Benzyl alcohol is relatively toxic in cats. Lactated Ringer's solution containing 1.5% benzyl alcohol can cause severe signs of toxicosis in this species

Clinical Effects

Antemortem

Clinical signs in cats include hyperesthesia, followed by depression, coma, and finally death. In humans, respiratory distress (gasping syndrome), CNS depression, seizures and hemolysis are regarded as highly suggestive of benzyl alcohol poisoning. Surprisingly, hemolysis has not been reported in cats. The clinical chemistry picture is dominated by the presence of anion gap metabolic acidosis.

Postmortem

There are no specific findings.

Differential Diagnoses

Differential diagnoses are as per ethanol.

Diagnostics

Apart from a history of exposure, the most effective method of confirming the diagnosis is detection of elevated levels of benzyl alcohol, benzoic acid, and/or hippuric acid in blood, serum, urine, or aqueous humor.

Management of Exposures

Treatment resembles that of ethanol poisoning. Hemodialysis has been used in humans, but its effectiveness remains unknown.

Higher Alcohols

These include butanols, pentanols, hexanols, heptanols, octanols, paraffinic alcohols, aliphatic alcohols, and amyl alcohol (n-pentanyl alcohol), among others.

Sources/Formulations

Higher alcohols are largely used in industrial settings as solvent for paints, lacquers and varnishes, natural and synthetic resins, gums, vegetable oils, and dyes and alkaloids. They are used as intermediates in the manufacture of pharmaceuticals and chemicals and employed in industries producing artificial leather, textiles, safety glass, rubber cement, shellac, raincoats, and photographic films. They are also used as fragrances and solvents in perfumes, cosmetics, and personal care products.

Kinetics

Generally speaking, the shorter-chain higher alcohols are well absorbed through skin, the respiratory tract, and the gastrointestinal tract. Glucuronidation is a common pathway of metabolism for many of these chemicals. Excretion in urine is usually the major route of excretion.

Mechanism of Action

The mechanism of action of the higher alcohols in the CNS is assumed to be similar to that of ethanol and the hydrocarbon solvents. Given that glucuronidation is important in the metabolism and excretion of these alcohols, it is likely that cats are significantly more sensitive to toxicity (cats have relatively inefficient glucuronidation of metabolites).

Butanols and amyl alcohols are irritants. Amyl alcohol exposure results in hearing impairment in humans. All of the higher alcohols will produce defatting injuries to the skin with repeated exposures. Most of these chemicals will produce dyschromatopsias (alterations in color vision) in humans.

Toxicity

As a general rule, as the alcohol's carbon chain lengthens, its toxicity decreases. Branched chain alcohols are generally more toxic than the straight chained alcohols of similar carbon number. Longer chain alcohols are absorbed more slowly, are less able to penetrate the skin, and are less likely to be inhaled.

Importantly, many of the higher alcohols have kinematic viscosities less than $19\,mm^2 \times s^{-1}$ and are thus significant aspiration hazards.

Clinical Effects

Antemortem

Acute exposure to higher alcohols may result in CNS depression, hypotension, nausea, vomiting, and diarrhea. Butanols and amyl alcohols are irritants. Most of these materials are significant aspiration hazards. If aspirated, hemorrhagic pneumonitis is common. Other effects resemble those of ethanol.

Postmortem

Postmortem effects resemble those in ethanol poisoning. Chemical hemorrhagic aspiration pneumonitis is likely.

Differential Diagnoses

Differential diagnoses are as per ethanol.

Diagnostics

A history of potential exposure is the most important diagnostic tool. Tests for the presence of these materials in biological samples are not routinely available. The presence of chemical pneumonitis is strongly suggestive of postingestion aspiration.

Management of Exposures

General symptomatic management as per ethanol poisoning is recommended.

Prognosis

Given their generally lower toxicity, for a given identical dose, the prognosis can usually be expected to be better than ethanol toxicity.

GLYCOLS

Ethylene Glycol

Synonyms include 1,2-dihydroxyethane; 1,2-ethandiol; 1,2-ethane-diol; 2-hydroxyethanol; ethylene alcohol; ethylene dihydrate; glycol; monoethylene glycol; MEG; Lutrol-9; Dowtherm Sr 1; Fridex; Norkool; Ramp; Tescol; Ucar 17.

Sources

Ethylene glycol is a ubiquitous household chemical found in adhesives, sealers, deicers, radiator coolants, hydraulic fluids, some brake fluids, cleaners, wood preservatives, grouting mixtures, inks, caulks, and paints. One of the most common sources of ethylene glycol poisoning in domestic animals is automotive radiator coolant.

Kinetics

Ethylene glycol is rapidly and nearly completely absorbed from the digestive tract. Peak blood concentrations occur within about 1–4 hours following ingestion. Ethylene glycol is oxidized by alcohol deydrogenase to glycoaldehyde and then subsequently converted to glycolic acid, glyoxylic acid, and oxalic acid (Figure 28.1). Glyoxylic acid is metabolized in intermediary metabolism to malate, formate, and glycine. Ethylene glycol, glycolic acid, calcium oxalate, and glycine (and its conjugate, hippurate) are excreted in urine.

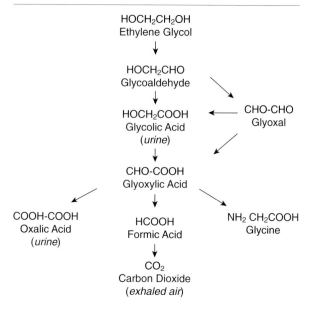

Figure 28.1. Metabolism of ethylene glycol.

Mechanism of Action

Ethylene glycol poisoning has three basic mechanisms of action: (1) CNS depression and inebriating effects that resemble those of the alcohols; (2) the metabolism to glycoaldehyde, glycolic acid, glyoxylic acid, oxalic acid, malate, formate, and glycine results in an anion gap metabolic acidosis; and (3) free calcium in the blood and tissues reacts with oxalic acid to form calcium oxalate, which then crystallizes out of solution in the proximal tubules of the kidney and in and around small blood vessels (particularly in the brain). This results in kidney failure.

Toxicity

The minimum lethal dosage of pure ethylene glycol in dogs is around 6.6 ml/kg. Cats are significantly more sensitive, with a minimum lethal dosage of around 1.5 ml/kg.

Clinical Effects

Signs

The ethylene glycol toxidrome occurs in three sequential stages. Stage 1 is the CNS depression phase. CNS depression begins soon after exposure, and lasts up to 12 hours after ingestion. This depression appears similar to ethanol intoxication but is typically more severe on a consumed volume-to-volume basis compared with ethanol consumption. The effects are due to unmetabolized ethylene glycol. Frequent urination and excessive thirst are common signs in dogs during this early stage. Cats typically do not develop this polydipsia.

Stage 2 is the cardiopulmonary phase. It is characterized by cardiorespiratory signs that typically consist of tachycardia, tachypnea, and hypotension or hypertension. After the glycoaldehyde metabolite forms at 4–12 hours post-consumption, anion gap metabolic acidosis develops and the following effects may occur: seizures, myoclonic jerks, cerebral edema (in some cases), and coma, gastrointestinal irritation (vomiting). Cerebral edema, deposition of calcium oxalate crystals in the walls of small blood vessels in the brain, and exposure of the metabolically active deep grey matter nuclei of the brain basal ganglia to ethylene glycol metabolites contribute to the CNS toxicity.

Significant cardiac arrhythmias may occur during this phase.

Significant pulmonary edema, pneumonitis, congestive heart failure, and circulatory shock may develop during this phase.

Metabolism of the glycoaldehyde to oxalic acid often results in the appearance of calcium oxalate crystal precipitates in the meninges, blood vessel walls, lung, myocardium, and associated tissue injury. The formation of calcium oxalate crystal precipitates in tissues may be associated with hypocalcemia. Death may occur during this stage in some cases.

Stage 3 is the renal failure phase. Kidney damage due to formation of calcium oxalate crystals in the renal tubules usually develops 24–72 hours after exposure. The subsequent decline in kidney function and oliguria exacerbate the anion gap metabolic acidosis and other serum chemistry disturbances.

Classically, the formation of calcium oxalate crystals in the kidneys has been claimed associated with the development of the "renal medullary rim" or "halo" sign in dogs. A renal medullary rim sign is detected by ultrasound and is a distinct hyperechoic line in the renal medulla parallel to the corticomedullary junction. However, more recent studies have demonstrated that the renal medullary rim sign is a nonspecific ultrasonographic sign that is present in a high proportion of dogs with apparently normal kidney function.

The following conditions characterize the third phase: flank pain, costovertebral angle tenderness, and oliguric renal failure. Prolonged, rarely permanent, kidney failure is distinguished by proteinuria, hematuria, crystalluria, and increased serum BUN and creatinine. Calcium oxalate crystals may appear in the urine as early as stage 1, but absence of these crystals does not rule out the diagnosis of ethylene glycol poisoning. Myopathy and bone marrow suppression may occur in some individuals

Laboratory Findings

Ethylene glycol test kits are available that will accurately detect blood ethylene glycol down to a level of 50 mg/dl. Unfortunately, cats may become significantly poisoned at blood levels below 50 mg/dl. Thus the test is not sufficiently sensitive enough to conclusively rule out ethylene glycol toxicosis in cats. Furthermore, in patients that present in the late stages of the toxicosis, blood ethylene glycol levels may fall below the limit of detection due to its catabolism. Two newer ethylene glycol test kits have been introduced, but both of these kits can give false positives in the presence of alcohols, so careful interpretation of the results is needed.

An osmolal gap, without metabolic acidosis, or an anion gap can be detected before significant metabolism of ethylene glycol occurs. As ethylene glycol is metabolized, the osmolal gap, if present, will decrease and an anion gap metabolic acidosis evolves. Patients who present late may have renal failure with normal osmolal and anion gaps and no acidosis or measurable ethylene glycol levels.

Isosthenuria, due to an osmotic diuresis produced by urinary excretion of unmetabolized ethylene glycol is common in the early stage of the toxicosis in dogs. Decrease in urine specific gravity may also occur in cats during this stage, but isosthenuria rarely develops. Calcium oxalate monohydrate crystals (clear, six-sided, prismlike crystals) can be detected within 3–6 hours postingestion in dogs. Urinary crystals can take many forms such as dumbbells, envelopes, and needles (most commonly). Importantly, the absence of urinary crystals, however, does not rule out poisoning. Urinary pH is usually decreased in ethylene glycol poisoning.

Many radiator fluid formulations that contain ethylene glycol also contain fluorescine (a fluorescent green or red dye, depending on pH). In occasional cases, the dye (which fluoresces with UV light exposure) may be detectable in the urine. It may also be useful to examine any vomitus, the mouth, the face, and the animal's paws with a Wood's lamp to determine whether they appear fluorescent.

Once oliguric or anuric renal failure has developed (typically 24–48 hours following ingestion), large increases in serum blood urea nitrogen (BUN) and creatinine will occur. Elevated serum potassium usually develops during this phase. About 50% of patients will also have decreased serum calcium due to the formation of calcium oxalate. Likewise, about 50% of patients will have elevated blood glucose.

During the period of recovery from renal failure, patients will typically be isosthenuric. Urinalysis during this phase will typically reveal calcium oxalate monohydrate crystals, hematuria, proteinuria, and glucosuria.

Differential Diagnoses

The most critical differential diagnosis in the early stages of the toxidrome is poisoning by the various alcohols. Hydrocarbon solvents, chemsols, marijuana, macrolide antiparasitics, and amitraz produce similar effects to the alcohols, as do most benzodiazepine, barbiturate, antipsychotic, antiseizure, and antidepressant human prescription drugs. During the later stages of the toxidrome, other causes of renal failure are the major differential diagnoses.

Diagnostics

Antemortem

The patient's history plus the presence of the typical clinical signs/laboratory findings of the ethylene glycol toxidrome plus detection of ethylene glycol in vomitus, urine, or blood are usually the best diagnostic clues. The level of ethylene glycol or its metabolites can be measured in most body fluids and in the gastric contents. Definitive diagnosis typically requires the determination of blood ethylene glycol. Aspirating stomach contents using a small-bore nasogastric tube can often yield useful samples if performed within about 30 to 60 minutes following ingestion. Samples of the material suspected of being ingested, preferably in the original container, are always particularly valuable. It is important to communicate other possible exposures to the testing lab since 2,3-butanediol, often found in the plasma of following ethanol ingestion, can be mistakenly identified as ethylene glycol when the analysis is performed by gas chromatography. Propylene glycol can also interfere with some ethylene glycol assays.

Recent studies have demonstrated usefulness of glycolic acid analysis in ethylene glycol poisoning cases. Measuring glycolic acid in ethylene glycol poisonings has certain advantages: findings correlate better with ethylene glycol toxicity than ethylene glycol levels, findings determine how much ethylene glycol has metabolized to glycolic acid, the presence of glycolic acid objectively indicates toxicity, and the test confirms that the metabolic acidosis was due to ethylene glycol poisoning rather than another cause.

Postmortem

Signs of gastritis or enteritis (gastric and intestinal mucosa is hemorrhagic and hyperemic) are typically present, as are pulmonary edema and hyperemia. The kidneys are usually swollen, tan-colored and have intermittent gray or yellow streaks at the corticomedullary junction.

Histologically, calcium oxalate crystals are found in and around the proximal convoluted tubules of the kidneys. In animals that survive, regenerating renal tubules may be seen. Similar crystals may be seen in the adventitia and perivascular spaces of the brain blood vessels.

Management of Exposures

Decontamination of the upper digestive tract either by inducing vomiting or dosing with activated charcoal has been proven to be ineffective. Aspiration of stomach contents with a small-bore nasogastric tube may be of some benefit and may yield valuable diagnostic samples if performed within about 30–60 minutes postingestion.

There are three critical objectives in the treatment of ethylene glycol poisoning: (1) prevention of conversion of ethylene glycol to its toxic metabolites, (2) correction of the anion-gap metabolic acidosis and maintenance of renal glomerular filtration rate, (3) adjunctive and supportive care. Except for hemodialysis, which is rarely available in veterinary practice, the older practices of increasing the excretion of ethylene glycol and its toxic metabolites by forced dieresis and/or urinary alkalinization have been proved to be ineffective. Furthermore, these techniques have been demonstrated to increase the serious complication rate and the death rate.

The single most important factor associated with survival and reduction of morbidity in ethylene glycol poisoning is preventing conversion of ethylene glycol to its toxic metabolites by the prompt administration of the specific antidote fomepizole (4-methylpyrazole). Fomepizole (loading dose of 15 mg/kg IV followed in 12 hours by 10 mg/kg every 12 hours for 4 doses) is the first choice antidote and is highly effective even in cases of massive poisonings and substantially reduces the risk of significant CNS and renal complications. Fomepizole is also highly effective following oral dosing. Fomepizole acts as a competitive inhibitor of the metabolism of ethylene glycol to glycolaldehyde metabolite and thus limits the formation of oxalate and associated tissue crystallization of calcium oxalate. Fomepizole greatly reduces the severity of the cardiopulmonary and renal failure stages of the poisoning. Fomepizole has a high therapeutic index and a very low risk of serious side effects. Fomepizole will not prevent the inebriation and CNS effects induced by unmetabolized ethylene glycol (and any other alcohols present) and may prolong this state in poisoned individuals.

The second choice antidote is ethanol. Ethanol can be administered as a 5% aqueous solution intravenously. The intravenous solution is hyperosmotic and can cause osmotic dehydration, hyponatremia, and venous irrita-

Table 28.1. Distilled alcoholic beverages and doses that can be administered by small-bore nasogastric tube to treat ethylene glycol exposure

Name of Alcoholic Beverage	Typical Proof	Typical Percent Ethanol by Volume	Typical Grams of Ethanol per 100 ml of Beverage	Typical ml/kg of Beverage Required for Loading Dose	Typical ml/kg of Beverage Required for Maintenance Dose
Brandy	40–60	20–30%	15.8–23.7	3.2–4.7 ml/kg	0.64–0.94 ml/kg
Cognac	80	40%	31.6	2.4	0.5 ml/kg
Gin	90–110	45–55%	35.6–43.5	1.7–2.1 ml/kg	0.3–0.4 ml/kg
Grain alcohol	190	95%	75.0	1 ml/kg	0.2 ml/kg
Rum	151	75.5%	59.6	1.3 ml/kg	0.25 ml/kg
Schnapps	30–100	15–50%	11.8–39.5	1.9–6.4 ml/kg	0.4–1.3 ml/kg
Tequila	80–100	40–50%	31.6–39.5	1.9–2.4 ml/kg	0.4–0.5 ml/kg
Vodka	80–100	40–50%	31.6–39.5	1.9–2.4 ml/kg	0.4–0.5 ml/kg
Whisky	80–100	40–50%	31.6–39.5	1.9–2.4 ml/kg	0.4–0.5 ml/kg

tion. Regardless of route of administration the objective is to rapidly achieve and maintain a blood ethanol concentration of at least 100 mg/dl in order to provide adequate competitive inhibition of ethylene glycol metabolism. To attain this goal, it is usual to administer a loading dose of 0.6 g/kg. A maintenance dose is chosen based upon the ethanol elimination rate (66–130 mg/kg/hour). Frequent blood ethanol determinations should be made. Any increase in the anion gap or decrease in blood bicarbonate concentration implies that the ethanol dose is insufficient to achieve competitive inhibition of ethylene glycol metabolism. The disadvantages of ethanol include further disturbance of blood electrolyte and glucose levels, increased CNS depression, ethanol-related toxicity such as hepatitis, pancreatitis, hypoglycemia and disulfiam-like reactions, increased cardiovascular/respiratory depression, and hypothermia. Overly aggressive treatment with ethanol should be avoided. Never administer ethanol to a hypothermic patient. Never administer ethanol to a significantly dehydrated patient or an animal in oliguric/anuric renal failure. Patients undergoing ethanol treatment require intensive monitoring, particularly for exacerbated cardiovascular/respiratory depression, hypothermia, dehydration and electrolyte disturbances.

In extreme circumstances where ethanol infusion is not possible, pharmaceutical-grade material can be administered orally or by small-bore nasogastric tube. The oral loading dose is 750 mg/kg body weight administered slowly over the first hour, with a maintenance dose of 150 mg/kg body weight per hour thereafter. Always administer the ethanol slowly to reduce the risk of vomiting. If there is a high risk of vomiting, secure the airway using a cuffed endotracheal tube.

If pharmaceutical-grade ethanol is not available, distilled alcoholic beverages can be administered by small bore nasogastric tube as summarized in Table 28.1.

Administration of thiamine hydrochloride (promotes the metabolism of ethylene glycol to ketoadipate), and the administration of vitamin B6 (pyridoxine; promotes the metabolism of ethylene glycol to glycine and ultimately to hippuric acid) may be beneficial.

Detailed discussion of the treatment of acute oliguric renal failure and anion-gap metabolic acidosis is beyond the scope of this chapter. However, reestablishment of a near-normal renal glomerular filtration rate by the use of intravenous crystalloids and/or diuretics, such as manitol, and/or vasopressors, such as dopamine, is often the most effective method of correcting the anion-gap metabolic acidosis and other electrolyte disturbances associated with ethylene glycol poisoning. Care must be taken to avoid exacerbating electrolyte disturbances such as hyperkalemia and/or hypernatremia. The administration of bicarbonate may be useful in the initial control of metabolic acidosis.

Regular monitoring of the patient's electrocardiogram and early correction of any arrhythmias that develop is recommended.

Prognosis

The prognosis for ethylene glycol poisoning in domestic animals is always guarded. Early aggressive treatment, particularly with fomepizole, is associated with an improved prognosis.

Propylene Glycol

Synonyms include 1,2-dihydroxypropane; 1,2-propylene glycol; 2,3-propanediol; isopropylene glycol; 1,2-propanediol; and trimethyl glycol.

Sources/Formulations

Propylene glycol is a ubiquitous ingredient in cosmetic and personal care products. It is also a "Generally Recognized as Safe" food additive, except in cat foods. In food, it is primarily used as a humectant. It can also be found in paints, cleaning agents, sealants, inks, and caulking agents. Propylene glycol is progressively replacing the use of ethylene glycol in radiator coolants, deicing solutions, and hydraulic fluids. It is also a ubiquitous excipient and solvent in pharmaceutical preparations.

Kinetics

Propylene glycol is rapidly and relatively completely absorbed from the gastrointestinal tract. Propylene glycol undergoes metabolic oxidation to pyruvic acid, acetic acid, lactic acid, and propionaldehyde. These metabolites are then consumed, primarily by the citric acid cycle. Propylene glycol is rapidly converted to proprionic acid, a volatile fatty acid, in the rumen. The volatile fatty acid is then rapidly absorbed and converted to glucose via gluconeogenesis. For this reason, administration of propylene glycol via an ororumen tube has been used as an emergency energy supplement in debilitated sheep and cattle.

Mechanism of Action

The CNS is the main target organ in acute propylene glycol toxicoses. The effects are similar to ethanol and the other alcohols. The rapid metabolism of propylene glycol to lactic acid may also result in metabolic acidosis.

A high level of dietary propylene glycol produces oxidative damage to erythrocytes and decreased red cell lifespan in cats. For this reason, propylene glycol is no longer used in cat feeds.

Toxicity

The median lethal dosage in dogs is about 9 ml/kg. Horses appear to be more sensitive to the toxicoses than dogs with poisoning being reported at dosages around 6 ml/kg.

Clinical Effects

CNS depression is the primary manifestation of acute propylene glycol poisoning. Other effects include anion gap metabolic acidosis and blood hyperosmolality and frequent urination due to osmotic dieresis. Propylene glycol does not cause direct damage to the kidneys.

Propylene glycol is a common diluent for injectable medications, most notably phenytoin. Toxicity following intravenous injection of pharmaceuticals containing high levels of propylene glycol may cause hypotension and cardiac arrhythmias.

Differential Diagnoses

Important differential diagnoses are similar to those of ethanol and ethylene glycol but also include other potential causes of anion gap metabolic acidosis.

Diagnostics

A history of consumption and the presence of anion gap metabolic acidosis are key diagnostic pointers. Detection of propylene glycol in vomitus or samples obtained by small-bore nasogastric aspiration, and/or in blood or other body fluids is usually conclusive. As always, samples of the ingested material are always particularly useful.

Management of Exposures

Antidotal therapy with fomepizole or ethanol is not required. Care is largely supportive. Intravenous bicarbonate and fluid therapy may be necessary to correct the acidosis and prevent dehydration.

Prognosis

Propylene glycol is normally unpalatable to domestic animals. Thus voluntary ingestions usually result in mild intoxication. Sere anion gap metabolic acidosis is indicative of a more guarded prognosis.

Butylene Glycol

Synonyms include 1,3-butanediol and 1,3-butylene glycol.

Sources/Formulations

Butylene glycol is commonly used in cosmetics and personal care products. Butylene glycol is a relatively common drug of abuse and has been sold in health food stores as a "supplement."

Kinetics

Butylene glycol is rapidly and nearly completely absorbed from the gastrointestinal tract. It is rapidly metabolized to acetoacetate and gamma-hydroxybutyrate.

Mechanism of Action

Gamma hydroxybutyrate is a CNS GABA agonist and this produces pronounced CNS depression and anesthetic/narcoticlike effects.

Clinical Effects

The primary effects resemble those of alcohol intoxication.

Differential Diagnoses

Differential diagnoses are similar to ethanol.

Diagnostics

Detection of the material in the ingested substance, stomach contents or body fluids, plus a history of exposure are the key diagnostic steps.

Management of Exposures

Management is largely supportive and is similar to ethanol poisoning.

Prognosis

The prognosis is dependent on the severity of the CNS depression. The presence of unconsciousness or significant cardiovascular/respiratory depression is always associated with a more guarded prognosis.

BRAKE FLUID AND CLUTCH FLUIDS

Sources

Brake fluid is a common household item. The main chemical constituents are high boiling point and high molecular weight polyalkylene glycol ethers. Some brands may also contain small amounts of ethylene and/or diethylene glycol. These products also contain small amounts of additives (e.g., corrosion inhibitors, antioxidants). These materials are usually mobile, water miscible liquids. Color ranges from colorless to amber; in some cases it may also contain dyes.

Kinetics

The main routes of exposure are ingestion and skin contact. In general, these materials are relatively poorly absorbed from the intestinal tract. Ingestion of large amounts can result in systemic effects.

Mechanism of Action

In general, brake fluids are considered to be of low toxicity, following oral and dermal exposure. Since these products are based on synthetic, polyalkylene glycol ethers, their acute toxicological properties are usually similar to those of the polyglycol ethers except that they do not produce damage to erythrocytes.

Brake fluids may cause eye irritation on accidental contact. The effects are likely to be only transient, however, and serious/permanent damage is considered unlikely.

Accidental skin contact is unlikely to cause significant irritation, although prolonged or repeated contact may cause dermatitis.

Exposure to high concentrations of mist or vapor is very unlikely because of the low vapor pressure of these products, but heating of the products may result in vapors capable of causing irritation of the respiratory tract.

Ingestion of small amounts is unlikely to cause systemic toxicity; transient gastrointestinal effects may, however, be experienced. Swallowing of larger amounts may result in nausea, vomiting and possibly signs of central nervous system depression. Kidney damage may also occur with some products, due to the presence of diethylene glycol.

The viscosity of the products is such that aspiration of product into the lung is unlikely.

Brake fluids contain small amounts of additives. Although some of these may be hazardous in their own right, the amount of each present, typically less than 1%, is unlikely to contribute significantly to the acute toxicity of the product.

Clinical Effects

Signs

Following ingestion, the main clinical signs will most commonly relate to gastrointestinal upset, i.e., salivation, vomiting, and diarrhea. If ingestion of large amounts has occurred, there is a possibility of central nervous system depression and/or kidney damage. In rare cases, kidney failure and death may result.

Laboratory Findings

Laboratory findings (if any) will most commonly reflect hemoconcentration. In very rare cases, evidence of kidney failure may be present (i.e., elevated blood urea nitrogen and creatinine, oliguria). Occasionally, the brake fluid may be visually detectable in the feces.

Differential Diagnoses

The most common differential diagnoses will be virtually any cause of acute diarrhea. If CNS depression is present, differential diagnoses are similar to those listed in the section on ethanol.

Diagnostics

A history of exposure and consumption is the most common method of diagnosis. Aspiration of stomach contents via small-bore nasogastric tube may yield valuable diagnostic samples if performed within about an hour following ingestion.

Management of Exposures

Management of ingestions is most commonly symptomatic and supportive. If the diarrhea is severe, fluid therapy may be required.

Contamination of the skin and coat is best managed by gentle washing in a body-temperature solution of dilute, mild, neutral hand-dishwashing detergent followed by rinsing with clean water. Several rinse/wash cycles over a 5–10 minute period may be required. Alternatives to dishwashing detergents include pharmaceutical-grade PEG 400, PEG 300, and polyvinyl pyrrolidone solutions.

Due to their skin barrier disruptive effect, the use of solvents, petroleum distillates (such as baby oil, Stoddard solvent, engine degreasers, naphthas, kerosene, petrol, diesel etc), mechanic's hand degreasers, strong cationic detergents, strong anionic detergents and abrasive materials is contraindicated in dermal decontamination. These materials are known to be ineffective and to increase systemic absorption.

Prognosis

Prognosis is usually good.

DETERGENTS

Sources

Detergents are ubiquitous materials in most households. There are four basic types.

Anionic Detergents

The detergent property of these materials is due to its anionic properties. The anion is neutralized with an alkaline or basic material to produce full detergency. There are three main groups: the alkyl aryl sulphonates, the long-chain (fatty) alcohol sulphates, and other sulphonates (olefine sulphates and sulphonates, alpha olefine sulphates and sulphonates, sulphated monoglycerides, sulphated ethers, sulphosuccinates, alkane sulphonates, phosphate esters, alkyl isethionates, sucrose esters).

These materials commonly contain water-softening agents such as sodium phosphate, sodium carbonate, and sodium silicate. Laundry detergents (liquid and powdered) and shampoos are the most common sources of these materials in the home.

Nonionic Detergents

The materials are ionically inert and are the largest and most chemically diverse member of the detergent chemical family. Typical nonionic detergents include alkyl and aryl polyether suphates, alcohols or sulfonates, polyglycol ethers, polyethylene glycol, and sorbitan monostearate. Common household sources of these materials include soaps, laundry detergents, and dishwashing detergents.

Cationic Detergents

The detergency of these materials is dependent on its cationic properties. However, these have poor detergency and are more commonly used as germicides, fabric softeners, and specialist emulsifiers; liquid potpourri products are also sources of cationic detergents. Typically, these materials are large halogenated (i.e., contain bromine, iodide, or chlorine) molecules. Common examples include benzethonium chloride, benzalkonium chloride, methyl benzethonium, cetylpyridinium chloride, and holgenated quarternary ammonium compounds.

Amphoteric Detergents

These contain both acidic and basic groups in their molecule and can act as cationic or anionic detergents, depending on the pH of the solution. These materials are commonly found in shampoos, skin cleaners, and carpet shampoo. They are very stable in strong acidic conditions and often used in conjunction with hydrofluoric acid in industrial settings.

Kinetics and Mechanism of Action

The main site of action of most of these materials is local i.e., at the site of contact. In most cases, this means the skin, the oral mucous membranes or the gastrointestinal tract. The systemic toxicity of most domestic detergents is usually relatively low. The notable exceptions to this generalization are the cationic detergents and those detergents that contain citronella extract (fragrance), pine oil extracts (fragrance), or phenol-based disinfectants (see relevant sections of this text).

Toxicity

In most circumstances, detergents formulated for general household use are specifically designed to have a low toxic potential. The exception to this is often machine dishwashing detergents, which are notoriously alkaline and capable of producing serious caustic burns to mucous membranes and the gastrointestinal tract.

As a general rule, ionic detergents are more irritating than nonionic detergents and anionic detergents are less irritating than cationic detergents. Household anionic detergents are rarely irritant or toxic, even following ingestion. Cationic detergents (particularly quarternary ammonium compounds) are irritating to the gastrointestinal tract, skin, and mucous membranes and may be potent systemic toxicants.

Clinical Effects

Signs

Repeated exposure of the skin to detergents results in a cumulative irritant dermatitis, typically due to defatting injury to the skin. Relevant clinical signs include thickening of the skin with weeping, cracking, scaling, and possibly blistering.

Splash injuries to the eyes with nonionic or anionic detergents usually produce transient signs of irritation. Splash injuries of the eyes by cationic detergents are potentially serious and may result in significant damage to the cornea and surrounding eye structures.

Ingestion of many ionic detergents often results in signs of gastrointestinal disturbance i.e., salivation, vomiting, nausea, diarrhea, and gastrointestinal distension.

Quarternary ammonium compounds are frequently corrosive to the mouth, and gastrointestinal tract and ingestion may result in serious vomiting (including vomiting of blood (appears like "coffee grounds" due to partial digestion in the stomach), diarrhea, vascular shock, collapse, and possibly death.

Ingestion of cationic detergents, particularly those containing quarternary ammonium compounds, is associated with a systemic toxidrome consisting of CNS and respiratory depression, fever, seizures, collapse, and coma.

Ingestion of anionic detergents may result in intravascular red cell hemolysis in patients with impaired liver function. This is thought to be due to the reduced metabolism and excretion of the detergent.

Laboratory Findings

Since most of the effects of detergent are local, few laboratory signs can be expected in most cases. Clinical pathology signs that reflect dehydration may occur in cases where significant diarrhea is present. Alkaline dishwashing detergents will cause coagulative to liquefactive necrosis at the sites of contact.

Differential Diagnoses

The most common differential diagnoses will be virtually any cause of acute diarrhea or cumulative skin irritation. Systemic cationic detergent poisoning (particularly quarternary ammonium compounds) may resemble several types of pesticide poisoning.

Diagnostics

A history of exposure and consumption is the most common method of diagnosis.

Management of Exposures

Splash injuries to the eyes should be initially treated by copious flushing of the affected eye(s) with water or a specialist eye flush solution for 10 to 15 minutes. Specialist treatment may be required, particularly for eye injuries due to cationic detergents or machine dishwashing detergents.

Washing with hand soaps (technically a mild anionic detergent) are generally effective at neutralizing and removing cationic detergents on the skin.

Administration of milk, egg whites, or water as diluents has been recommended for treatment of ingestion of anionic and cationic detergents provided there is no corrosive injury to the gastrointestinal tract. Induction of emesis is generally contraindicated because of the potential corrosive action of these materials. Activated charcoal use is also commonly recommended, although its efficacy is unknown. Simple aspiration of stomach contents using a fine-bore nasogastric tube may also be beneficial if performed within about 60 minutes postingestion.

Management of ingestions is most commonly symptomatic and supportive. If the diarrhea is severe or if vascular shock is present/likely, intravenous fluid therapy may be required. If significant damage to the mouth and/or esophagus has occurred, placement of a percutaneous esophageal gastric tube may be required for adequate nutritional support.

Prognosis

With ingestion of nonionic and anionic detergents, prognosis is usually good. With ingestion of cationic detergents, prognosis is often guarded.

ESSENTIAL OILS

Essential oils (see also herbal toxicities in Chapters 21) are fragrant hydrophobic plant extracts produced by distillation or solvent extraction of plant material. Common alternative names include "volatile oils," "votive oils," "ethereal oils," or simply as the "oil of" the plant material from which they were extracted, such as oil of clove. These oily plant extracts are considered "essential" if they carry a distinctive scent or essence, of plant source. These materials do not have any specific chemical properties other than their characteristic fragrances.

Sources and Toxicity

Common essential oils found in many household products and herbal medicine products are listed in Table 28.2.

Table 28.2. Common essential oils found in many household and herbal medicine products

Name of Essential Oil	Plant of Origin	Chemical Properties	Key Toxic Effects
Camphor oil	*Cinnamomum camphora*	Camphor, a terpinoid	Pure material is an aspiration hazard. Local irritant to skin, eye, and gastrointestinal tract; CNS manifestations may range from an altered mental status to seizures to coma.
Cardamom oil	*Elettaria cardamomum*	1,8-Cineole (eucalyptol) and alpha-terpinyl acetate	Pure material is an aspiration hazard. Low potential for toxicity.
Carnation oil	*Dianthus caryophyllus*	Eugenol, phenethyl alcohol, linalool, benzyl benzoate, (Z)-3-hexenyl benzoate and benzyl salicylate	Pure material is an aspiration hazard. Low potential for toxicity.
Carrot seed oil	*Daucus carota* (carrot)	50% carotol, a sesquiterpene alcohol	Pure material is an aspiration hazard. Like most sequiterpene-containing materials it is an irritant to the gastrointestinal tract, respiratory tract, skin. and eyes. Possibly CNS effects may occur at high doses.
Cedar oil	Cedar wood oils: *Juniperus* spp., *Cupressus* spp. Cedar leaf oil: *Thuja occidentalis*	30 % (+)-cedrol, alpha-cedrene, and other sesquiterpenes	Pure material is an aspiration hazard. Skin, eye, and gastrointestinal irritant. Long-term high exposure to vapor may result in lung and liver damage. Cedrol is a sedative.
Citral (syn = lemonal)	Present in the oils of several plants, including lemon myrtle (90–98%), *Listsea citrata* (90%), *Litsea cubeba* (70–85%), lemongrass (65–85%), lemon tea-tree (70–80%), *Ocimum gratissimum* (66.5%), *Lindera citriodora* (approx. 65%), *Calypranthes parriculata* (approx. 62%), petitgrain (36%), lemon verbena (30–35%), lemon ironbark (26%), lemon balm (11%), lime (6–9%), lemon (2–5%), and oranges	Bi-terpenoid	Pure material is an aspiration hazard. Low toxicity in lab animal studies. May produce contact hypersensitivity in some individuals.

DL-Limonene	Purified chemical substance from orange or lemon oils	Pure material is an aspiration hazard. Can have a phototoxic effect on bare skin. Citrus oil flea dips have been associated with poisoning in cats—clinical signs include hypersalivation, muscle tremors, ataxia, coma, and death.
Eucalyptus oil	*Eucalyptus globulus*	1,8-cineole and alpha-pinene (bicyclic terpene)	Poisoning affects the nervous system (loss of consciousness, hypoventilation, depression of reflexes, and convulsions), the gastrointestinal system (abdominal pain, vomiting, and diarrhea) and the respiratory system (respiratory depression, dyspnea, pneumonitis, and bronchospasm). Gastrointestinal effects are frequently the initial effects, although drowsiness may occur in a few minutes and coma within 10 minutes. The patient may vomit while drowsy or unconscious and aspiration is a major risk. Tachycardia and weak irregular pulse has been noted. Muscle weakness and ataxia may occur. Nephritis is rare but has been recorded. Both miosis and mydriasis can occur (miosis being more common). Central nervous system (CNS) depression or vomiting have been delayed up to 4 hours. Recovery or death is often within 24 hours. It is a mild skin irritant.
Lemon oil	*Citrus limon* (Lemon tree)	>90% d-limonene (a cyclic terpene).	Pure material is an aspiration hazard. Can have a phototoxic effect on bare skin. Citrus oil flea dips have been associated with poisoning in cats—clinical signs include hypersalivation, muscle tremors, ataxia, coma, and death.
Menthol	Purified chemical substance from peppermint or spearmint	Aromatic alcohol	Pure material is an aspiration hazard. Has low toxicity. Pure material is a moderate skin, eye, and gastrointestinal irritant.

Continued

Table 28.2. *Continued*

Name of Essential Oil	Plant of Origin	Chemical Properties	Key Toxic Effects
Oil of citronella	*Cymbopogon* sp. (Citronella grasses)	*Ceylon type:* (obtained from *Cymbopogon nardus* Rendle) consists of geraniol (18–20%), limonene (9–11%), methyl isoeugenol (7–11%), citronellol (6–8%), and citronellal (5–15%) *Java type:* (obtained from *Cymbopogon winterianus* Jowitt) consists of citronellal (32–45%), geraniol (11–13%), geranyl acetate (3–8%), limonene (1–4%)	Pure material is an aspiration hazard. Skin irritant in some individuals.
Oil of cloves	*Syzygium aromaticum*	60–90% eugenol, eugenyl acetate, caryophyllene	Pure material is an aspiration hazard. Large oral doses may produce vomiting, sore throat, seizure, sedation, pulmonary edema, vomiting of blood, decreased blood clotting, kidney failure, and liver damage or failure. May produce hypoglycemia. Undiluted clove oil has a high risk of causing contact dermatitis, skin irritation, and burns. Allergic reactions to clove, its component eugenol, have been reported, including possible severe reactions (anaphylaxis).
Oil of spearmint	*Mentha spicata*	R-Carvone, a terpinoid	Pure material is an aspiration hazard. Considered nontoxic. May be a gastrointestinal irritant.
Oil of wintergreen	*Gaultheria procumbens*	Menthyl salicylate and gaultherilene	Pure material is an aspiration hazard. See salicylate poisoning in the relevant section of this book.
Orange oil (syn = sweet orange)	*Citrus sinensis* (sweet orange tree)	>90% d-limonene (a cyclic terpene)	Pure material is an aspiration hazard. Can have a phototoxic effect on bare skin. Citrus oil flea dips have been associated with poisoning in cats—clinical signs include hypersalivation, muscle tremors, ataxia, coma, and death.

Pennyroyal oil	*Mentha pulegium*	Pulegone, menthone, iso-menthone, and neomenthone	Pure material is an aspiration hazard. Causes abortion in humans. Produces acute liver damage.
Peppermint oil	*Mentha × piperita*, a cross between the watermint (*Mentha aquatica*) and spearmint (*Mentha spicata*)	Menthol, an aromatic alcohol Carvone, a terpinoid	Pure material is an aspiration hazard. Peppermint oil is nontoxic and nonirritant in low concentrations. Pure material is irritant to the skin, mucous membranes, eyes, and gastrointestinal tract.
Pine oil	*Pinus sylvestris*	Mainly bicyclic terpene alcohols, but may also contain terpene hydrocarbons, ethers, and esters	Pure material is an aspiration hazard. Skin irritant at high concentration. Potential for contact hypersensitivity.
Sandalwood oil	*Santalum* sp.	Alpha and beta santalol, aromatic alcohols	Pure material is an aspiration hazard. Considered nontoxic and not irritating.
Sassafras oil	Brazilian sassafras oil, obtained from the trunkwood of *Ocotea pretiosa*, and Chinese sassafras oil from *Cinnamomum camphora*	>80% safrole, 5-menthoxy-eugenol, asarone, coniferaldehyde, camphone, and traces of thujone, anethole, apiol, and eugenol	Pure material is an aspiration hazard.. Safrole is carcinogenic and hepatotoxic. Irritant to skin, eyes, and gastrointestinal tract. CNS effects such as depression, hallucinations, and coma may occur.
Tea tree oil	*Melaleuca alternifolia*	Mixture of terpenoids and sesquiterpenoids, with terpinene-4-ol (36 %), gamme-terpinene (20 %), alpha-terpinene (8 %), and 1,8-cineole (4 %) as the major components	Pure material is an aspiration hazard. Can produce anaphylaxis in some individuals. Can be toxic in cats and dogs following topical exposure and ingestion. Toxidrome consists of ataxia, CNS depression, muscle tremors, coma. Evidence of liver damage has been reported in cats. Toxidrome following oral exposure resembles that of eucalyptus oil.

DIPHENYLMETHANE DIISOCYANATE ADHESIVES

Sources

Gorilla glue is the most common brand name. Similar products are marketed as polyurethane glues.

Toxicity and Treatment

As the glue dries, it will expand to 3–4 times its original volume. Thus, when the glue is swallowed, it will potentially cause an acute gastric obstruction. Surgical removal of the gastric foreign body is usually required.

DEICING SALTS

Sources

Common deicing salts may contain one or other of the following: calcium carbonate, calcium magnesium acetate, urea, potassium chloride, magnesium chloride, and sodium chloride.

Toxicity and Treatment

Calcium carbonate, calcium magnesium acetate, and urea are primarily gastric irritants and will produce vomiting and diarrhea. Sodium chloride can produce serious hypernatremia (muscle tremors, acidosis, seizures), and osmotic diuresis. Muscle weakness and cardiac rhythm/electrical abnormalities can result from ingestion of potassium chloride or magnesium chloride.

Treatment is symptomatic and supportive.

REFERENCES

Dart, R.C., Editor. 2003. *Medical Toxicology, 3rd ed.* Philadelphia: Lippincott Williams & Wilkins.

Gfeller, R.W. and Messonnier, S.P. 2003. *Handbook of Small Animal Toxicology and Poisonings.* St Louis: Mosby.

Gupta, R.C., Editor. 2007. *Veterinary Toxicology.* Basic and Clinical Principles. Amsterdam: Elsevier.

Osweiler, G.D. 1996. Toxicology. *The National Veterinary Medical Series.* Philadelphia: Lippincott Williams & Wilkins.

Peterson, M.E. and Talcott, P.A. 2006. *Small Animal Toxicology, 2nd ed.* Philadelphia: W.B. Saunders Co.

Rossoff, I.S. 2001. *Encyclopedia of Clinical Toxicology.* The Parthenon Publishing Group. Boca Raton, Florida: Boca Raton Group.

Metals and Minerals

29

Robert H. Poppenga

INTRODUCTION

Metals are intrinsic to nature and are ubiquitous in the environment of animals. While the form or valence of any given metal can be changed, metals themselves cannot be destroyed. The activities of man have resulted in the large-scale redistribution of metals in the environment. Perhaps the best example of this relates to lead, which originates as lead ore that is processed for numerous uses. The prior use of lead as an antiknock compound in gasoline and pigment in paints contributed to widespread environmental contamination before such uses were banned. Despite curtailment of lead use, it still poses significant risks for intoxication. Lead in old paints continues to cause adverse health effects in people and pets.

Metals can be categorized as those that play an essential role in biological processes (e.g., those that are nutritionally necessary such as iron, copper, zinc and selenium, among others) and those that do not (e.g., lead and mercury). It is important to point out that disease syndromes caused by deficiencies of nutritionally important metals are different in pathogenesis and clinical manifestations than those caused by exposure to excessive amounts of the same metal.

The toxicity of metals is sometimes harder to define than for other toxicants. One reason for this is that the form of a metal plays a critical role in how readily it is systemically absorbed resulting in intoxication. For example, elemental mercury, when ingested, is essentially unavailable for systemic absorption. In contrast, organic forms of mercury such as methyl mercury are highly bioavailable. The interaction of metals also plays an important role in the determination of toxicity. For example, high dietary calcium can decrease absorption of lead because lead uses calcium transport mechanisms for its uptake into the body. Other factors that can influence toxicity include animal age, gender, and the capacity of an individual for biotransformation of a metal.

The distribution and accumulation of metals in certain tissues in the body can mitigate damage. Lead can accumulate in bone where it is not available to affect target tissues such as the CNS. Also, metals can be sequestered in the body by cystine-rich proteins called *metallothioneins*. Metallothioneins are highly inducible by metals and are essential for metal homeostasis and detoxification of metals (Liu et al. 2008). The interaction of metals with sulfhydryl-containing groups like cystine is the basis for the efficacy of metal chelators, such as succimer or dimercaprol, which contain numerous sulfhydryl groups.

Although the periodic table is full of potentially toxic metals, the following discussion is limited to those few metals that most commonly intoxicate, or pose an intoxication risk for, companion animals. We do not discuss metals that are more frequently involved in livestock or wildlife intoxications such as selenium and mercury nor discuss copper accumulation in susceptible dog breeds. However, keep in mind that most metals, under appropriate circumstances, can poison animals and people.

Small Animal Toxicology Essentials, First Edition. Edited by Robert H. Poppenga, Sharon Gwaltney-Brant.
© 2011 John Wiley and Sons, Inc. Published 2011 by John Wiley and Sons, Inc.

Arsenic

Sources/Formulations

Historically, various forms of arsenic have been used as herbicides, insecticides, wood preservatives, growth promotants, and therapeutic agents. Arsenic is found in various valences and forms. There are trivalent and pentavalent inorganic and organic arsenic forms. The trivalent inorganic arsenic trioxide was formerly used as an insecticide and herbicide and as a source for other arsenicals (Ensley 2004). Pentavalent (arsenate, H_3AsO_4) and trivalent (arsenite, H_3AsO_3) forms of arsenic include sodium, potassium, and calcium salts. Paris green (copper acetoarsenite) and lead arsenate have been used as insecticides, and trivalent inorganic arsenic forms such as monosodium methanarsentate (MSMA) and disodium methanearsonate (DMSA) are used as herbicides. Pentavalent organic arsenicals such as sodium arsenilate and 3-nitro, 4-hydroxyphenylarsonic acid are used as feed additives for some livestock species.

Although arsenic is still utilized in some products, it is not as ubiquitous as it once was due to restrictions on its use and the availability of newer, more targeted pesticides. For example, its use as a wood preservative in the form of chromated copper arsenic (CCA) has been banned for residential use by the USEPA (http://www.epa.gov/oppad001/reregistration/cca/). Thiacetarsamide, a phenylarsenoxide previously used as a heartworm adulticide, is no longer commercially available in the U.S. although another organic arsenical, melarsomine, is available (Plumb 2005). According to the ASPCA Animal Poison Control Center, the highest number of arsenic-related calls involves the exposure of dogs and cats to ant or roach baits, which are typically inorganic forms of arsenic (Neiger 2004).

Kinetics

As for most metals, the bioavailability of arsenic is variable and depends on its form (organic vs. inorganic, solution vs. powder). The arsenic in solutions of organic arsenicals is almost completely absorbed from the GI tract (Neiger 2004). Alternatively, arsenic compounds of low solubility such as arsenic trioxide are absorbed less efficiently. Once absorbed, arsenic is widely distributed in the body and reaches its highest concentrations in the liver, spleen, kidney, lungs, and GI tract. Persistent residues are found in keratinized tissues such as skin, hair, and nails. Clearance of arsenic from the blood is multiphasic with the first phase having a 1- to-2 hour half-life. Forty to 70% of an absorbed dose is eliminated via the urine within the first 48 hours. To a large extent, inorganic arsenic is metab-olized in the liver by the addition of methyl groups prior to its elimination.

Toxicity

The toxicity of arsenic is quite variable and depends on its form, purity, solubility, particle size, valence, and species exposed, and the condition of the exposed individual (Neiger 2004). For example, trivalent arsenicals are 4 to 10 times more toxic than pentavalent arsenicals. The cat is considered to be one of the more sensitive species. A lethal oral dose of sodium arsenite is reported to be less than 5 mg/kg body weight. More generally, the range of lethal oral doses for sodium arsenite is 1 to 25 mg/kg body weight. Weak and debilitated animals are more susceptible to intoxication (Neiger 2007).

Mechanism of Action

The mechanism of toxic action is dependent on the form of arsenic. Trivalent inorganic arsenicals (i.e., arsenites) inhibit cellular respiration. They bind to sulfhydryl compounds, especially lipoic acid and α-keto oxidases. Lipoic acid, a tissue respiratory enzyme cofactor, plays an essential role in the tricarboxylic acid cycle (TCA). Tissues with high oxidative energy requirements (e.g., actively dividing cells such as those of the intestinal epithelium, kidney, liver, skin, and lungs) are more severely affected. Trivalent arsenic affects capillary integrity by an unknown mechanism. The gastrointestinal tract is most affected; capillary dilatation is followed by transudation of plasma into the gastrointestinal tract resulting in submucosal congestion and edema.

In contrast, pentavalent inorganic arsenicals (i.e., arsenates) appear to substitute for phosphate in oxidative phosphorylation. Uncoupling of oxidative phosphorylation produces a cellular energy deficit. Elevated body temperature is not characteristic of pentavalent arsenical poisoning as it is in poisonings by other oxidative uncouplers (e.g., nitrophenols).

The organic arsenicals also vary in terms of their mechanism of toxic action. Trivalent organic arsenicals appear to have a mechanism of toxic action similar to the inorganic arsenicals. However, pentavalent organic arsenicals (e.g., used as livestock feed additives) act on nerves by an unknown mechanism. They produce demyelination and eventual axonal degeneration, leading some researchers to believe that pentavalent organic arsenicals interfere with the B vitamins essential for maintenance of nervous tissue.

Although chronic arsenic exposure has been associated with various cancers in people, its ability to cause cancer is animals is uncertain (Neiger 2004). In humans, chronic exposure to arsenic induces characteristic changes in the skin including hyper- or hypopigmentation and hyperkeratosis.

Clinical Effects

Typically, arsenic intoxication in small animals is an acute illness. Signs can occur within minutes of exposure, with death occurring within several hours. Intoxication from chronic arsenic exposure is not well described in companion animals. However, there is one case report describing dermatitis in a German shorthaired pointer chronically exposed to arsenic (Evinger and Blakemore 1984). The source of exposure was from a container of 44% sodium arsenate that had been leaking into the dog's house.

Signs

Signs associated with acute arsenic intoxication generally develop in the following progression: intense abdominal pain, salivation, vomiting, staggering gait, diarrhea (often bloody), rapid and weak pulse, hypothermia, collapse, and death. Experimentally, long-term exposure of dogs to inorganic arsenic caused nonspecific signs such as anorexia and weight loss secondary to reduced food consumption (Neiger and Osweiler 1989).

Laboratory

There are no specific abnormalities noted from CBC or serum chemistry tests. Because arsenic can damage multiple organs, changes associated with liver or kidney dysfunction can be present if the animal survives for several days. Protein, red blood cells, and casts can be noted in the urine.

Differential Diagnoses

Other disease etiologies to consider include intoxication from other metals or metal salts (e.g., lead, copper, or zinc salts), ingestion of acid or alkaline caustics, ingestion of irritating plants (e.g., those containing insoluble calcium oxalates, castor bean), and infectious agents such as parvovirus.

Diagnostics

Antemortem

An antemortem diagnosis relies on a history of ingestion of arsenic, the occurrence of consistent clinical signs, and the detection of toxic concentrations of arsenic in vomitus or stomach contents, whole blood, or urine. Suspect sources of exposure can also be tested to confirm the presence of arsenic. The rapid elimination of the metal from the body makes the collection of appropriate samples as early as possible an important consideration. Most veterinary diagnostic laboratories can test for arsenic. It is important to point out that low-level concentrations of arsenic in blood or urine are not unusual and do not indicate arsenic intoxication. The interpretation of a given concentration of arsenic depends on an evaluation of the entire case and the timing of sample collection in relation to exposure.

Postmortem

Postmortem analysis of stomach contents, liver, kidney, or urine can confirm exposure. Again, the significance of detected concentrations, especially relatively low concentrations, needs to be interpreted in conjunction with other case variables. Postmortem lesions might be absent in cases of rapid death. Otherwise, severe gastrointestinal lesions consisting of reddening of the gastric mucosa and proximal small intestine, watery GI contents, and blood and sloughed mucosa in the feces are commonly noted. Other organ lesions are not specific for arsenic.

Management of Exposures

The rapidity of onset of clinical signs such as vomiting often precludes initiating decontamination procedures. Activated charcoal is unlikely to adsorb significant amounts of arsenic, although with significant exposures its administration is recommended (Ford 2006). Symptomatic animals need to be stabilized first. This might entail treatment for circulatory shock and hypotension and maintenance of body temperature. Renal and liver failure and electrolyte abnormalities might need to be addressed. Glucose and glycogen stores should be maintained parenterally with dextrose or parenteral alimentation solutions (Ford 2006).

Chelation therapy is typically indicated. Historically, dimercaprol (BAL or British anti-Lewisite) was the recommended chelator. It is a sulfhydryl-containing chelator that binds to arsenic and allows the arsenic-chelator complex to be eliminated. An alternative chelator, succimer, has several theoretical advantages over dimercaprol, including less toxicity and oral (vs. injectable) dosing form. It has been theorized that because succimer is hydrophilic it might not remove arsenic that has escaped the extracelluar space as efficiently as dimercaprol (Neiger 2004). However, available studies suggest that succimer is equal to or even superior to dimercaprol in increasing arsenic elimination (Ford 2006). If dimercaprol is used, monitoring for adverse reactions included pain at the injection site, vomiting, tremors, and seizures is required.

Table 29.I. Percentages of elemental iron found in common iron formulations

Iron Formulation	% Elemental Iron
Ionic Forms	
Ferrous chloride	28%
Ferrous fumarate	33%
Ferrous gluconate	12%
Ferrous lactate	19%
Ferrous sulfate	20%
Nonionic Forms	
Carbonyl iron	98%
Iron polysaccharide	46%

Although the administration of B-complex vitamins and amino acids has been recommended, the evidence for their efficacy is lacking. Parenteral antibiotic administration might be considered to prevent secondary bacterial infections of the GI tract. The use of GI protectants might also be indicated. Hemodialysis is not recommended in the absence of renal impairment (Ford 2006). Recovering animals should be fed a high-quality diet in small portions, which can be increased as time and circumstances permit.

Prognosis

The prognosis in symptomatic animals is always guarded, particularly in the absence of early intervention and intensive monitoring and treatment.

Iron

Sources/Forms

Iron is an element essential for life. Sources for readily ionizable iron include multivitamins and dietary mineral supplements (for geriatric use or use during pregnancy) (Hall 2007a). In humans, the most commonly reported iron intoxication occurs in children ingesting iron supplements.

There are a number of iron salts and formulations. The more common formulations and their respective percent elemental iron concentrations are provided in Table 29.1. Some insoluble forms of iron such as elemental iron and ferric oxide (i.e., rust) are not hazardous when ingested due to low bioavailability. One newer source of iron, a chelated iron called iron phosphate EDTA, is found in some slug and snail baits, which are advertised as being nontoxic to pets. However, there are many anecdotal reports of illness in dogs following ingestion of these products, possibly as a result of enhanced absorption of the chelated iron.

Kinetics

The kinetics of iron absorption are complex. Iron body stores are regulated at the site of absorption from the GI tract because the body is not able to actively excrete iron. From the GI tract, iron must first enter duodenal mucosal cells, possibly by a carrier-mediated process. Next the iron is either lost as the mucosal cells slough into the GI lumen or is bound to ferritin for later transfer to transferrin, a serum iron-binding transport protein. Serum transferrin concentrations greatly exceed amounts necessary to bind iron under normal physiological processes (normal binding capacity is 3 to 4 times the serum iron concentration). However, during intoxications the binding capacity is exceeded, allowing free iron to cause cell damage.

Toxicity

The toxicity of iron for dogs is believed to be similar to that for humans. Ingestion of less than 20 mg/kg body weight of elemental iron is not considered to cause more than mild gastric upset. Dosages of 20 to 60 mg/kg body weight cause mild to moderate intoxication, and dosages in excess of 60 mg/kg are associated with severe intoxication. Without early intervention, dosages of 100 mg/kg are potentially fatal. It is important to determine the dose or dosage of elemental iron ingested by approximating how much of a product was ingested, knowing the form and amount of iron per unit of product weight, and then multiplying the total by the percentage of elemental iron based upon the form (see Table 29.1).

Mechanism of Action

Free iron can cause direct or indirect tissue and cell damage. Iron acts as a free radical and can also generate free radicals. Free radicals have one or more unpaired electrons, which can initiate lipid peroxidation resulting in cell membrane damage. Tissues that have first contact with free iron are primarily affected although all tissues are susceptible to damage if exposed. The primary targets are the gastrointestinal, cardiovascular, and hepatic tissues. Iron also damages mitochondria, leading to loss of oxidative metabolism (Hall 2007a). Iron might have a direct negative inotropic effect on the myocardium (Perrone 2007).

Clinical Effects

Classically, the signs associated with iron intoxication follow more or less well-defined stages.

Signs

Initial clinical signs are due to GI upset (within 6 hours after ingestion). Bloody vomitus or stool can occur during this stage. The next stage (approximately 6 to 24 hours postexposure) mimics an apparent recovery as GI signs subside. The apparent recovery stage is followed by a worsening of signs that include vomiting, diarrhea, depression, GI hemorrhage, abdominal pain, circulatory shock, tremors, metabolic acidosis, coagulopathy, and in some cases, death. The last stage, 2 to 6 weeks after exposure, is characterized by GI obstruction secondary to fibrosing repair of prior GI damage.

Laboratory

Leukocytosis, hyperglycemia, metabolic acidosis, and normal-to-high AST, ALT, ALP, and serum bilirubin concentrations can occur. Iron-containing tablets or pills might be visualized by abdominal imaging.

Differential Diagnoses

A variety of diseases with a significant GI involvement needs to be considered. Such diseases include garbage intoxication, toxic plant ingestion (e.g., castor bean) gastric torsion, caustic ingestions, snake bite, heat prostration, and infectious (bacterial or viral) enteritis.

Diagnostics

Antemortem

A diagnosis relies on a history of exposure and occurrence of compatible clinical signs. Serum iron in excess of the total serum iron-binding capacity (TIBC) is consistent with exposure to excessive iron (Hall 2007b). If possible, TIBC should be determined at 2 to 3 hours and again at 5 to 6 hours postexposure. Analysis of vomitus or stomach contents might suggest a high iron exposure.

Postmortem

Postmortem tissue iron concentrations might help support a diagnosis of iron intoxication. Lesions in the liver tend to have a rather distinct periportal distribution because periportal regions of the liver are the first to be exposed to excessive free iron absorbed from the GI tract.

Management of Exposures

Early after exposure (within the first 2 hours), emesis can be induced or gastric lavage considered. Keep in mind that pill bezoars can form that makes gastric evacuation more challenging. Also many patients present with significant prior vomiting; in such cases induction of emesis is not warranted. In cases where pill bezoars might form, particu-

larly with large ingestions, emergency gastrotomy has been suggested (Hall 2007a). Although not used much in veterinary medicine currently, in human exposures, whole bowel irrigation using polyethylene glycol electrolyte lavage solution has shown some promise for removing iron tablets or pills. Activated charcoal does not bind iron and is not indicated.

Patient stabilization is a priority in symptomatic animals. Treating circulatory shock and metabolic acidosis is critical. Sucrafate might be useful in order to provide some GI protection.

Deferoxamine mesylate is an effective iron chelator. It combines with iron to form ferrioxamine, which is subsequently eliminated via the kidneys (Perrone 2007).

Deferoxamine given intravenously too rapidly can cause cardiac arrhythmias; it is a teratogen and should be used in pregnant animals only if the potential benefits outweigh the risks.

Prognosis

The prognosis is variable depending on the dosage ingested and availability of appropriate monitoring. In animals that recover from acute intoxication, owners should be instructed to watch for evidence of GI obstruction several weeks after discharge.

LEAD

The true incidence of lead intoxication of household pets is unknown but is likely to be of decreasing prevalence due to curtailment of lead paint use and resulting decreases in exposure. At least historically, a higher prevalence of intoxication is reported during warmer months. There is also a higher prevalence in young animals, most likely due to their increased susceptibility as a result of greater bioavailability of lead and a more permeable blood-brain barrier (Poppenga 2007). Additionally, the prevalence is higher in pets housed in older homes or buildings. Low socioeconomic status of a pet-owning family is more likely to be associated with a high blood-lead concentration in pets, although housing undergoing renovations in urban areas of "gentrification" is potentially hazardous. In one review of lead intoxication in cats, 84% of the cases involved exposure of the cats to old paint, most often as a result of home renovations (Knight and Kumar 2003).

Sources/Forms

Lead is used in an impressive array of products including tank linings, piping, radiation shielding, paint pigments, inks, lead ammunition (shot and bullets), ballast and weights, solder, linoleum, wine bottle foil, lubricants, bearings, alloys, storage batteries, ceramics, plastics, electronic devices, leaded glass, stained-glass framing, fishing gear, jewelry and small toys (Casteel 2004; Poppenga 2007). Wrappers used for imported candies have been found to contain high concentrations of lead as a result of the use of lead-contaminated inks (Medlin 2004). Animals can be intoxicated from lead-contaminated soils. For example, cats and birds can ingest lead-contaminated soil via grooming or foraging behavior, respectively. Pet and aviary birds are unlikely to be exposed to many sources of lead due to their being kept in home or cage environments. The more common sources of exposure for such birds are likely to be from paint (either from direct ingestion of lead-based paint flakes or secondary to paint dust contaminating the environment) or from ingestion of small lead-containing objects.

Because of the toxicity of lead for children and wild bird species, several former uses of lead have been eliminated or curtailed (e.g., in paints, gasoline, and ammunition). Lead has not intentionally been added to most paint since 1978, although it has been estimated by the Centers for Disease Control that 74% of privately owned housing in the United States built before 1980 still contains hazardous quantities of lead paint (Casteel 2004). Thus, animals kept in older homes have an increased risk of lead exposure from paint.

Kinetics

As for other metals, the bioavailability of lead following ingestion depends on its form. Elemental lead is less bioavailable than inorganic lead salts such as lead acetate or organic lead such as tetraethyl lead. Elemental lead is relatively insoluble in hard, basic water, but more soluble in acidic water. Therefore, elemental lead is more soluble, and therefore more bioavailable, in the acidic fluids of the proventriculus or ventriculus of birds and the stomach of mammals. Lead is actively transported across the GI tract using the same transport mechanisms used for calcium absorption. This absorption mechanism explains the greater bioavailability of lead in immature, rapidly growing animals with an increased need for calcium. Irrespective of the form of lead, a significant amount of ingested lead is excreted in the feces without being absorbed.

Approximately 90% of absorbed lead is found in red blood cells, with small amounts bound to albumin or found in plasma as free lead. Within red blood cells, lead is associated with the cell membrane, hemoglobin and possibly other cell components (Liu et al. 2008). Lead is widely distributed in soft tissues and bone serves as a

long-term storage site. The half-life of lead is multiphasic due to redistribution within various compartments of the body (Gwaltney-Brant 2004). For example, the half-life of lead in whole blood is approximately 35 days, whereas in brain it is approximately 2 years. Lead can persist in bone for years. Enhanced bone remodeling can release lead into the blood and cause adverse effects. Elimination of absorbed lead can occur via sloughing of renal tubular epithelial cells, via the bile or via pancreatic secretions (Gwaltney-Brant 2004).

Toxicity

Few studies have determined the acute or chronic toxicity of lead for many species, especially for pet birds. The risk for lead intoxication is influenced not only by the amount and form of lead ingested (see "Kinetics"), but species exposed, dietary factors, size of ingested lead particles and, in birds, the amount of grit in the ventriculus. The length of retention of lead particles in the GI tract varies among individuals within a given species and between species. Given the large number of variables that can affect the toxicity of lead, the availability of precise toxic or lethal doses is limited.

Mechanism of Action

Most cellular damage due to lead is caused by the ability of lead to substitute for a variety of polyvalent cations, especially calcium and zinc, in their binding sites (Garza et al. 2006). The role that metal ions play in biological systems are numerous and diverse. They serve as charge carriers, intermediates in catalyzed reactions, and structural elements in the maintenance of protein conformation. Metal transport, energy metabolism, apoptosis, ionic conduction, cell adhesion, inter- and intracellular signaling, diverse enzymatic processes, protein maturation, and genetic regulation can all be affected. Lead produces oxidative damage to lipids and proteins as a result of release of iron, disruption of antioxidant mechanisms, and direct oxidative damage.

The neurotoxicity of lead is most likely due to such diverse mechanisms as lipid peroxidation, excitotoxicity (i.e., cell damage secondary to receptor overstimulation due to excitatory neurotransmitters such as glutamate), alterations in neurotransmitter synthesis, storage and release, alterations in expression and functioning of receptors, interference with mitochondrial metabolism, interference with second messenger systems, and damage to astroglia and oligodendroglia.

The mechanism of lead-induced altered GI motility is not entirely clear, but it does not appear to be related to an effect of lead on peripheral nerves or calcium flux. Lead-induced relaxation may be due to stimulation of adenylate cyclase activity resulting in an increase in intracellular cyclic AMP (Boyer et al. 1985).

Lead causes anemia by increasing erythrocyte fragility, delaying erythrocyte maturation, and inhibiting heme synthesis. Heme synthesis is impaired as a result of aminolevulinic acid synthetase, δ-aminolevulinic acid dehydratase (ALAD), coproporphyrinogen decarboxylase, and ferrochelatase inhibition (Henritig 2002).

Clinical Effects

Signs

As discussed, the primary organ systems affected are the gastrointestinal, nervous, and hematopoietic. The most obvious and common signs reflect GI and CNS effects. Gastrointestinal signs often precede CNS signs and are predominant with chronic, low-level exposure. CNS signs are more frequently observed following acute exposures and are more common in younger animals. Common signs include vomiting, diarrhea, anorexia, abdominal pain, regurgitation due to megaesophagus, lethargy, hysteria, seizures, and blindness. In intoxicated cats central vestibular abnormalities such as vertical nystagmus and ataxia are reported (Poppenga 2007). In a review of lead intoxication of cats, the most common clinical signs reported were anorexia, vomiting, and seizures (Knight and Kumar 2003).

In pet birds, signs of intoxication can be nonspecific and limited to anorexia, weakness, and weight loss. Signs related to nervous system impairment include lethargy, weakness manifested as wing droop, leg paresis or paralysis, changes in phonation, head tilt, ataxia, blindness, circling, head tremors, and seizures (Locke and Thomas 1996). Gastrointestinal signs include regurgitation and decreased motility of the upper GI tract (esophagus, proventriculus, and ventriculus) resulting in impaction and greenish diarrhea, which stains feathers around the vent (Locke and Thomas 1996; Dumonceaux and Harrison 1994).

It is important to note that blood lead concentrations do not correlate with the occurrence or severity of clinical signs.

Laboratory

Diagnostic laboratory abnormalities are noted most frequently when the hematopoietic system is affected. The presence of 5 to 40 nucleated RBCs/100 WBCs without anemia strongly suggests lead exposure. However, the absence of nucleated RBC changes does not rule out the diagnosis. Red blood cell changes include anisocytosis, polychromasia, poikilocytosis, target cells, hypochromasia, and basophilic stippling. The latter is often difficult to detect. A neutrophilic leukocytosis might be noted. In cats, elevated AST and ALP values are reported. Urinalysis can reflect mild nonspecific renal damage, glucosuria, and hemoglobinuria.

Diagnostics

Antemortem

As mentioned, clinical signs associated with lead intoxication can be nonspecific, making a diagnosis more difficult. Radiographs might identify metallic objects in the GI tract. Obviously, detecting a metal density does not identify it as to type of metal. The absence of metal densities does not rule out metal exposure, because metal objects may have been passed or exposure to lead was from a nonradiodense form.

Diagnosis of lead exposure or intoxication is most directly made by measurement of lead in whole blood samples. In contrast to the diagnosis of zinc intoxication, serum or plasma are not appropriate samples for lead analysis, because lead associates with the red blood cell. Lead analyses are widely available through veterinary diagnostic laboratories. Fortunately, small sample sizes can be used; blood samples as small as 20 μl are often suitable. This is important when obtaining blood from small animals such as many caged birds. In general, any anticoagulant, including EDTA can be used to prevent samples from clotting, although there may be exceptions to this general rule; it is best to consult with the laboratory conducting the testing prior to sample collection. Whole blood lead concentrations consistent with lead exposure and/or intoxication are generally 0.20 ppm or greater (20 μg/dl or greater). There are no "normal" background blood lead concentrations in animals. Measurement of ALAD activity, blood zinc protoporphyrin, or free erythrocyte protoporphyrin concentrations are also good biomarkers of lead exposure, but these tests are not widely available.

Postmortem

Postmortem diagnosis relies on an antemortem history of compatible clinical signs, detection of metallic particles or other forms of lead in the GI tract, and measurement of liver or kidney lead concentrations. Reported diagnostic liver or kidney concentrations are variable, but values of 4 ppm wet weight or greater in either tissue are likely to be significant. There can be significant differences in liver and kidney tissue concentrations in the same animal; as a consequence it is often advisable to test both tissues.

Necropsy findings can include the observation of paint chips or lead objects in the gastrointestinal tract. Intranuclear inclusion bodies in hepatocytes or renal tubular epithelial cells (intracellular storage form of lead) are considered highly suggestive. Cerebrocortical lesions can include spongiosis, vascular hypertrophy, gliosis, neuronal necrosis, and demyelination.

Differential Diagnoses

With the exception of CBC changes, clinical signs associated with lead intoxication are nonspecific and a number of differential diagnoses need to be considered. In dogs, the following diseases can mimic lead intoxication: canine distemper, infectious encephalitides, epilepsy, bromethalin, methylxanthine or tremorgenic mycotoxin toxicoses, NSAID toxicosis, heatstroke, intestinal parasitism, intussusception, foreign body, pancreatitis, and infectious canine hepatitis. In cats, degenerative or storage diseases, hepatic encephalopathy, infectious encephalitides, and organophosphorous/carbamate, bromethalin, or methylxanthine toxicoses need to be considered.

Management of Cases

Case management focuses on evacuation of the GI tract, stabilization of the patient, and reduction of lead body burden. Typically, animals intoxicated by lead have not been exposed to a single dose of lead or developed signs immediately after a single exposure. Thus, gastric evacuation is not always indicated. The exception would be in those cases in which a metallic object is detected in the stomach. In those cases, gastric lavage or endoscopy can be considered. Because a significant amount of lead might remain in the GI tract beyond the stomach, decontamination of the GI tract can be useful. This is accomplished using saccharide or saline cathartics such as sorbitol or sodium or magnesium sulfate. The advantage of using sodium or magnesium sulfate lies in the potential to form lead sulfate, which has relatively low bioavailability. However, use of sodium sulfate in combination with chelators such as $CaNa_2EDTA$ or succimer has not been shown to be more effective than using a chelator alone. In pet birds, decontamination approaches include the use of emollient laxatives such as mineral oil, bulk laxatives such as psyllium, or cathartics such as sodium sulfate. Administration of 3 to 5 appropriately sized pieces of grit has been reported to aid in the passage of metal objects from the ventriculus (Dumonceaux and Harrison 1994). Saline lavage has been successful in removing lead particles from the proventriculus or ventriculus of lead-intoxicated birds (Loudis 2004).

If animals present with neurologic symptoms such as seizures, control with a benzodiazepine can be tried. Seizure activity might suggest the presence of cerebral edema. This should be treated using mannitol and dexamethasone.

Chelation therapy is universally recommended. The two chelators most commonly used are calcium disodium EDTA ($CaNa_2EDTA$) and succimer. In human medicine, succimer has largely replaced the use of $CaNa_2EDTA$ due to its efficacy, lack of adverse side effects and ability to be given orally.

If using EDTA, only the calcium salt should be used to avoid calcium chelation and resulting hypocalcemia (Casteel 2004; Poppenga 2007). There are several significant disadvantages to the use of $CaNa_2EDTA$. It is potentially nephrotoxic, which can either induce renal dysfunction or exacerbate concurrent lead-induced renal impairment. It has to be administered parenterally because oral administration of $CaNa_2EDTA$ enhances the absorption of lead from the GI tract. Repeated IM injections in birds can cause significant muscle damage. Additionally, $CaNa_2EDTA$ chelates important endogenous minerals such as zinc. Prolonged use of $CaNa_2EDTA$ is generally interrupted by intervals of no therapy to avoid adverse effects. Treatment periods of 5–10 days followed by a 3–5-day "rest" period are recommended. Assessment of renal function every 2–3 days during chelation therapy is also recommended.

Succimer (DMSA, dimercaptosuccinic acid) is a newer chelating agent that has several advantages over $CaNa_2EDTA$. It can be given orally, which avoids the need for repeated IM injections and potentially allows for in-home treatment, it does not increase elimination of other essential minerals such as zinc and it is not nephrotoxic. Succimer is more effective at removing lead from soft tissues compared to $CaNa_2EDTA$. Succimer decreases CNS lead concentrations more rapidly than $CaNa_2EDTA$ (Gwaltney-Brant 2004). In pet birds, succimer can be given orally by gavage or other direct means, although it has been effective when sprinkled on food (Hoogesteijn et al. 2003). As with $CaNa_2EDTA$ use, the length of treatment should be based on clinical improvement and determination of blood lead concentrations. Whole blood lead should be determined following chelation to assess the need for additional chelation therapy. However, 3 to 5 days should be allowed for remaining lead to reequilibrate to obtain an accurate assessment of lead status. Succimer has been used successfully in dogs and cats (Ramsey et al. 1996; Knight et al. 2001).

Table 29.2. Comparison of CaNa$_2$EDTA and succimer for the treatment of lead and zinc intoxications

	CaNa$_2$EDTA	Succimer
Tradenames	Calcium Disodium Versenate (3M) 200 mg/ml	Chemet (Sanofi-Synthelabo) 100 mg capsules
Routes of administration	Slow IV infusion, IM or SQ injection; dilution with saline or 5% dextrose needed if given IV	Oral
Advantages	Rapid absorption Can chelate lead and zinc	Oral administration Not nephrotoxic Does not chelate essential minerals such as zinc, manganese, and copper More rapid clinical improvement in lead intoxication More effective at removing lead from soft tissues
Disadvantages	Need for repeated IM injections Pain at injection site Potential nephrotoxicity and therefore need to monitor renal function regularly Chelation of essential minerals such as zinc, manganese, and copper with long-term use Potential to worsen CNS signs as a result of lead redistribution	Less effective chelation of zinc; efficacy uncertain in zinc intoxication Regurgitation noted in cockatiels

Clinical improvement is likely to be more rapid (within 24 hours) following succimer use compared to CaNa$_2$EDTA. Neurologic signs may initially worsen in animals treated with CaNa$_2$EDTA. This is most likely due to CaNa$_2$EDTA-induced mobilization of lead from bone in animals with chronic lead exposure, since acutely intoxicated animals would be expected to have lower bone lead concentrations. Combining CaNa$_2$EDTA and succimer does not appear to be more efficacious than CaNa$_2$EDTA or succimer alone. A comparison between CaNa$_2$EDTA and succimer is provided in Table 29.2.

Irrespective of what chelator is used, assessment of blood lead concentrations at the end of each rest period should dictate the length of time needed for chelation therapy. The goal is to chelate for the minimum amount of time necessary to resolve the intoxication (based upon resolution of clinical signs and a decline in blood lead concentrations).

D-penicillamine has also been used to chelate lead in animals, but its use is associated with a number of possible adverse effects and is currently not recommended for use in people (Van Alstine et al. 1993; Henritig 2002).

There is evidence in mammals that the efficacy of chelation is improved when thiamine or antioxidants such as ascorbic acid are used in conjunction with chelators. Such combinations have not been investigated in birds.

Prognosis

The prognosis is favorable with treatment, although it is guarded in animals presenting with uncontrollable seizures. Signs should improve significantly within 24 to 48 hours of initiating chelation therapy.

Zinc

Zinc intoxication is most commonly reported in small dogs and caged birds. Although cats are occasionally intoxicated based upon anecdotal reports, intoxication appears to be relatively uncommon in this species.

Sources/Forms

Metallic zinc is commonly used to galvanize metals, such as iron and steel, to provide protective coating. Until 1982, pennies consisted mainly of copper (95%) and zinc (4%), but the copper-clad pennies minted after 1982 contain 97% zinc and 2.5% copper (Barceloux 1999). Additionally, zinc is found in soil and may be present at high enough concentrations to result in avian poisonings. Zinc is also used in a variety of medical formulations, pigments, wood preservatives, insecticides, and rubber. Zinc oxide ointments and creams can be licked from the skin following topical application or cause intoxication if the products are chewed and the contents swallowed (Talcott 2004).

Kinetics

The rate of absorption depends on the amount and form of ingested zinc. The acidity of the stomach provides an excellent environment for the quick release and dissolution of zinc from metallic objects (Talcott 2004). Once absorbed, zinc is distributed widely to tissues, including pancreas, liver, kidney, bone, muscle, brain, retina, and skin. In tissues, especially the pancreas, liver, kidney, intestinal mucosa, and brain, zinc is bound to metallothionein. Metallothionein is a low molecular weight, cysteine-rich protein that has potent metal-binding capabilities. Zinc has a high binding affinity for metallothionein, which may play an integral role in zinc metabolism. The major route of excretion of zinc is via the feces.

Toxicity

Zinc is an essential metal, and animals and humans have the ability to regulate zinc effectively. Zinc is relatively nontoxic in mammals as judged by their tolerance to dietary concentrations greater than 100 times the minimum recommended daily zinc requirement (Leonard and Gerber 1989). If dietary exposure is excessive and homeostatic mechanisms fail, zinc toxicity can occur. Definite data on the toxicity of zinc in caged birds is lacking, although there is limited information available for certain avian and mammalian species. In dogs, the ingestion of one or two pennies is likely sufficient to cause intoxication. One report estimated that the toxic dose of zinc in the form of zinc oxide for dogs was 108 grams of zinc (Breitschwerdt et al. 1986).

Mechanism of Action

Zinc is required for a large number of physiological processes including bone formation, immunity, keratogenesis, reproduction, growth, vision, wound healing, brain development, normal functioning of the central nervous system, and many other physiological processes (Talcott 2004). Major pathophysiological mechanisms of zinc intoxication are attributed to direct and indirect toxic effects on the gastrointestinal tract, liver, kidney, pancreas, red blood cells, and brain, although specific mechanisms for many of these effects have not elucidated. In acute cases of zinc poisoning, particularly when zinc salts are ingested, local corrosive effects occur in the gastrointestinal tract followed by damage to the liver, kidney, and pancreas. The hemolytic anemia associated with zinc intoxication might be due to a direct damaging effect of zinc on red blood cell membranes. In birds, a major concern is chronic zinc toxicosis with resulting anemia. Anemia might be secondary to functional iron or copper deficiencies. Zinc has been shown to cause acute pancreatic, hepatic, and renal failure, although underlying specific pathophysiological mechanisms have not been described. Zinc toxicosis has been associated with brain damage that is most likely a combination of hypoxic and direct toxic effects.

Clinical Effects

Signs

In intoxicated dogs, the most common signs include anorexia, vomiting, diarrhea, lethargy, depression, pale mucous membranes, icterus, and orange-tinged feces. Often metallic objects are noted on abdominal radiographs, although the absence of such findings does not rule out zinc intoxication. Arrhythmias and ST-segment abnormalities have been reported (Talcott 2004).

In birds clinical signs of intoxication are variable and nonspecific. They include lethargy, anorexia, regurgitation, polyuria, polydipsia, hematuria, hematochezia, pallor, dark or bright green diarrhea, foul-smelling feces, paresis, seizures, and sudden death (Puschner and Poppenga 2009). However, zinc toxicosis was associated with sudden death in 7 of 21 psittacine birds evaluated in one study (Puschner et al. 1999). Therefore, any acute death in a caged bird needs to be evaluated for possible zinc poisoning. Excessive zinc exposure as a cause of feather picking is questionable.

Laboratory

In dogs, findings indicative of an oxidant-induced hemolytic anemia predominate. These include Heinz body formation, target cells, spherocytosis, hemoglobinemia, hemoglobinuria, and bilirubinemia. Regenerative changes such as nucleated RBCs, basophilic stippling, and polychromasia might be noted.

Diagnostics

Antemortem

Antemortem diagnosis relies on a history of ingestion of zinc, the occurrence of compatible clinical signs (e.g., hemolytic anemia in conjunction with a metallic object in the GI tract), and measurement of zinc in serum samples. Serum zinc concentrations typically exceed 5 ppm and are often much higher (for dogs and cats a serum zinc reference range is 0.7 to 2.0 ppm). Because many rubbers can leach zinc, it is important to use appropriate serum tubes (i.e., royal blue top) for sample collection and submission or scrupulously avoid contact of the blood/serum samples with rubber (e.g., a plastic-capped vial can be used to store and ship serum). Once exposure to zinc is stopped, follow-up determinations of serum zinc concentrations might be useful.

Postmortem

A postmortem diagnosis relies on antemortem findings and measurement of zinc concentrations in appropriate tissue samples. Liver is the most commonly tested sample, although kidney and pancreatic tissue samples can also be used.

Differential Diagnoses

Differential diagnoses include immune-mediated hemolytic anemia, *Babesia*, onion/garlic, naphthalene mothball, some mushroom and acetaminophen intoxications, snake and brown recluse spider bites, caval syndrome, overhydration, skunk spray, and numerous causes of gastrointestinal signs.

Management of Exposures

The most important intervention is rapid removal of any identified zinc object by endoscopy or laparotomy. Severe hemolytic anemias might require blood transfusions. In one case series of 19 dogs with zinc intoxication, all animals received either packed red blood cells or an oxygen-carrying solution (Oxyglobin®) (Gurnee and Drobatz 2007). Fluid therapy and diuresis are important to both maintain hydration and minimize renal damage from hemoglobinuria. Although CaNa$_2$EDTA and D-penicillamine can chelate zinc, their routine use is questionable, given the relatively rapid elimination of zinc. Once exposure to zinc is stopped, tissue and serum zinc concentrations drop rapidly. H$_2$-receptor blockers might help reduce stomach acidity and the rate of release of zinc from zinc objects, although rapid removal of the zinc object might make their use unnecessary.

Frequent evaluation of PCV and ECGs is warranted. Periodic assessment of renal function might also be prudent.

Prognosis

The prognosis is good to guarded. In one retrospective study in dogs (N = 19), 17 dogs receiving treatment survived (one was euthanized without treatment and one was discharged but returned the next day in severe respiratory distress) (Gurnee and Drobatz 2007). Rapid removal of the source of zinc should result in progressive improvement over 2 to 3 days. The mean hospital stay in the retrospective study was 2 days. Multiple organ failure, DIC, pancreatic disease, renal failure, and cardiopulmonary arrest are potential complications (Talcott 2004).

REFERENCES

Barceloux, D.G. 1999. Zinc. *J Toxicol—Clin Toxicol* 37:279–292.

Boyer, I.J., Cory-Slechta, D.A., DiStefano, V. 1985. Lead induction of crop dysfunction in pigeons through a direct action on neural or smooth muscle components of crop tissue. *J Pharmacol Exp Ther* 234:607–615.

Breitschwerdt, E.B., Armstrong, P.J., Robinette, C.L. 1986. Three cases of acute zinc toxicosis in dogs. *Vet Hum Toxicol* 28:109–117.

Casteel, S.W. 2004. Lead. In Peterson, M.E., Talcott, P.A., eds. *Small Animal Toxicology, 2nd ed.* St. Louis, Saunders Elsevier, pp. 795–805.

Dumonceaux, G. and Harrison, G.H. 1994. Toxins. In Ritchie, B.W., Harrison, G.J., Harrison, L.R., eds. *Avian Medicine: Principles and Application*. Delray Beach, Florida: Wingers Publishing, pp. 1030–1052.

Ensley, S. 2004. Arsenic. In Plumlee, K.H., ed. *Clinical Veterinary Toxicology*. Mosby, St. Louis, pp. 193–195.

Evinger, J.V. and Blakemore, J.C. 1984. Dermatitis in a dog associated with exposure to an arsenic compound. *J Am Vet Med Assoc* 84(10):1281–1282.

Ford, M. 2006. Arsenic. In Flomenbaum, N.E., Howland, M.A., Goldfrank, L.R. et al., eds. *Goldfrank's Toxicologic Emergencies*. New York, McGraw-Hill, pp. 1251–1264.

Garza, A., Vega, R., Soto, E. 2006. Cellular mechanisms of lead neurotoxicity. *Med Sci Monit* 12:RA57–65.

Gurnee, C.M., Drobatz, K.J. 2007. Zinc intoxication in dogs: 19 cases (1991–2003). *J Am Vet Med Assoc* 230(8): 1174–1179.

Gwaltney-Brant, S. 2004. Lead. In Plumlee, K.H., ed. *Clinical Veterinary Toxicology*. Mosby, St. Louis, pp. 204–210.

Hall, J.O. 2007a. Iron. In Peterson, M.E., Talcott, P.A., eds. *Small Animal Toxicology, 2nd ed.* St. Louis, Saunders Elsevier, pp. 777–784.

———. 2007b. Iron toxicity. In Tilley, L.P., Smith, F.W.K., eds. *Blackwell's Five Minute Veterinary Consult, 4th ed.* Ames, Iowa: Blackwell Publishing, p. 771.

Henritig, F.M. 2002. Lead. In Goldfrank, L.R., Flomenbaum, N.E., Lewin, N.A., eds., *Goldfrank's Toxicologic Emergencies*. Mew York: McGraw-Hill pp. 1200–1238.

Hoogesteijn, A.L., Raphael, B.L., Callem P. et al. 2003. Oral treatment of avian lead intoxication with meso-2,3-dimercaptosuccinic acid. *J Zoo Wildl Med* 34:82–87.

Knight, T.E., Kent, M., Junk, J.E. 2001. Succimer treatment of lead toxicosis in two cats. *J Am Vet Med Assoc* 218(12):1946–1948.

Knight, T.E., Kumar, M.S.A. 2003. Lead toxicosis in cats—A review. *J Feline Med and Surg* 5:249–255.

Leonard, A., Gerber, G.B. 1989. Zinc toxicity—Does it exist? *J Am Coll Toxicol* 8:1285–1290.

Liu, J., Goyer, R.A., Waalkes, M.P. 2008. Toxic effects of metals. In Klaassen, C.D., ed. *Casarett and Doull's Toxicology: The Basic Science of Poisons*. New York: McGraw Hill, pp. 931–979.

Locke, L.N., Thomas, N.J. 1996. Lead poisoning of waterfowl and raptors. In Fairbrother, A., Locke, L.N., Hoff, G.L., eds. *Noninfectious Diseases of Wildlife*. Ames: Iowa State University Press, Ames, pp. 108–117.

Loudis, B. 2004. Endoscope assisted gastric lavage for foreign body retrieval. *Association of Avian Veterinarians* 83–88.

Medlin, J. 2004. Sweet candy, bitter poison. *Environ Health Perspect* 112:A803.

Neiger, R.D. 2004. Arsenic. In Peterson, M.E., Talcott, P.A.(eds). *Small Animal Toxicology, 2nd ed.* St. Louis, Saunders Elsevier, pp. 592–602.

———. 2007. Arsenic. In Tilley, L.P., Smith, F.W.K., eds. *Blackwell's Five Minute Veterinary Consult, 4th ed.* Ames, Blackwell Publishing, p. 101.

Neiger, R.D. and Osweiler, G.D. 1989. Effect of subacute low level dietary sodium arsenite on dogs. *Fund Appl Toxicol* 13:439–451.

Perrone, J. 2007. Iron. In Flomenbaum, N.E., Howland, M.A., Goldfrank, L.S. et al., eds. *Goldfrank's Toxicologic Emergencies*. New York, McGraw-Hill, pp. 629–637.

Plumb, D.C. 2005. Thiacetarsamide sodium. In *Plumb's Veterinary Drug Handbook, 5th ed.* Ames, Blackwell Publishing, pp. 747–749.

Poppenga, R.H. 2007. Lead poisoning. In Tilley, L.P., Smith, F.W.K., eds. *Blackwell's Five Minute Veterinary Consult, 4th ed.* Ames, Blackwell Publishing, pp. 796–797.

Puschner, B. and Poppenga, R.H. 2009. Lead and zinc intoxication in companion birds. *Compend Contin Educ Vet* 31(1):E1–12.

Puschner, B., St. Leger, J., Galey, F.D. 1999. Normal and toxic zinc concentrations in serum/plasma and liver of psittacines with respect to genus differences. *J Vet Diagn Invest* 11:522–527.

Ramsey, D.R., Casteel, S.W., Fagella, A.M. et al. 1996. Use of orally administered succimer (meso-2,3-dimercaptosuccinic acid) for treatment of lead poisoning in dogs. *J Am Vet Med Assoc* 208(3):371–375.

Talcott, P.A. 2004. Zinc. In Peterson, M.E., Talcott, P.A., eds). *Small Animal Toxicology, 2nd ed.* St. Louis, Saunders Elsevier, pp. 1094–1100.

Van Alstine, W.G., Wickliffe, L.W., Everson, R.J. et al. 1993. Acute lead toxicosis in a household of cats. *J Vet Diagn Invest* 5:496–498.

Miscellaneous Toxicants

30

Michelle Mostrom

INTRODUCTION

This chapter discusses clinical signs and suggested treatments for a diverse group of compounds. In many cases, animals may not be observed consuming the toxic agent and owners report clinical signs with no known toxicant exposure. In other cases, an exposure may be recognized but a dose and the potential for intoxication is unknown. In a number of these instances, the veterinary clinical staff must treat the animal and developing clinical signs and not a textbook description of toxicity and therapy. Sorting through a complete history and evaluating the animal, particularly as clinical signs develop, may be the only approach available for a treatment regime and establishing a plausible diagnosis. A presumptive diagnosis can often be based on findings from the history and clinical observations (i.e., observing a toxicant in the vomitus or gastric lavage; smelling a hydrocarbon on animal breath, urine, or skin; history of training on plastic explosives and animals displaying seizures). The confirmatory diagnosis may be difficult to achieve due to lack of analytical testing procedures for a particular toxic agent. Contact your local state diagnostic laboratory or check on the American Association of Veterinary Laboratory Diagnosticians (AAVLD) website (http://www.aavld.org) and "Accreditation" link for diagnostic lab contact information to assist in veterinary toxicology analytical testing.

PETROLEUM-BASED PRODUCTS

Sources

Animals can be exposed to petroleum-based hydrocarbon products through inhalation, oral, ocular, or dermal routes in the house, hobby or work areas, garage, or outdoor environment. Generally pets will be exposed to refined petroleum products, such as fuels (gasoline, diesel, kerosene), paint thinners or pesticide carriers (petroleum distillates), degreasing and dry-cleaning compounds, and solvents. Petroleum products are complex chemical mixtures produced from the distillation of crude oil. Petroleum distillates are comprised of aliphatic and aromatic hydrocarbons and are usually liquids with a strong characteristic odor (e.g., diesel, gasoline, paint solvent, barbecue lighter fluids). Some petroleum products are in the form of flammable gases, such as methane, ethane, propane, and butane, which act more as simple asphyxiants. The aromatic hydrocarbons, benzene, toluene, ethyl benzene, and xylene (BTEX), are found in glues, quick-drying paints, lacquers, etc., and they are associated with more neurological signs and potential bone marrow toxicity. Although most hydrocarbons are of petroleum origin, some are wood-based such as turpentine and pine oil. Petroleum hydrocarbon–based products may contain additional compounds, such as surfactants, metals, and insecticides.

Small Animal Toxicology Essentials, First Edition. Edited by Robert H. Poppenga, Sharon Gwaltney-Brant.

Table 30.1. Petroleum hydrocarbon products listed by relative viscosity (lower to higher)*

	Saybolt Universal Seconds (SUS) at 100°F
Lighter fluid (naptha)	<32
Degreasers	<32
Carburetor cleaner	<32
Kerosene	32
Gasoline treatment	35
Diesel fuel 2D	32–45
Fuel oil 2	33–40
Mineral seal oil	36–42
Furniture polish	40
Turpentine	<60
Baby oil	70
No. 4 Fuel oil	80
Paint thinners	<100
Stoddard solvent (white spirits)	
Transmission fluids	<138
Heavy mineral oil	180
Machine Lubricant #10	160–235
Motor oil (10W30)	325
Tar, pine	200–300
Tar, road RT-6	250–400

*Adapted in part from 16 CFR Part 1700: http://www.cpsc.gov/businfo/frnotices/fr97/frpetdis.html

Table 30.2. Clinical signs related to petroleum hydrocarbon product ingestion

Inhalation	Aspiration pneumonia
	Dyspnea
	Coughing
	Bronchospasms
	Fever
	Cyanosis
	Depression
Dermal/ocular	Blisters
(grooming can lead to	Burns
oral exposure)	Inflammation
	Corneal ulcers
Oral	Salivation
	Pawing at mouth/shaking head
	Oral irritation/ulceration
	Severe vomiting
	Abdominal tenderness
	Diarrhea
	Anorexia
Systemic	Tachycardia/dysrhythmias
	Ataxia
	Tremors
	Weakness
	Depression
	Agitation
	Seizures
	Aspiration pneumonia
	Dyspnea/tachypnea
	Hepatic insult
	Renal degeneration

Mechanism

The dose or amount of exposure is generally difficult if not impossible to estimate unless observed. Petroleum products with lower viscosity (resistance to flow) and higher volatility (ability to vaporize) are more likely to result in inhalation or aspiration into lungs. Aspiration of a small amount of refined petroleum distillation products (<5 ml or 1 tsp) can lead to fatal aspiration pneumonia in pets. In general hydrocarbons with a viscosity of <35 SUS (Saybolt Universal Seconds, a measure of viscosity) pose a severe aspiration hazard because volatile products with a low surface tension diffuse into distal airways even when small quantities of fluid are ingested (see Table 30.1). Products with a viscosity of 35 to 100 SUS pose a moderate aspiration hazard. These products can cause vomiting and subsequent aspiration pneumonia. Products with a viscosity >100 SUS present a minimal aspiration hazard. Exposure to petroleum products results in clinical signs involving the respiratory, gastrointestinal, integumentary, and central nervous systems. Diverse clinical effects may occur. Some hydrocarbons may sensitize the myocardium to catecholamines and result in cardiac arrhythmias. Benzene, an aromatic hydrocarbon and carcinogen, can cause bone marrow depression and pancytopenia.

Clinical Effects

SIGNS

Clinical effects in animals generally occur 1 to 8 hours postexposure (see Table 30.2). When animals inhale petroleum products in enclosed spaces or while walking through spills, respiratory signs of coughing, aspiration pneumonia, fever, cyanosis, and depression may occur. Hydrocarbons can penetrate deep into the lung, causing bronchospasms, inflammation, and oxygen displacement

Table 30.3. Therapy recommendations for petroleum hydrocarbon product exposure

Clinical Sign	Recommendation	Dose
Respiratory	Oxygen	Based on blood gas data
	Positive end-expiratory pressure ventilation	
	Antibiotics	As needed
	Chest radiographs	
Bronchospasm	Beta-2 selective agonist (avoid epinephrine) e.g., terbutaline	Dogs: 0.003 to 0.005 mg/kg SC every 4 h Cats: 0.005 to 0.01 mg/kg SC every 4 h
Cardiac dysrhythmia	Electrocardiogram	
Dehydration	Crystalloid Fluids	As needed
Gastrointestinal irritation	Famotidine	0.25 mg/kg PO every 12 h
	Sucralfate	Dogs: 0.5 to 1 g PO every 8 to 12 h Cats: 0.25 g PO every 8 to 12 h
Seizures	Diazepam	0.5 to 2 mg/kg IV
Dermal contact	Mild detergents/cool water	
	Topical antibiotics	

in the alveolus leading to hypoxia. Direct contact with alveolar surfaces may cause hemorrhage, edema, and thrombosis leading to hypoxia, atelectasis, and pneumonitis. Cats and dogs breathing large amounts of petroleum solvents for several hours can suffer seizures and bronchitis.

Dermal contact can cause skin blisters and burns, severe buccal irritation, reduced respiratory function, and abdominal tenderness. Cats and dogs can be exposed to petroleum products through dermal contact and subsequent oral ingestion via grooming. After a heavy dermal exposure to hydrocarbons of lower viscosity (e.g., paint thinners, kerosene, Stoddard solvent, gasoline), systemic and dermal clinical signs may occur. Petroleum products can irritate the eyes producing inflammation, corneal damage, and ulcers.

Oral exposure in animals from direct contact with petroleum products may cause salivation, severe vomiting, oral ulcerations, abdominal tenderness, diarrhea, and anorexia. Systemic toxicity associated with petroleum exposures include tachycardia and dysrhythmias (originating from hypoxia or myocardial sensitization to catecholamines), ataxia, tremors, weakness, central nervous system (CNS) stimulation (agitation, seizures) or depression, tachypnea, fever, aspiration pneumonia, cyanosis, and hepatic and renal damage.

Management of Exposures

Treatment of petroleum hydrocarbon exposures is challenging because of a general lack of dose and toxicity information and proven treatment regimens. If the exposure involves small amounts of petroleum products with a high viscosity, sometimes just cage rest and observation for 12 to 24 hours is required.

Following ingestion of petroleum hydrocarbon products, avoid inducing emesis and performing gastric lavage to reduce the risk of aspiration. The use of an endotracheal tube cuff is not thought to be protective against aspiration. Administration of adsorbents (activated charcoal) is generally not effective in adsorbing hydrocarbons and can increase the risk of aspiration of petroleum product. However, if an animal ingested a large amount of petroleum product containing additional toxicants (insecticides, metals, chloride–containing compounds), the risk of gastric lavage and possible aspiration should be balanced against the toxicity. Do not use mineral oil to dilute the petroleum product. Treatment for aspiration pneumonia may be necessary, including monitoring chest radiographs, blood gases, and performing a CBC and serum biochemistries for hepatic and renal damage.

Animals with aspiration pneumonia should be hospitalized with intravenous fluids, oxygen therapy if needed, and cage rest (Table 30.3). In severe inhalation cases consider the use of positive end-expiratory pressure ventilation with caution because pneumothorax and pneumomediastinum could occur. Use of antibiotics may be indicated for secondary infections and bronchospasms treatment may be required using a beta-2 selective agonist (avoid epinephrine). Perform chest radiographs initially (preferably within 2 hours postexposure) and 2 to 4 days postexposure to check for pulmonary damage. Monitor a complete blood count (CBC) for hemoconcentration (increased packed cell volume and hemoglobin concentrations) and inflammatory responses and perform serum biochemistry to check for elevated blood urea nitrogen and hepatic enzyme levels associated with systemic toxicity. Check for hypoglycemia and monitor blood gases and oxygen saturation for pulmonary performance. Rapid progression of respiratory problems is a guarded prognosis. Respiratory signs may take days to almost two weeks or longer to resolve.

With evidence of buccal irritation, animals can be provided oral egg whites or milk. Oral protectants, such as sucralfate or famotidine, may be needed. Follow up with intravenous fluids and bland diets providing adequate nutrition. It is recommended that animals with abnormal cardiac rhythms should be monitored with electrocardiograms and treated appropriately. Seizures in animals can be treated with diazepam or barbiturates.

Dermal exposure to petroleum hydrocarbons should be treated by washing the animal with mild, nonsolvent-based detergents; note that petroleum distillates are not very miscible with water. Topical ointments or antibiotics may be required depending on skin irritation. Exposure to heavier chain hydrocarbons (asphaltenes or tar) may require clipping the hair coat. Animals may need an Elizabethan collar to prevent grooming and oral exposure. Flush eyes with warm water or saline for 15 minutes and stain for corneal ulcers if ocular exposure has occurred. Observe animals for at least 12 hours postexposure, particularly for respiratory effects, which may require oxygen supplementation and cage rest.

Diagnostics

Postmortem lesions may involve pulmonary congestion and edema, hepatic fatty change, renal degeneration, and necrosis (see Table 30.4). Ulcerations and the presence of an oily substance may be noted on oral and tracheal

Table 30.4. Postmortem lesions reported following ingestion or aspiration of petroleum hydrocarbons

Ulcerations in oral, gastrointestinal, or tracheal mucosa
Oily contents in gastrointestinal tract or lung
Pulmonary edema and congestion (lesions generally bilateral and caudoventral in lung)
Hepatic fatty change and centrilobular necrosis
Renal degeneration and necrosis

mucous membranes. The most severe clinical signs are associated with aspiration pneumonia, and the more volatile or highly refined products the greater the risk of aspiration and development of pulmonary edema.

Diagnosis will be based on history of exposure to petroleum products and compatible clinical signs. The characteristic odor of petroleum hydrocarbons can sometimes be detected in vomitus, gastrointestinal contents, urine, skin secretions, and on the breath. Although few diagnostic labs perform testing for petroleum hydrocarbons in gastrointestinal contents, it is recommended to save gastrointestinal contents in airtight, clean, glass containers and tissue samples (lung, liver, kidney) in aluminum foil and airtight containers; freeze samples. Contact a veterinary diagnostic laboratory for location of a lab to perform analysis, or commercial environmental labs may perform petroleum testing depending on the matrix.

A quick test for hydrocarbons in stomach contents involves mixing the contents vigorously with warm water and observing for petroleum products to rise to the surface as oily bubbles or oil film. This is not a definitive test because fatty acids can produce an oil film.

Differential Diagnoses

Differential diagnoses for clinical signs include organophosphates, caustic compounds, and trauma.

Avoid toxicosis by preventing animal access to petroleum product containers in the home, garage, and hobby areas. Where hydrocarbon spills occur, clean up immediately and prevent animal access to spill area.

FERTILIZERS

Sources

Fertilizers are typically based on N-P-K or nitrogen-phosphorus-potassium compounds and reported as numbers "5-10-5." These numbers represent percent by weight of ingredients in the fertilizer—for example. 5% nitrogen and potassium and 10% phosphorus. Fertilizers are used for agricultural, lawn and garden, and household plants. Formulations can be as granules, powders, liquids (concentrated or diluted), and solid sticks. The source of nitrogen is varied, including ammonium or potassium nitrate, urea, or organic in the form of blood meal (about 12% to 13% nitrogen), canola meal, and fish powder. Phosphorus sources can be inorganic, ammonium or potassium phosphate, or organic in the form of bone meal (containing about 12% phosphorus) or fish emulsions. Often potassium is added as potassium chloride or potash (salts of potassium carbonate, potassium oxide, or potassium chloride). Minor trace nutrients such as magnesium, boron, copper, molybdenum, cobalt, zinc, and iron, can be incorporated. Fertilizers with high iron concentrations (>1%) can cause iron intoxication and severe gastrointestinal irritation (see Chapter 29).

Fertilizers can include epsom salts (magnesium sulfate) and cocoa bean hulls and be incorporated with pesticides, herbicides, and fungicides. A history on ingestion of the particular product and listed ingredients is needed to evaluate exposure.

Clinical Effects

Signs

Clinical signs are dependent on the ingredients in the product. Typically, fertilizers are of low toxicity, and only gastrointestinal irritation is reported with ingestion (Table 30.5). Dogs are generally involved in exposures. Clinical signs of salivation, vomiting, diarrhea, and lethargy generally develop within 2 to 10 hours postexposure. Recovery occurs in 12 to 24 hours. Less common clinical signs reported are rash, pruritis, stiffness, tremors, and muzzle swelling in dogs. Dogs can be attracted to ingest large amounts of blood or bone meal and could develop severe gastroenteritis and possible pancreatitis. Fertilizers containing nitrates as the main nitrogen source may cause methemoglobinemia. The elimination half-life for nitrate in dogs is relatively long, 44.7 hours, with most absorbed nitrate eliminated in urine. In monogastrics, use of ammonium salts and urea as the nitrogen source produces gastrointestinal irritation. Death is not commonly reported with fertilizer ingestions in monogastrics.

Management of Exposures

Animals with recent fertilizer ingestion and no clinical signs should be induced to vomit (Table 30.6). Emesis should not be induced in animals with a history of vomiting. Often no additional therapy is required. If the animal is dehydrated or in shock, fluid therapy is recommended. Depending on clinical signs, additional therapy may be necessary for managing the animal. The appearance of congested mucous membranes and chocolate brown blood can indicate methemoglobinemia requiring oxygen therapy and methylene blue or ascorbic acid treatment. Check

Table 30.5. Fertilizer clinical signs

Reported	Vomiting
	Salivation
	Diarrhea
	Abdominal tenderness
	Polydipsia
	Lethargy
Less frequently reported	Urticarial rash
	Pruritis
	Seizures
	Stiffness
	Tremors
	Swollen muzzle
	Methemoglobinemia
	Pancreatitis
Calcium cyanamide ingestion	Skin irritation/ulceration
	Gastritis
	Rhinitis
	Tracheobronchitis
	Tachypnea
	Pulmonary edema
	Ataxia
	Hypotension and shock

Table 30.6. Treatment of fertilizer ingestion

Treatment	Recommendation	Dose
Emesis	Apomorphine	0.02 to 0.04 mg/kg IV, IM, or subconjunctival sac
	3% hydrogen peroxide	1 to 5 ml/kg PO (generally do not exceed 50 ml for dogs or 10 ml total for cat)
		Can repeat once after 15 min
Cathartic	Sorbital	3 ml/kg (70%) PO
Dehydration/shock	Crystalloid fluids	
Methemoglobinemia	Oxygen therapy	
	Methylene blue	1.5 mg/kg IV as a 10% solution in saline (monitor for Heinz bodies)
	Ascorbic acid in cats	30 mg/kg PO 4 times daily (slow in action)

appropriate chapters in this book for treatment of iron, herbicide, or insecticide toxicosis.

One compound used as a fertilizer is calcium cyanamide ($CCaN_2$). It can also be applied as a pesticide, defoliant, and fungicide. The compound is irritating to skin, eyes, and respiratory tract. Clinical signs can be skin irritation and ulcers, rhinitis, tracheobronchitis, and gastritis. Acute oral exposure may result in erythematous reaction in the face, dizziness, lethargy, vomiting, rapid breathing, pulmonary edema, hypotension, ataxia, shock, and possible hepatic insult.

Prognosis

The prognosis for recovery is generally good with fertilizer ingestion and treatment. However, additional ingredients of iron, herbicides, and insecticides may cause more severe clinical signs. Several of the Veterinary Diagnostic Laboratories are capable of testing stomach contents or product samples for fertilizers, herbicides and insecticides. Nitrate analysis can be performed on serum, feed, and ocular fluids by many veterinary labs.

Following application of fertilizer to plants, lawn, garden, or agricultural area, animals should be kept from contacting the area until dry or product has been incorporated into the soil. Fertilizers should be kept in containers and animals prevented access to the containers or storage areas.

MULCHES

Sources

A variety of mulches are used in gardens or landscapes. Inorganic mulches include lava rock, river stones, geotextile fabrics, and pulverized rubber. Organic mulches include shredded wood, bark or wood chips, conifer needles, leaves, grass clippings, newspapers, and straw, which are generally nontoxic unless consumed in large amounts and could cause gastrointestinal irritation or obstruction. With ingestion of organic mulches, consider exposure to possible pesticides or molds and mycotoxins. A popular mulch or organic fertilizer is cocoa bean mulch, which can be toxic to animals, particularly dogs attracted to the sweet, chocolate aroma. Cocoa bean mulch is made of cocoa bean shells and reportedly contains between 0.19 to 2.98% theobromine (approximately 860 to 13,500 mg theobromine/lb or 54 to 850 mg theobromine/oz). The concentrations of theobromine in cocoa bean mulch can be higher than concentrations

Table 30.7. Clinical signs in dogs consuming cocoa bean mulch

Commonly reported	Vomiting
	Muscle tremors
Less frequently reported	Tachycardia
	Hyperactivity
	Diarrhea

found in some chocolates. Unless "significant" amounts of cocoa bean mulch are ingested, many animals have no clinical signs. When large amounts of cocoa bean mulch are ingested by an animal, vomiting and muscle tremors can occur similar to signs from a methylxanthine toxicosis (Table 30.7).

Management of Cases

Treatment depends on the amount of mulch (particularly cocoa bean mulch) ingested, time elapsed since ingestion, and clinical signs observed. If a small amount was ingested, the animal should be observed for up to 24 hours for clinical signs. When larger amounts of cocoa bean mulch are ingested within a few hours of discovery (<3 to 4 hours), vomiting has not occurred, and the animal has normal mentation, emesis can be induced with 3% hydrogen peroxide or apomorphine (Table 30.8). If the dog is hyperexcitable or has seizures, gastric lavage should be performed with an endotracheal tube cuff in place. Hyperactivity or seizures can usually be controlled with diazepam. Repeated doses of activated charcoal should be given every 3 to 6 hr for up to 72 hr. Use a cathartic with the first dose of activated charcoal. Intravenous fluid therapy can increase urinary excretion of methylxanthines. Consider urinary bladder catheterization, which may reduce reabsorption of theobromine. Heart function should be monitored in dogs, particularly for premature ventricular contractions and persistent tachyarrhythmias; treatment with lidocaine (without epinephrine and not in cats) and beta-blockers may be required. Bradycardia is not reported as commonly as tachyarrhythmias. Death is not common with ingestion of cocoa bean mulches (see Chapter 24). Contact your state veterinary laboratory or the AAVLD website for information on diagnostic confirmation of theobromine in cocoa bean mulch or gastric contents.

Prevention includes recommending use of alternative mulches, such as pine or cedar mulches, where dogs have access to roam or exercise.

Table 30.8. Treatment of mulch/cocoa bean mulch (theobromine) ingestion

Treatment	Recommendation	Dose
Emesis	Apomorphine	0.02 to 0.04 mg/kg IV, IM, or subconjunctival sac
	3% hydrogen peroxide	1 to 5 ml/kg PO (generally do not exceed 50 ml for dogs or 10 ml total for cat)
		Can repeat once after 15 min
Adsorbent	Activated charcoal	2 to 5 g/kg body weight PO (1 g activated charcoal in 5 ml water)
Cathartic	Sorbital	3 ml/kg (70%) PO
Tremors	Diazepam	0.5 to 2 mg/kg IV
	Methocarbamol	50 to 220 mg/kg IV slowly
Seizures	Diazepam	0.5 to 2 mg/kg IV
	Phenobarbital	2 to 6 mg/kg IV slowly
Tachyarrhythmia	Propanolol	0.02 to 0.06 mg/kg IV slowly
	Metoprolol	0.04 to 0.06 mg/kg IV slowly
	Lidocaine	1 to 2 mg/kg IV slowly, and then infuse at 30 to 50 mcg/kg/min
Bradycardia	Atropine	0.01 to 0.02 mg/kg IV

COMPOST PILES

Sources

Compost piles may contain decomposing lawn, garden, and food products, especially fruit and vegetable wastes, leaves, and paper products. Generally meat, bones, dairy, and fat products are not added to compost but cannot be eliminated from consideration with ingestion of compost by pets. Dogs, as compared with cats, are more prone to scavenging and ingesting decaying products such as compost. A succession of bacterial populations occurs during composting, including growth of *Bacillus spp.* and perhaps *Staphylococcus* and *Streptococcus*, which could cause clinical signs of gastroenteritis. Yeast and mold populations aid in decomposition of compost materials. Mold growth of *Penicillium*, *Aspergillus*, and *Claviceps* on dairy, grain, bread, pasta, and walnut products could release tremorgenic mycotoxins that cause muscle tremors and seizures (see also Chapter 23). Chemicals may be added to compost to improve decomposition, such as nitrogen (inorganic as ammonium nitrate or organic as manure or blood meal) and lime (alkalinize the compost pile).

Toxicity

Expect typically low toxicity with ingestion of compost.

Clinical Effects

Clinical signs of gastroenteritis, vomiting, diarrhea, dehydration, and fever may occur within a few hours after consumption of compost (Table 30.9). Animals ingesting

Table 30.9. Clinical signs of compost ingestion

Bacterial	Vomiting
	Diarrhea
	Dehydration
	Fever
	Depression
	Shock
Botulism	Drooling
	Limb and tail weakness
	Poor reflexes of eyes and throat
	Respiratory paralysis
	Death
Tremorgenic mycotoxins (roquefortine and penitrem A)	Irritability
	Salivation
	Vomiting
	Ataxia
	Tachycardia
	Muscle tremors
	Panting
	Hyperthermia
	Nystagmus
	Seizures
	Death

a small amount of compost material may require only monitoring and treatment of clinical signs over 12 to 24 hours. Depending on the contents of the compost pile, *Salmonella* spp., *Escherichia Coli*, and *Clostridium* spp. (including *Clostridium botulinum*) could contribute to

Table 30.10. Treatment of compost ingestion (with potential of tremorgenic mycotoxins and botulism exposure)

Treatment	Recommendation	Dose
Emesis	Apomorphine	0.02 to 0.04 mg/kg IV, IM, or subconjunctival sac in the dog
Gastric lavage	Water at body temperature	10 mg/kg body weight by gravity installation; continue until lavage fluid runs clear
Adsorbent	Activated charcoal	2 to 5 g/kg body weight PO (1 g activated charcoal in 5 ml water)
Cathartic	Sorbital	3 ml/kg (70%) PO
Dehydration	Crystalloid fluids	As needed
Acid base imbalance	Sodium bicarbonate	As needed
Seizures	Diazepam	0.5 to 5 mg/kg IV (can be repeated at 10 min intervals up to 3 times)
	Phenobarbital	6 mg/kg IV to effect
	Pentobarbital	3 to 15 mg/kg IV slowly to effect
Muscle tremors	Methocarbamol	55 to 220 mg/kg IV to effect at a rate of no more than 2 ml/min
Botulism	Antitoxin	
	Artificial respiration	As required

more severe clinical signs of bloody diarrhea, endotoxic shock, and depression. Botulinum toxin ingestion may result in drooling; limb and tail weakness; poor reflexes in the eyes, throat, and legs; respiratory paralysis; and death. Dogs and cats are reported less sensitive to botulism than cattle, horses, and birds.

The tremorgenic mycotoxins, roquefortine and penitrem A, are readily absorbed following ingestion and within 30 minutes to several hours can cause irritability, muscle tremors (initially in the head and neck regions), weakness, panting, and eventually seizures, nystagmus, opisthotonus, recumbency, and death.

Management of Exposures

Clinical signs of tremors or central nervous system stimulation should be treated first. Tremors may be controlled by methocarbamol, a centrally acting muscle relaxant (Table 30.10). Diazepam may not be effective alone for treatment of seizures and phenobarbital may be needed. Pentobarbital is also effective controlling tremor and seizures in dogs with tremorgenic mycotoxin ingestion.

Treatment may include emesis if the animal has not already vomited and has normal CNS function. If animals exhibit tremors, induction of emesis is not recommended because vomiting may trigger seizures. Gastric lavage is recommended in large ingestions of compost, where vomiting has not occurred, and when animal is exhibiting clinical signs (tremors and central nervous system signs). A recommendation is use of a short-acting anesthesia for gastric lavage with a cuffed endotracheal tube in place to prevent aspiration pneumonia. Follow gastric lavage with activated charcoal and cathartic administration. Multiple doses of activated charcoal every 4 to 6 hours for up to 3 days may be necessary with tremorgenic mycotoxin ingestion due to excretion of toxins in bile with enterohepatic circulation. Monitor the animal with a complete blood count, serum biochemistry panel, determination of serum anion gap (increased lactate production from muscle tremors), urinalysis, and arterial blood gas measurements.

Animals with dehydration should be given fluids in conjunction with monitoring of electrolyte balance. With an acid-base imbalance sodium bicarbonate should be administered. Corticosteroids may be indicated for animals in shock.

Body temperature should be monitored for hyperthermia and body temperature regulated with the onset of tremors and seizures. In tremorgenic mycotoxin exposure, methocarbamol oral dosage may be required for several days to control tremors. The prognosis is good for recovery if gastric decontamination occurred and clinical signs are aggressively treated over the first 24 to 48 hours. If the animal had no gastrointestinal decontamination and ingested a large ingestion of tremorgenic material, the prognosis is poor.

If botulism is suspected, appropriate gastric lavage and activated charcoal therapy should be given soon after ingestion. Antitoxin treatment should be considered early in the course of therapy if a diagnosis of botulism is made based on clinical signs. Animals will require supportive care and possible artificial respiration. Prognosis is poor to guarded in animals showing clinical signs of botulism.

Diagnostics

A tentative diagnosis of compost pile ingestion is based on the history and compatible clinical signs. Stomach contents and suspect moldy material can be submitted for analysis of tremorgenic mycotoxins and botulism at a veterinary diagnostic laboratory. Contact the lab for submission information.

Differential Diagnoses

Differential diagnoses include methylxanthines, strychnine, bromethalin rodenticides, metaldehyde, illicit drug ingestion, tetanus toxoid, and a variety of human or veterinary drug ingestion. Prevention is through adequate enclosure of compost piles and decaying food material and restraint of animals from these areas.

CHARCOAL BRIQUETTES

Charcoal briquettes are of low toxicity and pose primarily a foreign body obstruction risk if swallowed. The solid cubes contain char dust that after ingestion could act as a gastrointestinal irritant causing vomiting. Clinical signs generally are self-limiting. Inhalation of charcoal dust can irritate ocular mucous membranes, nose, and throat (Table 30.11). Gently flush the eyes with saline or warm water and remove animals from the source of irritation. Quick lighting charcoal briquettes contain 10 to 20% hydrocarbon solvent, char dust, and limestone (<15%). Ingestion of the hydrocarbon-containing briquettes may cause vomiting, diarrhea, ataxia, lethargy, and possibly seizures if large amounts are ingested (see the section on petroleum-based products for therapy recommendations). Store product in a location where animals have no access.

FIRELOGS

Firelogs contain combustible products such as reclaimed sawdust, wood flour, paper pulp, and ground nut shells pressed into a log shape. The cellulosic material may be combined with petroleum-based wax (up to 65%) for quick ignition. The "green firelogs" can contain a vegetable or plant-based wax that dogs may be attracted to ingest in large amounts. Colorful firelogs can contain particulates mixed with a variety of chemicals (calcium or sodium chloride, potassium nitrate, copper sulfate, boric acid, or metals such as lead, arsenic, antimony, selenium). Chemicals such as coffee waste can be in java logs. Additional

chemicals in firelogs are oxidizing agents such as perborates and persulfates to improve viscosity and burning, nonporous extenders (silica, clay, coal dust), and fire retardants to extend burning time.

Firelog ingestion can cause gastroenteritis (see Table 30.11). Dogs may chew on logs when bored or can be attracted to the odor of wax-impregnated logs. Clinical signs of gastrointestinal irritation, such as vomiting, diarrhea, and constipation can occur. Animals may show depression, hypotension, and, rarely, renal failure. Treatment may consist of oral decontamination including emesis if ingestion is within 2 to 3 hours, vomiting has not occurred, and the animal has normal mentation. The use of activated charcoal and a cathartic are recommended. Depending on clinical signs, fluids and monitoring renal function should be considered. Prevention recommendation is to store firelogs in an area where animals have no access.

MATCHES

Match heads are made from potassium chlorate and regarded as having low toxicity with ingestion (see Table 30.11). Potassium chlorate is an oxidizing agent that can cause methemoglobinemia. If animals ingest a box or books of matches, clinical signs may develop including vomiting, abdominal pain, CNS depression, hypotension, cyanosis, hemolysis, and possibly methemoglobinemia. If treatment is required and ingestion has occurred within several hours, recommend oral decontamination with emesis. Supportive therapy may include gastrointestinal protectants (e.g., egg whites, milk) and fluids. If methemoglobinemia develops, treatment with oxygen and methylene blue (1% at 4 mg/kg in dogs or once at 1.5 mg/kg in cats IV) should be considered. The effective use of ascorbic acid treatment in cats (30 mg/kg PO 4 times daily) may be too slow for practical therapy.

FIREWORKS AND FLARES

Fireworks can contain oxidizing agents (potassium nitrate or chlorates), potassium perchlorates, heavy metal salts, and black powder (potassium nitrate or salt peter, charcoal, and sulfur) (see Table 30.11). Sparklers can contain potassium nitrate on a thin metal wand. Flares are made from metal nitrates or sodium nitrate, sulfur and hydrocarbons. The toxicity from ingestion of these products is generally low. Primarily gastrointestinal irritation is reported as vomiting (sometimes severe), abdominal pain, and salivation. Occasionally ulcerations may occur in the gastrointestinal tract and bloody feces are reported. Reports of hemolysis and seizures in affected animals are rare.

Table 30.11. Products involving ignition

Product	Chemical	Clinical Signs
Charcoal briquettes	Char dust (wood, coal, starch, lime)	Vomiting
	10–20% hydrocarbon solvent	Diarrhea
		Mucous membrane irritation
		Lethargy
Firelogs	Cellulose/lignin: sawdust, wood flour,	Vomiting (severe)
	coal dust, ground nut shells, silica	Diarrhea
	Petroleum-based wax	Constipation
	Vegetable/plant wax	Depression
	Potassium nitrate	Renal failure (rare)
	Sodium chloride	
	Heavy metals	
Match head	Potassium chlorate	Methemoglobinemia
Striking surface	Red phosphorus	Cyanosis
	Powdered glass	Vomiting
		Hypotension
		Depression
		Hemolysis
Sparklers	Potassium nitrate	Gastroenteritis
Fireworks	Oxidizing agents (potassium nitrate,	Vomiting (severe)
	chlorates)	Abdominal pain
	Potassium perchlorates (produces white	Bloody feces
	flash and noise)	Shallow breathing
		Methemoglobinemia
	Colors produced by heavy metal salts	Additional signs could be associated
	(mercury, antimony, copper, strontium,	with heavy metals
	lithium, barium, phosphorus)	
	Black powder:	
	75% potassium nitrate	Vomiting
	15% charcoal	Diarrhea
	10% sulfur	Methemoglobinemia
Watusi or dancing firecracker	Yellow phosphorus	Acute liver toxicity and organ failure
Signaling or Illuminating Flares	Metal nitrates or sodium nitrate	Gastroenteritis
	Hydrocarbons	Methemoglobinemia

Provide symptomatic care for clinical signs. If signs of methemoglobinemia occur (cyanosis, dyspnea, ataxia), treatment with oxygen and methylene should be considered.

Yellow phosphorus fireworks found in "dancing firecracker" or "Watusi" fireworks made in Asia are extremely toxic. Yellow phosphorus is readily absorbed from the gastrointestinal tract and is a general protoplasmic poison affecting multiple organ systems. While the United States restricts the use of yellow phosphorus in matches and fireworks, some of these products could find their way into the country. Reported clinical signs in humans following ingestion of these fireworks are acute hepatic injury and hepatic failure, upper-gastrointestinal hemorrhage, disseminated intravascular coagulation, bonemarrow depression, cerebral edema, and death. Treatment includes aggressive early decontamination of the gastrointestinal tract, monitoring hepatic function and acid-base balance, and providing fluids, glucose, and fresh frozen plasma. The administration of intravenous N-acetylcysteine did not appear to affect survival rates in human exposures.

EXPLOSIVES

Plastic Explosives

Sources

Plastic explosives (e.g., RDX, C-4, PE-4) are generally malleable solids that burn without exploding and are relatively insensitive to friction or impact; therefore, they are easily transported without undue precautions. Ingestion is usually by dogs undergoing training for military or police and accidental. In one report, a working dog ingested a small fragment of C-4 (the size of a grain of rice) and was treated with emesis of gastric contents but still developed systemic effects including generalized seizures.

The chemical cyclonite or cyclotrimethylenetrinitramine is a component in many plastic explosives (Table 30.12). Cyclonite crystals are colorless and insoluble in water. It has been reported that during manufacturing of cyclonite, human workers breathing the dust for several days developed "tonic-clonic spasms" that lasted for 5 to 10 minutes, occurred intermittently, and did not readily stop when the worker was removed from the work environment.

Kinetics

From experimental studies, plastic explosives appear to be slowly absorbed from the gastrointestinal tract. In a rat experiment, RDX was rapidly cleared from the plasma following absorption and distributed to tissues. C-4 is distributed widely to tissues, with kidneys having the highest concentration, followed by brain, heart, and lung.

Toxicity

An experimental estimate of a fatal dosage of PE-4 in a dog is 14 to 34 mg/kg body weight. Postmortem lesions are listed in Table 30.12. The lethal dosage of RDX for cats was reported to be 100 mg/kg. It appears from reported exposure cases that dogs display individual sensitivity to plastic explosive ingestion.

Clinical Effects

Signs

Clinical signs appear within minutes to several hours after ingestion. Animals that are clinically normal after a potential exposure to plastic explosives should be observed for a minimum of 4 to 6 hours. Clinical effects can be serious and severe, with early recognition of the ingestion and rapid treatment improving the outcome. Following ingestion of plastic explosives with cyclonite, clinical signs can appear rapidly and include lethargy, ataxia, confusion,

hyperesthesia, salivation, vomiting, tremors, and seizures that can become prolonged.

Management of Exposures

Because of the rapid onset of seizures, use of emetics (such as apomorphine) is controversial. Emesis is not indicated if the animal is showing neurological signs because of the potential for aspiration pneumonia, and vomiting may have already occurred following ingestion. Cyclonite appears to have a long retention time in the stomach; it is strongly recommended that gastric lavage be performed, preferably within several hours postexposure and with an endotracheal tube cuff in place (see Table 30.13). Activated charcoal should be given following lavage, either orally or by an orogastric tube. To protect against potential C-4 caustic action, gastrointestinal protectants were recommended during and after hospitalization. If the animal is salivating profusely consider using atropine.

Seizures may have durations of several minutes separated by periods of 10 to 30 minutes of initial calm that progresses to hyperesthesia and tremors. Convulsions can be controlled with sedatives such as diazepam and phenobarbital (which may be necessary for up to 6 hours). In the case of severe convulsions deep anesthesia may be needed for up to 6 to 8 hours. An oral maintenance phenobarbital therapy may be required for a period of days after the acute clinical signs abate to help control seizures and possibly stimulate cytochrome P450 enzyme activity and cyclonite metabolism. If animals go into respiratory arrest, mechanical ventilation may be required for a period of time. Dogs should be allowed to recover consciousness gradually, but resume anesthesia if convulsions reoccur. In one canine case, transient blindness and lack of menace response was reported for 12 hours after hospitalization; thiamine (8 mg/kg IM) was administered every 24 hours to help protect the CNS from insult.

Fluids (such as lactated ringers and dextrose saline drips) should be used to maintain hydration and for acidotic patients. In one case the dog developed facial and appendicular edema within 8 hours after hospitalization and was treated for hypoproteinemia with intravenous fresh frozen plasma followed by hydroxyethyl starch (1 ml/kg/hr). To help prevent pulmonary edema it is recommended to turn the dog every few hours while under sedation or anesthesia. Monitor a complete blood count for anemia and serum biochemistries for hepatic and renal functions and elevations in liver enzymes, bilirubin, and blood urea nitrogen. In one report, the blood biochemistry panel indicated liver damage three days after exposure to

Table 30.12. Explosives and clinical signs

Name	Chemical	Clinical Signs
RDX (syn. royal defense explosive)	Cyclonite (cyclotrimethylenetrinitramine)	Confusion Hyperesthesia
C-4	91% cyclonite 5.4% plasticizer 2.1% polyisobutylene 1.6% motor oil	Hyperventilation Lethargy Ataxia Tremors/facial twitches Seizures
PE-4	88% RDX (cyclonite) 12% plasticizer paraffin	Transient blindness Hyperthermia Hematuria Oliguria Proteinuria Salivation Vomiting Pale or congested mucous membranes Petechial rash Hepatic injury Anemia Urinary incontinence Renal damage Death
PETN (penthrite)	Pentaerythrityl tetranitrate	Vomiting Ataxia Collapse Bradycardia Dysrhythmia Depression Disorientation
TNT	2,4,6-trinitrotoluene	Methemoglobinemia Anemia Hepatic injury Splenomegaly Anorexia Skin irritation (skin yellow-orange color) Mucous membrane irritation Death
Dynamite	Nitroglycerin (glyceryl trinitrate) Nitrate salts Diatomaceous earth or sawdust	Methemoglobinemia Dyspnea Hypotension Depression Muscle weakness Anorexia Convulsions Death

Table 30.13. Treatment for explosive ingestion

Treatment	Recommendation	Dose
Emesis	Apomorphine	0.02 to 0.04 mg/kg IV, IM, or subconjunctival sac in the dog
Gastric lavage	Water at body temperature	10 mg/kg body weight
Adsorbent	Activated charcoal	2 to 5 g/kg body weight PO (1 g activated charcoal in 5 ml water)
Seizures	Phenobarbital	4 mg/kg, IV every 4 hr, 4 times for a total of 16 mg/kg total dose 3 mg/kg PO, every 12 hr as maintenance dose, and then tapering dose
	Diazepam	0.28 mg/kg rectally 0.34 mg/kg/hr, IV
	Propofol	0.4 mg/kg IV
Gastrointestinal protectant	Famotidine	0.57 mg/kg PO every 12 hr
	Sucralfate	28.5 mg/kg PO every 8 hr
	Omeprazole	1.15 mg/kg PO every 12 hr
Respiratory arrest	Oxygen Positive pressure ventilation	As needed
Fluids	Isotonic crystalloid	68.5 ml/kg/day IV reduced to 48 ml/kg/day IV
Hypoproteinemia	Fresh frozen plasma	10 ml/kg IV as a rate of 5 ml/kg /hr
Diuretic	Furosemide	1 mg/kg
Liver insult	Vitamin K Multivitamins	2 mg/kg PO every 24 hr IM
Salivation	Atropine	30 to 50 µg/kg subcutaneously
Methemoglobinemia	Oxygen therapy Methylene blue	1.5 mg/kg IV as a 10% solution in saline (monitor for Heinz bodies)

RDX and indicated a prolonged recovery. With hepatic damage, the dog was supplemented with vitamin K₁ and multivitamins. Urine protein and output should be monitored. Following rehydration the use of a diuretic is recommended to help accelerate elimination of metabolites in urine.

Table 30.14. Postmortem lesions reported following ingestion of plastic explosives

Generalized congestion
Pulmonary edema
Petechial hemorrhages in the pancreas
Hepatic congestion and enlargement
Renal congestion and hydropic degeneration

Diagnostics

Fragments of plastic explosives may be identified visually in gastric contents to help confirm exposure (Table 30.14).

Prognosis

Although clinical signs can be severe, with prompt treatment death is not common following accidental exposure.

Recovery occurs in about 48 hours. Prognosis is generally good with early detection of exposure and treatment, although renal toxicity was associated with one canine exposure. In this case of a 2-year-old Labrador dog ingesting cyclonite (C-4), the dog responded to treatment for seizures but subsequently developed polyuria/polydipsia and renal insufficiency characterized by a 70% reduction in glomerular filtration rate.

Pentaerythrityl Tetranitrate (PETN or Penthrite)

Sources

PETN is a nitroglycerin compound and high explosive. Dogs can be exposed to PETN during training in military or police work.

Clinical Effects

Signs

Initial clinical signs in a dog that chewed on a wrapped PETN container were gastrointestinal irritation, repeated vomiting, depression, mild disorientation, miosis, weakness, and ataxia (see Table 30.12). Depending on the time postingestion and clinical signs, gastric lavage may be effective; the animal may have vomiting frequently prior to hospitalization. In one report, a clinical exam of a dog following PETN ingestion revealed a slight bradycardia and blood pressure within normal range. The dog showed conscious proprioceptive deficits in the hindlimbs.

Laboratory

It is recommended to monitor serum biochemical changes for mild hepatic damage, including elevated bilirubin and increased levels in AST, ALT, ALP, and gamma glutamyl transferase (GGT). Monitor the heart rate with an electrocardiogram; an affected dog displayed a slight bradycardia and dysrhythmia (described as sinus arrhythmia with periods of sinus arrest).

Management of Exposures

Treatment may include fluids, the antiemetic metoclopramide (0.5 mg/kg IV,IM, PO q 6 to 8 h), and suppression of gastric acid production (e.g., omeprazole or rantidine (2 mg/kg q 12 hr). Multiple vitamins, particularly thiamine, B1, B6, and B12 were recommended. In a reported case of PETN ingestion, the dog was hospitalized for 7 days and showed gradual improvement of ataxia, normal heart rate, and incidence in nausea/vomiting. The bradycardia observed in this case was thought to be related to nitroglycerin induced increased vagal tone.

Diagnostics

Veterinary diagnostic laboratories do not routinely analyze for plastic explosives; the presumptive diagnosis is based on a history of exposure to plastic explosives and compatible clinical signs. In one case report, analysis of the dog's serum using a method based on ion mobility spectrometry detected fragments characteristic of PETN.

Dynamite

The primary ingredients of dynamite are nitroglycerin and nitrate salts. Potential effects of nitroglycerin ingestion include vomiting, bradycardia, dysrhythmia, and ataxia. The treatment is similar to exposure to PETN. Methemoglobinemia may result from the nitrate salts in dynamite. Treatment for methemoglobinemia includes oxygen and methylene blue (see Table 30.13).

2,4,6-trinitrotoluene or TNT

TNT or 2,4,6-trinitrotoluene is classified as a secondary explosive because it requires an initiating explosive for ignition. TNT is a crystalline substance with good chemical and thermal stability; it is practically insoluble in water and not affected by acids. It is affected by alkalis becoming a pink, red, or brown color and more sensitive. TNT may be mixed with other explosives such as RDX or HMX (high melting explosive). Workers handling TNT developed a canary yellow discoloration to their skin. Ingestion of TNT can cause methemoglobinemia, hepatic damage, irritated mucous membranes, sneezing, coughing, cyanosis, muscular pain, dysrhythmia, erythema, and pruritis (see Table 30.12). More chronic exposures in workers have resulted in anemia, peripheral neuritis, and splenic, hepatic, and renal damage. Treatment following ingestion includes oral decontamination, activated charcoal, and cathartic use (see Table 30.13). Monitor the CBC and serum biochemical panel for hepatic damage. If methemoglobinemia develops use oxygen and methylene blue with supportive therapy.

REFERENCES

Albretsen, Jay C. 2004. Fertilizers. In *Clinical Veterinary Toxicology*, edited by Konnie Plumlee, pp. 154–155. St. Louis: Mosby.

Bruchim, Y., Saragusty, J., Weisman, A., and Sterneim, D. 2005. Cyclonite (RDX) intoxication in a police working dog. *Vet Rec* 157:354–356.

Cope, Rhian B. 2007. Mushroom poisoning in dogs. *Vet Med* February:95–100.

De Cramer, K.G.M. and Short, R.P. 1992. Plastic explosive poisoning in dogs. *J S Afr Vet Assoc* 63(1):30–31.

Fishkin, Randi A., Stanley, Skye W., and Langston, Cathy E. 2008. Toxic effects of cyclonite (C-4) plastic explosive ingestion in a dog. *J Vet Emerg Crit Care* 18(5):537–540.

Naude, T.W. and Berry, W.L. 1997. Suspected poisoning of puppies by the mushroom *Amanita pantherina*. *J S Afr Vet Assoc* 68(4):154–158.

Oehme, Frederick W. and Kore, Anita M. 2006. Miscellaneous indoor toxicants. In *Small Animal Toxicology*, *2nd ed.*, edited by Michal Peterson and Patricia Talcott, pp. 986–995. St. Louis: Elsevier Saunders.

Osweiler, Gary D. 1996. *The National Veterinary Medical Series. Toxicology*, pp. 324–325. Media,Pennsylvania: Williams & Wilkins.

Potocnjak, D., Baric-Rafaj, R., Lemo, N., Matijatko, V., Kis I., Mrljak, V., and Harapin I. 2008. Poisoning of a dog with the explosive pentaerythrityl tetranitrate. *J Small Anim Pract* 49(6):314–318.

Raisbeck, Merl F. and Dailey, Rebecca N. 2006. Petroleum hydrocarbons. In *Small Animal Toxicology*, *2nd ed.*, edited by Michal Peterson and Patricia Talcott, pp. 986–995. St. Louis: Elsevier Saunders.

Appendices

Appendix 1
Drugs Used in Toxicology[a]

Drug	Indication	Species	Dosage
Acepromazine	Sedation for agitation caused by psychotropic drugs (e.g., amphetamines, phenylpropanolamine, pseudoephedrine)	Dogs:	0.025–0.2 mg/kg IM or IV (Start with low dose and titrate up to effect)
		Cats:	0.05–0.1 mg/kg IV, IM, SC
N-acetylcysteine (Mucomyst®, Acetadote®)	Management of acetaminophen toxicosis	Dogs and Cats:	Mucomyst®: Dilute to 5% solution; 140 mg/kg PO loading dose, and then 70 mg/kg q 4–6 h for 7 treatments; if hepatic enzymes elevated, continue for additional 10 treatments
			Acetadote®: 150 mg/kg in 3 ml/kg diluent IV over 1 h; and then 50 mg/kg IV in 7 ml/kg diluent over 4 h, and then 100 mg/kg in 14 ml/kg diluent over 16 h[h]
Activated charcoal[b]	Adsorption of toxicants (poor adsorption of many metals and minerals, small molecules [e.g., alcohols]). Generally administered with a cathartic—when administering multiple doses, cathartic is given every third dose	Dogs and Cats:	1–3 g/kg PO
Aluminum hydroxide	Antacid	Dogs:	5–15 ml PO q 12–24 h
		Cats:	2–10 ml PO q 24 h
Antivenin Crotalidae Polyvalent, Equine Origin	Management of crotalid snake envenomation (rattlesnake, copperhead, water moccasin)	Dogs and Cats:	Administer 1–5 rehydrated vials IV depending on severity of bite

Continued

Small Animal Toxicology Essentials, First Edition. Edited by Robert H. Poppenga, Sharon Gwaltney-Brant.
© 2011 John Wiley and Sons, Inc. Published 2011 by John Wiley and Sons, Inc.

Drug	Indication	Species	Dosage
Antivenin Crotalidae Polyvalent Immune FAB, Ovine origin (CroFab®)	Management of crotalid snake envenomation (rattlesnake, copperhead, water moccasin)	Dogs and Cats:	Dilute 1 vial in 250 ml sterile saline and infuse over 1 h; monitor for anaphylaxis; repeat as necessary[i]
Antivenin *Lactrodectus* (Lyovac)[c]	Management of envenomation by *Lactrodectus* (black widow spider)	Dogs and Cats:	Contents of 1 vial diluted in 2.5 ml of horse serum IM or further dilute in 10–50 ml of sterile saline and administer IV over 15 minutes
Apomorphine	Induction of emesis; may not be effective in cats: because they have few opioid receptors within their emetic center in the CNS	Dogs:	0.03 mg/kg IV or 0.04 mg/kg IM
			Alternatively a portion of tablet may be crushed in a syringe and dissolved with few drops of water and administered into the conjunctival sac. After sufficient vomiting occurs, rinse conjunctival sac free of unabsorbed apomorphine.
		Cats:	0.04 mg/kg IV or 0.08 mg/kg SC or IM
Atipamizole	Reversal of bradycardia, hypotension, and sedation from alpha agonists (e.g., amitraz, xylazine), imidazole decongestants	Dogs:	50 mcg/kg IM
Atropine	Test dose for suspected organophosphorus (OP) or carbamate toxicosis (TD)	Dogs and Cats:	TD: determine heart rate, and then administer 0.02 mg/kg IV; recheck heart rate—if rate increases >5 bpm, not an OP or carbamate toxicosis
	Treatment of bradycardia or excessive bronchial secretions from organophosphorus or carbamate toxicosis (XD)	Dogs and Cats:	XD: 0.2–0.5 mg/kg, give ¼ dose IV, rest IM or SC
	Treatment of bradycardia from cardiac depressant drugs (e.g., digoxin) (CD)	Dogs and Cats:	0.022–0.044 mg/kg IM, IV, SC prn
Bicarbonate, Sodium	Management of acidosis	Dogs and Cats:	mEq required = 0.5× body wt (kg) × (desired total CO_2 minus measured total CO_2); give ½ calculated dose over 3–4 h, and then recheck blood gases

Drug	Indication	Species	Dosage
Blood, whole (transfusion)	Replacement therapy for anemia	Dogs and Cats:	10–20 ml/kg IV
Buprenorphine	Management of pain	Dogs and Cats:	0.005–0.01 mg/kg IM, IV, SC q 6–12 h
Calcitonin, Salmon	Treatment of hypercalcemia caused by cholecalciferol toxicosis	Dogs:	4–6 IU/kg SC q 8–12 h
Calcium EDTA	Heavy metal chelator	Dogs and Cats:	25 mg/kg SC qid for 5 days
Chlorpromazine	Antiemetic	Dogs and Cats:	0.5 mg/kg IV, IM or SC q 6–8 h
	Sedation for agitation caused by psychotropic drugs (e.g., amphetamines, phenylpropanolamine, pseudoephedrine)	Dogs:	3 mg/kg PO q 12 h
			0.5 mg/kg IM or IV q 12 h
		Cats:	3 mg/kg PO q 24 h
			0.5 mg/kg IM or IV q 24 h
Cyproheptadine[d]	Assistance in management of serotonin syndrome and serotonergic effects of psychotropic drugs	Dogs:	mg/kg PO or per rectum q 6 h
		Cats:	2–4 mg per cat PO q 12–24 h
Dantrolene	Management of *Lactrodectus* (widow) spider bites; management of malignant hyperthermia from hops	Dogs:	1–5 mg/kg PO q 8 h or 1 mg/kg IV
		Cats:	0.5–2 mg/kg PO q 8 h or 1 mg/kg IV
Dapsone	Management of dermal necrosis from *Loxosceles* bits (recluse spiders)	Dogs and Cats:	1 mg/kg PO q 8–24 h
Deferroxamine	Chelator of iron	Dogs and Cats:	15 mg/kg/hour IV or 40 mg/kg IM q 4–8 h
Diazepam	Sedation for CNS stimulation; CAUTION: avoid use or use with caution with sympathomimetic (e.g., amphetamine) intoxication because paradoxical excitation may occur	Dogs:	0.1 mg/kg slow IV
	Management of seizures	Dogs and Cats:	0.2–5 mg/kg IV to effect

Continued

Drug	Indication	Species	Dosage
Digibind^e	Management of cardiac glycoside toxicosis (drugs, plants, toads) where life-threatening arrhythmias have not resolved with symptomatic therapy or serum potassium levels >5 mmol/l in the setting of severe digitalis intoxication^e	Dogs and Cats:	Dosage based on serum digoxin levels or amount of digoxin ingested (formulas on insert); if unknown exposure level, start with 1–2 vials^f
Dimercaprol (BAL)	Heavy metal chelator	Dogs and Cats:	2.5 mg/kg IM; repeat q 4h for 2 days, q 8h on 3rd day, and then q 12h for 10 d;
Diphenhydramine	Management of acute allergic reactions; antiemetic	Dogs:	2–4 mg/kg PO q 8–12h
			1 mg/kg IM, SC, IV q 8–12h
		Cats:	0.5 mg/kg PO q 12h
			2 mg/kg IM q 8h
Epinephrine	Systemic treatment of acute anaphylaxis		0.01–0.02 mg/kg IV, IM or SC
Esmolol	Management of ventricular arrhythmias; ultra–short-acting	Dogs and Cats:	Loading dose of 200–500 mcg/kg IV over 1 minute followed by constant rate IV infusion of 25–200 mcg/kg/minute
Ethanol	Management of ethylene glycol toxicosis; prevents formation of toxic metabolites	Dogs:	As 20% solution, administer 5.5 ml/kg IV q 6h for 5 treatments, and then q 8h for 4 treatments
		Cats:	As 20% solution, administer 5 ml/kg IV q 6h for 5 treatments, and then q 8h for 4 treatments
Flumazenil	Benzodiazepine antagonist used to aid in severe benzodiazepine overdose	Dogs and Cats:	0.01 mg/kg IV
Fomepizole	Management of ethylene glycol toxicosis; prevents formation of toxic metabolites	Dogs:	20 mg/kg IV, and then 15 mg/kg IV at 12 and 24h, and then 5 mg/kg at 36h and q 12h until no detectable EG in blood
		Cats:	125 mg/kg slow IV; then 31.25 mg/kg at 12, 24 and 36h

Drug	Indication	Species	Dosage
Furosemide	Diuretic for use in management of pulmonary edema secondary to inhalation toxicity	Dogs:	Up to 7.7 mg/kg IV or IM q 1–2 h as needed
		Cats:	Up to 4.4 mg/kg IV or IM q 1–2 h as needed
	Diuretic to enhance calcium excretion in hypercalcemia (e.g., cholecalciferol toxicosis)	Dogs and Cats:	2–4 mg/kg q PO, IV or IM 8–12 h
Glucagon	Manages severe cardiac arrhythmias (bradycardia, AV block) due to beta adrenergic blocker, calcium channel blocker, and tricyclic antidepressant overdoses	Dogs and Cats:	5–10 mg IV
H_2 blockers	Reduces gastric acid secretion	Dogs and Cats:	Cimetidine: 5–10 mg/kg PO, SQ, IM, IV q 6–8 h
		Dogs:	Famotidine: 0.5–1 mg/kg PO, IM, SQ, IV q 12–24 h
		Cats:	0.5 mg/kg PO, SC, IM, IV q 24 h
			Anecdotal reports of intravascular hemolysis when used IV in cats
		Dogs:	Ranitidine: 0.5–2 mg/kg PO, IV, IM q 8–12 h
		Cats:	2.5 mg/kg IV q 12 h or 3.5 mg/g PO q 12 h
3% Hydrogen peroxide	Induction of emesis	Dogs and Cats:	1 ml/lb to maximum of 45–50 ml[b]; can repeat once
Hydroxocobalamin	Management of cyanide toxicosis	Dogs:	75–150 mg/kg IV[k]
Intravenous Lipid Solution (20%; Liposyn®, Intralipids®)	Management of intoxication by highly lipid soluble compounds (e.g., ivermectin, moxidectin, baclofen, calcium channel blockers); emerging modality that some consider experimental; should be reserved for severe cases that are poorly responsive to other therapy	Dogs and Cats:	1.5 ml/kg IV administered over 10–20 minutes followed by 0.25 ml/kg/min IV for 1 hour; repeat dosing can be given at 3–4 hour intervals (or when serum no longer lipemic)[g]

Continued

Drug	Indication	Species	Dosage
Kaolin-pectin	Demulcent and putative adsorbent; CAUTION: many formulations now contain bismuth subsalicylate	Dogs:	1–5 ml/kg PO q 4–12 h
		Cats:	1–2 ml/kg PO q 4–12 h
Lactulose	Laxative and reduces blood ammonia levels; helpful in cases of liver insufficiency	Dogs:	15–30 ml PO q 6 h
		Cats:	0.25–1 ml PO q 8 h
Lidocaine	Management of ventricular arrhythmias	Dogs:	Bolus 2 mg/kg slow IV up to 8 mg/kg; or rapid IV 0.8 mg/kg/minute, and then CRI of 25–80 mcg/kg/min
		Cats:	Bolus 0.25–0.5 mg/kg slowly; repeat at 0.15–0,25 mg/kg in 5–20 minutes; CRI at 0.01–0.02 mg/kg min
Magnesium hydroxide	Reduces gastric acid	Dogs:	5–30 ml q 12–24 h
		Cats:	5–15 ml q 12–24 h
Mannitol	Osmotic diuretic for management of oliguric renal failure	Dogs and Cats:	0.25–0.5 gm/kg IV over 15–20 minutes
	Treatment of cerebral edema	Dogs and Cats:	0.5–1.5 g/kg IV over 10–20 minutes
Maropitant	Antiemetic	Dogs:	1 mg/kg SC q 24 h[h]
			2 mg/kg PO q 24 h
Methocarbamol	Management of muscle tremors, rigidity, convulsive activity (e.g., Permethrin, metaldehyde toxicoses)	Dogs and Cats:	55–220 mg/kg IV; administer half rapidly, wait for the animal to relax, and then administer remainder to effect; do not exceed 330 mg/kg/day
Methylene Blue	Treatment of methemoglobinemia; use with extreme caution, especially in cats:	Dogs:	4 mg/kg slow IV once
		Cats:	1–1.5 mg/kg IV once
Metoprolol	Management of tachycardia	Dog	5–50 mg PO q 8–12 h or
			0.2–0.4 mg/kg PO q 12 h
		Cats:	2–15 mg per cat PO q 12 h
Naloxone	Reversal of opioid toxicosis	Dogs:	0.04 mg/kg IV, IM or SC
		Cats:	0.05–0.1 mg/kg IV

Drug	Indication	Species	Dosage
Nitroprusside	Treatment of hypertension	Dogs:	Initial dose 1–2 mcg/kg/minute; increase incrementally q 3–5 min until desired BP attained
		Cats:	Initial dose 0.5 mcg/kg/minute; increase incrementally q 3–5 min until desired BP attained
Pamidronate (Aredia®)	Management of hypercalcemia due to intoxication by vitamin D or analogues	Dogs:	0.65–2 mg/kg in 0.9% NaCl slow IV over 2–3 hours; may repeat in 4–7 days if needed
D-Penicillamine	Copper or lead chelator	Dogs:	110 mg/kg/day PO divided qid for 1–2 weeks
		Cats:	125 mg q 12 h PO for 5 days
Pentobarbital	Management of seizures	Dogs:	3–15 mg/kg slow IV to effect
Phenobarbital	Management of seizures	Dogs and Cats:	3–6 mg/kg IV to effect
Pralidoxime Chloride	Treatment of organophosphorous insecticide intoxication	Dogs and Cats:	20 mg/kg IM, IV, SC q 8–12 h if no response after 3 doses, discontinue
Prednisone	Adjunct therapy in hypercalcemia due to vitamin D or analogue toxicosis	Dogs and Cats:	1–2 mg/kg PO q8–12 h
Propanolol	Management of tachycardia or other cardiac arrhythmias	Dogs and Cats:	0.02 mg/kg slow IV
Propofol	Management of seizures	Dogs and Cats:	0.1–0.6 mg/kg/minute
			3–6 mg/kg IV followed by CRI 8–12 mg/kg/h
Protamine Sulfate	Management of heparin overdoses	Dogs and Cats:	Administer 1–1.5 mg to antagonize each mg (100 units) heparin; slow IV
Pyridostigmine	Management of toxicosis from non-depolarizing neuromuscular blocking agents, botulism, atropine, avermectin, coral snake envenomation, and anticholinergics	Dogs:	0.5–3 mg/kg PO q 8–12 h
		Cats:	0.25 mg/kg/day

Continued

Drug	Indication	Species	Dosage
Pyridoxine	Used in management of seizures from penicillamine, *Gyromitra* mushroom, isoniazid, and hydrazines; adjunct therapy for ethylene glycol toxicosis	Dogs:	Administer milligram for milligram the dose of isoniazid/hydrazine; if not known, initial dosage 70 mg/kg IV[j]
SAMe	Hepatoprotectant	Dogs:	17–20 mg/kg/ day PO
		Cats:	200 mg/day PO
Silymarin	Hepatoprotectant	Dogs and Cats:	20–50 mg/kg/day PO
Succimer	Heavy metal chelator	Dogs and Cats:	10 mg/kg PPO q 8 h for 10 days; can be given rectally if patient is vomiting
Trientine	Chelator for copper hepatotoxicity	Dogs:	10–15 mg/kg PO q 12 h before meals
Vitamin K₁ (Phytonadione)	Treatment of anticoagulant rodenticide coagulopathy	Dogs and Cats:	3–5 mg/kg PO divided BID; treat for 7, 21, or 28 days according to type of rodenticide; check prothrombin time 48 h after last vitamin K
Xylazine	Emetic	Cats:	0.44 mg/kg IM
Yohimbine	Reversal of bradycardia, hypotension and sedation from alpha agonists (e.g., amitraz, xylazine), imidazole decongestants	Dogs:	0.11 mg/kg IV

Sources:

[a]Unless otherwise indicated, dosages come from Plumb, Donald C. 2005. *Plumb's Veterinary Drug Handbook, 5th ed.* Ames, Iowa: Blackwell Publishing Professional.

[b]DeClementi, Camille. 2007. Prevention and treatment of poisoning. In *Veterinary Toxicology*, edited by Ramesh C. Gupta, pp. 1139–1158. San Diego: Academic Press-Elsevier.

[c]Merck & Co, Inc. 2005. Antivenin (*Lactrodectus mactans*), Equine origin, product insert.

[d]Gwaltney-Brant, Sharon. 2004. Antidepressants. In *Clinical Veterinary Toxicology*, edited by Konnie H. Plumlee, pp. 286–291. St. Louis: Mosby.

[e]Smithkline Beecham Corporation. 2009. Digibind product information.

[f]Dalefield, Rosalind R. and Oehme, Frederick W. Antidotes for specific poisons. In *Small Animal Toxicology, 2nd ed.*, edited by Michael E. Peterson and Patricia A. Talcott, pp. 459–474. St. Louis: Saunders.

[g]Gwaltney-Brant, Sharon. 2010. Newer Antidotal Therapies. Proceedings of the CVC Baltimore, Baltimore, Maryland.

[h]Cumberland Pharmaceuticals. 2008. Acetadote package insert.

[i]Savage Labs. 2008. CroFab package insert.

[j]Villar D, Knight MW, Holding J, Barret GH, Buck WB. 1995. Treatment of acute isoniazid overdose in dogs. *Veterinary and Human Toxicology* 37(5):473–477.

[k]Borron, Stephen W, Stonerook, Michael, Reid, Frances. 2006. Efficacy of hyroxocobalamin in the treatment of acute cyanide poisoning in adult beagle dogs. *Clinical Toxicology* 44(Suppl 1):5–15.

Appendix 2
Additional Toxic Plants and Associated System-Based Effects

GASTROINTESTINAL

African milk bush (*Synadenium grantii*)

Ageratum, floss-flower (*Ageratum* spp)

Alder buckthorn (*Rhamnus* spp)

Amaryllis (*Amaryllis* spp)

Anemone, Pasque flower, windflower, meadow anemone, crowfoot (*Anemone* spp)

Apricot, peach, plum, bitter almond, cherry, choke cherry (*Prunus* spp)

Arnica (*Arnica montana*)

Aucuba, Japanese aucuba, Japanese laurel, spotted laurel (*Aucuba japonica*)

Azalea (*Rhododendron* spp)

Baby's breath (*Gypsophilia paniculata*)

Barberry, pipperidge (*Berberis* spp)

Bird-of-paradise (*Caesalpinia* spp)

Bittersweet, woody nightshade, wild nightshade (*Solanum dulcamara*)

Black bryony (*Tamus communis*)

Black laurel, mountain laurel (*Leucothoe davisiae*)

Black locust (*Robinia pseudo-acacia*)

Black nightshade (*Solanum nigrum*)

Bleeding heart, Dutchman's breeches, squirrel corn, stag-gerweed (*Dicentra* spp)

Blood lily, powderpuff lily (*Haemanthus multiflorus*)

Blue cohosh (*Caulophyllum thalictroides*)

Box, common box, boxwood (*Buxus sempervirens*)

Bluebell (*Hyacinthoides non-scripta*)

Broom (*Cytisus* spp)

Buttercup, meadow buttercup, crowfoot, lesser spearwort (*Ranunculus* spp)

Caladium (*Caladium* spp)

Calla lily (*Zantedeschia* spp)

Candelabra aloe, octopus plant, torch plant, Barbados aloe, medicinal aloe (*Aloe* spp)

Candelabra cactus, false cactus, mottled spurge, dragon bones (*Euphorbia lactea*)

Castor bean (*Ricinus communis*)

Ceriman, Swiss cheese plant, fruit-salad plant, split-leaf philodendron, Mexican breadfruit (*Monstera* spp)

Chenille plant, red-hot cattail (*Acalypha hispida*)

Cherry laurel (*Prunus laurocerasus*)

Chinaberry tree (*Melia azederach*)

Chinese evergreen (*Aglaonema* spp)

Chinese lantern, winter cherry, Cape gooseberry (*Physalis alkekengi*)

Chinese yam, cinnamon vine (*Dioscorea batatas*)

Christmas rose, black hellebore (*Helleborus* spp)

Common bean (*Phaseolus vulgaris*)

Common tansy (*Tenacetum* spp)

Coral bean, coral tree (*Erythrina* spp)

Corn plant (Dracaena spp)

Crinum lily, spider lily, swamp lily (*Crinum* spp)

Croton (*Codiaeum variegatum*)

(*Croton tiglium*)

Crown of thorns (*Euphorbia milii*)

Daffodil, trumpet narcissus, jonquil (*Narcissus* spp)

Death camas (*Zigadenus* spp)

Devil's ivy, ivy arum, pothos, hunter's robe, taro vine (*Epipremnum aureum*)

Dieffenbachia, dumb cane (*Dieffenbachia* spp)

Dogbane, Indian hemp (*Apocynum cannabium*)

Easter lily, star-gazer lily, tiger lily (*Lilium* spp, hyb)

Continued

Small Animal Toxicology Essentials, First Edition. Edited by Robert H. Poppenga, Sharon Gwaltney-Brant.
© 2011 John Wiley and Sons, Inc. Published 2011 by John Wiley and Sons, Inc.

GASTROINTESTINAL *Continued*

Elder, dwarf elder, Danewort (*Sambucus ebulus*)

Elephant's ear (*Alocasia* spp)

English ivy, Irish ivy, common ivy (*Hedera helix*)

Eucalyptus, blue gum, cider gum, silver dollar, Australian fever tree (*Eucalyptus* spp)

Euonymus, spindle (*Euonymus* spp)

Euphorbium (*Euphorbia resinifera*)

European mistletoe (*Viscum album*)

False hellebore, white hellebore (*Veratrum* spp)

Firethorn (*Pyracantha* spp)

Fishtail palm (*Caryota mitis*)

Flamingo flower (*Anthurium* spp)

Four o'clock (*Mirabilis jalapa*)

Foxglove, common foxglove, long purples, dead men's fingers (*Digitalis purpurea*)

Gloriosa lily, glory lily, climbing lily (*Gloriosa superba*)

Golden chain tree (*Laburnum anagyroides*)

Golden corydalis, bulbous corydalis, scrambled eggs, fitweed, fumitory (*Corydalis* spp)

Goosefoot, nephthytis, African evergreen, arrowhead vine (*Syngonium* spp)

Greater celandine (*Chelidonium majus*)

Green earth star (*Cryptanthus acaulis*)

Guelder-rose, high-bush cranberry (*Viburnum* spp)

Herb-Paris (*Paris quadrifolia*)

Holly, yaupon, possum-haw (*Ilex* spp)

Horse-chestnut, buckeye (*Aesculus* spp)

Horseradish, red cole (*Armorica rusticana*)

Hyacinth, garden hyacinth, Dutch hyacinth (*Hyacinthus orientalis*)

Hydrangea, hills of snow, French hydrangea, hortensia (*Hydrangea macrophylla*)

Iris, crested iris, dwarf iris, fleur-de-lis, blue flag, butterfly iris, poison flag, yellow iris (*Iris* spp)

Jack-in-the-pulpit (*Arisaema triphyllum*)

Jerusalem cherry, Christmas cherry, winter cherry, Natal cherry (*Solanum pseudocapsicum*)

Kaffir lily (*Clivia miniata*)

Kalanchoë, Palm-Beach-bells, feltbush, velvet elephant ear, devil's backbone, lavender-scallops (*Kalanchoe* spp)

Kingcup, marsh marigold (*Caltha palustris*)

Lantana, shrub verbena, yellow sage, bunchberry (*Lantana camara*)

Larkspur (*Delphinuim* spp)

Laurel, bay laurel, sweet bay (*Laurus nobilis*)

Lily of the palace, naked lady, amaryllis (*Hippeastrum* spp)

Lily-of-the-valley (*Convallaria majalis*)

Lobelia, cardinal flower, blue lobelia (*Lobelia* spp)

Lords-and-ladies, cuckoo pint, Adam-and-Eve (*Arum maculatum*)

Lupin, lupine, bluebonnet (*Lupinus* spp)

Macadamia nut (*Macadamia integrifolia*)

Male-fern (*Dryopteris filix-mas*)

Marigold, African marigold, French marigold, bog marigold, Aztec marigold (*Tagetes* spp)

Marsh marigold, kingcup (*Caltha palustris*)

May apple, mandrake (*Podophyllum* spp)

May lily (*Maianthemum bifolium*)

Meadow saffron, autumn crocus (*Colchicum autumnale*)

Mescal bean, mountain laurel, frijolito, Eve's necklace (*Sophora* spp)

Mezereon, spurge olive (*Daphne* spp)

Milkweed, butterfly weed (*Asclepias* spp)

Mock azalea, rusty-leaf (*Menziesia ferruginea*)

Monk's-hood (*Aconitum* spp)

Mountain laurel, dwarf laurel (*Kalmia* spp)

Netted vriesea (*Vriesea fenestralis*)

Nettle, stinging nettle, noseburn (*Urtica* spp, *Cnidoscolus* spp, *Tragia* spp)

Night-blooming jessamine, Chinese inkberry (*Cestrum nocturnum*)

Nightshade (*Solanum* spp)

Oak (*Quercus* spp)

Old man's beard, traveler's joy, virgin's bower (*Clematis* spp)

Oleander (*Nerium oleander*)

Oregon grape, trailing mahonia (*Mahonia* spp)

Ornamental pepper (*Capsicum annuum*)

Oyster plant, boat lily, Moses in a boat (*Rhoeo spathacea*)

Peace lily, white sails, white anthurium, spathe flower, Mauna Loa (*Spathiphyllum* spp) very low toxicity

Pencil tree, milkbush, Indian tree, rubber euphorbia, finger tree, naked lady (*Euphorbia tirucalli*)

Periwinkle (*Vinca* spp)

Persian violet, alpine violet, sowbread (*Cyclamen* spp)

Peyote, mescal, mescal buttons (*Lophophora williamsii*)

Pheasant's eye (*Adonis* spp)

Philodendron, sweetheart plant, panda plant, parlor ivy (*Philodendron* spp)

Physic nut (*Jatropha curcas*)

Pieris (*Pieris japonica*)

Pineapple, pineapple tree (*Ananas comosus*)

Pink quill (*Tillandsia cyanea*)

Plumbago, Cape plumbago, Cape leadwort, Ceylon leadwort (*Plumbago* spp)

Poinsettia, Christmas star (*Euphorbia pulcherrima*) very low toxicity

Pokeweed, pokeberry, pokesalad (*Phytolacca americana*)

Potato (*Solanum tuberosum*)

Primrose, German primrose, poison primrose (*Primula* spp)

Privet, wax-leaf ligustrum (*Ligustrum* spp)

Pulsatilla (*Pulsatilla* spp)

Red bryony, white bryony (*Bryonia* spp)

Rhododendron (*Rhododendron* spp)

Rhubarb, garden rhubarb, pie plant, water plant, wine plant (*Rheum rhubarbarum*)

Rosary pea, prayer bean, jequerity, precatory bean (A*brus precatorius*)

Rowan, mountain ash, service tree, whitebeam (*Sorbus* spp)

Sago palm, leatherleaf palm, Japanese fern palm (*Cycas revoluta*, *Cycas* spp)

Sandbox tree, monkey pistol (*Hura crepitans*)

Savin (*Juniperus sabina*)

Schefflera, umbrella tree, rubber tree, starleaf (*Schefflera* spp)

Sea onion (*Urginea maritima*)

Sensitive plant, shame plant, touch-me-not, action plant, humble plant (*Mimosa pudica*)

Snowdrop (*Galanthus nivalis*)

Solomon's seal (*Polygonatum* spp)

Sorrel, wood sorrel (*Oxalis* spp)

Spider lily, crown-beauty, sea daffodil, basket flower, alligator lily (*Hymenocallis* spp)

Spurge, creeping spurge, donkeytail (*Euphorbia myrsinites*)

Squill, starry hyacinth, autumn scilla, hyacinth scilla, Cuban lily, Peruvian jacinth, hyacinth of Peru, bluebell (*Scilla* spp)

Star-of-Bethlehem, summer snowflake, dove's dung, nap-at-noon (*Ornithogalum* spp)

Sweet-flag (*Acorus calamus*)

Tobacco, tree tobacco (*Nicotiana* spp)

Tomato (*Lycopersicon lycopersicum*)

Tuberous begonia (*Begonia tuberhybrida*)

Tulip (*Tulipa* spp, hyb)

Tung oil tree (*Aleurites* spp)

Urn plant (*Aechmea fasciata*)

Water hemlock, cowbane (*Cicuta* spp)

Weeping fig, Java willow, Benjamin tree, small-leaved rubber plant (*Ficus benjamina*)

White cedar (*Thuja occidentalis*)

White mustard, charlock (*Sinapis* spp)

White snakeroot (*Eupatorium rugosum*)

Wild radish (*Raphanus rhaphinistrum*)

Wild rosemary (*Ledum palustre*)

Wisteria, Chinese kidney bean (*Wisteria sinensis*)

Wormwood, sagewort, sagebrush (*Artemisia* spp)

Yellow allamanda, Nani Ali'i, flor de barbero (*Allamanda cathartica*)

Yellow oleander, Mexican oleander (*Thevetia* spp)

Yesterday-today-and-tomorrow (*Brunfelsia calycina*)

Yew, Japanese yew (*Taxus* spp)

Zamia (*Macrozamia* spp)

Zephyr lily, rain lily, fairy lily, fire lily (*Zephyranthes* spp)

Zulu potato, climbing onion (*Bowiea volubilis*)

CENTRAL AND PERIPHERAL NERVOUS SYSTEM

Pinpoint pupils

Azalea (*Rhododendron* spp)

Black laurel, mountain laurel (*Leucothoe davisiae*)

California poppy (*Eschscholzia californica*)

Herb-Paris (*Paris quadrifolia*)

Kaffir lily (*Clivia miniata*)

Mountain laurel, dwarf laurel (*Kalmia* spp)

Opium poppy (*Papaver somniferum*)

Pieris (*Pieris japonica*)

Poppy (*Papaver* spp)

Rhododendron (*Rhododendron* spp)

Wild rosemary (*Ledum palustre*)

Dilated pupils

Angel's trumpet (*Brugmansia* spp)

Aralia, Balfour aralia, dinner plate aralia, Ming aralia, geranium-leaf aralia, wild coffee, coffee tree (*Polyscias* spp)

Bittersweet, woody nightshade, wild nightshade (*Solanum dulcamara*)

Black nightshade (*Solanum nigrum*)

Candelabra cactus, false cactus, mottled spurge, dragon bones (*Euphorbia lactea*)

Christmas rose, black hellebore (*Helleborus* spp)

Corn plant (*Dracaena* spp)

(*Croton tiglium*)

Deadly nightshade (*Atropa belladonna*)

English ivy, Irish ivy, common ivy (*Hedera helix*)

Euphorbium (*Euphorbia resinifera*)

Hemlock (*Conium maculatum*)

Henbane (*Hyoscyamus niger*)

Jerusalem cherry, Christmas cherry, winter cherry, Natal cherry (*Solanum pseudocapsicum*)

Jimsonweed, thorn-apple, moonflower (*Datura stramonium*)

Continued

CENTRAL AND PERIPHERAL NERVOUS SYSTEM *Continued*

Milkweed, butterfly weed (*Asclepias* spp)

Morning glory, bindweed, pearly gates (*Ipomoea* spp)

Pencil tree, milkbush, Indian tree, rubber euphorbia, finger tree, naked lady (*Euphorbia tirucalli*)

Peyote, mescal, mescal button (*Lophophora williamsii*)

Potato (*Solanum tuberosum*)

Sandbox tree, monkey pistol (*Hura crepitans*)

Schefflera, umbrella tree, rubber tree, starleaf (*Schefflera* spp)

Tomato (*Lycopersicon lycopersicum*)

Tung oil tree (*Aleurites* spp)

Yew, Japanese yew (*Taxus* spp)

Hyperexcitability, muscle twitches

Azalea (*Rhododendron* spp)

Black laurel, mountain laurel (*Leucothoe davisiae*)

Coffee (*Coffee arabica*)

Deadly nightshade (*Atropa belladonna*)

Golden chain tree (*Laburnum anagyroides*)

Golden corydalis, bulbous corydalis, scrambled eggs, fitweed, fumitory (*Corydalis* spp)

Henbane (*Hyoscyamus niger*)

Horse-chestnut, buckeye (*Aesculus* spp)

Jimsonweed, thorn-apple, moonflower (*Datura stramonium*)

Marijuana (*Cannabis sativa*)

Mezereon, spurge olive (*Daphne mezereum*)

Mock azalea, rusty-leaf (*Menziesia ferruginea*)

Mountain laurel, dwarf laurel (*Kalmia* spp)

Pieris (*Pieris japonica*)

Rhododendron (*Rhododendron* spp)

Wild rosemary (*Ledum palustre*)

Yesterday-today-and-tomorrow (*Brunfelsia calycina*)

Hallucination, behavioral changes

Angel's trumpet (*Brugmansia* spp)

Christmas rose, black hellebore (*Helleborus* spp)

Deadly nightshade (*Atropa belladonna*)

Golden chain tree (*Laburnum anagyroides*)

Henbane (*Hyoscyamus niger*)

Jimsonweed, thorn-apple, moonflower (*Datura stramonium*)

Madagascar periwinkle (*Catharanthus rocus*)

Male-fern (*Dryopteris filix-mas*)

Marijuana (*Cannabis sativa*)

Mescal bean, mountain laurel, frijolito, Eve's necklace (*Sophora* spp)

Morning glory, bindweed, pearly gates (*Ipomoea* spp)

Nutmeg (*Myristica fragrans*)

Peyote, mescal, mescal buttons (*Lophophora williamsii*)

Trembling, ataxia, weakness, depression

Ageratum, floss-flower (*Ageratum* spp)

Amaryllis (*Amaryllis* spp)

Aralia, Balfour aralia, dinner plate aralia, Ming aralia, geranium-leaf aralia, wild coffee, coffee tree (*Polyscias* spp)

Azalea (*Rhododendron* spp)

Bittersweet, woody nightshade, wild nightshade (*Solanum dulcamara*)

Black nightshade (*Solanum nigrum*)

Bleeding heart, Dutchman's breeches, squirrel corn, staggerweed (*Dicentra* spp)

Blue cohosh (*Caulophyllum thalictroides*)

Bluebell (*Hyacinthoides non-scripta*)

Box, common box, boxwood (*Buxus sempervirens*)

Chinaberry tree (*Melia azederach*)

Coral bean, coral tree (*Erythrina* spp)

Corn plant (Dracaena spp)

Daffodil, trumpet narcissus, jonquil (*Narcissus* spp)

Easter lily, star-gazer lily, tiger lily (*Lilium* spp)

Foxglove, common foxglove, long purples, dead men's fingers (*Digitalis purpurea*)

Gloriosa lily, glory lily, climbing lily (*Gloriosa superba*)

Golden corydalis, bulbous corydalis, scrambled eggs, fitweed, fumitory (*Corydalis* spp)

Hemlock (*Conium maculatum*)

Horse-chestnut, buckeye (*Aesculus* spp)

Horsetail (*Equisetum* spp)

Hound's-tongue (*Cynoglossum officinale*)

Jerusalem cherry, Christmas cherry, winter cherry, Natal cherry (*Solanum pseudocapsicum*)

Kalanchoe, Palm-Beach-bells, feltbush, velvet elephant ear, devil's backbone, lavender-scallops (*Kalanchoe* spp)

Lantana, shrub verbena, yellow sage, bunchberry (*Lantana camara*)

Larkspur (*Delphinuim* spp)

Lobelia, cardinal flower, blue lobelia (*Lobelia* spp)

Lupin, lupine, bluebonnet (*Lupinus* spp)

Macadamia nut (*Macadamia integrifolia*)

Mescal bean, mountain laurel, frijolito, Eve's necklace (*Sophora* spp)

Mezereon, spurge olive (*Daphne mezereum*)

Milkweed, butterfly weed (*Asclepias* spp)

Mimosa, silk tree (*Albizia julibrissin*)

Monk's-hood (*Aconitum* spp)

Mountain laurel, dwarf laurel (*Kalmia* spp)

Nettle, stinging nettle, noseburn (*Urtica* spp, *Cnidoscolus* spp, *Tragia* spp)

Opium poppy (*Papaver somniferum*)

Pieris (*Pieris japonica*)

Poppy (*Papaver* spp)

Red bryony, white bryony (*Bryonia* spp)

Rhododendron (*Rhododendron* spp)

Sage palm, leatherleaf palm, Japanese fern palm (*Cycas revoluta*, *Cycas* spp)

Schefflera, umbrella tree, rubber tree, starleaf (*Schefflera* spp)

Tobacco, tree tobacco (*Nicotiana* spp)

Water hemlock, cowbane (*Cicuta* spp)

White snakeroot (*Eupatorium rugosum*)

Wild rosemary (*Ledum palustre*)

Yesterday-today-and tomorrow (*Brunfelsia calycina*)

Zamia (*Macrozamia* spp)

Zephyr lily, rain lily, fairy lily, fire lily (*Zephyranthes* spp)

Paralysis

Angel's trumpet (*Brugmansia* spp)

Azalea (*Rhododendron* spp)

Black laurel, mountain laurel (*Leucothoe davisiae*)

Blood lily, powderpuff lily (*Haemanthus multiflorus*)

Broom (*Cytisus* spp)

Coral bean, coral tree (*Erythrina* spp)

Coyotilla, tullidora (*Karwinskia humboldtiana*)

Death camas (*Zigadenus* spp)

False hellebore, black hellebore (*Veratrum* spp)

Hemlock (*Conium maculatum*)

Kaffir lily (*Clivia miniata*)

Larkspur (*Delphinuim* spp)

Lily of the palace, naked lady, amaryllis (*Hippeastrum* spp)

Meadow saffron, autumn crocus (*Colchicum autumnale*)

Monk's-hood (*Aconitum* spp)

Mountain laurel, dwarf laurel (*Kalmia* spp)

Persian violet, alpine violet, sowbread (*Cyclamen* spp)

Pieris (*Pieris* spp)

Rhododendron (*Rhododendron* spp)

Wild rosemary (*Ledum palustre*)

Convulsions

Amaryllis (*Amaryllis* spp)

Angel's trumpet (*Brugmansia* spp)

Aralia, Balfour aralia, dinner plate aralia, Ming aralia, geranium-leaf aralia, wild coffee, coffee tree (*Polyscias* spp)

Black locust (*Robinia pseudo-acacia*)

Bleeding heart, Dutchman's breeches, squirrel corn, staggerweed (*Dicentra* spp)

Box, common box, boxwood (*Buxus sempervirens*)

Broom (*Cytisus* spp)

Candelabra cactus, false cactus, mottled spurge, dragon bones (*Euphorbia lactea*)

Castor bean (*Ricinus communis*)

Common tansy (*Tenacetum* spp)

(*Croton tiglium*)

Chinaberry tree (*Melia azederach*)

English ivy, Irish ivy, common ivy (*Hedera helix*)

Euphorbium (*Euphorbia resinifera*)

Golden chain tree (*Laburnum anagyroides*)

Golden corydalis, bulbous corydalis, scrambled eggs, fitweed, fumitory (*Corydalis* spp)

Meadow saffron, autumn crocus (*Colchicum autumnale*)

Mediterranean thistle (*Atractylis gummifera*)

Milkweed, butterfly weed (*Asclepias* spp)

Mimosa, silk tree (*Albizia julibrissin*)

Pencil tree, milkbush, Indian tree, rubber euphorbia, finger tree, naked lady (*Euphorbia tirucalli*)

Persian violet, alpine violet, sowbread (*Cyclamen* spp)

Sago palm, leatherleaf palm, Japanese fern palm (*Cycas revoluta*, *Cycas* spp)

Sandbox tree, monkey pistol (*Hura crepitans*)

Schefflera, umbrella tree, rubber tree, starleaf (*Schefflera* spp)

Sea onion (*Urginea maritima*)

Spurge, creeping spurge, donkeytail (*Euphorbia myrisinites*)

Squill, starry hyacinth, autumn scilla, hyacinth scilla, Cuban lily, Peruvian jacinth, hyacinth of Peru, bluebell (*Scilla* spp)

Snowdrop (*Galanthus nivalis*)

Tobacco, tree tobacco (*Nicotiana* spp)

Tung oil tree (*Aleurites* spp)

Water hemlock, cowbane (*Cicuta* spp)

White cedar (*Thuja occidentalis*)

Yellow jessamine, Carolina jessamine (*Gelsemium sempervirens*)

Yesterday-today-and-tomorrow (*Brunfelsia calycina*)

Zamia (*Macrozamia* spp)

Zulu potato, climbing onion (*Bowiea volubilis*)

Unconsciousness/coma

Ageratum, floss-flower (*Ageratum* spp)

Amaryllis (*Amaryllis* spp)

Azalea (*Rhododendron* spp)

Black laurel, mountain laurel (*Leucothoe davisiae*)

California poppy (*Eschscholzia californica*)

Calla lily (*Zantedeschia* spp)

Continued

CENTRAL AND PERIPHERAL NERVOUS SYSTEM *Continued*

Cherry laurel (*Prunus laurocerasus*)

Chinaberry tree (*Melia azederach*)

Deadly nightshade (*Atropa belladonna*)

English ivy, Irish ivy, common ivy (*Hedera helix*)

Hemlock (*Conium maculatum*)

Henbane (*Hyoscyamus niger*)

Horseradish, red cole (*Armorica rusticana*)

Jimsonweed, thorn-apple, moonflower (*Datura stramonium*)

Lobelia, cardinal flower, blue lobelia (*Lobelia* spp)

Mescal bean, mountain laurel, frijolito, Eve's necklace (*Sophora* spp)

Mezereon, spurge olive (*Daphne mezereum*)

Mountain laurel, dwarf laurel (*Kalmia* spp)

Opium poppy (*Papaver somniferum*)

Poppy (*Papaver* spp)

Potato (*Solanum tuberosum*)

Sago palm, leatherleaf palm, Japanese fern palm (*Cycas revoluta, Cycas* spp)

Sandbox tree, monkey pistol (*Hura crepitans*)

Sorrel, wood sorrel (*Oxalis* spp)

Spurge (*Euphorbia* spp)

Sweet-flag (*Acorus calamus*)

Tobacco, tree tobacco (*Nicotiana* spp)

Water hemlock, cowbane (*Cicuta* spp)

White snakeroot (*Eupatorium rugosum*)

Wild rosemary (*Ledum palustre*)

Yew, Japanese yew (*Taxus* spp)

Zamia (*Macrozamia* spp)

CARDIOVASCULAR

Amaryllis (*Amaryllis* spp)

Angel's trumpet (*Brugmansia* spp)

Aralia, Balfour aralia, dinner plate aralia, Ming aralia, geranium-leaf aralia, wild coffee, coffee tree (*Polyscias* spp)

Arnica (*Arnica montana*)

Avocado (*Persea americana*)

Azalea (*Rhododendron* spp)

Black laurel, mountain laurel (*Leucothoe davisiae*)

Black locust (*Robinia pseudo-acacia*)

Broom (*Cytisus* spp)

Castor bean (*Ricinus communis*)

Christmas rose, black hellebore (*Helleborus* spp)

(*Croton tiglium*)

Common bean (*Phaseolus vulgaris*)

Common tansy (*Tenacetum* spp)

Daffodil, trumpet narcissus, jonquil (*Narcissus* spp)

Day-blooming jessamine (*Cestrum diurnum*)

Deadly nightshade (*Atropa belladonna*)

Death camas (*Zigadenus* spp)

Dogbane, Indian hemp (*Apocynum cannabium*)

English ivy, Irish ivy, common ivy (*Hedera helix*)

Euonymus, spindle (*Euonymus* spp)

False hellebore, white hellebore (*Veratrum* spp)

Foxglove, common foxglove, long purples, dead men's fingers (*Digitalis purpurea*)

Hemlock (*Conium maculatum*)

Henbane (*Hyoscyamus niger*)

Horseradish, red cole (*Armorica rusticana*)

Jimsonweed, thorn-apple, moonflower (*Datura stramonium*)

Kalancho, feltbush, velvet elephant ear, devil's backbone, lavender-scallops (*Kalanchoe* spp)

Licorice (*Glycyrrhiza glabra*)

Lily of the palace, naked lady, amaryllis (*Hippeastrum* spp)

Lily-of-the-valley (*Convallaria majalis*)

Lobelia, cardinal flower, blue lobelia (*Lobelia* spp)

Lupin, lupine, bluebonnet (*Lupinus* spp)

Macadamia nut (*Macadamia integrifolia*)

Monk's-hood (*Aconitum* spp)

Morning glory, bindweed, pearly gates (*Ipomoea* spp)

Mountain laurel, dwarf laurel (*Kalmia* spp)

Nettle, stinging nettle, noseburn (*Urtica* spp, *Cnidoscolus* spp, *Tragia* spp)

Night-blooming jessamine (*Cestrum nocturnum*)

Oleander (*Nerium oleander*)

Periwinkle (*Vinca* spp)

Pieris (*Pieris japonica*)

Potato (*Solanum tuberosum*)

Privet, wax-leaf ligustrum (*Ligustrum* spp)

Rhododendron (*Rhododendron* spp)

Saffron crocus, meadow saffron (*Crocus sativus*)

Schefflera, umbrella tree, rubber tree, starleaf (*Schefflera* spp)

Sea onion (*Urginea maritima*)

Silk vine (*Periploca graeca*)

Snowdrop (*Galanthus nivalis*)

Squill, starry hyacinth, autumn scilla, hyacinth scilla, Cuban lily, Peruvian jacinth, hyacinth of Peru, bluebell (*Scilla* spp)

Star-of-Bethlehem, summer snowflake, dove's dung, nap-at-noon (*Ornithogalum* spp)

Tobacco, tree tobacco (*Nicotiana* spp)

Tulip (*Tulipa* spp, hyb)

Wild rosemary (*Ledum palustre*)

Yellow oleander (*Thevetia peruviana*)

Yew, Japanese yew (*Taxus* spp)

Zephyr lily, rain lily, fair lily, fire lily (*Zephyranthes* spp)

Zulu potato, climbing onion (*Bowiea volubilis*)

Respiratory

Dyspnea, cyanosis

Apricot, peach, plum, bitter almond, cherry, choke cherry (*Prunus* spp)

Arnica (*Arnica montana*)

Bleeding heart, Dutchman's breeches, squirrel corn, staggerweed (*Dicentra* spp)

Box, common box, boxwood (*Buxus sempervirens*)

Caladium (*Caladium* spp)

California poppy (*Eschscholzia californica*)

Calla lily (*Zantedeschia* spp)

Ceriman, Swiss cheese plant, fruit-salad plant, split-leaf philodendron, Mexican breadfruit (*Monstera* spp)

Cherry laurel (*Prunus laurocerasus*)

Day-blooming jessamine (*Cestrum diurnum*)

Devil's ivy, ivy arum, pothos, hunter's robe, taro vine (*Epipremnum aureum*)

Dieffenbachia, dumb cane (*Dieffenbachia* spp)

Elephant's ear (*Alocasia* spp)

False hellebore, white hellebore (*Veratrum* spp)

Flamingo flower (*Anthurium* spp)

Golden corydalis, bulbous corydalis, scrambled eggs, fitweed, fumitory (*Corydalis* spp)

Goosefoot, nephthytis, African evergreen, arrowhead vine (*Syngonium* spp)

Lords-and-ladies, cuckoo pint, Adam-and-Eve (*Arum maculatum*)

Marijuana (*Cannabis sativa*)

Nettle, stinging nettle, noseburn (*Urtica* spp, *Cnidoscolus* spp, *Tragia* spp)

Philodendron, sweetheart plant (*Philodendron* spp)

Potato (*Solanum tuberosum*)

Tulip (*Tulipa* spp, hyb)

Respiratory depression or paralysis

Angel's trumpet (*Brugmansia* spp)

Barberry, pipperidge (*Berberis* spp)

Bittersweet, woody nightshade, wild nightshade (*Solanum dulcamara*)

Box, common box, boxwood (*Buxus sempervirens*)

Broom (*Cytisus* spp)

Coral bean, coral tree (*Erythrina* spp)

Deadly nightshade (*Atropa belladonna*)

False hellebore, white hellebore (*Veratrum* spp)

Gloriosa lily, glory lily, climbing lily (*Gloriosa superba*)

Golden chain tree (*Laburnum anagyroides*)

Hemlock, poison hemlock (*Conium maculatum*)

Henbane (*Hyoscyamus niger*)

Jimsonweed, thorn-apple, moonflower (*Datura stramonium*)

Larkspur (*Delphinium* spp)

Lupin, lupine, bluebonnet (*Lupinus* spp)

Meadow saffron, autumn crocus (*Colchicum autumnale*)

Milkweed, butterfly weed (*Asclepias* spp)

Monk's-hood (*Aconitum* spp)

Opium poppy (*Papaver somniferum*)

Oregon grape, trailing mahonia (*Mahonia* spp)

Red bryony, white bryony (*Bryonia* spp)

Rhododendron (*Rhododendron* spp)

Tobacco, tree tobacco (*Nicotiana* spp)

Yew, Japanese yew (*Taxus* spp)

RENAL

Barberry, pipperidge (*Berberis* spp)

Black locust (*Robinia pseudo-acacia*)

Castor bean (*Ricinus communis*)

Day-blooming jessamine (*Cestrum diurnum*)

Easter lily, star-gazer lily, tiger lily (*Lilium* spp)

Gloriosa lily, glory lily, climbing lily (*Gloriosa superba*)

Licorice (*Glycyrrhiza glabra*)

Oregon grape, trailing mahonia (*Mahonia* spp)

Red bryony, white bryony (*Bryonia* spp)

Saffron crocus, meadow saffron (*Crocus sativus*)

White cedar (*Thuja occidentalis*)

Wild radish (*Raphanus rhaphinistrum*)

Calcium oxalate crystalluria

Caladium (*Caladium* spp)

Calla lily (*Zantedeschia* spp)

Ceriman, Swiss cheese plant, fruit-salad plant, split-leaf philodendron, Mexican breadfruit (*Monstera* spp)

Chinese evergreen (*Aglaonema* spp)

Continued

RENAL *Continued*

Devil's ivy, ivy arum, pothos, hunter's robe, taro vine (*Epipremnum aureum*)

Goosefoot, nephthytis, African evergreen, arrowhead vine (*Syngonium* spp)

Lord-and-ladies, cuckoo pint, Adam-and-Eve (*Arum maculatum*)

Schefflera, umbrella plant, rubber plant, starleaf (*Schefflera* spp)

Sorrel, wood sorrel (*Oxalis* spp)

Sweet-flag (*Acorus calamus*)

Hematuria, azotemia

Barberry, pipperidge (*Berberis* spp)

Black locust (*Robinia pseudo-acacia*)

Castor bean (*Ricinus communis*)

Garlic (*Allium* spp)

Onion (*Allium* spp)

Oregon grape, trailing mahonia (*Mahonia* spp)

Rosary pea (*Abrus precatorius*)

LIVER DAMAGE

Amaryllis (*Amaryllis* spp)

Borage (*Borago officinalis*)

Comfrey (*Symphytum officinale*)

Common ragwort, tansy ragwort (*Senecio jacobaea*)

Crotalaria (*Crotalaria* spp)

Daffodil, trumpet narcissus, jonquil (*Narcissus* spp)

Day-blooming jessamine (*Cestrum diurnum*)

Dusty miller, cineraria, butterweed, Cape ivy, German ivy, Natal ivy, parlor ivy, water ivy, wax vine (*Senecio* spp)

Fiddleneck, tarweed (*Amsinckia* spp)

Heliotrope (*Heliotropium* spp)

Hound's-tongue (*Cynoglossum officinale*)

Lantana, shrub verbena, yellow sage, bunchberry (*Lantana camara*)

Oak (*Quercus* spp)

Purple viper's-bugloss, calamity Jane, Patterson's curse (*Echium lycopsis*)

Rhubarb, garden rhubarb, pie plant, water plant, wine plant (*Rheum rhubarbarum*)

Sago palm, leatherleaf palm, Japanese fern palm (*Cycas revoluta, Cycas* spp)

Snowdrop (*Galanthus nivalis*) (*Solanum malacoxylon*)

White cedar (*Thuja occidentalis*)

Wild radish (*Raphanus rhaphinistrum*)

Zamia (*Macrozamia* spp)

EMACIATION, ASCITES, EDEMA OF DEPENDENT EXTREMITIES; JAUNDICE; HEPATOENCEPHALOPATHY

Borage (*Borago officinalis*)

Comfrey (*Symphytum officinalis*)

Common ragwort, tansy ragwort (*Senecio jacobaea*)

Crotalaria (*Crotalaria* spp)

Dusty miller, cineraria, butterweed, Cape ivy, German ivy, Natal ivy, parlor ivy, water ivy, wax vine (*Senecio* spp)

Fiddleneck, tarweed (*Amsinckia* spp)

Heliotrope (*Heliotropium* spp)

Hound's-tongue (*Cynoglossum officinale*)

Purple viper's-bugloss, calamity Jane, Patterson's curse (*Echium lycopsis*)

CONTACT DERMATITIS, EYE IRRITANTS, ALLERGENS

African blue lily, blue African lily (*Agapanthus orientalis*)

African milk bush (*Synadenium grantii*)

Anemone, Pasque flower, windflower, meadow anemone, crowfoot (*Anemone* spp)

Aralia, Balfour aralia, dinner plate aralia, Ming aralia, geranium-leaf aralia, wild coffee, coffee tree (*Polyscias* spp)

Arnica (*Arnica* spp)

Baby's breath (*Gypsophilia paniculata*)

Black bryony (*Tamus communis*)

Buttercup, meadow buttercup, crowfoot, lesser spearwort (*Ranunculus* spp)

Calla lily (*Zantedeschia* spp)

Candelabra cactus, false cactus, mottled spurge, dragon bones (*Euphorbia lactea*)

Ceriman, Swiss cheese plant, fruit-salad plant, split-leaf philodendron, Mexican breadfruit (*Monstera* spp)

Chenille plant, red-hot cattail (*Acalypha hispida*)

Chinese evergreen (*Aglaonema* spp)

Chinese lantern, winter cherry, Cape gooseberry (*Physalis akekengi*)

Chinese yam, cinnamon vine (*Dioscorea batatas*)

Chrysanthemum, marguerite, ox-eye daisy (*Chrysanthemum* spp, hyb)

Croton, ornamental (*Codiaeum variegatum*)

(*Croton tiglium*)

Crown of thorns (*Euphorbia milii*)

Daffodil, trumpet narcissus, jonquil (*Narcissus* spp)

Devil's ivy, ivy arum, pothos, hunter's robe, taro vine (*Epipremnum aureum*)

Dieffenbachia, dumb cane (*Dieffenbachia* spp)

Dog-tooth violet, trout lily, avalanche lily (*Erythronium* spp)

English ivy, Irish ivy, common ivy (*Hedera helix*)

Eucalyptus, blue gum, cider gum, silver dollar, Australian fever tree (*Eucalyptus* spp)

Euphorbium (*Euphorbia resinifera*)

European mistletoe (*Viscum album*)

Garlic, onion (*Allium* spp)

Geranium, zonal geranium, ivy geranium (*Pelargonium* spp)

Great lettuce, garden lettuce (*Lactuca* spp)

Green earth star (*Cryptanthus acaulis*)

Horseradish, red cole (*Armorica rusticana*)

Iris, yellow iris, crested iris, dwarf iris, fleur-de-lis, blue flag, poison flag (*Iris* spp)

Laurel, bay laurel, sweet bay (*Laurus nobilis*)

Lords-and-ladies, cuckoo pint, Adam-and-Eve (*Arum maculatum*)

Male-fern (*Dryopteris filix-mas*)

Marigold, African marigold, French marigold, bog marigold, Aztec marigold (*Tagetes* spp)

Netted vriesea (*Vriesea fenestralis*)

Old man's beard, traveler's joy, virgin's bower (*Clematis* spp)

Ornamental pepper (*Capsicum annuum*)

Oyster plant, boat lily, Moses in a boat (*Rhoeo spathacea*)

Peace lily, white sails, white anthurium, spathe flower, Mauna Loa (*Spathiphyllum* spp)

Pencil tree, milkbush, Indian tree, rubber euphorbia, finger tree, naked lady (*Euphorbia tirucalli*)

Peruvian lily, lily of the Incas (*Alstroemeria* spp)

Philodendron, sweetheart plant, panda plant, parlor ivy (*Philodendron* spp)

Piggyback plant, pickaback plant, thousand mothers, youth-on-age (*Tolmiea menziesii*)

Pink quill (*Tillandsia cyanea*)

Plumbago, Cape plumbago, Cape leadwort, Ceylon leadwort (*Plumbago* spp)

Poinsettia, Christmas star (*Euphorbia pulcherrima*)

Poison ivy, poison oak, poison sumac (*Rhus* spp)

Primrose, German primrose, poison primrose (*Primula* spp)

Pulsatilla (*Pulsatilla* spp)

Red bryony, white bryony (*Bryonia* spp)

Sneezeweed (*Helenium* spp)

Spurge, creeping spurge, donkeytail (*Euphorbia myrsinites*)

Tulip (*Tulipa* spp, hyb)

Tung oil tree (*Aleurites* spp)

Urn plant (*Aechmea fasciata*)

Weeping fig, Java willow, Benjamin tree, small-leaved rubber plant (*Ficus benjamina*)

White cedar (*Thuja occidentalis*)

Yellow allamanda, Nani Ali'i, flor de barbero (*Allamanda cathartica*)

Primary photosensitization

Bishop's weed, Queen Anne's lace (*Ammi majus*)

Dahlia (*Dahlia* spp)

Dutchman's breeches (*Thamnosma texana*)

Marigold, African marigold, French marigold, bog marigold, Aztec marigold (*Tagetes* spp)

St. John's wort (*Hypericum perforatum*)

SUDDEN DEATH

False hellebore, white hellebore (*Veratrum* spp)

Foxglove (*Digitalis purpurea*)

Hemlock, poison hemlock (*Conium maculatum*)

Kalanchoe, feltbush, velvet elephant ear, devil's backbone, lavender-scallops (*Kalanchoe* spp)

Laburnum, golden chain tree (*Laburnum anagyroides*)

Oleander (*Nerium oleander*)

Yellow oleander, Mexican oleander (*Thevetia* spp)

Yew, Japanese yew (*Taxus* spp)

Appendix 3
Plants Not Reported to Be Toxic

Achira (*Canna edulis*)
Achyranthes Verschaffelti (*Iresine herbstii*)
Acorn Squash (*Curcurbita pepo cv acorn*)
African Violet (*Saintpaulia ionantha*)
Algaroba (*Ceratonia sUiqua*)
Aluminum Plant (*Pilea cadierei*)
Alumroot (*Heuchera sanguinea*)
American Rubber Plant (*Peperomia obtusifolia*)
Anthericum Comosum (*Chlorophytum comosum*)
Antirrhinum Multiflorum (*Antirrhinum glandulosum*)
Apple Leaf Croton (*Polyscias balfouriana marginai*)
Arabian Gentian (*Exacum affine*)
Aregelia (*Neoregelia carolinae*)
Artillery Plant (*Pilea callitrichoides*)
Aspidium Falcatum (*Cyrtomium falcatum*)
Aubepine (*Crataegus oxyacantha*)
Autumn Olive (*Elaeagnus spp.*)
Baby Rubber Plant (*Peperomia obtusifolia*)
Baby Tears (*Helxine soleirolii*)
Bachelors Buttons (*Centaurea cyanus*)
Ball Fern (*Davallia bullata mariesii*)
Ball Fern (*Davallia fojeensis plumosa*)
Bamboo (*Phylostachys aurea*)
Bamboo Palm (*Chamaedorea erumpens*)
Bamboo Vine (*Smilax laurifolia*)
Banana (*Musa acuminata*)
Banana Squash (*Curcurbita maxima cv banana*)
Begonia Species
Belmore Sentry Palm (*Howeia spp.*)
Big Shellbark Hickory (*Carya spp.*)
Bignonia (*Jacaranda procera*)
Bitter Pecan (*Carya spp.*)

Bitternut (*Carya spp.*)
Black Haw (*Crataegus oxyacantha*)
Black Hawthorn (*Crataegus oxyacantha*)
Blaspheme Vine (*Smilax laurifolia*)
Bloodleaf Plant (*lresine herbstii*)
Blooming-Sally (*Epilobium angustijloium*)
Blue Bead (*Clintonia borealis*)
Blue Daisy (*Felicia amelloides*)
Blue Echeveria (*Echeveria derenbergii*)
Blue-Dicks (*Brodiaea capitata*)
Blue-Eyed Daisy (*Arctotis grandis*)
Bluebottle (*Centaurea cyanus*)
Blunt-Leaved Peperomia (*Peperomia obtusifolia*)
Blushing Bromeliad (*Neoregelia carolinae*)
Bold Sword Fern (*Nephrolepis exalta bostoniensi compacta*)
Boston Fern (*Nephrolespis exalta bostoniensi compacta*)
Boston Sword Fern (*Nephrolespis exaltata*)
Bottle Palm (*Beaucarnea recurvata*)
Bottlebrush (*Callistemon spp.*)
Brazilian Orchid (*Sophronitis spp.*)
Bride's-Bonnet (*Clintonia uniflora*)
Bristly Greenbrier (*Smilax hispida*)
Brodiaea Pulchella (*Brodiaea capitata*)
Broom Hickory (*Carya spp.*)
Bullbrier (*Smilax rotundifolia*)
Bur Gourd (*Cucumis anguria*)
Burro's Tail (*Sedum morganianum*)
Buttercup Squash (*Curcurbita maxima cv buttercup*)
Butterfly Ginger (*Hedychium coronarium*)
Butterfly Iris (*Spuria spp.*)
Butterfly Lily (*Hedychium coronarium*)

Small Animal Toxicology Essentials, First Edition. Edited by Robert H. Poppenga, Sharon Gwaltney-Brant.
© 2011 John Wiley and Sons, Inc. Published 2011 by John Wiley and Sons, Inc.

Butterfly Orchid (*Oncidium spp.*)
Butterfly Tulip (*Calochortus gunnisonii*)
Button Fern (*Pellaea rotundifolia*)
Caeroba (*Jacaranda procera*)
Calathea Insignis (*Maranta insignis*)
Calathea Lancifolia (*Maranta insignis*)
California Cobra Plant (*Darlingtonia californica*)
California Pitcher Plant (*Darlingtonia californica*)
Callistemon Bradyandrus (*Callistemon spp.*)
Callistemon Citrinus (*Callistemon spp.*)
Callistemon Viminalis (*Callistemon spp.*)
Calochortus Nuttalli (*Calochortus gunnisonii*)
Camellia (*Camellia japonica*)
Canada Hemlock (*Fsuga canadensis*)
Canary Date Palm (*Pheonix canariensis*)
Candle Plant (*Plectranthus coleoides (Marginatus)*)
Candycorn Plant (*Hypocyrta nummularia*)
Canna Lily (*Canna generalis*)
Cantebury-Bell (*Gloxinia perennis*)
Cape Jasmine (*Fabernaemontana*)
Cape Primrose (*Streptocarpus spp.*)
Carob (*Ceratonia siliq*)
Carob Tree (*Ceratonia sUiqua*)
Carob Tree (*Jacaranda procera*)
Caroba (*Jacaranda procera*)
Carobinha (*Jacaranda procera*)
Carolina Hemlock (*Tsuga spp.*)
Carrion Flower (*Smilax herbacea*)
Carrot Fern (*Davallia bullata mariesii*)
Carrot Fern (*Davallia fejeensis plumosa*)
Casaba Melon (*Cucumis melo*)
Cast Iron Plant (*Aspidistra elatior*)
Cat Brier (*Smilax glabra*)
Cat Ear (*Calochortus gunnisonii*)
Cattleya Labiata (*Cattleya trianaei*)
Cattleya Labiata Var Mossiae (*Cattleya mossiae*)
Cattleya Labiata Var Mossiae (*Cattleya trianaei*)
Celosia Globosa (*Celosia cristata*)
Celosia Plumosa (*Celosia cristata*)
Chamaedorean Humilis (*Chamaedorea erumpens*)
Chaparral Snapdragon (*Antirrhinum coulteranum*)
Chenille Plant (*Echeveria derenbergii*)
Chestnut (*Castanea spp.*)
Chicken-Gizzard Plant (*lresine herbstii*)
Chickens and Hens (*Echeveria agavoides*)
Chickens and Hens (*Echeveria elegans*)
Chicks and Hens (*Echeveria imbricata*)
Chicks and Hens (*Echeveria secunda*)
Chin-Lao-Shu (*Smilax glabra*)
China Aster (*Callistephus spp.*)

China Root (*Smilax glabra*)
Chinese Plumbago (*Ceratostigma willmottianum*)
Chlorophytum Bichetii (*Anthericum bichetii*)
Chlorophytwn
Sternbergianum (*Chlorophytum comosum*)
Chocolate Solider Plant (*Episcia dianthiflora*)
Christmas Dagger Fern (*Polystichym spp.*)
Christmas Orchid (*Cattleya trianaei*)
Christmas Palm (*Veitchia merrillii*)
Cinnamon Jasmine (*Hedychium coronarium*)
Cinquefoil (*Potentilla spp.*)
Cirrhopetalum
Appendeculatum (*Bulbophyllum appendeculatum*)
Clearweed (*Pilea pumila*)
Cliff Brake Fern (*Pellaea rotundifolia*)
Club Moss (*Selaginelia kraussiana*)
Cocks Comb (*Celosia cristata*)
Cocktail Orchid (*Cattleya forbesii*)
Coffee Plant (*Coffea arabica*)
Collinia Elegans (*Chamaedorea erumpens*)
Color-Band Cryptanthus (*Cryptanthus "It"*)
Columnar Cactus (*Cephalocereus*)
Common Camellia (*Camellia japonica*)
Common Catbrier (*Smilax rotundifolia*)
Common Garden Canna (*Canna generalis*)
Common Greenbrier (*Smilax rotundifolia*)
Common Snapdragon (*Antirrhinum majus*)
Common Staghorn Fern (*Platycerium bifurcatum*)
Confederate Jasmine (*Trachelospermum jasminoides*)
Coolwort (*Pilea pumila*)
Copper Rose (*Echeveria derenbergii*)
Copperlead (*Acalypha wilkesiana macafeana*)
Coral Ardisia (*Ardisia crenulata*)
Coral Bells (*Heuchera sanguinea*)
Coral Berry (*Ardisia crispa*)
Cornflower (*Centaurea cyanus*)
Crape Myrtle (*Lagerstroemia spp.*)
Crataegus Phaenopyrum (*Crataegus oxyacantha*)
Crataegus spp. (*Crataegus oxyacantha*)
Creeping Charlie (*Lysimachia nummularia*)
Creeping Charlie (*Pilea nummulariifolia*)
Creeping Charlie (*Plectranthus australis*)
Creeping Gloxinia (*Asarina erubscens*)
Creping Gloxinia (*Maurandia spp.*)
Creeping Mahonia (*Mahonia spp.*)
Creeping Pilea (*Pilea depressa*)
Creeping Rubus (*Rubus pedatus*)
Creeping Zinnia (*Sanvitalia spp.*)
Crepe Myrtle (*Lagerstroemia spp.*)
Crimson Bottlebrush (*Callistemon spp.*)

Crimson Cup (*Neoregelia carolinae*)

Crisped Feather Fern (*Nephrolepis exalta bostoniensis compacta*)

Crossandra (*Crossandra undulifolia infundibuliformis*)

Cucumber (*Cucumis sativus*)

Cushion Aloe (*Hawthoria spp.*)

Cushion Moss (*Selagenella kraussiana brownii*)

Cushon Aloe (*Haworthia subfasciata*)

Cyrtudeira Reptans (*Episcia reptans*)

Dainty (*Davallia bullata maries;i*)

Dainty (*Davallia fejeensis plumosa*)

Dainty Rabbits-Foot Fern (*Davallia bullata mariesii*)

Dainty Rabbits-Foot Fern (*Davallia fejeensis plumosa*)

Dallas Fern (*Nephrolepis exalta bostoniensis compacta*)

Dancing Doll Orchid (*Oncidium jlexuosum*)

Dancing Doll Orchid (*Oncidium lanceanum*)

Dancing Doll Orchid (*Oncidium sphacelatum*)

Davallia Bullata Mariessi (*Davallia fejeensis plumosa*)

Davallia Trichomanoides (*Davallia bullata mariesii*),

Desert Trumpet (*Eriogonum umbellatum*)

Dichelostemma Pulchellum (*Brodiaea capitata*)

Dichorisandra Reginae (*l'radescantia reginae*)

Dinteranthus Vanzylii (*Lithops vanzylii*)

Duffii Fern (*Nephrolepis exalta*)

Duffy Fern (*Nephrolepis exalta*)

Dwarf Boston Fern (*Nephrolepis exalta bostoniensis compacta*)

Dwarf Date Palm (*Pheonix roebelenii*)

Dwarf Feather Fern (*Nephrolepis exalta bostoniensis compacta*)

Dwarf Palm (*Chamaedorea erumpens*)

Dwarf Rose -Stripe Star (*Cryptanthus rose us pictus*)

Dwarf Royal Palm (*Veitchia merrillii*)

Dwarf Whitman Fern (*Nephrolepis exalta bostoniensis compacta*)

Earth Star (*Cryptanthus acaulis*)

Easter Cattleya (*Cattleya mossiae*)

Easter Daisy (*l'ownsendia sericea*)

Easter Lily Cactus (*Echinopsis multiplex*)

Easter Orchid (*Cattleya mossiae*)

Edible Banana (*Musa acuminata*)

Edible Canna (*Canna edulis*)

Elephant-Ear Begonia (*Begonia scharfiii*)

Emerald-Ripple Peperomia (*Peperomia caperata*)

English Hawthorn (*Crataegus oryacantha*)

Epidendrum Atropurpeum (*Epidendrum cocholeastum*)

Epidendrum Ibaguense (*Epidendrum cochloeastum*)

Epidendrum Prismatocarpum (*Epidendrum cochleastum*)

Episcia spp. (*Episcia dianthiflora*)

False Aralia (*Dizygotheca elegantissima*)

Fairy Fountain (*Celosia cristata*)

Fan Tufted Palm (*Rhapis spp.*)

Feather Fern (*Nephrolepis exalta bostoniensis compacta*)

Feathered Amaranth (*Celosia cristata*)

Fiery Reed Orchid (*Epidendrum cochleasrum*)

Fig-Leaf Gourd (*Cucurbita ficifolia*)

Figleaf Palm (*Fatsia japonica*)

Fingernail Plant (*Neoregelia carolinae*)

Fire Weed (*Epilobium angustifloium*)

Fish Tail Fern (*Cyrtomium falcarum*)

Flame African Violet (*Episcia reptans*)

Flame of the Woods (*Ixora coccinea*)

Flame Violet (*Episcia reptans*)

Florida Butter-Fly Orchid (*Epidendrum tampense*)

Fluffy Ruffles (*Nephrolepis exalta 6 bostoniensis compacta*)

Forster Sentry Palm (*Belmoreana howea Jorsteriana*)

Fortunes Palm (*TrachycarpusJortuneij*)

Freckle Face (*Hypoestes sanguinolenta*)

Friendship Plant (*Pilea involucrata*)

Frosty (*Episcia reptans*)

Garden Marigold (*Calendula officinalis*)

Garden Snapdragon (*Antirrhinum majus*)

German Violet (*Exacum affine*)

Gherkins (*Cucumis sativus*)

Ghost Leafless Orchid (*Polyrrhiza lindenii*)

Ghost Plant (*Graptopetalum paraguayense*)

Giant Aster (*Townsendia sericea*)

Giant Holly Fern (*Polystichum munitum*)

Giant White Inch Plant (*Tradescantia albiflora "Albo-vittata"*)

Gibasis Geniculata (*Tradescantia multiflora*)

Globe Thistle (*Echinops spp.*)

Gloxinia (*Sinningia spp.*)

Gold Bloom (*Calendula officina/is*)

Gold-Fish Plant (*Hypocyrta nummularia*)

Golden Aster (*Callistephus spp.*)

Golden Bells (*Forsythia spp.*)

Golden Lace Orchid (*Haemaria discolor*)

Golden Shower Orchid (*Oncidium flexuosum*)

Golden Shower Orchid (*Oncidium sphacelatum*)

Good Luck Palm (*Chamaedorea erumpens*)

Grape Hyacinth (*Muscari armeniacum*)

Grape Hyacinth (*Muscari spp.*)

Grape Ivy (*Cissus rhombifolia*)

Great Willow-Herb (*Epilobium angustiforium*)

Green-Ripple Peperomia (*Peperomia caperata*)

Greenbrier (*Smilax glabra*)

Hagbrier (*Smilax hispida*)

Hardy Baby Tears (*Nertera grandensis*)

Hardy Gloxinia (*Incarvillea spp.*)
Haw Apple (*Crataegus oxyacantha*)
Haworthia (*Haworthia subJasciata*)
Haws (*Crataegus oxyacantha*)
Hawthorn (*Crataegus oxyacantha*)
Hedgehog Gourd (*Cucumis dipsaceus*)
Hellfetter (*Smilax hospida*)
Hemlock Tree (*Tsuga spp.*)
Hen-and-Chickens Fern (*Asplenium bulbiferum*)
Hens and Chicks (*Echeveria imbricata*)
Hens and Chicks (*Echeveria secunda*)
Hens and Chickens (*Echeveria agavoides*)
Hens and Chickens (*Echeveria elegans*)
Hickory (*Carya spp.*)
Hindu Rope Plant (*Hoya carnosa "compacta"*)
Holligold (*Calendula officinalis*)
Holly Fern (*Cyrtomium jalcatum*)
Hollyhock (*Althaea rosea*)
Honey Locust (*Glenditsia triacanthos*)
Honey Plant (*Hoya carnosa "compacta"*)
Honeydew Melons (*Cucumis melo*)
Honeysuckle Fuchsia (*Fuchsia triphylla*)
Hookera Pu1chella (*Brodiaea capitata*)
Horse Brier (*Smilax rotundifolia*)
Hoya Carnosa "Exotica" (*Hoya carnosa "compacta"*)
Hoya Carnosa "Krinkle Kur!" (*Hoya carnosa "compacta"*)
Hoya Carnosa ,Variegata, (*Hoya carnosa "compacta"*)
Hoya "Mauna Loa" (*Hoya spp.*)
Hubbard Squash (*Curcurbita maxima cv hubbard*)
Hypocyrta spp. (*Hypocyrta nummularia*)
Ice Plant (*Aptenia cordifolia*)
Ice Plant (*Lampranthus spp.*)
Imbricata sword fern (*Polystichum munitum*)
Irish Moss (*Helxine soleirolii*)
Iron Cross Begonia (*Begonia masoniana*)
Iron Tree (*Ixora coccinea*)
Ivy Peperomia (*Peperomia griseoargentea*)
Ivy-Leaf Peperomia (*Peperomia griseoargentea*)
Jackson Brier (*Smilax lanceolata*)
Jacob's Ladder (*Smilax herbacea*)
Japanese Aralia (*Fatsia japonica*)
Japanese Holly Fern (*Cyrtomium jalcatum*)
Japanese Moss (*Helxine soleirolii*)
Japanese Pittosporurn (*Pittosporum tobira*)
Jasmine (*Jasminium rex*)
Jewel Orchid (*Haemaria discolor*)
Joseph's Coat (*Alternanthera amoena*)
Joseph's Coat (*Iresine herbstii*)
Jungle Geranium (*Ixora javanica*)
Kaempferis (*Kaempferia pulchra*)

Kahali Ginger (*Hedychium gardneranum*)
Kenilworth Ivy (*Cybalaria muralis*)
KentiaPalm (*Howeia spp.*)
Kenya Violet (*Saintpaulis spp.*)
Kharoub (*Ceratonia siliqua*)
King Nut (*Carya spp.*)
King of the Forest (*Anoectochilus setaceus*)
King-and-Queen Fern (*Asplenium bulbiferum*)
Kuang-Yen pa-Hsieh (*Smilax glabra*)
Lace Flower Vine (*Episcia dianthiflora*)
Lace Orchid (*Odontoglossum crispum*)
Lace Orchid (*Odontoglossum grande*)
Ladies Ear Drops (*Fuchsia spp.*)
Lady Lou (*Episcia reptans*)
Lady Palm (*Rhapis flabelliformis*)
Ladys Ear Drops (*Fuchsia spp.*)
Lagerstroemia Indica (*Lagerstroemia spp.*)
Lance Dracaena (*Pleomele thaliodes*)
Lance Pleumele (*Pleomele thalioides*)
Large Lady Palm (*Rhapsis excelsa*)
Laurel-Leaved Greenbrier (*Smilax laurifolia*)
Leather Peperomia (*Peperomia crassifolia*)
Leng-Fen Tu'an (*Smilax glabra*)
Leopard Lily (*Lachenalia spp.*)
Leopard Orchid (*Oncidium flexuosom*)
Leopard Orchid (*Oncidium lanceanum*)
Leopard Orchid (*Oncidium sphacelatum*)
Lesser Snapdragon (*Antirrhinum orontium*)
Lily of the Valley Orchid (*Odontoglossum crispum*)
Lily of the Valley Orchid (*Oncidium lanceanum*)
Linden (*filia americana*)
Lipstick Plant (*Aeschynathus pulcher*)
Little Zebra Plant (*Haworthia subfasciata*)
Little Zebra Plant (*Hawthoria spp.*)
Little-Fantasy Peperomia (*Peperomia caperata*)
Living Rock Cactus (*Pleiospilos bulusii*)
Living Stones (*Lithops vanzylii*)
Locust Pods (*Ceratonia siliqua*)
Lou-Lang-T'ou (*Smilax glabra*)
Luther (*Harald*)
Madagascar Jasmine (*Stephanotis floribunda*)
Magnolia Bush (*Magnolia stellata*)
Mahonia Aquifolium (*Mahonia acquifolium*)
Malabar Gourd (*Cucurbita ficilolia*)
Malaysian Dracaena (*Pleomele reflexa*)
Manila Palm (*Veitchia merrillii*)
Mapleleaf Begonia (*Begonia cleopatra*)
Maranta (*Prayer plants*)
Marbled Fingernail (*Neoregelia carolinae*)
Mariposa Lily (*Calochortus gunnisonii*)

Maroon (*Echeveria derenbergii*)

Mary-Bud (*Calendula officinalis*)

May Bush (*Crataegus oxyacantha*)

Measles Plant (*Hypoestes sanguinolenta*)

Melons (*Cucumis melo*)

Metallic Leaf Begonia (*Begonia metallica*)

Mexican Firecracker (*Echeveria spp.*)

Metallic Peperomia (*Peperomia metallica*)

Mexican Rosettes (*Echeveria spp.*)

Mexican Snowball (*Echeveria spp.*)

Miniature Date Palm (*Phoenix roe belen;;*)

Minature Fish Tail (*Chamaedorea erumpens*)

Minature Maranta (*Calathea micans*)

Miniature Marble Plant (*Neoregelia carolinae*)

Mistletoe Cactus (*Thipsalis cassutha*)

Mockernut Hickory (*Carya spp.*)

Mosaic Plant (*Fittonia verschaffeltii*)

Mosaic Vase (*Guzmania lingulata*)

Moss Agate (*Episcia reptans*)

Moss Campion (*Silene acaulis*)

Moss Fern (*Selaginella spp.*)

Moss Phlox (*Phlox subulata*)

Moss Rose (*Portulaca spp.*)

Mossy Campion (*Silene acaulis*)

Mother Fern (*Asplenium bulbiferum*)

Mother Spleenwort (*Asplenium bulbiferum*)

Mother-of-Pearl Plant (*Graptopetalum paraguayense*)

Mountain Camellia (*Stewartia*)

Mountian Grape (*Mahonia spp.*)

Mulberry Bush (*Morus spp.*)

Mulberry Tree (*Morus spp.*)

Musa Paradisiaca (*Musa acuminata*)

Muscari Armeniacum (*Muscari spp.*)

Muscari spp. (*Muscari armeniacum*)

Muskmelon (*Cucumis melo*)

Narrow-Leaved Pleomele (*Pleomele angustifolia*)

Natal Plum (*Carissa grandiflora*)

Neanthe Bella Palm (*Chamaedorea elegans "Bella"*)

Neanthebella (*Chamaedorea erumpens*)

Nematanthus spp. (*Hypocyrta nummularia*)

Neoregelia (*Neoregelia carlinae*)

Nepbrolepsis (*Nephrolepis exalta*)

Nerve Plant (*Fittonia verschaffeltii*)

New Silver & Bronze (*Pilea sp. "Silver Tree"*)

Night-Blooming Cereus (*Hylocereus undatus*)

Odontoglossum spp. (*Odontoglossum grande*)

Old Man Cactus (*Cephalocereus senilis*)

Old World Orchid (*Bulbophyllum appendeculatum*)

Orange Star (*Guzmania lingulata*)

Oregon Grape (*Mahonia acquifolium*)

Ossifragi Vase (*Neoregelia carolinae*)

Paddy's Wig (*Helxine soleirolii*)

Painted Lady (*Echeveria derenbergii*)

Palm Lily (*Yucca elephantipes*)

Pampus Grass (*Cortaderia selloana*)

Panamiga (*Pilea involucrata*)

Pansy Orchid (*Miltonia roezlii alba*)

Paradise Palm (*Howea spp.*)

Parlor Palm (*Chamaedorea erumpens*)

Parlor Plant (*Hoya carnosa*)

Parsley Fern (*Asplenium bulbiforum*)

Peace Begonia (*Begonia rex "Peace"*)

Peacock Plant (*Kaempferia pulchra*)

Pearl Plant (*Haworthia subfasciata*)

Pearl Plant (*Hawthoria spp.*)

Pearly Dots (*Haworthia subfasciata*)

Pearly Dots (*Hawthoria spp.*)

Peperomia Fosteri (*Peperomia dahlstedtii*)

Peperomia Hederifolia (*Peperomia griseoargentea*)

Peperomia Peltifolia (*Peperomia argyreia*)

Peperomia Rotundifolia (*Peperomia nummulariifolia*)

Peperomia Sandersii (*Peperomia argyreia*)

Pepper-Face (*Peperomia obtusifolia*)

Persian Violet (*Exacum affine*)

Pheasant Plant (*Cryptanthus zonatus*)

Piggy-Back Plant (*Tolmiea menziesii*)

Pigmy Date Palm (*Pheonix roebelenii*)

Pignut (*Carya spp.*)

Pignut Hickory (*Carya spp.*)

Pilea Microphylla (*Pilea callitrichoides*)

Pilea Mucosa (*Pilea callitrichoides*)

Pink Brocade (*Episcia "Pink Brocade"*)

Pink Pearl (*Begonia semperflorens "Pink Pearl"*)

Pink Polka Dot Plant (*Hypoestes sanguinolenta*)

Pink Starlite (*Crypthanthus rose us pictus "Pink Starllite"*)

Pirliteiro (*Crataegus oxyacantha*)

Pitaya (*Hylocereus undatus*)

Plantanus Orientalis (*Plantanus acerifolia*)

Plantanus Occidentalis (*Plantanus acerifolia*)

Platinum Peperomia (*Peperomia griseoargentea*)

Platycerium Alicicome (*Platycerium bifurcatum*)

Plumbago Larpentiae (*Ceratostigma plumbaginoides*)

Plush Plant (*Echeveria derenbergii*)

Polka Dot Plant (*Hypoestes sanguinolenta*)

Polystichum Falcatum (*Crytomium falcatum*)

Pony Tail (*Beaucarnea recurvata*)

Porcelain Flower (*Hoya carnosa "compacta"*)

Sego Lily (*Calochortus gunnisonii*)

Shagbark Hickory (*Carya spp.*)

Shan Ku'ei-Lai (*Smilax glabra*)

Shellbark Hickory (*Carya spp.*)

Shiny Leaf Smilax (*Smilax glabra*)

Shrimp Cactus (*Schlumbergera russelliana*)

Silver Bell (*Ralesia carolina*)

Silver Berry (*Elaeagnus spp.*)

Silver Heart (*Peperomia maremorata*)

Silver-Leaf Peperomia (*peperomia griseoargentea*)

Silver Nerve Plant (*Fittonia verschaffeltii argyroneura*)

Silver Pink Vine (*Hoya purpureafusca*)

Silver Star (*Cryptanthus lacerdae*)

Silver Table Fern (*Pteris ensiformis "virtoriae"*)

Silver Tree Panamiga (*Pilea sp. "Silver Tree"*)

Slender Deutzia (*Deutzia gracilis*)

Small-Fruited Hickory (*Carya spp.*)

Smilax Tamnoides Vas Hispida (*Smilax hispida*)

Speckled Wood Lily (*Clintonia umbeliulata*)

Spice Orchid (*Epidendrum cochleastum*)

Spider Ivy (*Chlorophytum comosum*)

Spider Plant (*Chlorophytum comosum*)

Spotted Laurel (*Aucuba japonica variegata*)

Squarenut (*Carya spp.*)

Squirrels Foot Fern (*Davallia spp.*)

Star Jasmine (*Frachelospermum jasminoides*)

Star Lily (*Leucocrinum montanum*)

Star Plant (*Haworthia subfasciata*)

Star Plant (*Hawthoria spp.*)

Star Tulip (*Calochortus gunnisonii*)

Star Window Plant (*Haworthia subfasciata*)

Star Window Plant (*Hawthoria spp.*)

Strawberry (*Fragaria spp.*)

Striped Blushing Bromeliad (*Neoregelia carolinae*)

Sugar-Pods (*Ceratonia siliqua*)

Sulfur Flower (*Eriogonum umbeliatum*)

Summer Hyacinth (*Galtonia spp.*)

Sunflower (*Helianthus annuus*)

Swamp Hickory (*Carya spp.*)

Swedish Ivy (*Plectranthus australis*)

Sweet William (*Phlox diuaricata*)

Sweetheart Hoya (*Hoya kerui*)

Sweetheart Peperomia (*Peperomia verschaffeltii*)

Sword Fern (*Nephrolepis exalta bostoniensis compacta*)

Swordfern (*Polystichum munitum*)

Tahitian Bridal Veil (*Tradescantia multiflora*)

Tailed Orchid (*Masdevallia veichiana*)

Tall Feather Fern (*Nephrolepis exalta bostoniensis compacta*)

Tall Mahonia (*Mahonia spp.*)

Teasel Gourd (*Cucumis dipsaceus*)

Texas Sage (*Salvia coccinea*)

Thea Japonica (*Camellia japonica*)

Thimble Cactus (*Mammillaria fragilis*)

Thorn Apple (*Carateagus oxyacantha*)

Ti Hu-Ling (*Smilax glabra*)

Tiger Orchid (*Odontoglossum crispum*)

Tiger Orchid (*Odtongolossum grande*)

Toad Spotted Cactus (*Stapelia variegata*)

Torch Lily (*Kniphofia spp.*)

Tous-Les-Mois (*Canna edulis*)

Trailing Peperomia (*Peperomia "nummularifoliaj"*)

Tree Cactus (*Cephalocereus*)

Tree Gloxinia (*Kohleria lindeniana*)

Tropical Moss (*Selaginella spp.*)

True Cantelope (*Cucumis melo*)

TuFu-Ling (*Smilax glabra*)

Tulip Poplar (*Liriodendron tulip/era*)

Tulip Tree (*Liriodendron tulip/era*)

Turban Squash (*Cucurbita maxima cv turbaniformis*)

TurfLily (*Liriope muscari*)

Umbrella Plant (*Eriogonum umbellatum*)

Urbinia Agavoides (*Echeveria agavoides*)

Usambara Violet (*Saintpaulia confusa*)

Variegated Laurel (*Aucuba japonica variegata*)

Variegated Oval Leaf Peperomia (*Peperomia obtusifolia "Variegata"*)

Variegated Philodendron Leaf Peperomia (*Peperomia scandens*)

Variegated Wandering Jew (*Tranescantia jluminsis "Variegata"*)

Variegated Wax Plant (*Hoya carnosa variegata*)

Velvet Plant (*Gynura*)

Venus Fly Trap (*Dionaea muscipula*)

Verona Fern (*Nephrolepis exalt a bostoniensis compacta*)

Verona Lace Fern (*Nephrolepis exalta bostoniensis compacta*)

Vining Peperomia (*Peperomia dahlstedtii*)

Violet Slipper Gloxinia (*Sinningia spp.*)

Waftle Plant (*Hemigraphis exotica*)

Walking Anthericum (*Chlorophytum comosum*)

Washington Hawthorn (*Crataegus oxyacantha*)

Water Hickory (*Carya spp.*)

Watermelon Begonia (*Pellionia daveauana*)

Waternelon Begonia (*Peperomia argyreia*)

Waternelon Peperomia (*Peperomia argyreia*)

Waternelon Pilea (*Pilea cadierei*)

Wax Plant (*Hoya carnosaz "compactsz"*)

Wax Rosette (*Echeveria derenbergii*)

Weeping Bottlebrush (*Callistemon spp.*)

Weeping Sargent Hemlock (*Fsuga canadensis pendula*)

Weisdornbluten Osaycantha (*Crataegus oxyacantha*)
West Indian Gherkin (*Cucumis anguria*)
Western Sword (*Polystichum munitum*)
White Ginger (*Hedychium coronarium*)
White-Edged Swedish Ivy (*Plectranthus coleoides "Marginatus"*)
White-Heart Hickory (*Carya spp.*)
Whitman Fern (*Nephrolepis exalta bostoniensis compacta*)

Wild Buckwheat (*Eriogonum umbellatum*)
Wild Hyacinth (*Brodiaea capitata*)
Wild Lantana (*Abronia fragrans*)
Wild Sarsaparilla (*Smilax glauca*)
Wild Strawberry (*Fragaria spp.*)
Willow-Herb (*Epilobium angustifloium*)
Windmill Palm (*FrachycarpusJortuneij*)
Winter Cattleya (*Cattleya trianaei)j*

Index

Small Animal Toxicology Essentials, First Edition. Edited by Robert H. Poppenga, Sharon Gwaltney-Brant.
© 2011 John Wiley and Sons, Inc. Published 2011 by John Wiley and Sons, Inc.

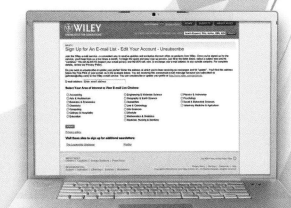
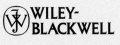